Physical Education and Sport: Performance Analysis and Monitoring

Physical Education and Sport: Performance Analysis and Monitoring

Editor: Claudia Dalton

MURPHY & MOORE
www.murphy-moorepublishing.com

www.murphy-moorepublishing.com

MURPHY & MOORE

Cataloging-in-Publication Data

Physical education and sport : performance analysis and monitoring / edited by Claudia Dalton.
p. cm.
Includes bibliographical references and index.
ISBN 978-1-63987-721-8
1. Physical education and training. 2. Sports. 3. Performance. 4. Athletic ability--Testing.
5. Athletes--Rating of. 6. Sports sciences. I. Dalton, Claudia.
GV206 .P49 2023
613.7--dc23

Murphy & Moore Publishing
1 Rockefeller Plaza,
New York City,
NY 10020, USA

ISBN 978-1-63987-721-8

Contents

Preface

I am honored to present to you this unique book which encompasses the most up-to-date data in the field. I was extremely pleased to get this opportunity of editing the work of experts from across the globe. I have also written papers in this field and researched the various aspects revolving around the progress of the discipline. I have tried to unify my knowledge along with that of stalwarts from every corner of the world, to produce a text which not only benefits the readers but also facilitates the growth of the field.

Physical education refers to a learning process that focuses on the knowledge, behaviors, and attitudes that are essential for students to lead a healthy and active lifestyle. It promotes physical literacy among individuals. Physical activity in the form of sports contributes in enhancing the strength, coordination, control, endurance, balance, and flexibility in an individual's body. It also promotes the health, capability, and well-being of participants. Sport performance analysis is a process that involves systematic observation, which gives valid, reliable and detailed information about the performance of players. Athletes and coaches obtain objective information using sport performance analysis techniques. Recent technological advancements have made it possible for teams to carefully monitor athlete performance throughout all competitions and sessions, which enables a better understanding of training techniques and this is advantageous to both athletes and coaches. This book outlines the concepts of performance analysis and monitoring within physical education and sports in detail. It consists of contributions made by international experts. This book will serve as a reference to a broad spectrum of readers.

Finally, I would like to thank all the contributing authors for their valuable time and contributions. This book would not have been possible without their efforts. I would also like to thank my friends and family for their constant support.

Editor

1

Secular Trends of Physical Fitness in Twenty-Five Birth Cohorts of Slovenian Children

*Žan Luca Potočnik, Gregor Jurak and Gregor Starc**

Laboratory for Physical and Motor Development Diagnosis, Faculty of Sport, University of Ljubljana, Ljubljana, Slovenia

***Correspondence:**
Gregor Starc
gregor.starc@fsp.uni-lj.si

In Slovenia, the national SLOfit surveillance system of the somatic and motor development of children and youth has been enabling researchers to observe the developmental trends of the entire population of school-aged children since 1987. The national database currently incorporates over 7.2 million sets of measurements of eight fitness tests and three anthropometric measurements. Since 1991, as in the rest of the world, in Slovenia, there is a common perception that the physical fitness of contemporary children is in decline and below the level of the physical fitness of the previous generation's childhood fitness. Our paper examines the trends of physical fitness in 26 birth cohorts of 7–10-year-olds. The analysis shows that the secular trends of physical fitness in boys and especially in girls have been positive and that the level of physical fitness of recent birth cohorts exceeds the national average of physical fitness of the 1989–2019 period. At the same time, the analysis reveals that the distribution of physical fitness has been changing from almost normal in the cohorts born in the first half of the 1980s, toward positively skewed in the subsequent cohorts born before the year 2000, and bimodal distribution in the later cohorts, indicating growing inequality and polarization of the motor development of children.

Keywords: physical fitness, children, secular trends, cohort, SLOfit

INTRODUCTION

There is a common perception that the physical fitness of children has declined over the last few generations due to growing sedentary behavior, lack of habitual physical activity, and the easy availability of energy-rich food. This perception, however, is based on a great deal of anecdotal and lay speculation since the evidence, deriving from longitudinal cohort studies of secular trends in physical fitness is scarce and the existing evidence inconclusive. The assessments of the secular trends of physical fitness of children have been distinctly understudied and have been mostly derived from temporal studies, relying mostly on cross-sectional designs, usually comparing only individual or joint age-groups of children at two or three time-points, predominantly comparing data on relatively small samples of one or several age-groups, and using a variety of different test batteries (1–14). Some studies of secular trends have been focusing only on the components of in aerobic fitness (15–17), while others focused only on the components muscular fitness (18–22).

We were unable to identify any study that used the cohort design of population data for the assessment of the secular trends in general physical fitness, which is why there is a lack of evidence on the actual secular trends of distribution of physical fitness comparing one generation of children to the other at multiple time points.

When studying secular trends of physical fitness, it is not sufficient to observe only the changes in the central tendency but also the changes in its distribution among the observed groups. We were, however, unable to identify any study of secular trends in physical fitness that addressed the problem of secular changes in its distribution; this is mainly due to a lack of national monitoring systems for the development of physical fitness that could regularly provide population data or at least nationally representative large datasets on the annual level.

In recent years, Hungary (23), Portugal (24), and Finland (25) have introduced national monitoring systems for the assessment of children's somatic development and functional capacity, but several years of measurements are required before they will be able to assess the secular trends of children's physical fitness in at least a few age groups of schoolchildren, since none of the systems covers the entire age-span of the school-going population. In Slovenia, however, the SLOfit national surveillance system for somatic and motor development of children and youth, implemented in 1982 (26), already enables the analyses of secular trends of childhood physical fitness of several generations on the population level.

The purpose of this study is not merely to analyze temporal trends bit to assess the actual secular trends of general physical fitness of Slovenian children (between ages 7 and 10) in 26 birth cohorts, born from 1983 until 2008, on the population data of the 1991–2019 period. In addition, the analysis attempts to assess whether the statistical distribution of physical fitness remained normal throughout generations with the entire population experiencing similar trends, or the distribution became skewed due to growing differences, reflected in the polarization of results at both extremes.

MATERIALS AND METHODS

Participants

The analysis included 1,953,847 measurements of children (girls $n = 953{,}001$, boys $n = 1{,}000{,}847$) from 26 birth cohorts. Children from every birth cohort were measured annually at ages 7, 8, 9, and 10. The oldest cohort was born between January 1, and December 31 in 1983 and the youngest in 2008. In 2019, the youngest cohort was in primary school grade 5. The number of boys and girls in individual birth cohorts at age 10 are visible in **Figure 1**. After the breakup of Yugoslavia, Slovenia experienced a decrease in natality rates, which was reversed after 2003 and is also reflected in the number of children measured. The average response rate was around 94%, ranging from 88.7% in the 1986 birth cohort to 97.7% in the 2008 cohort. The difference in response rates between girls and boys was negligible and did not exceed 0.3% on the average.

Instruments

Physical Fitness Assessment

The SLOfit test battery was used to assess the level of physical fitness of every child. This battery includes three anthropometric measurements (height, weight, and triceps skinfold thickness) and eight fitness tests (arm plate tapping, standing broad jump, backwards obstacle course, sit-ups in 60 s, stand and reach, bent-arm hang, 60-m dash, and 600-m run) (27).

Since each fitness test indicates a specific component of physical fitness, we used the Physical Fitness Index (PFI) based on the results of all fitness test as a single indicator of general physical fitness. A similar approach, utilizing a single indicator (Physical Fitness Indicator) based on the percentage of change of physical fitness, was utilized in two recent studies of physical fitness trends in Chinese populations (10, 13). In our case, PFI provides information about the percentile ranking of every child in the population of all Slovenian children in the 1989–2019 period ($N > 7.2$ million). To calculate the PFI, percentile scores of all eight fitness tests were calculated for each age-group, separate for boys and girls. Then, the mean percentile value of the eight fitness tests was calculated, each test contributing equally to PFI. The results of fitness tests were not adjusted to weight, height, triceps skinfold thickness, or BMI. The mean of eight fitness tests for every child was again ranked, and percentile score of PFI established on the entire population of the Slovenian children in the 1989–2019 period. In this way, the results of all individual tests for every child were ranked against the results of all children of same age and sex from 1989 onwards.

Procedure

The SLOfit national surveillance system of somatic and motor development is a part of the Slovenian educational system. Its primary purpose is to provide teachers insight into the status of the somatic and motor development of their pupils to better plan and implement the PE lessons and other curricular and extracurricular sporting activities. All primary and secondary schools in Slovenia are required to organize and carry out annual assessments of the somatic and motor development for all children, with parental consent. The physical fitness tests are administered annually every April in the children's schools by physical education teachers according to the uniform national protocol and standardized equipment (27). All the schools in Slovenia send children's measurement results to the Laboratory for Physical and Motor Development Diagnosis at the Faculty of Sport, University of Ljubljana, where the data are cleaned, analyzed, and evaluated; feedback reports sent back to schools. The results of every child are rigorously checked using specially designed software, with all the ambiguities communicated back to the PE teachers and subsequently corrected. All PE teachers in Slovenia are educated at the Faculty of Sport and are thoroughly trained in the SLOfit measurements and data management, which are also regulated by the education legislation at the national level. In this way, the SLOfit system has been able to limit the individual influences of the observers on the results and sustain a high and homogeneous level of quality of data collection through the years.

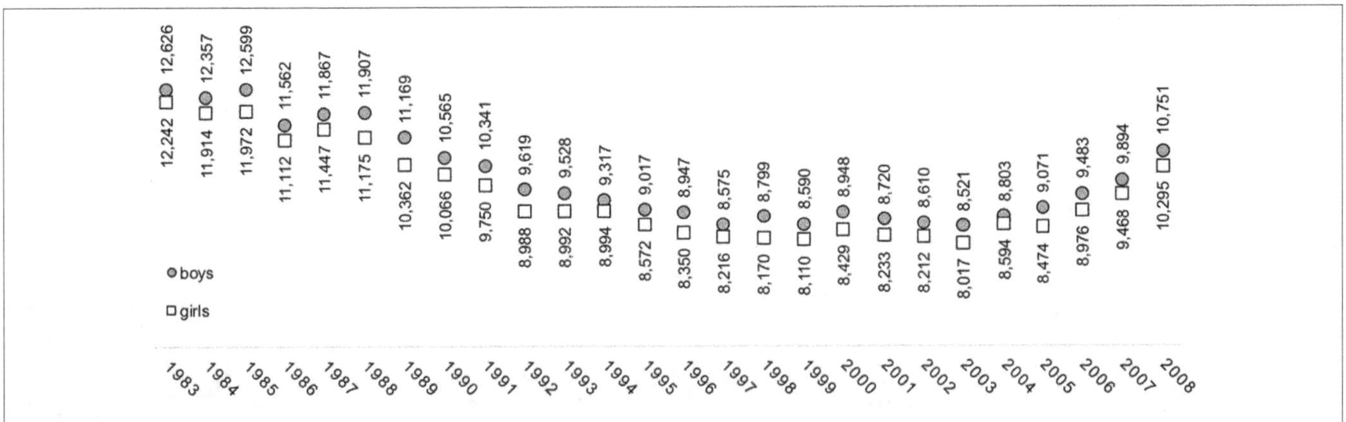

FIGURE 1 | The number of boys and girls in the analyzed birth cohorts at age 10.

The longitudinal cohort data with repeated measures were obtained from the SLOfit database to perform an exploratory analysis of secular trends of physical fitness. The selected age-span between 7 and 10 was used to minimize the effects of pubertal growth on physical fitness. Prior to the implementation of the 9-year primary school in the 1999/2000 school year, children in Slovenia had been entering primary school at age 7, but with the 9-year primary school, the admission age was changed to 6. The cohorts born before 1991, therefore, have data available only from age 7 onwards, which is why the data from age 6 was not included in the analysis.

Statistical Analysis

The SPSS 26.0 for Mac statistical package was used to carry out the data analysis (Armonk, NY: IBM Corp.). The Kolmogorov–Smirnov test and Levene's test were used to determine the nature of the data. They provided scores below 0.05, whereby a decision was made to produce non-parametric statistics. The Generalized Linear Models (GLMs) method was used (28) to compare the secular trends of physical fitness in 26 birth cohorts. We used the AIC method of goodness of fit to construct the comparison model. GLMs with linear variable response distribution were selected, with model-based estimator of co-variance matrix. Wald Chi-square statistics with confidence interval type, and maximum likelihood estimation method was used to build the interaction model between the birth cohorts as a factor and PFI as dependent response variable to assess the secular trends in boys and girls. No tests for random effects were performed. Since PFI is a percentile value, calculated separately for every age and sex, we did not include the two variables in the model as covariates. Results were considered significant if $P < 0.05$. To assess the secular changes in the distribution of PFI in different birth cohorts, we produced histograms, and visually inspected the shape of distribution separately in boys and girls.

RESULTS

Tables 1, **2** show the statistics of the GLMs for boys and girls, respectively, which show significant differences in physical fitness between the youngest birth cohorts and the majority of older birth cohorts. They show that after the decline of physical fitness in the birth cohorts from the 1990s, the trends improved in the cohorts from the 2000s.

For boys, there was no significant difference in PFI between the 2008, 1983, 1986, and 2006 cohorts, while all other cohorts, except for the 2007 birth cohort, had significantly lower PFI than the 2008 reference cohort ($P < 0.005$) (**Figure 2**). The 2000 birth cohort in boys experienced the poorest development of physical fitness while the first cohort that again exceeded the average national PFI of the 1989–2019 period was the 2004 birth cohort.

For girls, the positive secular trend of PFI was much more pronounced and started improving in the 1991 birth cohort (**Figure 2**), but there were significant differences in PFI between the 2008 birth cohort and all other birth cohorts except for the cohort born in 2007 ($P < 0.010$). All the birth cohorts of girls until 2001 were below the average national PFI of the 1989–2019 period, but all younger birth cohorts achieved the level of PFI above the national average. The lowest level of PFI in girls was observed in the 1990 birth cohort.

Although the analysis refutes the commonsensical speculations of declining general physical fitness and evidence about the positive secular trend, the changes in the distribution of PFI tell another interesting story (**Figure 3**). Namely, with every generation of boys and girls after 1983, the distribution of PFI deviated from the normal one toward the bimodal distribution with pronounced extremes, which evidence about a worrying trend of increasing inequality and polarization of physical fitness development in recent cohorts. More evidence of growing inequality is the growth of the share of children at both extremes of the distribution, specifically, those with poor physical fitness below the 5th percentile of the 1989–2019 period, and those with extraordinary physical fitness above 95th percentile (**Figure 4**). For boys and girls, the share of children with extremely low PFI was growing with every birth cohort until the year 2000 but has afterwards started to decline, although it is still higher than in the generations born in the 1980s. In contrast, the share of children with extremely high PFI has been growing with almost every generation, which has been especially expressed in girls. The share of girls with extremely high PFI in the most recent five generations has doubled in comparison with

GLMs statistics for boys.

Birth cohort	*B*	SE	95% Wald CI		Hypothesis test	
			Lower	Upper	Wald Chi-Square	Sig.
(Intercept)	51.057	0.1466	50.769	51.344	121,269.658	0.000
1983	−0.094	0.2046	−0.495	0.307	0.213	0.645
1984	−0.591	0.2044	−0.991	−0.190	8.352	0.004
1985	−0.925	0.2031	−1.323	−0.527	20.752	0.000
1986	−0.092	0.2063	−0.496	0.313	0.198	0.657
1987	−1.247	0.2048	−1.648	−0.845	37.064	0.000
1988	−0.850	0.2054	−1.253	−0.448	17.145	0.000
1989	−1.717	0.2086	−2.126	−1.308	67.755	0.000
1990	−1.830	0.2114	−2.244	−1.416	74.920	0.000
1991	−2.031	0.2123	−2.447	−1.615	91.479	0.000
1992	−1.391	0.2162	−1.814	−0.967	41.356	0.000
1993	−2.145	0.2169	−2.570	−1.720	97.795	0.000
1994	−2.454	0.2177	−2.881	−2.028	127.115	0.000
1995	−2.084	0.2183	−2.512	−1.657	91.178	0.000
1996	−2.387	0.2181	−2.814	−1.959	119.734	0.000
1997	−2.398	0.2194	−2.828	−1.968	119.427	0.000
1998	−2.893	0.2198	−3.324	−2.463	173.215	0.000
1999	−2.898	0.2205	−3.330	−2.466	172.747	0.000
2000	−3.095	0.2174	−3.522	−2.669	202.646	0.000
2001	−1.969	0.2192	−2.398	−1.539	80.695	0.000
2002	−2.368	0.2193	−2.798	−1.938	116.598	0.000
2003	−1.704	0.2200	−2.135	−1.272	59.936	0.000
2004	−0.747	0.2181	−1.175	−0.320	11.735	0.001
2005	−1.123	0.2166	−1.548	−0.699	26.900	0.000
2006	−0.256	0.2137	−0.675	0.163	1.432	0.231
2007	0.642	0.2113	0.228	1.056	9.226	0.002
2008	0[a]					

[a] 2008 is a reference cohort.

the 1983 generation, but overall, the overall share of boys and girls at both extremes rose by more than 70 per cent from 1983 to 2007 birth cohorts.

DISCUSSION

Our findings suggest that children in Slovenia have been experiencing positive trends of general physical fitness development, which was much more pronounced in girls than in boys. In this sense, our results do not reflect the negative global temporal trends of children's physical fitness (29, 30).

Furthermore, our findings suggest that the distribution of PFI in different birth cohorts changed from almost normal into bimodal due to growing differences in the development of children, evidencing that a part of the population did not experience the same favorable development.

The average level of general physical fitness in Slovenian children has been increasing with almost every generation of boys who were born since the year 2000, and especially with almost every generation of girls, born in the post-Yugoslav period from 1991 onwards, which is in concordance and probably related to the recent finding that the trends of overweight and obesity among Slovenian children and youth have been in decline from 2010 onwards (31).

Although we were unable to identify any other study that compared the secular trends of general physical fitness between different generations, the findings of our study show the opposite trends than the majority of recent studies of secular and temporal trends from other countries (4, 5, 7–11, 13, 18, 21). Nevertheless, we identified two recent studies that showed somewhat similar results to our analysis. A study among the Portuguese school children established the positive trend of certain components of physical fitness in the period between 1993 and 2013 (6), but the secular trends in our study are most similar to the trends among German children, who experienced a slight positive increase in numerous physical fitness components in the 2003–2017 period (14). The similarity of our results with the secular trends in Germany was also observed in the more expressed positive trend among girls, which was in opposition to the findings of the above-mentioned recent studies in which the trends of physical fitness were most often more negative among girls than boys.

TABLE 2 | GLMs statistics for girls.

Birth cohort	B	SE	95% Wald CI		Hypothesis test	
			Lower	Upper	Wald Chi-Square	Sig.
(Intercept)	53.822	0.149	53.529	54.115	129,716.781	0.000
1983	−4.294	0.208	−4.701	−3.886	426.668	0.000
1984	−4.132	0.208	−4.540	−3.725	395.143	0.000
1985	−5.506	0.207	−5.913	−5.099	704.600	0.000
1986	−4.902	0.210	−5.314	−4.490	544.259	0.000
1987	−5.820	0.209	−6.229	−5.411	777.780	0.000
1988	−5.707	0.210	−6.119	−5.295	737.415	0.000
1989	−7.015	0.215	−7.436	−6.593	1,063.253	0.000
1990	−7.432	0.216	−7.856	−7.008	1,178.927	0.000
1991	−6.628	0.218	−7.055	−6.200	922.504	0.000
1992	−5.354	0.223	−5.790	−4.918	579.157	0.000
1993	−5.794	0.223	−6.230	−5.358	677.419	0.000
1994	−5.811	0.222	−6.246	−5.376	685.885	0.000
1995	−5.500	0.224	−5.939	−5.061	603.873	0.000
1996	−4.644	0.224	−5.083	−4.204	428.686	0.000
1997	−4.242	0.225	−4.683	−3.802	356.548	0.000
1998	−4.072	0.226	−4.515	−3.629	324.899	0.000
1999	−4.704	0.227	−5.149	−4.260	429.917	0.000
2000	−3.873	0.224	−4.312	−3.435	299.629	0.000
2001	−3.783	0.225	−4.224	−3.342	282.201	0.000
2002	−2.851	0.225	−3.291	−2.411	161.055	0.000
2003	−1.709	0.226	−2.151	−1.266	57.272	0.000
2004	−0.585	0.223	−1.021	−0.149	6.916	0.009
2005	−1.710	0.223	−2.147	−1.273	58.758	0.000
2006	−0.272	0.219	−0.702	0.158	1.534	0.215
2007	0.314	0.216	−0.110	0.738	2.109	0.146
2008	0[a]					

[a] *2008 is a reference cohort.*

Despite the established positive secular trends of physical fitness in Slovenia, the changes in the distribution of PFI suggest a growing inequality in the opportunities for physical activity and polarization of physical fitness in the population, which could be connected to socio-economic reasons as was already evidenced in the studies of Danish children (2, 15) in which children from different socio-economic conditions experienced different trends of development. The almost normal distribution of physical fitness in the Slovenian cohorts, born in the first half of the 1980s who spent their pre-school period of life without computers and other screen technology, was rapidly changing into a positively skewed distribution with every new generation, resulting in growing numbers of children with low levels of physical fitness and diminishing numbers of children with high levels of physical fitness. In the 2010/2011 school year, Slovenia launched a national intervention program, Healthy Lifestyle, which provided two additional lessons of physical education per week to more than 30,000 children and significantly improved the perception of physical activity as a prerequisite of healthy development in the general public and also in schools that were not involved in the program. In the last decade, a large number of schools in Slovenia have also implemented other forms of "super-standard PE," resulting in increased time available for professionally guided physical activity within school settings. The Healthy Lifestyle program and other forms of additional PE were increasingly available to the cohorts of children born after the year 2000 and probably contributed to the improvement of physical fitness, but they did not add to the normalization of its distribution even if they have helped to improve the overall population median. In these cohorts, the positively skewed distribution of physical fitness became bimodal with a tendency toward negative skewness, evidencing the possibility to decrease the number of children with low physical fitness and increasing the number of children with excellent levels of physical fitness.

The methodology of our study differs substantially from the other existing studies of secular trends of physical fitness; it is also larger in scale and broader in scope than the previous studies, which make the direct comparison with other studies difficult but at the same time introduces a new perspective on the intra-generational change in physical fitness of children. By using a single indicator of physical fitness, incorporating most components of cardiorespiratory,

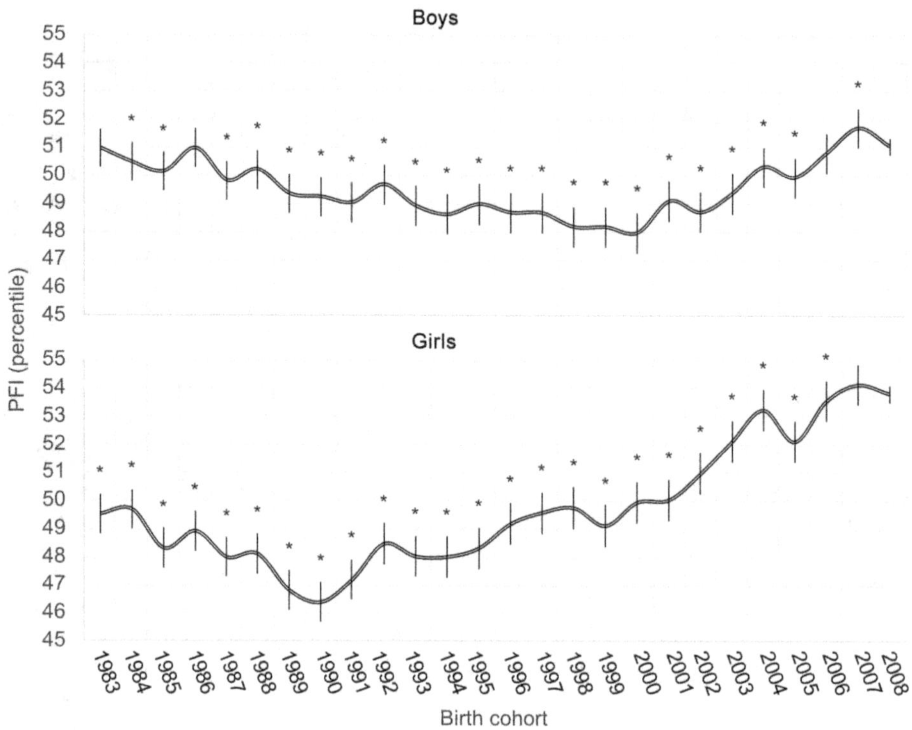

FIGURE 2 | Secular trends of physical fitness in boys and girls (*significant difference from the reference birth cohort of 2008).

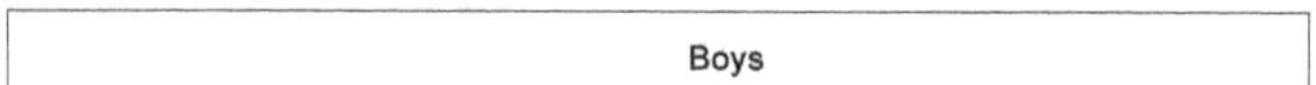

FIGURE 3 | Distribution of PFI in boys and girls (mean percentile, CI, *significant difference from the reference birth cohort of 2008).

muscular, and neuro-motor physical fitness, we attempted to surpass the limitations of looking only at a certain component of physical fitness. By looking at the physical fitness of individual birth cohorts throughout several years (7–10), we also attempted to avoid the limitations of looking only at a status of physical fitness of a cohort at only one time-point, which can be strongly influenced by individual differences in physical maturation. In comparison to the existing studies, our study does not focus only on the central tendency of the trend but also looks at the changes in the distribution of physical fitness, identifying a problem of growing inequality of physical fitness development.

The main strength of our study is its robustness due to the population data, its small probability bias due to high response rates, well-established test battery, highly qualified PE teachers performing the measurements, as well as its uniform measurement protocol and cohort design. However, it also has certain limitations. It uses one indicator of physical fitness as the aggregate of cardiorespiratory, muscular, and neuro-motor fitness, which can mask the negative trends in individual dimensions of physical fitness on behalf of positive trends in another dimension (for secular trends of individual fitness tests see **Supplementary Figures 1–8**). The analyzed data also do not enable the inclusion of various covariates that could reveal the causes of improved secular trends. The results are convincing and confirm that the physical fitness of children in

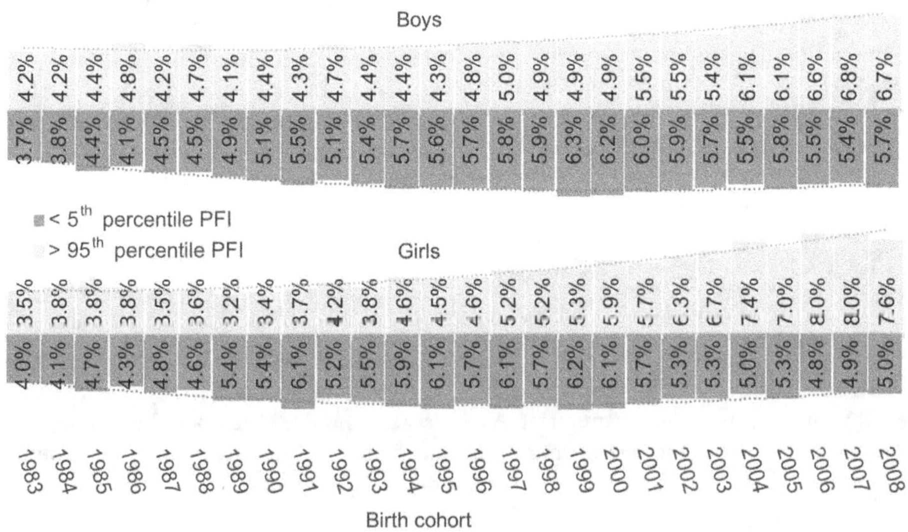

FIGURE 4 | Share of children above 95th and below 5th percentile of PFI per birth cohort.

Slovenia is improving, but they do not provide the answers about which environmental factors are the main cofounders and mediators of this improvement. Future research should, therefore, focus on studying the secular trends of physical fitness with different socio-economic indicators as covariates and should differentiate between children who were involved in interventions and sports training programs and those that were not. Although significant emphasis is placed on the assurance of the quality of data due to the high competence level of the PE teachers in measurement procedures, by standardized measurement conditions, and rigorous centralized data cleaning procedures, there are a large number of tests, a large number of schools, and a large number of children in a long period, which can compromise the quality of the data to some extent.

Lastly, the observed positive secular trends were studied only on the population of children between their ages 7 and 10 and do not provide information on the further development of their physical fitness in adolescence in adulthood.

CONCLUSION

Our study attempted to assess the secular trends of physical fitness and changes in its distribution in 23 birth cohorts of Slovenian children. Our primary research questions attempted to determine whether the negative temporal trends, evidenced in the majority of other studies, have also been evident in the population of Slovenian children and whether the changes in the central tendency of physical fitness change were equally distributed throughout every cohort.

The PFI of Slovenian children, as an indicator of physical efficiency, encompassing cardiorespiratory, muscular, and neuromotor fitness, shows that the secular trends of physical fitness of children in Slovenia are positive and that the recent generations of girls are experiencing strong emancipation through participation in regular physical activity and sport. Their level of physical fitness is superior to that of their mothers, born more than 20 years ago. The most recent cohorts of boys also managed to reach the physical fitness level of their fathers despite the unfavorable, sedentary environment in which they have been living. This positive trend is in contrast to observed temporal global trends (29, 30, 32) but simultaneously confirms that the contemporary generations of children in Slovenia are in fact among the most physically active children in the world (33) and have been also experiencing declining trends of overweight and obesity (31), which is directly reflected in the level of their physical fitness.

In contrast, the positive trend has not been experienced by the entire population of children, and with every generation, the share of children at the extremes of the distribution curve has been growing.

Our findings suggest that the high quality level of physical education teaching in Slovenia, supported by evidence data, exceptional school sports infrastructure, and additional hours of PE, provided by the Healthy Lifestyle intervention or at the initiative of schools, provided more favorable conditions for the development of physical fitness of children. However, the findings also suggest that the problem of growing inequality in physical fitness development should be considered and effective solutions found to provide better opportunities for development to the children at the negative end of the distributional curve.

ETHICS STATEMENT

The studies involving human participants were reviewed and approved by National Medical Ethics Committee of the Republic of Slovenia (ID 102/03/15). Written informed consent to participate in this study was provided by the participants' legal guardian/next of kin.

AUTHOR CONTRIBUTIONS

GS and ŽP conceptualized and designed the study, performed the statistical analysis, and wrote the first draft of the manuscript. ŽP organized the database. GJ wrote sections of the manuscript. All authors contributed to manuscript revision, read, and approved the submitted version.

program under Grant Agreement No. 774548. The content of this document reflects only the authors' views and the European Commission is not liable for any use that may be made of the information it contains. ŽP, GS, and GJ are also funded by the Slovenian Research Agency through the research program P5-014—Bio-psycho-social context of kinesiology.

ACKNOWLEDGMENTS

The authors wish to thank the schools, teachers, children, and their parents who generously agreed to be involved in the SLOfit system and the Ministry of Education, Science, and Sport of the Republic of Slovenia for funding the annual data analysis of the SLOfit measurements.

REFERENCES

Malina RM. Secular trends in growth, maturation and physical performance: a review. *Anthropological Review.* (2004) 67:3–31.

Wedderkopp N, Froberg K, Hansen HS, Andersen LB. Secular trends in physical fitness and obesity in Danish 9-year-old girls and boys: Odense School Child Study and Danish substudy of the European Youth Heart Study. *Scand J Med Sci Sports.* (2004) 14:150–5. doi: 10.1111/j.1600-0838.2004.00365.x

Malina RM. Physical fitness of children and adolescents in the United States: status and secular change. *Med Sport Sci.* (2007) 50:67–90. doi: 10.1159/000101076

Runhaar J, Collard D, Singh A, Kemper H, Van Mechelen W, Chinapaw M. Motor fitness in Dutch youth: differences over a 26-year period (1980-2006). *J Sci Med Sport.* (2010) 13:323–8. doi: 10.1016/j.jsams.2009. 04.006

Dos Santos FK, Prista A, Gomes TNQF, Daca T, Madeira A, Katzmarzyk PT, et al. Secular trends in physical fitness of Mozambican school-aged children and adolescents. *Am J Hum Biol.* (2015) 27:201–6. doi: 10.1002/ajhb.22638

Costa AM, Costa MJ, Reis AA, Ferreira S, Martins J, Pereira A. Secular trends in anthropometrics and physical fitness of young Portuguese school-aged children. *Acta Med Portuguesa.* (2017) 30:108–14. doi: 10.20344/amp.7712

Venckunas T, Emeljanovas A, Mieziene B, Volbekiene V. Secular trends in physical fitness and body size in Lithuanian children and adolescents between 1992 and 2012. *J Epidemiol Commun Health.* (2017) 71:181– 7. doi: 10.1136/jech-2016-207307

Aaberge K, Mamen A. A Comparative Study of Fitness Levels among Norwegian Youth in 1988 and 2001. *Sports.* (2019) 7:50. doi: 10.3390/sports7020050

Colley RC, Clarke J, Doyon CY, Janssen I, Lang JJ, Timmons BW, et al. Trends in physical fitness among Canadian children and youth. *Health Rep.* (2019) 30:3–13. doi: 10.25318/82-003-x201901000001-eng

Dong Y, Lau PW, Dong B, Zou Z, Yang Y, Wen B, et al. Trends in physical fitness, growth, and nutritional status of Chinese children and adolescents: a retrospective analysis of 1.5 million students from six successive national surveys between 1985 and 2014. *Lancet Child Adolesc Health.* (2019) 3:871– 80. doi: 10.1016/S2352-4642(19)30302-5

Gaya AR, Mello JB, Dias AF, Brand C, Cardoso VD, Nagorny GAK, et al. Temporal trends in physical fitness and obesity among Brazilian children and adolescents between 2008 and 2014. *J Hum Sport Exerc.* (2019). 15:549– 58. doi: 10.14198/jhse.2020.153.07

Shigaki GB, Batista MB, Paludo AC, Vignadelli LFZ, Serassuelo Junior H, Ronque ERV. Secular trend of physical fitness indicators related to health in children. *J Hum Growth Dev.* (2019) 29:381–9. doi: 10.7322/jhgd.v29.9537

Bi C, Zhang F, Gu Y, Song Y, Cai X. Secular Trend in the Physical Fitness of Xinjiang Children and Adolescents between 1985 and 2014. *Int J Environ Res Public Health.* (2020) 17:2195. doi: 10.3390/ijerph17072195

Hanssen-Doose A, Niessner C, Oriwol D, Bös K, Woll A, Worth Population-based trends in physical fitness of children and adolescents in Germany, 2003-2017. *Eur J Sport Sci.* (2020). doi: 10.1080/17461391.2020.1793003. [Epub ahead of print].

Møller NC, Wedderkopp N, Kristensen PL, Andersen LB, Froberg K. Secular trends in cardiorespiratory fitness and body mass index in Danish children: the European Youth Heart Study. *Scand J Med Sci Sports.* (2007) 17:331– 9. doi: 10.1111/j.1600-0838.2006.00583.x

Stratton G, Canoy D, Boddy L, Taylor S, Hackett A, Buchan I. Cardiorespiratory fitness and body mass index of 9-11-year-old English children: a serial cross-sectional study from 1998 to 2004. *Int J Obes.* (2007) 31:1172–8. doi: 10.1038/sj.ijo.0803562

Sandercock G, Voss C, McConnell D, Rayner P. Ten year secular declines in the cardiorespiratory fitness of affluent English children are largely independent of changes in body mass index. *Arch Dis Child.* (2010) 95:46– 7. doi: 10.1136/adc.2009.162107

Tyler R, Mackintosh KA, Palmer A, Jones A, Brophy S, Stratton G. Ten-year secular changes in selected health and fitness parameters of 10-11years old Swansea school children-2003-2013. *Adv Obes Weight Manag Control.* (2015) 3:267–71. doi: 10.15406/aowmc.2015.03.00072

Fraser BJ, Blizzard L, Tomkinson GR, Lycett K, Wake M, Burgner D, et al. The great leap backward: changes in the jumping performance of Australian children aged 11- 12-years between 1985 and 2015. *J Sports Sci.* (2019) 37:748–54. doi: 10.1080/02640414.2018.1523672

Kocić J, Stojanović D, Stanković S, Petrović L, Ignjatović A, Savić Z, et al. Muscle strength test performance changes over time in Serbian children. *Acta Med Medianae.* (2019) 58:154–60. doi: 10.5633/amm.2019.0223

Sandercock GR, Cohen DD. Temporal trends in muscular fitness of English 10-year-olds 1998-2014: An allometric approach. *J Sci Med Sport.* (2019) 22:201–5. doi: 10.1016/j.jsams.2018.07.020

Pinoniemi BK, Tomkinson GR, Walch TJ, Roemmich JN, Fitzgerald JS. Temporal trends in the standing broad jump performance of Sorić M, Jurak G, Durić S, Kovač M, Strel J, Starc G. Increasing United States children and adolescents. *Res Q Exerc Sport.* (2020). doi: 10.1080/02701367.2019.1710446. [Epub ahead of print].

Csányi T, Finn KJ, Welk GJ, Zhu W, Karsai I, Ihász F, et al. Overview of the Hungarian national youth fitness study. *Res Q Exerc Sport.* (2015) 86:S3–S12. doi: 10.1080/02701367.2015.1042823

Henriques-Neto D, Minderico C, Peralta M, Marques A, Sardinha LB. Test- retest reliability of physical fitness tests among young athletes: the FITescola®battery. *Clin Physiol Funct Imaging.* (2020) 40:173–82. doi: 10.1111/cpf.12624

Joensuu L, Syväoja H, Kallio J, Kulmala J, Kujala UM, Tammelin TH. Objectively measured physical activity, body composition and physical fitness: cross-sectional associations in 9-to 15-year-old children. *Eur J Sport Sci.* (2018) 18:882–92. doi: 10.1080/17461391.2018.1457081

Jurak G, Kovač M, Sember V, Starc G. 30 Years of SLOfit: its legacy and perspective. *Turk J Sports Med.* (2019) 54:23–7. doi: 10.5152/tjsm.2019.148

Strel J, Ambrožič F, Kondrič M, Kovač M, Leskošek B, Štihec J, et al. *Sports Educational Chart.* Ljubljana: Ministry of Education and Sport (1997).

Liang K-Y, Zeger SL. Longitudinal data analysis using generalized linear models. *Biometrika.* (1986) 73:13–22. doi: 10.1093/biomet/73.1.13

Tomkinson GR. Global changes in anaerobic fitness test performance of children and adolescents (1958-2003). *Scand J Med Sci Sports.* (2007) 17:497–507. doi: 10.1111/j.1600-0838.2006.00569.x

Tomkinson GR, Lang JJ, Tremblay MS. Temporal trends in the cardiorespiratory fitness of children and adolescents representing 19 high-income and upper middle-income countries between 1981 and 2014. *Br J Sports Med.* (2019) 53:478–86. doi: 10.1136/bjsports-2017-097982

Sori´c M, Jurak G, Duri´c S, Kova˘c M, Strel J, Starc G. Increasing trends in childhood overweight have mostly reversed: 30 years of continuous surveillance of Slovenian youth. *Sci Rep.* (2020) 10:11022. doi: 10.1038/s41598-020-68102-2

Tomkinson GR, Olds TS. Secular changes in pediatric aerobic fitness test performance: the global picture. *Med Sport Sci.* (2007) 50:46– 66. doi: 10.1159/000101075

Sember V, Starc G, Jurak G, Golobič M, Kovač M, Samardžija PP, et al. Results from the Republic of Slovenia's 2016 Report Card on Physical Activity for Children and Youth. *J Phys Activ Health.* (2016) 13(11 Suppl 2):S256– S64. doi: 10.1123/jpah.2016-0294

2

Performance Advantages of Left-Handed Cricket Batting Talent

Jonathan D. Connor[1], David L. Mann[2], Miguel-Angel Gomez[3], Anthony S. Leicht[1] and Kenji Doma[1]*

[1] Sport and Exercise Science, James Cook University, Townsville, QLD, Australia, [2] Department of Human Movement Sciences, Vrije Universiteit Amsterdam, Amsterdam, Netherlands, [3] Faculty of Physical Activity and Sports Sciences, Polytechnic University of Madrid, Madrid, Spain

Correspondence:
Jonathan D. Connor
jonathan.connor@jcu.edu.au

The purpose of this study was to examine performance advantages associated with batting stance, in the form of left- vs. right-handed dominant stance, and orthodox vs. reverse stance, of talented junior cricket batters within age-restricted competitions. Data were sourced from the national male younger age competition (YAC; Under-17; $n = 237$) and older age competition (OAC; Under-19; $n = 302$), as well as female YAC (Under-15; $n = 234$) and OAC (Under-18; $n = 260$) over a 4-year period. Left-hand dominant (LHD) batters were consistently overrepresented in the male YAC (Right: 69.2%; Left: 30.8%) and OAC (Right: 68.2%; Left: 31.8%) compared with the expected general population distribution. Male LHD batters exhibited a significantly ($p < 0.05$) higher batting aggregate (YAC: 116.82 ± 84.75 vs. 137.84 ± 89.74; OAC: 117.07 ± 89.00 vs. 146.28 ± 95.99), scored more runs (YAC: 19.65 ± 12.32 vs. 23.96 ± 14.71; OAC: 19.27 ± 12.61 vs. 23.98 ± 14.15), spent more time batting (YAC: 45.33 ± 25.89 min vs. 54.59 ± 28.62 min; OAC: 39.80 ± 21.79 min vs. 49.33 ± 27.41 min), and scored more boundary-4s per game (YAC: 1.83 ± 1.40 vs. 2.44 ± 1.87; OAC: 1.76 ± 1.32 vs. 2.19 ± 1.83), across both YAC and OAC groups with small effect sizes. No overrepresentation was present for either female group (YAC, Right: 88.5%/Left: 11.5%; OAC, Right: 90.0%/Left: 10.0%). Female LHD batters exhibited significantly higher batting aggregate (68.97 ± 53.17 vs. 102.96 ± 73.48), batting average (13.24 ± 10.88 vs. 17.75 ± 12.28), and spent more time batting per game (25.52 ± 15.08 vs. 37.75 ± 26.76 min), but only at the OAC level with small-moderate effects sizes. Finally, there were few performance advantages identified to batting with a reverse stance, with further work needed to clarify any potential biomechanical benefits. Team selection practices may exploit the left-handed advantage by over-selecting talented left-handed junior cricketers. Practical implications for coaches include creating practice environments that negate the negative frequency-dependent selection, such as providing more practice opportunities for their players against left-handed opponents.

Keywords: handedness, laterality, frequency dependence, talent identification and development, talent selection

INTRODUCTION

The overrepresentation of left-handers, compared with the expected distribution seen in the general population, has been well established within interactive time-restrictive skills (Hagemann, 2009; Harris, 2010; Loffing, 2017). The most prominent explanation for the left-hander's advantage has been the *negative frequency-dependent hypothesis* (Raymond et al., 1996; Grouios, 2004). This hypothesis presumes that athletes in interactive sports are much more likely to play and practice against right-handed opponents. As a result, these athletes develop both greater familiarity and highly specific skills to anticipate the action outcomes of their right-handed opponents via attunement to crucial perceptual information (Loffing and Hagemann, 2014). While a greater proportion of left-handers are commonly observed in high-level sports (~30%) compared to the general population incidence (~10–15%), a specific left-handed performance advantage during competition has not been clearly reported (Grouios et al., 2000; Loffing, 2017).

Evidence of a relative advantage for anticipating the actions of a right-handed (or footed) opponent has been reported across a number of interactive tasks including predicting left- and right-handed serves in volleyball (Loffing et al., 2012b), predicting kicking direction from left- and right-footed opponents in soccer (McMorris and Colenso, 1996) and predicting left- and right-handed serves in tennis (Loffing et al., 2009). Loffing et al. (2012a) concluded that the performance advantage for left-handers may be attributed to more highly skilled visual perception, stemming from more frequent encounters with right-handers (Loffing et al., 2012b). Unsurprisingly, handedness has also been reported as a potentially influential factor in team selection, with Brooks et al. (2004) finding that the most successful teams at the 2003 Cricket World Cup had nearly 50% representation of left-handed cricket batsmen.

Additional explanations for the prominence of left-handers within elite sporting teams have also included potential advantages afforded by sport-specific rule constraints and innate technical advantages (Grondin et al., 1999). For instance, Raymond et al. (1996) suggested that a greater frequency of left-handers may result from the constraints (e.g., rules) within the performance environment. For example, baseball batters who bat left-handed may have tactical or strategic advantages in that (i) their stance places them closer to first base toward which they must run and (ii) their momentum at the end of the swing is already directed toward first base (as opposed to toward third base for batters with a right-handed stance). Similarly, the leg-before-wicket rule in cricket may advantage cricket batters who bat left-handed. In the familiar situation of facing a right-handed bowler, it is much more challenging for a left-handed batter to be dismissed leg-before-wicket due to particularities in where the ball must bounce to be adjudicated as "out." However, potential advantages of handedness within interactive sporting tasks remain in development (Mann et al., 2017). Mann et al. (2016) examined the prevalence of left-handedness in elite cricket batters and found not only an increased frequency of left-hand dominant (LHD) stance cricket batters, but also a tendency for batters (particularly left-handers) to adopt a "back-to-front" batting stance. The reverse stance hypothesis was therefore proposed as a potential technical advantage when holding a cricket bat with the dominant hand positioned further away from the hitting end of the bat (Mann et al., 2016). Interestingly, this stance was more common in LHD stance batters and it is unknown as to what degree either factor influences performance.

While there is evidence that left-handedness—and perhaps a "reversed stance"—may be advantageous at the elite level of competition (Mann et al., 2016), much less is known about the age, gender, or performance level at which these advantages might emerge, particularly as other talent selection bias has been previously highlighted in cricket (Connor et al., 2019). If the *negative frequency-dependent hypothesis* were apparent, then it might be reasonable to expect the advantage of the left-handed cricket batters to increase over time due to a progressive accrual of experience competing against right vs. left-handed opponents. Loffing et al. (2012a) reported a moderate positive impact of left-handedness on tennis performance, which decreased over a time span of years for males, and was almost entirely absent in professional female tennis players. These results suggest that a left-hander's advantage may primarily happen within lower performance levels and be a rarity at the elite level. Alternately, others have shown that the magnitude of some performance advantages increases and can become increasingly more important, along the developmental pathway (Weissensteiner et al., 2008). Therefore, development of a handedness advantage at the junior level may be important for future performance, yet remains to be confirmed.

The aim of this study was to examine the magnitude of performance advantages associated with batting stance, in the form of left- vs. right-handed dominant stance, and orthodox vs. reverse stance, in junior cricket players within age-restricted competitions. Both male and female players were examined to account for any potential sex differences in performance due to handedness (Loffing, 2017). We hypothesized that the magnitude of the performance advantage, associated with batting handedness (left vs. right) and batting stance (orthodox vs. reverse), would be larger for both male and female cricket batters participating in the older age competition (OAC).

MATERIALS AND METHODS

Participants and Procedures

Playing data for all male younger-age cricketers who competed at the Annual National Junior championships in Australia between 2012 and 2015 were obtained from an open source online database[1] (excluding male Under-17, which included data from 2013 to 2015) and confirmed via the National Sporting body's database. Players were then separated into whether they competed in the younger age competition (YAC; male Under-17 and female Under-15) or the OAC (male Under-19 and female Under-18). Batting handedness was determined by the players throwing hand, in line with previous work (Cairney et al., 2018). Players were included and categorized as batters if they (1) were

[1] www.nationalchamps.com.au

listed by the coach as a batter in the top seven positions and (2) batted in these positions during at least three innings of the tournament. In total, 237 YAC and 302 OAC-19 males, and 234 YAC and 260 OAC female players met the criteria. This research received institutional approval from James Cook University (H6267) and was conducted in accordance with the National Statement on Ethical Conduct in Human Research (2007).

Data Analysis

Measures of batting performance were collated from the tournament database. Two measures of absolute performance were recorded: (i) *batting aggregate*, representing the total number of runs scored at the tournament, and (ii) *number of innings batted*. Relative measures included (i) *batting average* (i.e., number of runs scored divided by number of dismissals), (ii) *runs per innings* (i.e., number of runs scored divided by number of innings), (iii) *strike rate* (i.e., runs scored per 100 balls), (iv) *boundary-4s per game* (i.e., average number of "fours" scored per innings), (v) *boundary-6s per game* (i.e., average number of "sixes" scored per innings), and (vi) *time per innings* (i.e., average time spent batting per innings). Finally, the percentage of innings was recorded where the batter was (i) *not dismissed* (i.e., not outs), and where the batter had scored (ii) *ducks* (i.e., scores of 0 runs per player) and (iii) *centuries* (i.e., scores of 100 runs or more per player). Participant's batting handedness was recorded as either right-hand dominant (RHD) or LHD. Batting stance was also recorded as being *orthodox* (dominant hand placed on the bottom of the bat) if the dominant hand matched the batting handedness (e.g., left-handed batter, LHD) or *reversed* (dominant hand placed on top off the bat) if the dominant hand did not match the batting handedness (e.g., right-handed batter, LHD).

Statistical Analysis

All data were analyzed using the Statistical Package of Social Sciences (SPSS, version 25, IBM Corp., Armonk, NY, United States) with the alpha level set at ≤ 0.05 and descriptive information expressed as mean $\pm$ standard deviation. First, any over- or underrepresentation of left-handedness, when compared with the proportions expected from the general population (RH = 85%; LH = 15%; Raymond et al., 1996; Johnston et al., 2009; Medland et al., 2009), was determined using chi-squared goodness-of-fit tests. Measures of batting performance measures were compared between groups (e.g., left- and right-handed stances; orthodox and reverse stances) using separate one-way MANOVAs for each group. Effect sizes (95% confidence interval) were calculated using Cohen's *d*, and reported as 0.2, 0.5, and 0.8 as small, moderate, and large, respectively (Cohen, 1988).

RESULTS

Representation

There was a significant overrepresentation of LHD cricket batters compared with the general population at both the YAC and OAC male level (**Table 1**). For females, there was no significant overrepresentation of LHD cricket batters at either the YAC or OAC level when compared to the left-handedness expected of the general population (**Table 2**).

Batting Performance—Males

Irrespective of their age group, when compared to RHD cricket batters, LHD male batters had significantly higher batting aggregates, runs per innings, time spent batting, and boundary-4s (small ES, **Table 2**). LHD in the YAC group had a significantly higher batting average ($p < 0.05$), whereas the advantage in the OAC group for LHD batters was marginal ($p = 0.07$). LHD batters also exhibited significantly less ducks in the YAC group only, and significantly more centuries scored in the OAC group ($p < 0.05$). All other variables across both YAC and OAC groups were similar, including the number of matches, innings, boundary-6s, and strike rate, with all exhibiting a small ES (**Table 2**).

Batting Performance—Females

There was no significant difference between LHD and RHD batters for each performance measure at the YAC level (all small ES, **Table 3**). At the OAC level, LHD exhibited significantly greater batting aggregate, batting average, average runs per game, and batting time ($p < 0.05$; small-moderate ES, **Table 3**). No other differences were observed between LHD and RHD batters at the OAC level for number of matches or innings, boundary-4s and -6s scored, strike rate, non-dismissals, and ducks or centuries scored (small ES, **Table 3**).

Batting Stance

Younger age competition reverse stance male cricket batters had significantly greater batting time (small-moderate ES) compared with orthodox stance batters ($p < 0.05$) while no other significant differences between batting variables were evident between the different stances (trivial to small-moderate ES, **Table 4**). The OAC reverse stance batters also had significantly greater batting time as well as greater boundary-4s (small-moderate ES, **Table 4**) compared with orthodox stance batters ($p < 0.05$). There were no other significant differences evident between the different stances for OAC level (trivial to small-moderate ES, **Table 4**).

Female cricket batters with a reverse batting stance in the YAC group exhibited significantly greater batting aggregate and batting time ($p < 0.05$; small ES, **Table 5**). Batting average was also greater for reverse stance female batters ($p < 0.05$). No other differences were evident between reverse and orthodox stance for the YAC group. There were also no significant differences between stances for any performance measure at the OAC level (trivial to small-moderate ES, **Table 5**).

DISCUSSION

The purpose of this study was to examine the magnitude of performance advantages associated with various batting stances, within an interactive striking task. We found that LHD cricket batters were overrepresented in competition for junior males, but not for females. Furthermore, male LHD batters in both groups scored more runs and batted for longer periods of time when compared with their right-handed counterparts. For

TABLE 1 | Number (and percentage) of left- and right-hand dominant male and female batters.

	Competition level	Right-handed batting stance	Left-handed batting stance	χ^2	*p*-Value
Male	YAC	164 (69.2%)	73 (30.8%)	19.58	<0.001
	OAC	206 (68.2%)	96 (31.8%)	22.14	<0.001
Female	YAC	207 (88.5%)	27 (11.5%)	0.96	0.33
	OAC	234 (90.0%)	26 (10.0%)	1.96	0.16

General population left-handedness = 15%.

TABLE 2 | Mean (±standard deviation) batting performances measures for left- and right-handed male batters during the YAC and OAC and effect size calculations between batters with associated 95% confidence interval (CI).

		Right-handed batting stance	Left-handed batting stance	Effect size (95% CI)	*p*-Value
Matches	YAC	6.26 ± 1.56	5.99 ± 1.58	0.17 (− 0.11, 0.45)	0.22
	OAC	5.80 ± 1.43	5.83 ± 1.63	0.02 (− 0.26, 0.22)	0.86
Innings	YAC	5.65 ± 1.63	5.85 ± 1.51	0.12 (− 0.40, 0.16)	0.39
	OAC	5.77 ± 1.53	5.71 ± 1.46	0.04 (− 0.20, 0.28)	0.74
Batting aggregate	YAC	116.82 ± 84.75	137.84 ± 89.74	0.24 (− 0.49, 0.00)	<0.05
	OAC	117.07 ± 89.00	146.28 ± 95.99	0.32 (− 0.60, −0.04)	<0.05
Batting average	YAC	22.78 ± 14.41	27.63 ± 17.09	0.32 (− 0.56, −0.07)	<0.05
	OAC	23.76 ± 17.02	28.19 ± 17.62	0.26 (− 0.54, 0.02)	0.07
Runs per innings	YAC	19.65 ± 12.32	23.96 ± 14.71	0.33 (− 0.57, −0.08)	<0.01
	OAC	19.27 ± 12.61	23.98 ± 14.15	0.36 (− 0.64, −0.08)	<0.05
Batting time (per game)	YAC	45.33 ± 25.89	54.59 ± 28.62	0.35 (− 0.59, −0.10)	<0.01
	OAC	39.80 ± 21.79	49.33 ± 27.41	0.40 (− 0.68, −0.12)	<0.01
Boundary-4s (per game)	YAC	1.83 ± 1.40	2.44 ± 1.87	0.39 (− 0.64, −0.15)	<0.01
	OAC	1.76 ± 1.32	2.19 ± 1.83	0.29 (− 0.56, 0.00)	<0.05
Boundary-6s (per game)	YAC	0.24 ± 0.38	0.26 ± 0.38	0.05 (− 0.29, 0.19)	0.69
	OAC	0.21 ± 0.35	0.26 ± 0.35	0.17 (− 0.44, 0.11)	0.25
Strike rate	YAC	57.11 ± 21.84	58.86 ± 18.25	0.08 (− 0.33, 0.16)	0.50
	OAC	59.43 ± 22.68	60.75 ± 20.67	0.06 (− 0.34, 0.22)	0.67
Non-dismissal (%)	YAC	12.07 ± 15.54	8.87 ± 12.99	0.09 (− 0.15, 0.33)	0.47
	OAC	15.45 ± 18.59	13.72 ± 15.35	0.10 (− 0.18, 0.38)	0.29
Ducks scored	YAC	11.58 ± 11.37	7.25 ± 13.21	0.34 (0.06, 0.62)	<0.05
	OAC	10.31 ± 14.21	7.521 ± 1.41	0.21 (− 0.04, 0.45)	0.09
Centuries scored	YAC	1.88 ± 8.07	3.18 ± 5.90	0.20 (− 0.47, 0.08)	0.17
	OAC	1.29 ± 4.71	3.29 ± 7.57	0.35 (− 0.59, −0.10)	<0.05

female LHD cricket batters, only the OAC group scored more runs and spent more time batting compared with their right-handed counterparts. Reverse stance batters exhibited some performance advantages over orthodox stance batters, including greater batting time (YAC and OAC) and boundary-4s (OAC) for males, and greater runs scored and batting time for female cricket batters (YAC). These findings demonstrate evidence of a small left-handed advantage in cricket batting, with limited performance advantage for either orthodox or reverse batting stance at the youth representative level.

Left-handed male cricket batters were found to be more prevalent in junior elite competition when compared to the proportion expected from the general population (**Table 1**). Similar findings have been reported at the elite level for males, whereby batting records from the 2003 cricket World Cup showed that the most successful teams in the competition had close to 50% representation of left-handed batsmen (Brooks et al., 2004). Mann et al. (2016) investigated left- and right-handedness among the greatest elite male cricket batters to have played the game, and reported comparable proportions to this study (left-handers = 33%; right-handers = 67%). Additionally, Mann et al. recorded the handedness of inexperienced cricket batters, finding levels comparable to the general population (left-handers = 15.2%; right-handers = 84.8%). Collectively, the current and prior findings confirm an overrepresentation of left-handed cricket batters at the elite junior and senior levels (Mann et al., 2016; Loffing, 2017).

Hagemann (2009), in his review of advantages according to handedness, reported that overrepresentations commonly occur in sporting tasks that involve the anticipation of an opponent's action. There has also been further suggestion that left-handedness is particularly evident during more temporally demanding sporting tasks such as tennis, cricket batting, or baseball batting (Loffing et al., 2010, 2012b; Loffing, 2017), although the exact temporal demand threshold at which a handedness advantage becomes apparent is unclear. It is thought

TABLE 3 | Mean (±standard deviation) batting performances measures for left- and right-handed female batters during the YAC and OAC and effect size calculations between batters with associated 95% confidence interval (CI).

		Right-handed batting stance	Left-handed batting stance	Effect size (95% CI)	*p*-Value
Matches	YAC	7.54 ± 0.51	7.40 ± 0.50	0.28 (− 0.13, 0.69)	0.18
	OAC	7.50 ± 0.65	7.56 ± 0.58	0.08 (− 0.48, 0.32)	0.69
Innings	YAC	6.46 ± 1.65	6.60 ± 1.32	0.09 (− 0.50, 0.32)	0.67
	OAC	6.22 ± 1.32	6.67 ± 1.41	0.34 (− 0.74, 0.07)	0.10
Batting aggregate	YAC	76.96 ± 63.48	92.24 ± 63.02	0.24 (− 0.65, 0.17)	0.25
	OAC	68.97 ± 53.17	102.96 ± 73.48	0.61(− 1.01, −0.20)	<0.01
Batting average	YAC	15.01 ± 13.03	17.00 ± 12.15	0.15 (− 0.57, 0.26)	0.47
	OAC	13.24 ± 10.88	17.75 ± 12.28	0.41(− 0.81, 0.00)	<0.05
Runs per innings	YAC	11.25 ± 8.23	13.57 ± 8.09	0.28 (− 0.69, 0.13)	0.18
	OAC	10.66 ± 7.84	14.54 ± 8.89	0.49 (− 0.89, −0.08)	<0.05
Batting time	YAC	21.64 ± 12.50	24.76 ± 12.90	0.25 (− 0.66, 0.17)	0.24
	OAC	25.52 ± 15.08	37.75 ± 26.76	0.73 (− 1.13, −0.32)	<0.01
Boundary-4s	YAC	1.22 ± 1.08	1.43 ± 1.08	0.20 (− 0.61, 0.22)	0.35
	OAC	0.74 ± 0.75	1.00 ± 1.02	0.34 (− 0.74, 0.07)	0.10
Boundary-6s	YAC	0.03 ± 0.11	0.02 ± 0.07	0.03 (− 0.39, 0.44)	0.90
	OAC	0.02 ± 0.06	0.00 ± 0.03	0.21 (− 0.20, 0.61)	0.31
Strike rate	YAC	56.61 ± 23.60	63.33 ± 22.34	0.29 (− 0.70, 0.13)	0.18
	OAC	50.19 ± 20.33	50.75 ± 12.91	0.03 (− 0.43, 0.37)	0.89
Non-dismissals (%)	YAC	19.28 ± 17.80	17.44 ± 16.72	0.10 (− 0.31, 0.52)	0.62
	OAC	16.43 ± 15.82	15.22 ± 12.54	0.08 (− 0.32, 0.48)	0.70
Ducks scored	YAC	0.15 ± 0.17	0.16 ± 0.14	0.06 (− 0.46, 0.34)	0.68
	OAC	0.14 ± 0.14	0.14 ± 0.16	0.00 (− 0.41, 0.41)	0.98
Centuries scored	YAC	0.00 ± 0.02	0.00 ± 0.00	0.00 (− 0.40, 0.40)	0.47
	OAC	0.00 ± 0.03	0.00 ± 0.00	0.00 (− 0.41, 0.41)	0.63

TABLE 4 | Mean (±standard deviation) batting performances measures for orthodox and reverse stance during the male YAC and OAC and effect size calculations between batters with associated 95% confidence interval (CI).

		Orthodox batting stance	Reverse batting stance	Effect size (95% CI)	*p*-Value
Matches	YAC	6.21 ± 1.55	6.04 ± 1.62	0.11 (− 0.21, 0.42)	0.50
	OAC	5.83 ± 1.44	5.75 ± 1.64	0.05 (− 0.21, 0.31)	0.71
Innings	YAC	5.69 ± 1.59	5.73 ± 1.62	0.03 (− 0.34, 0.29)	0.85
	OAC	5.82 ± 1.52	5.53 ± 1.43	0.19 (− 0.59, −0.06)	0.16
Batting aggregate	YAC	121.44 ± 90.45	142.90 ± 96.54	−0.23 (− 0.55, 0.08)	0.15
	OAC	120.99 ± 86.07	131.45 ± 89.08	−0.12 (− 0.38, 0.14)	0.37
Batting average	YAC	24.71 ± 17.50	26.59 ± 16.51	−0.11 (− 0.42, 0.21)	0.50
	OAC	23.83 ± 15.03	25.89 ± 16.71	−0.13 (− 0.40, 0.13)	0.32
Runs per innings	YAC	19.97 ± 13.13	23.45 ± 13.43	−0.26 (− 0.58, 0.05)	0.10
	OAC	20.29 ± 12.42	23.31 ± 15.46	−0.23 (− 0.49, 0.04)	0.09
Batting time (per game)	YAC	41.14 ± 23.53	48.58 ± 25.00	−0.31 (− 0.63, 0.00)	<0.05
	OAC	46.45 ± 25.73	54.02 ± 30.43	−0.28 (− 0.54, −0.02)	<0.05
Boundary-4s (per game)	YAC	1.84 ± 1.53	2.07 ± 1.39	−0.15 (− 0.47, 0.16)	0.35
	OAC	1.90 ± 1.42	2.41 ± 1.99	−0.32 (− 0.59, −0.06)	<0.05
Boundary-6s (per game)	YAC	0.21 ± 0.34	0.29 ± 0.38	−0.23 (− 0.54, 0.09)	0.16
	OAC	0.24 ± 0.38	0.26 ± 0.41	−0.04 (− 0.30, 0.23)	0.78
Strike rate	YAC	59.48 ± 22.46	61.13 ± 20.61	−0.07 (− 0.39, 0.24)	0.64
	OAC	57.73 ± 21.06	57.48 ± 19.89	0.01 (− 0.25, 0.28)	0.93
Non-dismissal (%)	YAC	16.02 ± 18.34	10.78 ± 14.21	0.30 (− 0.02, 0.61)	0.06
	OAC	12.71 ± 15.54	8.90 ± 13.17	0.25 (− 0.01, 0.52)	0.06
Ducks scored	YAC	0.11 ± 0.13	0.08 ± 0.10	0.21 (− 0.11, 0.52)	0.20
	OAC	0.10 ± 0.14	0.07 ± 0.11	0.24 (− 0.02, 0.51)	0.07
Centuries scored	YAC	0.02 ± 0.06	0.03 ± 0.08	0.15 (− 0.46, 0.17)	0.36
	OAC	0.02 ± 0.05	0.03 ± 0.07	0.22 (− 0.49, 0.04)	0.10

TABLE 5 | Mean (±standard deviation) batting performance measures for orthodox and reverse stance during the female YAC and OAC tournaments and effect size calculations between batters with associated 95% confidence interval (CI).

		Orthodox batting stance	Reverse batting stance	Effect size (95% CI)	*p*-Value
Matches	YAC	7.55 ± 0.51	7.36 ± 0.49	0.37 (− 0.04, 0.78)	0.08
	OAC	7.49 ± 0.66	7.60 ± 0.55	−0.17 (− 0.53, 0.19)	0.36
Innings	YAC	6.44 ± 1.64	6.80 ± 1.29	−0.23 (− 0.64, 0.19)	0.28
	OAC	6.25 ± 1.31	6.37 ± 1.50	−0.09 (− 0.45, 0.27)	0.62
Batting aggregate	YAC	75.79 ± 62.60	103.08 ± 67.59	−0.43 (− 0.85, −0.02)	<0.05
	OAC	72.24 ± 57.47	76.60 ± 53.07	−0.08 (− 0.44, 0.28)	0.68
Batting average	YAC	14.82 ± 13.00	18.78 ± 12.02	−0.45 (− 0.72, 0.11)	<0.05
	OAC	13.83 ± 11.58	13.38 ± 8.10	0.04 (− 0.32, 0.40)	0.83
Runs per innings	YAC	11.11 ± 8.18	14.82 ± 8.09	−0.31 (− 0.87, −0.04)	0.15
	OAC	11.09 ± 8.29	11.17 ± 6.58	−0.01 (− 0.37, 0.35)	0.96
Batting time (per game)	YAC	21.38 ± 12.48	27.15 ± 12.22	−0.46 (− 0.88, −0.05)	<0.05
	OAC	26.99 ± 16.93	26.58 ± 19.02	0.02 (− 0.34, 0.38)	0.90
Boundary-4s (per game)	YAC	1.21 ± 1.07	1.55 ± 1.12	−0.31 (− 0.72, 0.10)	0.14
	OAC	0.77 ± 0.81	0.78 ± 0.68	−0.02 (− 0.37, 0.34)	0.93
Boundary-6s (per game)	YAC	0.03 ± 0.11	0.02 ± 0.07	0.08 (− 0.33, 0.49)	0.70
	OAC	0.02 ± 0.06	0.01 ± 0.03	−0.02 (− 0.20, 0.52)	0.39
Strike rate	YAC	56.66 ± 24.10	62.91 ± 16.60	−0.27 (− 0.68, 0.15)	0.21
	OAC	49.42 ± 18.65	54.99 ± 24.10	−0.28 (− 0.64, 0.08)	0.12
Non-dismissal (%)	YAC	19.27 ± 17.98	17.52 ± 14.73	0.10 (− 0.31, 0.51)	0.64
	OAC	16.45 ± 15.78	15.34 ± 13.72	0.07 (− 0.29, 0.43)	0.70
Ducks scored	YAC	0.15 ± 0.17	0.13 ± 0.12	0.12 (− 0.29, 0.54)	0.20
	OAC	0.14 ± 0.14	0.17 ± 0.16	0.22 (− 0.58, 0.14)	0.07
Centuries scored	YAC	0.00 ± 0.02	0.00 ± 0.00	0.15 (− 0.26, 0.57)	0.36
	OAC	0.00 ± 0.03	0.00 ± 0.00	0.10 (− 0.26, 0.46)	0.10

that the *negative frequency* effect may influence the acquisition of perceptual or strategic skills required to outperform a left-handed opponent (Schorer et al., 2012). Specifically, a greater proportion of practice time would likely be spent against right-handed opponents, which may afford better attunement to the perceptual information available from right-handers. This may result in increased difficulty when responding to or anticipating the actions of left-handers (Schorer et al., 2012), given the fewer experiences practicing against skillful left-handers (compared with right-handers).

This study also highlighted a number of performance advantages for left-handed male cricket batters, irrespective of their elite age level competition (**Tables 2, 3**). LHD batters had greater run scoring metrics (e.g., batting aggregate, batting average, runs per innings), batted for a longer period of time, and struck more boundary-4s. It should be noted that while there was a significant difference between these measures, there were also small effect sizes between LHD and RHD batters. No differences between strike rate, boundary-6s, and non-dismissals suggest that LHD batters do not score at a faster rate, nor are they dismissed by the opposition any less often than RHD (e.g., see **Table 2**). Some studies have also reported performance metric advantages for left-handers in other interceptive striking sports such as tennis and baseball (Grondin et al., 1999; Loffing et al., 2010), though there has been far less reported evidence for interactive sports which do not involve a striking implement (Baker and Schorer, 2013; Tirp et al., 2014; Cingoz et al., 2018). Rather than being explained by innate factors, the superiority of left-handers during sporting tasks can be explained due to a combination of tactical or strategic factors (Grouios et al., 2000; Loffing et al., 2012a). One of these crucial factors is the negative frequency effect of left-handers, which highlights the advantage left-handers possess due to their unfamiliarity of their competitors. Schorer et al. (2012) intervention study further supported the importance of familiarity and practice against left-handers, which reported that correctly anticipating the actions of left- or right-handers was dependent on whether participants had been practicing against a left- or right-handed opponent. The findings of these studies have important practical implications for coaches and athletes. In order to minimize the negative frequency effect of left-handers, training environments should be designed in an effort to provide greater opportunities for athletes to practice against left-handed competitors.

Interestingly, the prevalence of left-handedness in female cricket batters at the YAC and OAC level corresponded with levels expected within the general population (**Table 3**) with differences in performance metrics between LHD and RHD batters at the OAC level only. These findings support Loffing (2017) examination of left-handed overrepresentation in sports that have significant temporal demands, which are reportedly greater in the men's game due to faster bowling speeds (Felton et al., 2019). The performance advantage observed for OAC LHD batters may therefore be explained due to increased temporal demands within the older age group competition compared with the younger age group competition (Pyne et al., 2006; Connor et al., 2018). One other possible explanation for the contrasting differences in left-handedness prevalence and performance advantages is the degree to which there is competition for selection. Selection pressures within the "talent system" increase as selection between athletes becomes more competitive. In their review of other selection biases (i.e., relative age effects), Musch and Grondin (2001) described how selection biases increased, as the size of the playing pool from which players were selected from also increased. The 2018/19 cricket participation census released by Cricket Australia highlighted the vast difference between the percentage of male (~70%) and female players (~30%) participating in cricket. Therefore, a smaller population pool from which to select players may attenuate certain biases, such as handedness, and the performance advantage they afford male cricketers. Loffing (2017) highlighted similar findings in racket sports, which reported an overrepresentation of left-handers compared to the general population in elite male competition, but not the female competition. It is currently unclear whether the reduced handedness bias is due to potentially less selection pressures or the temporal demands of the sport. Further research is required to investigate laterality in female competitions.

Finally, to better understand any potential left-handed advantage, moderating factors such as the adoption of a "reversed" stance (Mann et al., 2016) were also analyzed in the current study. The reversed-stance advantage hypothesis (Mann et al., 2016) proposed an explanation for certain performance advantages above and beyond the negative frequency-dependent effects available to all left-handers. Their findings highlighted that professional cricket batsmen were seven times more likely to adopt a reversed stance than inexperienced batsmen. The current study provided some preliminary evidence for reverse stance batters having limited performance advantage at the talent pathway level. One explanation for these small performance advantages may be due to a potential technical advantage imposed by having a dominant hand on the top of the bat handle, rather than the bottom. The role of the top hand is thought to be primarily responsible for guiding the path of the bat in order to intercept the ball (Stretch et al., 1995, 1998). Therefore, it may be more advantageous for the dominant hand to be placed on top of the bat handle (reverse stance) rather than the bottom when attempting to forcefully contact the ball. However, more empirical work is required on the reverse-stance before any practical recommendations can or should be made to coaches, practitioners, and learners.

There are some limitations to consider within this study. First, handedness was compared to the expected distribution within the general sporting population, which may not accurately reflect the exact percentage of amateur level cricketers who are left-handed. Future studies would benefit from analyzing a sample of amateur or recreational level players within the population being investigated (Mann et al., 2016). Analysis was also specific to cricket batters and may not generalize to cricket bowlers. The use of frequencies and counts for those variables in the current study should be analyzed as independent measures for predictive (e.g., counts used via linear regression) and association (e.g., frequencies used via Crosstabs Commands) models in future work. Second, cricketers in this study were categorized based on whether they competed in a younger age or older age national competition, which relies on chronological age cutoffs. Previous research has highlighted that selection in these competitions can heavily bias the sample population toward relative older players (Connor et al., 2019). Finally, the nature of this study does not allow for the analysis of explanatory factors of various batting stances. Rather, it is an examination of batting stance and its impact on real-world sporting performance. Further investigations seeking to explore the mechanisms underpinning batting stance could focus on potential biomechanical differences across various skill levels Stretch et al., 1995; Sarpeshkar and Mann, 2011).

CONCLUSION

The current study has demonstrated a small left-handed performance advantage for cricket batters at the junior national representative level. This advantage was evident for both male and female batters despite overrepresentation of left-handers being evident in the male pathway system only. Highly competitive and large talent selection pools, coupled with temporally demanding sporting tasks, are proposed to explain the increased representation of left-handers in elite junior cricket. The lower frequency of female left-handers (in this case, compared with right-handers) would mean that there are also less practice opportunities against left-handers, which may partially explain the left-hander's performance advantage for female cricket. Further, this study provided evidence for the reverse stance hypothesis contributing a limited performance advantage to cricket batting. Together, these findings highlight the emergence of selection and performance biases occurring at the male and female youth representative level. Practical implications for coaches include creating practice environments that minimize the negative frequency effect, such as providing more practice opportunities against left-handed opponents. Future performance analysis research is encouraged to examine whether selecting a greater number of left-handers increases the likelihood of winning matches.

ETHICS STATEMENT

The study was conducted according to the ethical guidelines of the authors' affiliated institution. Written informed consent from the participants' legal guardian/next of kin was not required to participate in this study as analyzed data were archival data available in the public domain.

AUTHOR CONTRIBUTIONS

JC contributed to the conception and design of the work, writing of the manuscript, and analysis and interpretation of data. DM, AL, and KD contributed to the writing and critiquing of the manuscript and interpretation of data. M-AG contributed to the critiquing of the manuscript, data analysis, and interpretation of the data. All authors contributed to the article and approved the submitted version.

REFERENCES

Baker, J., and Schorer, J. (2013). The Southpaw advantage?-lateral preference in mixed martial arts. *PLoS One* 8:e79793. doi: 10.1371/journal.pone.0079793

Brooks, R., Bussiere, L. F., Jennions, M. D., and Hunt, J. (2004). Sinister strategies succeed at the cricket World Cup. *Proc. R. Soc. Lond. Ser. B Biol. Sci.* 271(Suppl._3), S64–S66.

Cairney, J., Chirico, D., Li, Y. C., Bremer, E., and Graham, J. D. (2018). Are Canadian-born major league baseball players more likely to bat left-handed? A partial test of the hockey-influence on batting hypothesis. *PLoS One* 13:e0195252. doi: 10.1371/journal.pone.00195252

Cingoz, Y. E., Gursoy, R., Ozan, M., Hazar, K., and Dalli, M. (2018). Research on the relation between hand preference and success in karate and taekwondo sports with regards to gender. *Adv. Phys. Educ.* 8:308. doi: 10.4236/ape.2018.83027

Cohen, J. (1988). "The effect size index," in *Statistical Power Analysis For The Behavioral Sciences*, ed. J. Cohen (New York, NY: Lawrence Erlbaum Associated Publishers), 20–26.

Connor, J. D., Farrow, D., and Renshaw, I. (2018). Emergence of skilled behaviors in professional, Amateur and junior cricket batsmen during a representative training scenario. *Front. Psychol.* 9:2012. doi: 10.3389/fpsyg.2018.02012

Connor, J. D., Renshaw, I., and Doma, K. (2019). Moderating factors influence the relative age effect in Australian cricket. *PeerJ* 7:e6867. doi: 10.7717/peerj.6867

Felton, P., Lister, S., Worthington, P. J., and King, M. A. (2019). Comparison of biomechanical characteristics between male and female elite fast bowlers. *J. Sports Sci.* 37, 665–670. doi: 10.1080/02640414.2018.1522700

Grondin, S., Guiard, Y., Ivry, R. B., and Koren, S. (1999). Manual laterality and hitting performance in major league baseball. *J. Exper. Psychol. Hum. Percept. Perform.* 25:747. doi: 10.1037/0096-1523.25.3.747

Grouios, G. (2004). Motoric dominance and sporting excellence: training versus heredity. *Percept. Mot. Skills* 98, 53–66. doi: 10.2466/pms.98.1.53-66

Grouios, G., Tsorbatzoudis, H., Alexandris, K., and Barkoukis, V. (2000). Do left-handed competitors have an innate superiority in sports? *Percept. Mot. Skills* 90, 1273–1282. doi: 10.2466/pms.2000.90.3c.1273

Hagemann, N. (2009). The advantage of being left-handed in interactive sports. *Attent. Percept. Psychophys.* 71, 1641–1648. doi: 10.3758/app.71.7.1641

Harris, L. J. (2010). In fencing, what gives left-handers the edge? Views from the present and the distant past. *Laterality* 15, 15–55.

Johnston, D. W., Nicholls, M. E., Shah, M., and Shields, M. A. (2009). Nature's experiment? Handedness and early childhood development. *Demography* 46, 281–301. doi: 10.1353/dem.0.0053

Loffing, F. (2017). Left-handedness and time pressure in elite interactive ball games. *Biol. Lett.* 13:20170446. doi: 10.1098/rsbl.2017.0446

Loffing, F., and Hagemann, N. (2014). Skill differences in visual anticipation of type of throw in team-handball penalties. *Psychol. Sport Exerc.* 15, 260–267. doi: 10.1016/j.psychsport.2014.01.006

Loffing, F., Hagemann, N., and Strauss, B. (2009). The serve in professional men's tennis: effects of players' handedness. *Intern. J. Perform. Analys. Sport* 9, 255–274. doi: 10.1080/24748668.2009.11868482

Loffing, F., Hagemann, N., and Strauss, B. (2010). Automated processes in tennis: do left-handed players benefit from the tactical preferences of their opponents? *J. Sports Sci.* 28, 435–443. doi: 10.1080/02640410903536459

Loffing, F., Hagemann, N., and Strauss, B. (2012a). Left-handedness in professional and amateur tennis. *PLoS One* 7:e49325. doi: 10.1371/journal.pone.0049325

Loffing, F., Schorer, J., Hagemann, N., and Baker, J. (2012b). On the advantage of being left-handed in volleyball: further evidence of the specificity of skilled visual perception. *Attent. Percept. Psychophys.* 74, 446–453. doi: 10.3758/s13414-011-0252-1

Mann, D. L., Loffing, F., and Allen, P. M. (2017). The success of sinister right-handers in baseball. *N. Engl. J. Med.* 377, 1688–1690. doi: 10.1056/nejmc1711659

Mann, D. L., Runswick, O. R., and Allen, P. M. (2016). Hand and eye dominance in sport: are cricket batters taught to bat back-to-front? *Sports Med.* 46, 1355–1363. doi: 10.1007/s40279-016-0516-y

McMorris, T., and Colenso, S. (1996). Anticipation of professional soccer goalkeepers when facing right-and left-footed penalty kicks. *Percept. Mot. Skills* 82, 931–934. doi: 10.2466/pms.1996.82.3.931

Medland, S. E., Duffy, D. L., Wright, M. J., Geffen, G. M., Hay, D. A., Levy, F., et al. (2009). Genetic influences on handedness: data from 25,732 Australian and Dutch twin families. *Neuropsychologia* 47, 330–337. doi: 10.1016/j.neuropsychologia.2008.09.005

Musch, J., and Grondin, S. (2001). Unequal competition as an impediment to personal development: a review of the relative age effect in sport. *Dev. Rev.* 21, 147–167. doi: 10.1006/drev.2000.0516

Pyne, D. B., Duthie, G. M., Saunders, P. U., Petersen, C. A., and Portus, M. R. (2006). Anthropometric and strength correlates of fast bowling speed in junior and senior cricketers. *J. Strength Condition. Res.* 20:620. doi: 10.1519/00124278-200608000-00025

Raymond, M., Pontier, D., Dufour, A.-B., and Møller, A. P. (1996). Frequency-dependent maintenance of left handedness in humans. *Proc. R. Soc. Lond. Ser. B Biol. Sci.* 263, 1627–1633. doi: 10.1098/rspb.1996.0238

Sarpeshkar, V., and Mann, D. L. (2011). Biomechanics and visual-motor control: how it has, is, and will be used to reveal the secrets of hitting a cricket ball. *Sports Biomech.* 10, 306–323. doi: 10.1080/14763141.2011.629207

Schorer, J., Loffing, F., Hagemann, N., and Baker, J. (2012). Human handedness in interactive situations: negative perceptual frequency effects can be reversed! *J. Sports Sci.* 30, 507–513. doi: 10.1080/02640414.2012.654811

Stretch, R. A., Buys, F. J., Toit, E. D., and Viljoen, G. (1998). Kinematics and kinetics of the drive off the front foot in cricket batting. *J. Sports Sci.* 16, 711–720. doi: 10.1080/026404198366344

Stretch, R. A., Buys, F. J., and Viljoen, G. (1995). The kinetics of the drive off the front foot in cricket batting: hand grip force. *South Afri. J. Res. Sport Phys. Educ. Recreat.* 18, 83–93.

Tirp, J., Baker, J., Weigelt, M., and Schorer, J. (2014). Combat stance in judo-laterality differences between and within competition levels. *Intern. J. Performa. Analys. Sport* 14, 217–224. doi: 10.1080/24748668.2014.11868716

Weissensteiner, J., Abernethy, B., Farrow, D., and Müller, S. (2008). The development of anticipation: a cross-sectional examination of the practice experiences contributing to skill in cricket batting. *J. Sport Exerc. Psychol.* 30, 663–684. doi: 10.1123/jsep.30.6.663

3

Trends in Neuromotor Fitness in 10-to-12-Year-Old Dutch Children: A Comparison between 2006 and 2015/2017

Manou Anselma [1], Dorine C. M. Collard [2], Anniek van Berkum [1], Jos W. R. Twisk [3], Mai J. M. Chinapaw [1] and Teatske M. Altenburg [1]*

[1] Amsterdam UMC, Vrije Universiteit Amsterdam, Department of Public and Occupational Health, Amsterdam Public Health Research Institute, Amsterdam, Netherlands, [2] Mulier Instituut, Utrecht, Netherlands, [3] Amsterdam UMC, Vrije Universiteit Amsterdam, Department of Epidemiology and Biostatistics, Amsterdam Public Health Research Institute, Amsterdam, Netherlands

***Correspondence:**
Manou Anselma
m.anselma@amsterdamumc.nl

Children with a low level of neuromotor fitness are less skilled to participate in sports activities. Moreover, lower levels of neuromotor fitness are related to adiposity, lower cardiovascular health, and poor self-esteem in children. The aim of this paper was to determine neuromotor fitness in 10–12-year-old Dutch children over a 10-year period. Test scores measured in 2015/2017 ($N = 533$ in 2015, $N = 941$ in 2017) were compared with scores of same-aged children measured in 2006 ($N = 1986$). Neuromotor fitness was assessed using the MOPER fitness test battery, including speed and agility, strength, flexibility, and coordination and upper-limb speed. Data were analyzed using multilevel linear regression models and tobit regression analyses in case of skewed distributions with an excess of zeros. Analyses were stratified by age and gender, and adjusted for level of urbanization. Children in 2015/2017 performed significantly worse on speed and agility ($\beta = 0.8$ to 1.1 s), significantly better on coordination/upper-limb speed ($\beta = -1.0$ to -0.6 s), and–except for 12-year-old girls–significantly worse on flexibility vs. children in 2006 ($\beta = -3.4$ to -1.8 cm). Additionally, upper-body strength was significantly worse among 10-year olds ($\beta = -3.2$ to -2.5 s) while leg strength was significantly worse among 11-year-olds in 2015/2017 vs. 2006 ($\beta = -1.8$ to -1.7 cm). Trunk strength was worse among 11- and 12-year old boys ($\beta = 1.1$ to 1.2 s). In line with a previously observed downward trend in neuromotor fitness among children (1980–2006), we found worse scores on speed and agility, and flexibility in 2015/2017 vs. 2006, stressing the need for interventions aimed at improving neuromotor fitness in order to promote physical activity and future health.

Keywords: physical activity, secular trend, youth, neuromotor fitness, MOPER fitness test

INTRODUCTION

Physical fitness is defined as "a set of attributes that people have or achieve", which are health- and skill-related attributes that aid performing physical activity (1). Health-related physical fitness consists of aerobic and neuromotor fitness. Neuromotor fitness comprises the components flexibility, coordination, muscle strength, muscle endurance, and speed of movement (1). Better fitness in children is associated with improved future health (2, 3). There is strong evidence for an inverse relationship between neuromotor fitness components and adiposity, cardiovascular health, bone health, and self-esteem (3). Furthermore, children with low levels of neuromotor fitness can experience difficulties with participating in sports activities as they do not have the physical skills required for the complex movements in sports (4). Children who do not participate in sports are also less likely to participate in sports through adolescence and into adulthood (5, 6), thereby increasing the risk for negative health outcomes at all ages (2, 7, 8). Therefore, it is worrisome that worldwide declining trends in childhood physical fitness scores are observed. A systematic review showed a decline in aerobic fitness scores in 6–19-year-old children from 27 countries between 1970 and 2003 (9). Studies on neuromotor fitness showed similar results (10–14). Lower muscular fitness scores in children were observed in different studies on various tests: 10-year-old English children scored lower on handgrip, sit-ups and bent-arm hang in 2008 vs. 1998 (12); Canadian children scored lower on sit-and-reach and handgrip in 2007/2009 vs. 1981 (11); Lithuanian 11–18-year-old children scored lower on standing broad jump, sit-and-reach, and bent-arm hang in 2012 vs. 1992 (14); and Czech children aged 8–9 and 12–13 scored lower on standing broad jump and sit-ups in 2013 vs. 1986 (13). Lower neuromotor fitness scores were also observed on bent-arm hang, sit-and-reach, 10 × 5 meter run, leg-lift, and plate-tapping in a large sample of Dutch 9–12-year-olds in 2006 vs. 1980 (10). However, it is unknown how this trend developed since 2006, as no data on neuromotor fitness of Dutch children have been published since.

The current paper compares neuromotor fitness scores of the same sample measured in 2006 with scores of 10–12-year-old Dutch children measured in 2015 and 2017, to gain insight in neuromotor fitness trends in the Netherlands in the last decade. As the last decade has seen many interventions aiming to improve physical activity of children in the Netherlands (15, 16), the current study can provide insight into the effectiveness of these efforts on neuromotor fitness of children and required future policy directions.

MATERIALS AND METHODS

Recruitment & Participants

For this study, data from three different studies were combined: baseline data collected in 2006 from the "iPlay" -study (10), data from a cross-sectional study in 2015, and baseline data collected in 2017 from the "Kids in Action" project. The iPlay-study included 2,208 children (aged 9–12 years) from 40 primary schools throughout the Netherlands. The original focus of the iPlay-study was to develop and evaluate a program to prevent sport and physical activity related injuries. More details on the study protocol and results are reported elsewhere (10, 17). The cross-sectional study performed in 2015 included 1000 children (aged 9–12 years) from 18 primary schools in and around the city of 's Hertogenbosch, the Netherlands. The original focus of this study was to determine the neuromotor fitness levels of children in order to indicate which children had a low fitness level. The Kids in Action study included 656 children (aged 9–12 years) from eight primary schools in and around Amsterdam, the Netherlands. The original focus of Kids in Action was to engage 9–12-year-old children from a low socioeconomic neighborhood in the co-creation of interventions to improve their physical activity and dietary behavior. The eight participating schools were located in neighborhoods of low socioeconomic position (18). In all three studies recruitment of children was conducted via schools. In 2015 and 2017, the MOPER test was conducted as part of a regular physical education class and therefore all children attending the respective physical education class participated in the test. In 2006 all children in grades 7 and 8 were eligible to participate in the study, and those who participated in the study took part in the fitness test. In 2017, four intervention schools were approached and all schools participated. Control schools were contacted ($N = 22$) until four schools agreed to participate (19). Parents of eligible children received a letter containing information on the study and a form to decline their child's participation (passive consent; participation rate 99.1%). In 2015, the MOPER test was conducted as part of the physical education class at 18 primary schools by the "care sport connector" working at the schools. The care sport connector links sports to several other sectors such as care and education. Data from all children participating in those physical education classes were obtained. Because the MOPER test was used as a student monitoring system in school, informed consent was not obtained. In 2006, 520 primary schools were invited to participate in the iPlay-study of which 40 primary schools were included. Parents of eligible children from grades 7 and 8 received a letter containing information on the study and a form to decline their child's participation (passive consent; participation rate: 99.9%). As the three studies only included a small number of children under the age of 10 and over the age of 12 years, these children were not included in the analysis. The Medical Ethics Committee of the VU Medical Center approved the iPlay (2006.129) and Kids in Action (2016.366) study.

Measurements

Procedures

All three studies used the same, standardized protocol of the Motor Performance (MOPER) fitness test (20). The MOPER fitness test consists of eight items in total: 10 × 5 meter run, leg-lifting while laying down, plate-tapping, bent-arm hang, sit-and-reach, arm pull, standing high jump, and a 6-min run test. The MOPER fitness test is considered a valid and reliable measurement tool in children aged 9–18 years (21). The average test-retest coefficient was 0.57 for the high-jump and at least 0.74 for the other items in 9–11-year old boys and girls (21). Assessment of structural validity showed low correlations between test items—correlation coefficients ranging from 0.1 to 0.4—indicating that each item measures a unique characteristic of children's neuromotor fitness (21). In the "Kids in Action" study, the arm-pull test was interchanged for a hand-grip test and in both the "Kids in Action" and "iPlay" study, the 6-min run test was not conducted for practical reasons. Therefore, these tests were not included in the analysis. **Table 1** presents a description of the included items of the MOPER fitness test and their metric units.

TABLE 1 |

Item	Characteristic	Description	Unit
1. 10 × 5 meter run	Speed and agility	10 times running between 2 lines with a five meters distance as fast as possible, 2 attempts	s
2. Plate-tapping with one hand	Coordination and upper limb speed	Tapping two plates alternately with the dominant hand 50 times as fast as possible, 2 attempts	s
3. Bent-arm hang	Upper body strength	Hanging from a horizontal bar with bended arms as long as possible, 1 attempt	s
4. Standing high jump	Explosive leg strength	Jumping up from a standing position as high as possible, 2 attempts	cm
5. Leg-lifting while laying down	Trunk and leg strength	Lifting outstretched legs 10 times while laying on back as fast as possible, 1 attempt	s
6. Sit-and-reach	Flexibility	Reaching from sitting position with outstretched legs and arms as far as possible, 3 attempts	cm

The MOPER test was conducted during a physical education lesson in the school's gym. In 2006 the MOPER was conducted at the beginning of the school year (September), in 2015 and 2017 at the end of the school year (April-May). The children had no previous experience with the test and were not familiarized with the test items. Trained researchers, physical education teachers and/or sports instructors conducted the tests. The participating children were divided into groups of two to four children and they performed the test items one by one. The participants performed the MOPER test bare foot and were encouraged by the instructors to perform optimally.

Covariates

Children's age and gender were obtained prior to the MOPER test. Urbanization was included as a confounder as it has been associated with neuromotor fitness in children (22). Data on the degree of urbanization of the school's neighborhood was obtained from Statistics Netherlands (23). The classification of population density in a neighborhood was divided into five categories: extremely high density (>2,500 addresses per km^2), high density (1,500–2,000 addresses per km^2), moderate density (1,000–1,500 addresses per km^2), low density (500–1,000 addresses per km^2), and extremely low density (<500 addresses per km^2).

Statistical Analyses

Descriptive characteristics and fitness test data were analyzed using means, standard deviations or medians and 25th-75th percentiles, and frequencies. For the fitness data first assumptions of normality, linearity, homoscedasticity and the absence of multicollinearity were checked.

The data collected in 2015 and 2017 were combined to increase the sample size. The comparison between the 2006 and 2015/2017 fitness test scores was made using multilevel linear regression analyses for normally distributed variables. The multilevel analyses accounted for the hierarchical structure results within schools (24), e.g., due to different physical activity programs or culture between schools. The residuals of two tests were not normally distributed. The "leg-lifting" scores were log-transformed resulting in a normal distribution of the residuals, and therefore multilevel linear regression analyses were used. Due to the skewed distribution and excess of zeros, differences in "bent-arm hang" were analyzed using tobit regression analysis. All analyses were stratified by age and gender, to provide insight in possible age- and gender-specific trends. Analyses were adjusted for the degree of urbanization of the school's neighborhood. Betas (β) and 95% confidence intervals (CI) are reported; the betas of the log-transformed data have to be interpreted as a ratio. *Post-hoc* power calculations showed that the sample size is sufficient to detect a difference of 3-8% as statistically significant. The statistical analyses were conducted using IBM SPSS Statistics 22.0.

RESULTS

Children were on average 10.8 (SD = 0.7) years old (51% girls) in 2006 and 11.0 (SD = 0.8) years old (52% girls) in 2015/2017. In the 2006 sample, 41% of children attended a school in a high or extremely high density neighborhood, while this was 62% in the 2015/2017 sample.

Table 2 (girls) and **Table 3** (boys) provide the results of all fitness tests (mean and standard deviation, median and interquartile range, beta and confidence interval), stratified by age. Both girls and boys in all age categories performed significantly worse on the "10 × 5 meter run" in 2015/2017 vs. 2006 and significantly better on "plate-tapping". Girls and boys in 2015/2017 ran about 1 s (β ranging from 0.8 to 1.1 s, depending on age and gender) slower than girls and boys in 2006, and were almost a second (β ranging from −1.0 to −0.6 s) faster on "plate-tapping". "Sit-and-reach" scores were significantly worse in 2015/2017 vs. 2006 in girls (β ranging from −3.4 to −1.8 cm) and boys (β ranging from −2.8 to −2.3 cm), except for 12-year-old girls. Girls and boys in all age categories performed worse in 2015/2017 vs. 2006 on the "bent-arm hang" test, but this was only significant in 10-year-old girls (β = −3.2 s) and boys (β = −2.5 s). 11-year-old girls (β = −1.8 cm) and boys (β = −1.7 cm) scored significantly worse on "standing high jump" in 2015/2017 vs. 2006.

11- and 12-year-old boys scored significantly worse on "leg-lifting" in 2015/2017 vs. 2006 (β of log-transformed data = 1.1 and 1.2 s). In girls, no significant differences were found.

DISCUSSION

This study investigated differences in neuromotor fitness in Dutch 10–12-year-old children in 2006 vs. 2015/2017. Children scored worse in most age and gender categories in 2015/2017 on speed and agility ("10 × 5 meter run") and flexibility ("sit-and-reach"). 10-year olds scores worse on upper body strength ("bent-arm hang") and 11-year-olds on explosive leg strength ("standing

TABLE 2 | MOPER fitness test scores for girls in 2006 and 2015/2017, stratified by age.

Girls	10-year-olds			11-year-olds			12-year-olds		
	2006	**2015/2017**	**%**	**2006**	**2015/2017**	**%**	**2006**	**2015/2017**	**%**
10x5 meter run (s)[1] x̄ (SD)	20.1 (1.5)	21.2 (1.8)	+4.9	19.9 (1.5)	20.9 (2.0)	+5.0	19.8 (1.6)	20.7 (2.1)	+4.5
β (95% CI)[2]	**1.0 (0.6; 1.4)*** **			**0.9 (0.6; 1.3)*** **			**0.8 (0.3; 1.4)** **		
n	372	222		516	329		109	213	
Bent-arm hang (s)[3,4] x̃ (IQR)	6.0 (3.0–14.0)	5.0 (1.0–10.0)	−16.7	6.0 (2.0–13.0)	4.0 (1.0–10.0)	−33.3	6.0 (2.0–12.0)	4.0 (1.0–11.0)	−33.3
β (95% CI)[2]	**−3.2 (−5.2; −1.1)** **			−0.8 (−2.4; 0.7)			−0.8 (−3.3; 1.6)		
n	372	224		521	330		109	213	
High jump (cm)[3] x̄ (SD)	35.8 (6.3)	34.6 (6.4)	−3.4	37.3 (6.3)	35.2 (6.5)	−5.6	37.5 (6.4)	36.4 (6.3)	−2.9
β (95% CI)[2]	−0.6 (−2.2; 0.9)			**−1.8 (−2.9; −0.8)** **			−1.4 (−3.0; 0.7)		
n	373	224		520	330		109	213	
Leg-lifting (s) [1,4,5] *x̃* (IQR)	16.3 (13.9–19.1)	14.8 (13.2–17.6)	−9.2	16.5 (14.2–19.9)	15.9 (13.9–20.0)	−3.6	16.3 (13.8–21.0)	15.4 (13.3–18.3)	−5.5
β (95% CI)[2]	1.0 (0.9–1.1)			1.0 (1.0–1.1)			1.0 (0.9–1.1)		
n	369	223		519	330		107	212	
Sit-and-reach (cm)[3] x̄ (SD)	30.4 (6.0)	28.4 (7.1)	−6.6	30.2 (6.2)	26.8 (7.3)	−11.3	29.1 (6.6)	28.1 (7.7)	−3.4
β (95% CI)[2]	**−1.8 (−3.2; −0.4)***			**−3.4 (−4.4; −2.4)*** **			−1.1 (−3.0; 0.7)		
n	373	224		515	330		109	213	
Plate-tapping (s) [1] x̄ (SD)	15.2 (1.8)	14.6 (2.0)	−3.9	14.4 (1.8)	13.7 (2.0)	−4.9	14.1 (1.7)	13.2 (1.8)	−6.4
β (95% CI)[2]	**−0.8 (−1.3; −0.3)** **			**−0.7 (−1.1; −0.4)*** **			**−0.9 (−1.4; −0.3)** **		
n	372	224		521	330		109	213	

*[1] A lower value indicates a better test score [2] 2015/2017 vs. 2006 [3] A higher value indicates a better test score [4] Data not normally distributed, therefore the median (x̃) and interquartile range (IQR) (25th-75th percentiles) are provided [5] Data have been log-transformed, therefore the β should be interpreted as a ratio. Bold is significant, by *$p < 0.05$, **$p < 0.01$, ***$p < 0.001$.*

high-jump"). In contrast, children in 2015/2017 performed better on coordination/upper limb speed ("plate-tapping") vs. 2006.

In contrast to a Dutch study comparing neuromotor fitness scores of children between 2006 and 1980 (10), the current study found no significant differences on trunk and leg strength ("leg-lifting") and improved scores on coordination and upper limb speed ("plate-tapping") in 2015/2017 vs. 2006 in most age and gender groups. A possible explanation for the improved "plate-tapping" scores could be the increase in computer use and gaming (25). Playing certain video games can promote fine motor skills and movement coordination (26), which may have contributed to children's improved "plate-tapping" scores. The item "leg-lifting" showed only worse scores in 11- and 12-year-old boys. In 2006 vs. 1980 all age and gender categories scored significantly worse on upper body strength ("bent-arm hang"), while in the current study significant worse scores were only found in 10-year olds in 2015/2017 vs. 2006. Lastly, in 2006 vs. 1980 children in all age and gender categories scored significantly better on explosive leg strength ("standing high-jump"), while the current study only found significantly worse scores in 11-year-olds.

Previous studies evaluating motor fitness of children over a longer time period showed mixed results. Several studies in Europe and Canada observed worse scores on most items of the motor fitness tests over the past two decades (11, 12, 27). In contrast, one study in Portuguese children demonstrated better scores on speed, trunk strength, and flexibility in 2013 compared to 1993, and no changes in explosive leg strength (28). The authors contributed the improvements to more access to and participation in organized sports of Portuguese children over this time period. The Dutch study comparing neuromotor fitness scores of children between 2006 and 1980, found worse neuromotor fitness scores in 2006 on upper body strength, flexibility, speed and agility, trunk and leg strength, and coordination and upper limb speed (10). The current study again shows significantly worse scores in 2015/2017 vs. 2006 on speed and agility, and flexibility in boys aged 10–12 years and girls aged 10 and 11 years. The declines on these test-items were small, for example only about 1 s on the "10 × 5 meter run," but differences are comparable to and in some instances larger than reported in the study comparing scores from 2006 to 1980 in the Netherlands (10). Our finding that the downward trend in certain neuromotor fitness scores from 1980 to 2006 has continued from 2006 to 2015/2017, may have important implications for physical activity enjoyment and participation and as a result future health (29).

The downward trend over the last decades in children's neuromotor fitness may be related to downward trends in children's motor competence (30). A study funded by the Dutch ministry showed lower levels of motor competence (balancing, swinging on a rope, aiming at a high target, catching and throwing a small ball via the wall and playing tennis against a wall) in Dutch children from 2006 vs. 2016 (31). The Dutch government responded to these alarming results by implementing several policies to improve children's motor competence (32), such as the recent adoption of an amendment that obligates Dutch primary schools to provide at least 2 h of physical education per week (33). In the past decade a number of Dutch policies have focused on improving physical activity and/or motor competence

TABLE 3 | MOPER fitness scores for boys in 2006 and 2015/2017, stratified by age.

Boys	10-year-olds			11-year-olds			12-year-olds		
	2006	**2015/2017**	**%**	**2006**	**2015/2017**	**%**	**2006**	**2015/2017**	**%**
10 × 5 meter run (s)[1] $\bar{x}$ (SD)	19.7 (1.5)	20.7 (2.2)	+5.1	19.4 (1.6)	20.4 (2.2)	+5.1	19.2 (1.5)	20.1 (2.0)	+4.7
β (95% CI)[2]	**0.9 (0.4; 1.4)****			**1.0 (0.5; 1.5)*****			**1.1 (0.5; 1.6)*****		
n	366	205		459	298		153	204	
Bent-arm hang (s)[3,4]	9.0 (4.0–20.0)	5.0 (1.0–10.0)	−44.4	9.0 (4.0–18.0)	7.0 (2.0–16.0)	−22.2	10.0 (4.0–21.0)	7.0 (1.0–15.8)	−30.0
$\tilde{x}$ (IQR) β (95% CI)[2]	**−2.5 (−5.0; −0.0)***			−1.5 (−3.5; 0.6)			−2.9 (−5.9; 0.1)		
n	365	205		458	298		153	204	
High jump (cm)[3] $\bar{x}$ (SD)	36.8(5.8)	35.8(6.3)	−2.7	38.6(6.5)	36.8(6.7)	−4.7	39.6(6.5)	39.2(7.0)	−1.0
β (95% CI)[2]	−0.8 (−2.2; 0.5)			**−1.7 (−3.0; −0.4)****			−0.5 (−2.1; 1.2)		
n	367	205		460	298		153	204	
Leg-lifting (s)[1,4,5] $\tilde{x}$ (IQR)	16.4 (14.2–20.0)	15.8 (13.4–19.8)	−3.7	16.7 (13.9–21.4)	16.8 (13.9–21.0)	+0.6	16.4 (13.9–20.8)	17.2 (13.5–22.3)	+4.9
β (95% CI)[2]	1.0 (0.9–1.1)			**1.1 (1.0-1.2)***			**1.2 (1.0-1.4)***		
n	363	205		449	298		147	203	
Sit-and-reach (cm)[3] $\bar{x}$ (SD)	27.0 (6.4)	24.6 (6.5)		25.4 (6.9)	22.7 (6.8)	−10.6	25.5 (7.1)	23.6 (6.6)	−7.5
β (95% CI)[2]	**−2.3 (−3.4; −1.2)*****		−8.9	**−2.8 (−4.0; −1.6)*****			**−2.3 (−4.1;−0.5)***		
n	365	205		459	298		153	204	
Plate-tapping (s)[1] $\bar{x}$ (SD)	15.6 (1.9)	14.6 (1.9)	−6.4	14.8 (1.8)	14.0 (2.0)	−5.4	14.1 (1.9)	13.4(1.8)	−5.0
β (95% CI)[2]	**−1.0 (−1.4; −0.6)*****			**−0.7 (−1.1; −0.3)****			**−0.6 (-1.1; −0.2)***		
n	367	205		59	298		153	204	

*[1] A lower value indicates a better test score [2] 2015/2017 vs. 2006 [3] A higher value indicates a better test score [4] Data not normally distributed, therefore the median ($\tilde{x}$) and interquartile range (IQR) (25th-75th percentiles) are provided. [5] Data have been log-transformed, therefore the β should be interpreted as a ratio. Bold is significant, by *$p < 0.05$, **$p < 0.01$, ***$p < 0.001$.*

of children. Practical implications of our results are that upper-body strength and flexibility need specific attention in physical education or physical activity interventions. Implementing internationally standardized tests as part of the school curriculum could provide more insight in time trends and risk groups, and consequently lead to better tailored interventions. Future research has to determine the effects of implemented policies on children's neuromotor fitness and motor competence, as well as physical activity levels and health indicators.

A major strength of this study is the large sample size, including 1986 children in the 2006 sample and 1,474 in the 2015/2017 sample. The use of the same fitness test items and a standardized measurement protocol further strengthens this study as non-standardization of tests has been a problem in previous studies (11). Lastly, the current study compares neuromotor fitness levels in children in 2015/2017 vs. 2006 and such recent data was not available yet. A major limitation of this study is that no data was available at both the individual and school level on potential covariates such as physical activity level, socioeconomic position, cultural background, and BMI, while these could have influenced the results. The schools neighborhoods for example differed in the percentage of people with a non-Western background, with ~11.4% in 2006 and 23.1% in 2015/2017 (34). We adjusted for the degree of urbanization of the school's neighborhood, as that was the only data available. Unfortunately, we could also not adjust for BMI. A previous study including the 2006 MOPER data showed that even when children with overweight and obesity were excluded from the analyses, most declines in children's neuromotor fitness scores from 1980 to 2006 remained significant (10). This suggests that the inferior neuromotor fitness scores found in current generations are not only due to the higher prevalence of overweight, however, we could not verify this in the current study.

CONCLUSIONS

The current study found that the previously observed downward trend in most components of neuromotor fitness among 10–12-year old Dutch children from 1980 to 2006 continued from 2006 to 2015/2017. Persistent low scores were found on most strength components and worsened scores on speed and agility and flexibility (with the exception of 12-year-old girls for the latter item) in 2015/2017 vs. 2006. This downward trend in neuromotor fitness can have important implications on physical activity enjoyment and participation and thereby future health. Therefore, improving children's neuromotor fitness from an early age should be a larger public health priority and be reflected as such in local and national policy.

ETHICS STATEMENT

The iPlay (2006.129) and Kids in Action (2016.366) study were approved by the Medical Ethics Committee of the VU Medical Center. Written informed consent for participation was not provided by the participants' legal guardians/next of kin because: in 2015, the MOPER test was used as a student monitoring system in school and therefore informed consent was not obtained; in 2006 and 2017, parents of eligible children received a letter containing information on the study and a form to decline their child's participation.

AUTHOR CONTRIBUTIONS

TA, MC, and MA designed the 2017 study. MA coordinated and led data collection in 2017 with AB assisting the data collection. DC and MC designed the 2006 study with DC coordinating and leading data collection. AB conducted the data cleaning and assisted in the first draft of this manuscript. MA wrote the manuscript with DC, MC, and TA providing critical input and feedback. JT assisted with the data analysis. All authors contributed to the article and approved the submitted version.

ACKNOWLEDGMENTS

We would like to thank all researchers and physical education teachers who helped with the administration of the tests and the children for their enthusiastic participation. We would like to thank D. van den Oever for sharing the data collected in 2015.

REFERENCES

Caspersen CJ, Powell KE, Christenson GM. Physical activity, exercise, and physical fitness: definitions and distinctions for health-related research. *Public Health Rep.* (1985) 100:126–31.

Janssen I, Leblanc AG. Systematic review of the health benefits of physical activity and fitness in school-aged children and youth. *Int J Behav Nutr Phys Act.* (2010) 7:40. doi: 10.1186/1479-5868-7-40

Smith JJ, Eather N, Morgan PJ, Plotnikoff RC, Faigenbaum AD, Lubans DR. The health benefits of muscular fitness for children and adolescents: a systematic review and meta-analysis. *Sports Med.* (2014) 44:1209–23. doi:10.1007/s40279-014-0196-4

Hardy LL, Reinten-Reynolds T, Espinel P, Zask A, Okely AD. Prevalence and correlates of low fundamental movement skill competency in children. *Pediatrics.* (2012) 130:e390–8. doi: 10.1542/peds.2012-0345

Perkins DE, Jacobs J, Barber B, Eccles J. Childhood and adolescent sports participation as predictors of participation in sports and physical fitness activities during young adulthood. *Youth Soc.* (2004) 35: 495–520.

Gallant F, O'Loughlin JL, Brunet J, Sabiston CM, Belanger M. Childhood sports participation and adolescent sport profile. *Pediatrics.* (2017) 140:e20171449. doi: 10.1542/peds.2017-1449

Hallal PC, Victora CG, Azevedo MR, Wells JC. Adolescent physical activity and health: a systematic review. *Sports Med.* (2006) 36:1019–30. doi: 10.2165/00007256-200636120-00003

Warburton DER, Bredin SSD. Health benefits of physical activity: a systematic review of current systematic reviews. *Curr Opin Cardiol.* (2017) 32:541–56. doi:10.1097/HCO.0000000000000437

Tomkinson GR, Olds TS. Secular changes in pediatric aerobic fitness test performance: the global picture. *Med Sport Sci.* (2007) 50:46–66. doi: 10.1159/000101075

Runhaar J, Collard DC, Singh AS, Kemper HC, van Mechelen W, Chinapaw M. Motor fitness in Dutch youth: differences over a 26-year period (1980- 2006). *J Sci Med Sport.* (2010) 13:323–8. doi: 10.1016/j.jsams.2009.04.006

Tremblay MS, Shields M, Laviolette M, Craig CL, Janssen I, Connor Gorber S. Fitness of Canadian children and youth: results from the 2007-2009 Canadian Health Measures Survey. *Health Rep.* (2010) 21:7–20.

Cohen DD, Voss C, Taylor MJ, Delextrat A, Ogunleye AA, Sandercock GR. Ten-year secular changes in muscular fitness in english children. *Acta Paediatr.* (2011) 100:e175–7. doi: 10.1111/j.1651-2227.2011.02318.x

Mullerova D, Langmajerova J, Sedlacek P, Dvorakova J, Hirschner T, Weber Z, et al. Dramatic decrease in muscular fitness in the czech schoolchildren over the last 20 years. *Cent Eur J Public Health.* (2015) 23 (Suppl):S9–13. doi: 10.21101/cejph.a4069

Venckunas T, Emeljanovas A, Mieziene B, Volbekiene V. Secular trends in physical fitness and body size in Lithuanian children and adolescents between 1992 and 2012. *J Epidemiol Community Health.* (2017) 71:181–7. doi:10.1136/jech-2016-207307

European Commission and WHO Regional Office for Europe. *Netherlands Physical Activity Factsheet. European Union Member States Factsheets on Health-Enhancing Physical Activity.* European Commission and WHO Regional Office for Europe (2015). Available online at: https://www.euro.who. int/ data/ assets/pdf_file/0011/382574/netherlands-eng.pdf

European Commission and WHO Regional Office for Europe. *Netherlands Physical Activity Factsheet 2018. Physical Activity Factsheets for the 28 European Union Member States of the WHO European Region.* European Commission and WHO Regional Office for Europe (2018).

Collard DC, Chinapaw MJ, Verhagen EA, Bakker I, van Mechelen W. Effectiveness of a school-based physical activity-related injury prevention program on risk behavior and neuromotor fitness a cluster randomized controlled trial. *Int J Behav Nutr Phys Act.* (2010) 7:9. doi: 10.1186/1479-5868-7-9

Municipality of Amsterdam. *Gebiedsanalyse 2016 Noord West Stadsdeel Noord.* Municipality of Amsterdam (2016). p. 1–10. Available online at: https:// docplayer.nl/45710584-Gebiedsanalyse-2016-noord-west-stadsdeel- noord. html

Anselma M, Altenburg TM, Emke H, van Nassau F, Jurg M, Ruiter RAC, et al. Co-designing obesity prevention interventions together with children: intervention mapping meets youth-led participatory action research. *Int J Behav Nutr Phys Act.* (2019) 16:130. doi: 10.1186/s12966-019- 0891-5

Leyten C, Kemper HCG, Verschuur R. *De Moper Fitheidstest: Handleiding en Prestatieschalen 9 t/m 11 Jarigen.* Haarlem: BV Uitgeverij De Vrieseborch (1982).

Leyten C. *De Moper Fitheidstest: Onderzoeksverslag - 9 t/m 11 Jarigen.* Haarlem: BV Uitgeverij De Vrieseborch (1982).

Chillon P, Ortega FB, Ferrando JA, Casajus JA. Physical fitness in rural and urban children and adolescents from Spain. *J Sci Med Sport.* (2011) 14:417–23. doi: 10.1016/j.jsams.2011.04.004

Statistics Netherlands (CBS). *Kerncijfers Wijken En Buurten 2004-2018.* (2018). Retrieved from https://www.cbs.nl/nl-nl/dossier/nederland- regionaal/wijk-en-buurtstatistieken/kerncijfers-wijken-en-buurten-2004- 2018 (accessed November 13, 2020).

Twisk JWR. *Applied Multilevel Analysis: A Practical Guide.* Cambridge University Press (2006). p. 1–182. Available online at: https:// www.onderwijsinspectie.nl/ documenten/rapporten/2018/04/20/peil- bewegingsonderwijs-einde-basis-speciaal-basisonderwijs-2016-2017

Bucksch J, Sigmundova D, Hamrik Z, Troped PJ, Melkevik O, Ahluwalia N, et al. International trends in adolescent screen-time behaviors from 2002 to 2010. *J Adolesc Health.* (2016) 58:417–25. doi: 10.1016/j.jadohealth.2015.11.014

Borecki L, Tolstych K, Pokorski M. *Computer Games and Fine Motor Skills.* Dordrecht, Springer (2013).

Ignasiak Z, Sławińska T, Malina RM. Short term secular change in body size and physical fitness of youth 7–15 years in Southwestern Poland: 2001– 2002 and 2010–2011. *Anthropol Rev.* (2016) 79:311. doi: 10.1515/anre-20 16-0023

Costa AM, Costa MJ, Reis AA, Ferreira S, Martins J, Pereira A. Secular trends in anthropometrics and physical fitness of young portuguese school-aged children. *Acta Med Port.* (2017) 30:108–14. doi: 10.20344/ amp.7712

Fransen J, Deprez D, Pion J, Tallir IB, D'Hondt E, Vaeyens R, et al. Changes in physical fitness and sports participation among children with different levels of motor competence: a 2-year longitudinal study. *Pediatr Exerc Sci.* (2014) 26:11–21. doi: 10.1123/pes.20 13-0005

Robinson LE, Stodden DF, Barnett LM, Lopes VP, Logan SW, Rodrigues LP, et al. Motor competence and its effect on positive developmental trajectories of health. *Sports Med.* (2015) 45:1273–84. doi: 10.1007/s40279-015- 0351-6

Inspection of education. *Peil.Bewegingsonderwijs.* Ministry of Education Culture and Science [Ministerie van Onderwijs Cultuur en Wetenschap] (2018).

Ministry of Public Health Well-being and Sports. *National Sports Agreement.* Dutch: Nationaal Sportakkoord (2018).

Sport and Strategie. *"The Obligated Two Hours of PE is Necessary to Intervene at Schools".* (2020). Retrieved from https://www.sportenstrategie. nl/overheid/ de-verplichte-twee-uur-gym-is-nodig-om-in-te-grijpen-op- scholen/ (accessed March 03, 2020).

Central bureau of statistics (CBS). *Population; Key Figures.* (2020). Retrieved from https://opendata.cbs.nl/statline/portal.html?_la=nl&_catalog=CBS& tableId=37296ned&_theme=61 (accessed April 23, 2020).

4

Positional In-Match Running Demands of University Rugby Players in South Africa

*Cameron Donkin[1], Ranel Venter[1], Derik Coetzee[2] and Wilbur Kraak[1]**

[1] Department of Sport Science, Stellenbosch University, Stellenbosch, South Africa, [2] Department of Sport and Exercise Sciences, University of the Free State, Bloemfontein, South Africa

Correspondence:
Wilbur Kraak
kjw@sun.ac.za

The implementation of the Varsity Cup rugby competition among South African universities has sparked interest in university rugby cultures around the country. The Varsity Cup has established itself as one of the most important rugby competitions for full-time students. The development of specific conditioning programs for rugby players requires a thorough understanding of the game and the unique demands of playing positions. Therefore, the study aimed to investigate the in-match running demands of South African university rugby players by using GPS during match play for primary and secondary positional groups. Rugby players (n = 40) from two universities were assessed during match play (n = 17) over a competitive season by using GPS. Players were grouped into two primary positional groups, forwards (n = 22) and backs (n = 18), and five secondary positional groups, tight forwards (n = 14), loose forwards (n = 8), half backs (n = 5), inside backs (n = 6), and outside backs (n = 7). The GPS analysis provided the following match-play movements: total distance, high-speed meters, maximum velocity, match intensity, the number of accelerations and decelerations, and velocity zone. Halfbacks recorded the highest total distance (6620.9 $\pm$ 784.4 m; p = 0.02) and match intensity (77.7 $\pm$ 11.6 m/min; p = 0.01). Outside backs recorded the highest maximum velocity (8.385 $\pm$ 1.242 m/s; p = 0.00). Loose forwards registered the highest number of accelerations (385.5 $\pm$ 122.1) and decelerations (378.7 $\pm$ 108.1). Backs and their specific subgroups play at and within high velocity thresholds, significantly higher (p = 0.01) than that of the forwards. Forwards tend to be involved in a higher amount of accelerations and decelerations during match play, suggesting that forward play is at close quarters to the opposition. During university rugby matches, the backs covered greater distances and speeds than the forwards, whereas the forwards achieved more accelerations and decelerations than backs. Results from the study can assist Varsity Cup strength and conditioning coaches to prepare players for the position-specific demands of the competition.

Keywords: GPS, rugby union, positional groups, student athletes, performance analysis

INTRODUCTION

Rugby union ("rugby"), as an intermittent, high-intensity, collision sport that is popular globally, is characterized by physically intense phases of play and displays of speed, skill, and strength (Lindsay et al., 2015). In South Africa, rugby is enjoyed by players of all ages (Harris and Wise, 2011). Universities in South Africa have become part of an inter-university competition (Varsity Cup) that allows students to compete against one another on a semi-professional level. The Varsity Cup (VC) rugby competition in South Africa has become the most innovative and stimulating competitions in South Africa in terms of ideas (rules and law changes) and match play. The VC has expanded since it commenced in 2008 and has developed into a high-intensity, physically high-demanding competition at a university level. Furthermore, all the players are full-time students and have a full academic program. Nine university teams partake in a round-robin format to determine the top four university teams that would progress to knockout rounds. Teams play an equal number of matches both home and away over the 9-week round-robin format with one bye before the knockout stages of the competition. Limited information on the management of players to perform on all the demands of being a student athlete in South Africa has been published. However, since the onset of professionalism in rugby in 1995, the demands of the game have increased. The game became more intense, with players becoming heavier, and the backs particularly became taller (Quarrie and Hopkins, 2007; Vahed et al., 2014). The number of impacts and impacts at high speed (McLellan et al., 2011; Owen et al., 2015) and increased ball-in-play time (Schoeman and Coetzee, 2014) contributed to the changing demands of the sport. These increases could predominantly be attributed to changes in laws and improved match analysis, equipment technology, and player conditioning (Quarrie and Hopkins, 2007).

Along with increased demands on players, the demands differ per position played (Duthie et al., 2003; Austin et al., 2011; Cahill et al., 2013; Tee and Coopoo, 2015; Tee et al., 2017). Players are generally separated into two primary positional groups, namely, backs and forwards, and further subdivided into secondary positional groups discussed later in the "Materials and Methods" section (Duthie et al., 2003). All players are required to perform core actions/activities, such as tackling and rucking, during a match (Duthie et al., 2003), but the technical and tactical demands on players are different for the playing positions (Owen et al., 2015; Tee et al., 2018). Technically, backs focus on handling, passing, kicking, and running, whereas forwards focus on body position in contact and ball carrying. Tactically backs may aim to beat the defense using skillful moves and speed, where forwards may look to physically beat opponents to gain field advantage. To determine these position-specific characteristics, it is often difficult due to the dynamic movement of opposition players; accurate methods to quantify in-match running demands are required. Rugby as a sport takes place in a complex dynamic setting (Rothwell et al., 2017). In such a system, recorded player data for specific metrics become dependent on the actions of the opposition, known as the ecological and dynamic systems approach (Vilar et al., 2012). Although not a focus of this specific study, the understanding of the dynamic systems approach can assist in the understanding of recorded metrics as well as specific skill acquisition (Vilar et al., 2012; Rothwell et al., 2017). To develop specific conditioning programs and recovery strategies for rugby players, a thorough understanding of the game and the unique demands of different playing positions is essential (Venter et al., 2011).

A modern method used to quantify these positional demands is through global positioning systems (GPS). Research on players' primary positional demands (Cunniffe et al., 2009) revealed that the total distances covered by elite rugby players per game by forwards were 6,680 m, and by backs, 7,227 m. Other studies confirmed that forwards accumulated 5,850 m (Cahill et al., 2013), 6680 m (Cunniffe et al., 2009), and 5,370 m (Cunningham et al., 2016) of total running distance. The backs accumulated total running distances of 6,545 m (Cahill et al., 2013), 7,227 m (Cunniffe et al., 2009), and 6,230 m (Cunningham et al., 2016). Austin et al. (2011) reported that the total distances covered by secondary positional groups during the Super Rugby tournament were as follows: front row (4,662 ± 659 m); back row (5,262 ± 131 m); inside backs (6,095 ± 213 m); and outside backs (4,774 ± 1,017 m). Yamamoto et al. (2017) found in a study on Japanese professional rugby players that the distance covered for the front row was 5604.0 m, second and third row forwards 5690.2 m, scrumhalf's 7001.0 m, and backs 6072.3 m. However, little research has been carried out that quantified the running demands of university rugby players per positional group. Particular attention should be paid to the specific physical requirements of players in different positions to ensure that they receive adequate training (Tee et al., 2017) and individualized recovery.

GPS uses wearable microtechnology to record geographic positions over time and create a movement profile for players (Owen et al., 2015). Using this form of player movement analysis, individual external player loads can indicate specific positional demands of these players. The purpose of any rugby-specific physical training program should be to optimally prepare players for the demands of match play (Owen et al., 2015; Tee et al., 2018). This can be achieved by maximizing training specificity through the manipulation of training activities to simulate or exceed the skill and physical demands of the match (Tee et al., 2018). Tee et al. (2018) noted that physical preparation should not be done in isolation but with all the subsequent components for performance. Training sessions should be based around a combination of physical and mental aspects of the game that emulate match specificity, such as moving at high velocities and making decisions based on stimuli, such as defenders (Tee et al., 2018). The purpose of the current study was to give strength and conditioning coaches an indication of the match-specific positional running demands of South African university rugby players to develop and execute specific training sessions to maximize performance. Performance profiling of players participating in university rugby is necessary to establish normative values; the performance profiles can assist strength and conditioning coaches in monitoring players' readiness for competition. Additionally, teams with the means to monitor training sessions can maximize performance and minimize injury risk through analyzing player load. Repeated exposure to high-speed running, accelerations, and decelerations will increase both injury risk and player load. Therefore, the current study aimed to investigate the in-match running demands of South African university rugby players by using GPS during match play for primary and secondary positional groups.

MATERIALS AND METHODS

Participants

A total of 40 male rugby players from two South African universities competing in the 2018 VC rugby competition volunteered to participate in the study (**Table 1**). A total of 17 matches were played by the two teams against different teams and each other, both home and away for the competition duration. All players were informed about the purpose of the study and gave informed consent before participating in the study. The participants' demographic information is shown in **Table 1**. Data were excluded from the study if a participant played less than 60 min or the GPS device lost signal. A total of 271 observations were included based on the inclusion and exclusion criteria.

Players were categorized according to their playing positions and divided into primary positional groups described by Cahill et al. (2013) and Owen et al. (2015), namely, forwards (loose-head prop, hooker, tight-head prop, locks, blind-side flanker, open-side flanker, and eighth man) and backs (scrum-half, fly half, left winger, inside center, outside center, right winger, and fullback). The grouping was assumed to accurately reflect similar match demands for the playing positions and allow comparison with previous research. The secondary positional grouping subdivided the team into five groups, similar to the study by Owen et al. (2015). The five secondary positional groups for the current study consist of the tight forwards (loose head prop, hooker, tight-head prop, and locks), loose forwards (blind-side flanker, open-side flanker, and eighth-man), half backs (scrumhalf and fly half), inside backs (inside and outside centers), and outside backs (right- and left-wingers and fullbacks). The current study grouped the scrum and fly halves into one group called the half backs. The two positions were combined because the studies by Quarrie et al. (2013) and Tee and Coopoo (2015) reported no significant differences between the two playing positions. **Table 2** presents the in-match running demands variables used in the current study. Only three velocity zones were measured as these zones were seen to best describe the running demands of rugby players, where velocity zones 1 and 2 represented low-velocity movements such as walking. The Health Sciences Research Ethics Committee (HSREC) (UFS-HSD2017/0062) at the University of the Free State approved the study.

TABLE 2 | In-match running demands variables used in the study.

Variables	Description
Total distance (m)	Total distance describes the total number of meters covered by a player during the match. The metric is measured by the displacement of the GPS unit over time.
High-speed meters (m)	High-speed meters refer to distance covered at high speed. For the purpose of the current study, all meters ran above 5.56 m/s were registered as high-speed meters. Similar to total distance, the time between displacements of different samples when recording data indicates the type of meterage registered.
Maximum velocity (m/s)	Represents the maximum velocity achieved by a player during the match. Maximum velocity is registered at the peak of the player's running performance.
Match intensity (m/min)	Measured as meters covered per minute, this metric represents an internal calculation of the GPS software that determines the meters ran over the duration of the match and equates it as match intensity. Cummins et al. (2013) similarly referred to relative distance (with reference to match intensity) as a calculated workload based on the overall distance covered per minute.
Number of accelerations (n) and decelerations (n)	Accelerations and decelerations indicate a change in speed over the established velocity zones. Accelerations are registered because of increases in speed through the velocity zones and decelerations are recorded because of decreases in speed through the velocity zones.
Velocity zones	Velocity zones 3 (4.44–5.56 m/s), 4 (5.57–6.94 m/s), and 5 (>6.95 m/s) were indicative of the total distance covered within the velocity zones.

Data Collection Procedure

Players from the two universities were fitted with Catapult Minimax X4 10 Hz GPS units for the matches (Catapult;

TABLE 1 | Demographic information of participants per positional group.

Positional group	n	Age (years) M ± SD	Height (cm) M ± SD	Weight (kg) M ± SD	Observations n
Combined	40	20.77 ± 0.44	179.55 ± 1.21	91.52 ± 0.83	271
Forwards	22	20.75 ± 0.61	183.34 ± 1.04^	101.24 ± 1.13^	147
Backs	18	20.78 ± 0.06	177.02 ± 0.75	85.05 ± 0.52	124
Tight forwards	14	20.84 ± 1.36	183.10 ± 7.7^{cde}	107.05 ± 8.83^{cde}	94
Loose forwards	8	20.65 ± 2.58	183.58 ± 5.63^{cde}	95.43 ± 6.57^{cde}	53
Half-backs	5	20.72 ± 1.48	175.22 ± 5.87	81.10 ± 7.68	36
Inside backs	6	20.67 ± 1.62	178.33 ± 4.05	88.43 ± 7.43	36
Outside backs	7	20.95 ± 1.57	177.50 ± 5.01	85.60 ± 8.64	52

^denotes significant differences in weight between primary positional groups. [a] denotes significant differences when comparing tight forwards to other secondary positional groups. [b] denotes significant differences when comparing loose forwards to other secondary positional groups. [c] denotes significant differences when comparing half backs to other secondary positional groups. [d] denotes significant differences when comparing inside backs to other secondary positional groups. [e] denotes significant differences when comparing outside backs to other secondary positional groups ($p \leq 0.05$).

Melbourne, Australia). These two universities made use of the Catapult Minimax X4 10 Hz GPS units with the same velocity zones allowing for comparisons to be made on players' performance. It should also be noted that the use of GPS units during matches is not common within the VC setting. The GPS units fitted into specialized neoprene vests designed specifically for positioning and securing of the unit on the player's upper back. The GPS unit was switched on before the start of the warm-up and switched off after the match. The warm-up and half-time data were excluded and discarded. The data were analyzed to identify information regarding player demands as presented in **Table 3** during match play in primary and secondary positional groups. Data were extracted and divided into the relative periods from the GPS units, using the Catapult Open Field (version 1.21.1) software (Catapult; Melbourne, Australia). Data were extracted as a csv file for further clean-up in a Microsoft Excel spreadsheet before being analyzed by the Statistica 13 data processing package (version 13.0.159.8) (Dell Inc., Round Rock, TX, United States).

Data Analysis

The Statistica 13 software package was used to process the data. Participant information was described by using descriptive statistics (mean [M] ± standard deviation [SD]). Mixed model ANOVA was used with "player" and "player*period" as random effects, and "position," "period," and "position*period" as fixed effects. Fisher least significant difference (LSD) testing was used for *post-hoc* testing. Normality assumptions were evaluated by inspecting normal probability plots and were mostly found to be acceptable. Participants were grouped according to primary and secondary positional groups. The position*period effect was found to be not significant in all cases, so the results for the position effect are reported.

RESULTS

Results for all recorded metrics and per positional group are presented in **Table 3**. When comparing the primary positional groups, backs recorded significantly higher totals for high speed meters (p = 0.01), maximum velocity (p = 0.01), and velocity zones 3 (p = 0.01), 4 (p = 0.01), and 5 (p = 0.01). No significant differences were observed for the total distance covered and the number of accelerations and decelerations.

When comparing secondary positional groups, significant differences were observed for all metrics except for the number of accelerations and decelerations between the different subgroups. Half backs covered the highest total distance, significantly more (p = 0.02) than tight forwards. The outside backs covered the most high-speed meters (556.450 m), significantly more than all secondary positional groups (p = 0.01). The outside backs recorded the highest maximum velocity (8.385 ± 1.242 m/s), significantly different (p = 0.01) from the tight forward, loose forward, and half back positions. Tight forwards recorded the lowest maximum velocity (6,066 ± 1,079 m/s) and were significantly lower (p = 0.01) than all secondary positional groups. Half backs recorded the highest match intensity (77.7 ± 11.6

TABLE 3 | Positional demands for different variables per match during the 2018 Varsity Cup tournament (mean ± standard deviation).

Positional groups	Total distance (m)	High-speed meters (m)	Maximum velocity (m/s)	Match intensity (m/min)	Accelerations (n)	Decelerations (n)	VZ^{3} (4.45–5.56 m/s)	VZ^{4} (5.57–6.94 m/s)	VZ^{5} (>6.95 m/s)
Forwards	5734.4 ± 693.7	158.1 ± 30.8	6.598 ± 0.944	68.6 ± 9.5	363.8 ± 132.2	358.5 ± 117.7	197.4 ± 48.0	65.15 ± 24.5	27.9 ± 12.7
Backs	6261.6 ± 745.2	459.2 ± 58.7*	7.865 ± 1.001*	72.9 ± 11.4	367.9 ± 114.3	361.7 ± 96.4	305.3 ± 65.4*	158.3 ± 40.6*	71.5 ± 30.8*
Tight Forwards	5352.9 ± 798.6	69.7 ± 22.2	6.066 ± 1.079	66.8 ± 10.4	342.2 ± 142.3	338.4 ± 127.3	259.9 ± 43.7	61.2 ± 18.2	8.5 ± 7.8
Loose Forwards	6115.9 ± 588.8	246.4 ± 39.4	7.129 ± 0.809^{a}	70.4 ± 8.5	385.5 ± 122.1	378.7 ± 108.1	529.5 ± 52.2^{a}	199.2 ± 30.6^{a}	47.2 ± 17.5^{a}
Half Backs	6620.9 ± 784.4^{a}	349.3 ± 54.5^{a}	7.279 ± 0.866^{a}	77.7 ± 11.6^{ab}	366.0 ± 115.5	362.8 ± 98.8	760.6 ± 88.7^{abcd}	291.3 ± 46.4^{a}	58.0 ± 18.6^{a}
Inside Backs	6084.6 ± 779.4	471.9 ± 55.8^{abc}	7.930 ± 0.895^{abc}	71.2 ± 11.3	363.3 ± 116.2	356.5 ± 98.6	573.9 ± 57.5^{a}	321.1 ± 37.6^{a}	150.9 ± 31.9^{ab}
Outside Backs	6079.5 ± 671.7	556.5 ± 65.8^{abc}	8.385 ± 1.242^{abc}	69.7 ± 11.4	374.5 ± 111.2	365.9 ± 91.8	497.0 ± 49.8^{a}	336.6 ± 37.8^{ab}	219.9 ± 41.9^{abc}

^{*,a,b,c,d,e} *indicates significant differences.* **indicates differences for primary positional groups.* ^{a,b,c,d,e} *indicates differences for secondary positional groups.*

m/min), significantly higher than tight forwards and outside backs ($p = 0.01$).

Half backs recorded the highest distance within velocity zone 3 (760.6 ± 88.7 m), significantly higher than all secondary positional groups ($p = 0.00$). Outside backs recorded the highest distance within velocity zones 4 (336.6 ± 37.8 m), significantly different ($p = 0.01$) from tight and loose forwards, and 5 (219.9 ± 41.9 m), significantly different from tight forwards, loose forwards, and half backs ($p = 0.01$).

DISCUSSION

The current study aimed to investigate the in-match running demands of South African university rugby players by using GPS during match play for primary and secondary positional groups. To the authors' knowledge, no studies that assessed the in-match running demands of South African university rugby players have been conducted to date, which makes it difficult to draw comparisons.

The findings of the current study were similar to studies by McLellan et al. (2011) and Austin and Kelly (2014) (both elite-level rugby leagues), and Reardon et al. (2015) (elite rugby). All these studies reported that backline players achieved a greater total distance covered than the forwards during matches. Results differed only in the number of meters ran where younger players were participants. Venter et al. (2011) analyzed under-19 players, but their findings differed from the trend where front row forwards covered the most distance followed by the outside backs. Austin and Kelly (2014), however, found that players from both positional groups recorded higher total distance averages than those seen in similar studies. This could be attributed to the fact that their study involved elite rugby league players, who played with only 13 players on a regulation-sized field. The current study supported earlier findings by Austin et al. (2011) on Super 14 rugby players where backline players covered greater distances than forwards.

In the current study, the half backs recorded the highest total distance covered, with the tight forwards recording the least total distance in meters. This result was contrary to the findings of Quarrie et al. (2013), where outside backs achieved the greatest total distance (5,950 ± 755 m), followed by half backs (5,756 ± 915 m). This finding could be attributed to differences in sampling and grouping of players or the increased ball in playtime of the modern game. Austin et al. (2011) reported similar results to the findings of the current study. The study found that the inside backs achieved the greatest total distances; however, the study made use of four positional groups and combined the half backs and inside backs (Austin et al., 2011). The results for total distances covered vary to some degree between studies published in the literature. Discrepancies, such as sampling, competition level, age, and period of playing time in the case of Venter et al. (2011) could have influenced the results. Uncontrollable elements, such as the tactical planning of coaches and player fitness, would also affect the accuracy of results during match play. Teams could have further been influenced by tournament laws, such as the VC where players must overcompensate while other players in the team must sit out during the power play. Because of a lack of studies conducted on the student athlete population and the VC competition itself, strong inferences cannot be made that the law changes influenced the total distances covered. The results of the players also do not differ greatly from what has already been reported in the literature.

Limited literature is available on high-speed meters covered for primary positional groups. Players in the study by Reardon et al. (2015) covered more high-speed meters than the current study. These higher totals were possible because the participants were elite rugby players. Possible reasons for the large differences could be the inability of the tight forwards to reach the minimum speed to register high-speed meters and the number of contact events involving the tight forwards. Our findings were similar to those reported by Reardon et al. (2015) for secondary positional groups where outside backs recorded the highest and tight forwards the lowest high-speed meters. Jones et al. (2015), however, noted that the inside backs covered the most and the tight forwards covered the least distance for meters at high speed. Both studies indicate that they made use of professional players for their data collection, where player level, competition laws, and coaching tactics may affect the results of recorded data. Players exposed to high-speed meters during training may be able to cope with match loads better when experiencing constant exposure to high-speed meters. In the study by Reardon et al. (2015), the teams might have played a more running-oriented game that allowed the forwards to register more meters covered but still have the outside backs covering more meters at high speeds. Jones et al. (2015) possibly recorded teams where the tactic was to use the inside backs group to control the attacks through the middle of the field. Line breaks and higher numbers of phases could have contributed to the high number of meters by inside backs.

The maximum velocity of the primary positional groups was significantly different for the full match, whereas literature reported that the backs attained the highest scores. Our results conform to current literature (Duthie et al., 2006; Reardon et al., 2015; Tee and Coopoo, 2015) at different competition levels. The results of the current study followed a trend indicating some consistency in recorded results. Differences in results could be determined by playing level and game plans where teams play to their strengths. The maximum velocity of different playing positions of the current followed similar trends within published literature. Reardon et al. (2015) reported individual positions maximum velocities, where outside backs' positions (wingers and fullbacks) registered maximum velocities of 8.34 and 7.99 m s^{-1}, respectively. Inside backs registered 8.05 m s^{-1} (Reardon et al., 2015), which were lower than that of the outside backs, and it corresponds with the results of the current study. Owen et al. (2015) noted that forwards, because of their size and weight, were not physically able to move at high speeds, unlike the lighter smaller backline players. Forwards are also tactically used for their physicality and not necessarily speed. Another possible reason is the forwards' involvement in set pieces and phase play, which is generally slow, while backs are often already moving when they receive the ball. Another notable point is the space within which both positional groups operate in. Backs are in more open playing field, while forwards are used physically in slower phase play.

The backs recorded a higher match intensity average for the duration of the match when compared to the forwards, similar to Cunniffe et al. (2009) and Reardon et al. (2015). These high averages may be attributed to the player level because the participants were professional players. Tee and Coopoo (2015), however, reported results that differed from other studies; their study revealed that there was no statistical difference between the forwards and backs. The difference between the two groups, population fitness and game plan, may have resulted in such close scores. The inside backs and loose forwards recorded the second and third highest averages in the current study. This might be a result of the physical demands of each position, where the loose forwards are involved in rucking, tackling, and defensive work regularly compared to the inside backs and outside backs who cover more distance in single bouts and at greater speeds, but less frequently. Limited research has been conducted on match intensity, especially regarding the secondary positional groups. A possible explanation might be the practicality of the information, where coaches and researchers might not see the use of the data because they could analyze the total distance recorded. Match intensity combined with match analysis statistics might be able to distinguish player work rate during matches. Coaches could analyze a player's effectiveness on the field after seeing a high match intensity recording from a GPS unit. Similarly, match intensity may offer an indication of player intensity during training providing an indication of intensity rather than only volume as in the case with total distance.

Limited information on the number of accelerations and decelerations in rugby has been published. The current study recorded higher acceleration and deceleration counts compared to previous research by Owen et al. (2015). However, only one-half of match play was recorded in the Owen et al. study to increase the sample size. This large difference in the number of accelerations and decelerations from the current study could be attributed to the inclusion and exclusion criteria used. Delaney et al. (2018) noted that the average velocity of most team sports was between 1.3 and 2.3 m/s (low intensity), which could question the ability of the players to accelerate and decelerate. Rugby as a stop-start, high-impact sport requiring players to accelerate and decelerate numerous times within matches was highlighted by the study on Super Rugby players by Owen et al. (2015).

The constant effort to move contributes to fatigue during play, affecting the ability to perform (Hewit et al., 2011). Dalen et al. (2016) focused on accelerations and decelerations among

TABLE 4 | Practical applications and recommendations based on recorded match demands.

Position	Results	Practical application
Forwards	Covered less total distance, lower maximum velocity, lower match intensity, and completed less accelerations and decelerations.	Focus on increasing overall fitness to improve total distance and match intensity scores. Expose the groups to a series of high-intensity running protocols and construct games and drills that expose the forwards to extensive or prolonged running at a higher match intensity. Contact at higher match intensities could also be integrated into training to add more positional specificity of game demands to the conditioning of the position.
Backs	Covered more total distance, attained a higher maximum velocity, had a higher match intensity, and completed more accelerations and decelerations.	Focus on increasing overall fitness. Focus on ability to accelerate and decelerate safely and effectively from high velocity. Repeat exposure to high-intensity and high-speed running to avoid detraining effects. The implementation of repeat speed, maximal aerobic speed running, and high-intensity gameplay to further expose players that could result in overreaching on running demands.
Tight forwards	Covered the least total distance, attained the lowest maximum velocity, lowest match intensity, and lowest accelerations and decelerations.	Focus on increasing overall fitness. Focus on improving ability to perform repeated outs of high intensity to assist with increasing match intensity. Maximal aerobic speed running and drills ensuring players are overloaded adequately to meet running demands during training. Variations in work-to-rest ratios and metabolic training such as tempo or lactate running could be used.
Loose forwards	Highest number of accelerations and decelerations. High total distance, maximum velocity, and match intensity.	Focus on overall fitness. Implement acceleration and deceleration strategies to expose players to high braking and acceleration loads. Repeat speed training to further expose players to forces of acceleration and deceleration to stimulate adaptations assisting the management of braking and accelerating forces on the body.
Half backs	Highest total distance Highest match intensity	Focus on overall running fitness. Implement work-to-rest ratios within training to maximize running efficiency. Expose players to high training intensities to simulate match conditions through repeat speed, maximal aerobic speed, and overspeed running.
Inside backs	High match intensity, maximum velocity, and total distance	Focus on overall fitness. Focus on maintaining high running velocity over longer distances. Repeated bouts of high intensity running or repeat speed, while adjusting the work to rest ratios stimulating adaptations for consistent high-speed running.
Outside backs	Highest maximum velocity	Focus on overall fitness. Focus on high speed running to expose players to longer periods of high-intensity running. Maximal speed running and repeat speed ability through varied rest periods during training can be implemented. The focus may be aimed at the quality of the speed meters covered rather than the distance.

soccer players and highlighted the physical strain of accelerating and decelerating on players. Metrics such as acceleration, deceleration, mass, and velocity provide player load (Dalen et al., 2016). It is unclear whether there are trends within published literature in the number of accelerations and decelerations. It is difficult to compare literature because researchers analyze different aspects of accelerating and decelerating, such as Hewit et al. (2011); Owen et al. (2015), and Delaney et al. (2018) who reported on the forcefulness of accelerating and decelerating. Assessing the number of accelerations and decelerations may indicate match demands on players for soft tissue injury management strategies or adapted training to cope with the demands of matches.

The backs and back secondary groups outperformed both the forwards and forward secondary groups in terms of distance covered in all three zones for the duration of the match; this agrees with researched literature. Reardon et al. (2015) reported that scrumhalves and fly halves covered less distance when compared to half backs of the current study. The experimental law changes in VC should be considered, where teams may play within these velocity zones to outpace opponents and benefit from the extra points on offer for scoring. Reardon et al. (2015) did, however, report on all meters covered >5.0 m/s, lower velocities than the current study. Cahill et al. (2013) reported that scrumhalves registered higher than the reported meters in the current study, which can be attributed to the groupings of positions because scrumhalves were identified as individual positions. Quarrie et al. (2013), however, reported values of non-significant or higher recorded metrics for fly half players when viewing individual position results; this could justify the selected positional groups of the current study. As mentioned by Cahill et al. (2013); Owen et al. (2015), and Tee et al. (2017), scrumhalf and fly half positions are constantly involved in set and phase play, often as the link between the forwards and backs providing context to the roles of the position.

The limitations of this study were GPS units that malfunctioned, reducing the number of valid data points, small sample size, and recording only 17 matches. The study has highlighted the following limitations: (1) small sample size due to GPS malfunction, players and teams not meeting the GPS or minimum time requirements, and only recording two teams over one competitive season; (2) lack of normative values for velocity thresholds; (3) lack of normative values for velocity thresholds for both primary and secondary positional groups, as well as the use of absolute thresholds over individualized thresholds; (4) tactical substitutions of players further reducing sample size; (5) no consistent data on valid inclusion times for player data; and (6) no contact data recorded, which may have impacted the results seen for some metrics.

Practical Implications

The coaching staff in a university rugby environment can identify player demands during match play and focus efforts on these areas during training. **Table 4** represents the positional recommendations for primary and secondary positional groups based on match-recorded data. Season and session planning may be taken into consideration, or for priority matches and examination periods. Recorded data on player running demands may also provide an indication of player ability during match play, which could be paired with training data. Similarly, the coaching staff may plan or cancel sessions based on player load data, where specific session running demands could increase player injury risk. Coaching sessions that may have yielded superior or inferior results than expected could lead to changes in the planning of player training sessions. This form of player monitoring would ideally enhance the management of player loads. The possibility of individualized player profiles or primary and secondary positional profiles can assist teams with regard to accuracy in which they prepare and execute training. Adjustments to velocity zones for the different positional groups can be done to accurately represent player ability during training. The recorded data reported here, paired with video analysis, could provide an even better indication of player movement and tactical impacts on playing positions for the future of rugby at a university level in South Africa.

CONCLUSION

The major findings of the study note that backs covered higher speed meters and achieved higher maximum velocities than forwards for primary positional groups. The halfbacks covered the highest total distance and the most distance within velocity zone 3, and the outside back covered the highest high-speed meters among all secondary positional groups. Although the VC competition had a variety of law changes, many of the results remained significantly unchanged as seen in previous research listed in the "Discussion" section. As mentioned before, the involvement of the half back positions during a match may indicate the importance of conditioning in those specific positions for players to be able to handle the specific match loads. It is also important to note that no impact data have been recorded, where such data might better describe the lower totals of the tight forwards group involved in the set phases of play. Recorded data of the current study might serve as a stepping stone to in-match running demands in the South African university rugby context and stimulate further research on other aspects of this unique population and a changing game. It must be noted that only two universities were part of the study, and the results do not represent the whole university rugby population. Further research should be aimed at developing training programs catering to the demands of match play during training. These programs should be tailored to a specific metric, such as total distance or high-speed meters, and the implications thereof. Further research on player wellness during training demands spikes or increased loads to simulate match conditions, which leads to another avenue to explore, namely, player management.

ETHICS STATEMENT

The studies involving human participants were reviewed and approved by Research Ethics Committee (HSREC) (UFS-HSD2017/0062) at the University of the Free State approved the study. The patients/participants provided their written informed consent to participate in this study.

AUTHOR CONTRIBUTIONS

CD collected the data and drafted the manuscript. All authors contributed to the article and approved the submitted version.

ACKNOWLEDGMENTS

We would like to thank the players and coaching staff of the University of Free State and the University of Johannesburg for their participation in the study; and Prof. Martin Kidd from the Centre for Statistical Consultation, Stellenbosch University, for assisting with the statistical analysis.

REFERENCES

Austin, D., Gabbett, T., and Jenkins, D. (2011). The physical demands of Super 14 rugby union. *J. Sci. Med. Sport* 14, 259–263. doi: 10.1016/j.jsams.2011.01.003

Austin, D. J., and Kelly, S. J. (2014). Professional rugby league positional match-play analysis through the use of global positioning system. *J. Strength Cond. Res.* 28, 187–193. doi: 10.1519/jsc.0b013e318295d324

Cahill, N., Lamb, K., Worsfold, P., Headey, R., and Murray, S. (2013). The movement characteristics of English Premiership rugby union players. *J. Sports Sci.* 31, 229–237. doi: 10.1080/02640414.2012.727456

Cummins, C., Orr, R., O'Connor, H., and West, C. (2013). Global positioning systems (GPS) and microtechnology sensors in team sports: a systematic review. *Sports Med.* 43, 1025–1042. doi: 10.1007/s40279-013-0069-2

Cunniffe, B., Proctor, W., Baker, J. S., and Davies, B. (2009). An evaluation of the physiological demands of elite rugby union using global positioning system tracking software. *J. Strength Cond. Res.* 23, 1195–1203. doi: 10.1519/jsc.0b013e3181a3928b

Cunningham, D., Shearer, D. A., Drawer, S., Eager, R., Taylor, N., Cook, C., et al. (2016). Movement demands of elite U20 international rugby union players. *PLoS One* 11:e0153275. doi: 10.1371/journal.pone.0153275

Dalen, T., Ingebrigtsen, J., Ettema, G., Hjelde, G. H., and Wisløff, U. (2016). Player load, acceleration, and deceleration during forty-five competitive matches of elite soccer. *J. Strength Cond. Res.* 30, 351–359. doi: 10.1519/jsc.0000000000001063

Delaney, J. A., Cummins, C. J., Thornton, H. R., and Duthie, G. M. (2018). Importance, reliability, and usefulness of acceleration measures in team sports. *J. Strength Cond. Res.* 32, 3485–3493. doi: 10.1519/jsc.0000000000001849

Duthie, G., Pyne, D., and Hooper, S. (2003). Applied physiology and game analysis of rugby union. *Sports Med.* 33, 973–991. doi: 10.2165/00007256-200333130-00003

Duthie, G. M., Pyne, D. B., Marsh, D. J., and Hooper, S. L. (2006). Sprint patterns in rugby union players during competition. *J. Strength Cond. Res.* 20, 208–214. doi: 10.1519/00124278-200602000-00034

Harris, J., and Wise, N. (2011). Geographies of scale in international rugby union. *Geograph. Res.* 49, 375–383. doi: 10.1111/j.1745-5871.2011.00714.x

Hewit, J., Cronin, J., Button, C., and Hume, P. (2011). Understanding deceleration in sport. *Strength Condition. J.* 33, 47–52. doi: 10.1519/ssc.0b013e3181fbd62c

Jones, M. R., West, D. J., Crewther, B. T., Cook, C. J., and Kilduff, L. P. (2015). Quantifying positional and temporal movement patterns in professional rugby union using global positioning system. *Eur. J. Sport Sci.* 15, 488–496. doi: 10.1080/17461391.2015.1010106

Lindsay, A., Draper, N., Lewis, J., Gieseg, S. P., and Gill, N. (2015). Positional demands of professional rugby. *Eur. J. Sport Sci.* 15, 480–487. doi: 10.1080/17461391.2015.1025858

McLellan, C. P., Lovell, D. I., and Gass, G. C. (2011). Performance analysis of elite rugby league match play using global positioning systems. *J. Strength Cond. Res.* 25, 1703–1710. doi: 10.1519/jsc.0b013e3181ddf678

Owen, S. M., Venter, R. E., Du Toit, S., and Kraak, W. J. (2015). Acceleratory match play demands of a Super Rugby team over a competitive season. *J. Sports Sci.* 33, 2061–2069. doi: 10.1080/02640414.2015.1028086

Quarrie, K. L., and Hopkins, W. G. (2007). Changes in player characteristics and match activities in Bledisloe Cup rugby union from 1972 to 2004. *J. Sports Sci.* 25, 895–903. doi: 10.1080/02640410600944659

Quarrie, K. L., Hopkins, W. G., Anthony, M. J., and Gill, N. D. (2013). Positional demands of international rugby union: evaluation of player actions and movements. *J. Sci. Med. Sport* 16, 353–359. doi: 10.1016/j.jsams.2012.08.005

Reardon, C., Tobin, D. P., and Delahunt, E. (2015). Application of individualized speed thresholds to interpret position specific running demands in elite professional rugby union: a GPS study. *PLoS One* 10:e0133410. doi: 10.1371/journal.pone.0133410

Rothwell, M., Stone, J. A., Davids, K., and Wright, C. (2017). Development of expertise in elite and sub-elite British rugby league players: a comparison of practice experiences. *Eur. J. Sport Sci.* 17, 1252–1260. doi: 10.1080/17461391.2017.1380708

Schoeman, R., and Coetzee, D. F. (2014). Time-motion analysis: discriminating between winning and losing teams in professional rugby. *South Afr. J. Res. Sport Phys. Educ. Recreat.* 36, 167–178.

Tee, J. C., Ashford, M., and Piggott, D. (2018). A tactical periodization approach for rugby union. *Strength Condition. J.* 40, 1–13. doi: 10.1519/ssc.0000000000000390

Tee, J. C., and Coopoo, Y. (2015). Movement and impact characteristics of South African professional rugby union players. *South Afr. J. Sports Med.* 27, 33–39.

Tee, J. C., Lambert, M. I., and Coopoo, Y. (2017). Impact of fatigue on positional movements during professional rugby union match play. *Int. J. Sports Physiol. Perform.* 12, 554–561. doi: 10.1123/ijspp.2015-0695

Vahed, Y., Kraak, W., and Venter, R. (2014). The effect of the law changes on time variables of the South African Currie Cup Tournament during 2007 and 2013. *Int. J. Perform. Anal. Sport* 14, 866–883. doi: 10.1080/24748668.2014.11868764

Venter, R. E., Opperman, E., and Opperman, S. (2011). The use of global positioning system (GPS) tracking devices to assess movement demands and impacts in under-19 rugby union match play: sports technology. *Afr. J. Phys. Health Educ. Recreat. Dance* 17, 1–8. doi: 10.1016/j.humov.2016.05.007

Vilar, L., Araújo, D., Davids, K., and Button, C. (2012). The role of ecological dynamics in analysing performance in team sports. *Sports Med.* 42, 1–10. doi: 10.2165/11596520-000000000-00000

Yamamoto, H., Takemura, M., Kaya, M., and Tsujita, J. (2017). Physical demands of elite rugby union match-play using global positioning system. *Football Sci.* 14, 15–23.

5

Can Functionalised Play Make Children Happy? A Critical Sociology Perspective

Annika Frahsa [1,2]* *and Ansgar Thiel* [1,2]

[1] *Institute of Sport Science, University of Tüebingen, Tuebingen, Germany,* [2] *Interfaculty Research Institute for Sport and Physical Activity, University of Tüebingen, Tuebingen, Germany*

Correspondence:
Annika Frahsa
annika.frahsa@uni-tuebingen.de

The functionalisation of play basically stems from the diagnosis of a global childhood inactivity crisis, the so-called "children's obesity pandemic." Hence, in the context of the activity-related guidelines, children's play appears no longer to be unproductive and purpose-free. It is rather considered an anti-obesity tool that will help children to meet physical activity recommendations. It is questionable whether such a functionalised tool can also provide what has been called the salience of the pleasures of free-play for children. Furthermore, a "normalization" of functionalised practices of play, in turn, could stigmatize children who do not or cannot adhere to these practices. Based upon this background, this paper will take a critical sociology perspective to analyse the functionalisation and medicalisation of children's play in an individualized, mediatized, and pedagogised society. In this sense, the paper aims to pay attention to how the primary goal of play in the sense of "simply make children happy" has given way to the goal of making them healthy and functional.

Keywords: children's play, individualization, functionalization, digitalization, child health, medicalisation, physical activity monitoring

INTRODUCTION

Play has been perceived as so important to optimal child development that it has been recognized by the United Nations High Commission for Human Rights. According to the UN Convention on the Rights of the Child, every child has the right "to rest and leisure, to engage in play and recreational activities" (1). At the same time, current research reports a decline in play among children in the Global North, particularly for middle-class, female, younger, and ethnic-minority children (2).

Historical analyses have highlighted that childhood play is a natural human trait, but its extent depends on socio-cultural conditions in which people live. During many historical eras, such as post-hunter-gatherer societies, in the ages of agriculturalization, or following the industrial revolution, children had only limited opportunities to play because they had to spend most of the daytime working (3). Playing nevertheless occurred, whenever possible, sometime intertwined with labor, without parental or generally adult supervision and direction. Children's play tended to be free and spontaneous; in rural regions it took place in fields, streams, and farmyards, in urban regions it tended to be located in vacant lands and parks (4). However, it was not until the Age of Enlightenment, with the discovery of childhood as an independent phase of life, that children's play was recognized as a human developmental necessity (5).

Children's play, as we know it today, is a phenomenon of modern society. Authors such as Chudacoff (4) have identified the mid-1950s as "golden age" of children's play in North America and potentially the Global North in general. After World War II, children tended to be free from long working hours. Generally, children's play was positively attributed, which was also reflected in the development of supportive environments, such as parks and other playgrounds. However, this "golden age" did not last long. Starting already in the mid 1950s, children's play has been continuously declining. Part of this decline has been attributed to the role of adults and their control and supervision of children's activities (3).

In the following, we will take up the challenge of understanding and explaining this decline and its consequences for public health. Understanding and explaining changes in play requires a broader perspective. Thus, we will apply a critical sociological lens to analyze occurring changes in play. We follow an understanding of children's play as *free play,* as an "activity that is freely chosen and directed by the participants and undertaken for its own sake, not consciously pursued to achieve ends that are distinct from the activity itself" (3). Our central assumption is that free play of children has been increasingly replaced by playful activities which are functionalized in the sense that they are aimed at fulfilling a purpose that is outside the activity. Hence, we argue against the background of the notion that children's leisure lives are reframed (6) in the sense that the basic intention of play to "simply make children happy" (7) has given way to the goal of making them healthy and functional.

In building our argument, we will first provide a critical reflection about four recent trends in today's society that have had an impact on children's play: (i) individualization, pedagogisation, and protection, (ii) indoor- and setting-orientation (iii) mediatisation and digitalization, as well as (iv) medicalisation. Following the critical reflection of those trends, we will discuss the potential consequences of functionalisation to the pleasures linked to free play. We will conclude the paper by arguing for a more holistic understanding of free play to be integrated into physical activity promotion and monitoring in public health.

TRENDS IN CHILDREN'S PLAY

Individualization, Pedagogisation, and Protection

In principle, modern meritocratic societies are characterized by the fact that social advancement is not *per se* predetermined by social background. However, the chances of professional success are—among other factors—limited by qualifications and skills, which have to be developed. In this sense, children find themselves in a "state of permanent endangerment" (8). This has consequences, both at the micro- and at the macro-level (9). At the macro-level, the development of talents in each individual has become a central goal of education policy. Hence, the design of learning environments has increasingly focused on a methodically and didactically professionalized promotion of individual strengths and self-development (10). We observe that this pedagogical aspiration has been extended to the earliest childhood, for example, in foreign language courses for 3-months-old babies or special toys for highly gifted toddlers. We call this a "pedagogisation" that also impacts the way in which a child's social sphere is organized at the micro-level. Children's life worlds have become "pedagogised" in order to limit the risks of uncertain biographies and to offer children and adolescents the best possible start in life.

One consequence is that performance pressure already starts in early childhood. The pedagogisation of children's life worlds also causes so-called "helicopter parents" to hovering over their children, eagerly trying to support them wherever they can in order to solve their problems and promote their success (11, 12).

With regard to the spatial structure of these life-worlds, childhood in today's societies tends to be characterized by functionalized "islands." Children and adolescents commute between separate islands throughout the day, from daycare or school to selected enrichment activities, including individual and collective extracurricular sporting, cultural, and leisure opportunities (2). This island structure of the children's life worlds makes children's life dependent on continous parental support. If parents want to provide their children with the broadest possible support for development, they have to transport them from one island to another: from school to the sports club, to the music school, and even to the playdate with friends. Consequently, parents take control over both children's everyday and leisure-time activities as well as their everyday and leisure-time mobility.

As a result of these societal processes of individualization and pedagogisation, time and significance given to schooling and other adult-directed school-like or enrichment activities have increased (3, 13). Increases in time spent at school, pre-school, and kindergarten have come along with decreases in break times. Play tends to take place within structured settings such as P.E. and supervised breaks, daycare and after school care in clubs or recreation centers. Due to the fact that these scheduled activities do not necessarily provide links between each other, children mostly do not have relationships to other children that go beyond the functionalized islands. Furthermore, the pedagogisation of children's lifestyles considerably restricts the opportunities to autonomously explore social spaces in between the specialized islands. Consequently, the time children spend play freely has continuously decreased over the last decades. Data indicates that the time children spent in free play decreased by about 25% in the USA, already between the 1980s and late 1990s (14). Instead, children's games have become functionalised. To promote children's development in the best possible way, they serve a predetermined purpose, take place at a fixed location, and are instructed by professionals (15).

At the same time, parent-children interaction with regard to children's play has changed. For the 1990s, Valentine and McKendrick showed that, due to adult restrictions and parental rules, children's freedom declined significantly for outdoor play and travel in their neighborhoods (16, 17). Several studies have provided more insights on parenting styles to free play, particularly free unsupervised outdoor play. Parenting styles have become of interest to popular media as well as research, and multiple hyper-parenting styles have been identified (18). The already mentioned "helicopter parents" tend to be overly involved and protective parents who supervise their children's activities and often intervene in their children's affairs and make decisions for them (12, 19, 20). Janssen (18) referred to further parental styles, introduced by other authors, that hinder children's autonomy: "Little emperor" parents focus on providing all material goods available to and craved by children. "Tiger moms" strive for extraordinary achievement among their children. Finally, parents characterized by "concerted cultivation" provide children with a plethora of extracurricular activities aimed at giving the children socio-cultural advantages compared to their peers.

Hyper-parenting styles have influenced children's outdoor play (21). Studies showed that more fear for children's safety is linked to less free play (21–25). In this regard, the desire to prevent potentially risky situations is a main barrier toward the exploration of unknown spaces by the children. Consequently, games that had been perceived as normal in earlier generations are now considered dangerous (26). Fear and danger might either lead parents to eliminate children's play, such as to completely forbid unsupervised outdoor play, or to modify play by putting it under parental supervision, accompanying children in every while playful activity or limiting play to the own backyard (27).

Mediatisation and Digitalization

The consequences of individualization and pedagogisation for children's play are amplified by mediatisation and digitalization. It is not only that parents can use media and digital gadgets to constantly supervise their children's play and their locations (28). In today's Global North, the children's world itself is shaped by information and communication technologies. Due to the digitalization of life-worlds, socio-spatial conditions of growing up have fundamentally changed. Internet-based communication technologies have become a natural part of everyday life. According to Statista, almost every adolescent over 11 owns a smartphone in Germany (29). For some adolescents, smartphones have become so important for coping with everyday life that they perceive these devices as a parts of their own body (30).

With regard to the structures of everyday communication, instant messaging (e.g., WhatsApp, Snapchat, iMessage, or Hangout) has become much more important for the communication with peers than phone calls (31), potentially also more important than face-to-face communication. Digitalization boosts the individualization of everyday communication (9). Communication via WhatsApp or Snapchat does not rely on instantly responding to messages, as it is the case with analog face-to-face communication. Messages are read and answered, when it suits the recipients. Digitalization also impacts social relationships. Emotions are expressed by emoticons and emojis. Facial expressions and nonverbal gestures, fundamentally important for analog communication, play a minor role in digitalized communication.

In a digitalized society, adolescents do not communicate less. However, it is different *how* they communicate. Social negotiation processes play a less important role. In many cases, it is no longer important to "read" body language. The social restrictions of digitalized everyday communication may lead to deficits in adolescents' development of social skills which are relevant for playing games in analog worlds (32). The shift toward digital activities might also minimize positive effects associated with offline events, such as opportunities to increase social capital, build and enlarge networks as well as transform relationships to a deeper level (33).

On the other hand, the internet enables us to transcend concrete geographic space. The ability to communicate virtually independent of time of day and location provides the opportunity to create virtual "meeting places" (34). In this sense, digitalized communication offers participation and inclusion in an otherwise fragmented lifeworld by creating a second "virtual" reality, including new playgrounds and meeting places. At the same time, certain multiplayer online role-playing games might allow for digital social interaction and positive effects on social capital (35). Those might result in new friendships that can deepen through shared interest whereas non-playing offline friends might get neglected.

The trend toward digitalization will ultimately result in a, at least partly, transfer of play into virtual playfields or arenas. Especially virtual playfields are nowadays increasingly used to promote physical activity among children.

Medicalisation

One consequence of individualization and mediatisation of children's play is the trend toward creating games for children to serve health-related purposes. Behind the development of exergames or serious games is the idea that children who tend to be inactive can be motivated to exercise via playful and enjoyable activities. The WHO, for example, states that "for children who are currently inactive, progressive increase in activity to reach the target through additional time for free active play will have health benefits" (36). With similar intent, a clinical report by the Committee on Psychosocial Aspects of Child and Family Health and the Council on Communications and Media of the American Academy of Pediatrics (37) emphasizes the health-related benefits of play even aims aim to provide information "to write a prescription for play at well visits to complement reach out and read" (37).

This "medicalization of play" basically stems from the diagnosis of a global childhood inactivity crisis, the so-called "children's obesity pandemic." Hence, in the context of the activity-related guidelines, children's play is primarily discussed to tackle the problem of inactivity (38–40). In this regard, the Active Healthy Kids Global Alliance developed a matrix for national report cards on children's core physical activity, initiated by Active Healthy Kids Canada in 2004 (39). The matrix considers "active play" as one indicator of core physical activity (41). So far, Active Healthy Kids research working groups from 49 countries have adopted the procedure and presented national report cards. For Germany, Demetriou et al. (38) have very recently presented the German report card and concluded that <25% of children and adolescents play actively for several hours per day.

The flipside of this well-meant trend is that children's play no longer appears to be unproductive and purpose-free. It is rather considered an anti-obesity tool that will help children reach the recommended 60 min of physical activity per day (36). Data already has indicated that functionalised play could become a privileged and exclusive support activity for some children only. Middle-class children in England participate to a higher degree in functionalised play activities, such as extracurricular sporting and leisure activities, than working-class children, even though parents of both classes value such activities in similar ways (2). A relevant factor in this regard is the ability to incorporate functionalised play into the life-worlds of families. Since this transfer seems to work better in middle-class families, functionalised playing activities in these families can compensate the loss of free unstructured play to a higher degree than working-class families in England (2). Hence, a "normalization" of functionalised practices of play could stigmatize children who do not or cannot adhere to these practices (42).

Furthermore, it is questionable whether a functionalised anti-obesity tool can also provide what Sutton-Smith has called the salience of the pleasures of free play for children (7).

CAN FUNCTIONALIZED PLAY PROVIDE THE PLEASURES OF CHILDREN'S FREE PLAY?

Data already indicates that the restriction of free play may have a negative impact on the general well-being of children (43, 44). Free play is an activity that is (a) voluntary, (b) open and uncertain, (c) separated from everyday life, (d) unproductive and self-sufficient, (e) regulated, and (f) fictional (45).

First, *voluntary participation* is indispensable for play, one cannot really be forced to play. Play only takes place "when the players have a desire to play, and play the most absorbing, exhausting game in order to find diversion, escape from responsibility and routine" (45). Play thus represents a space of action sought for its own sake. Play enables the actors to satisfy their current needs for action and to experience the joy of immediate activity. Play is an activity that is motivated by the quality of life, excitement, satisfaction, and joy experienced in the course of action. People can become absorbed in play, fully immerse themselves in the activity, receive intensive feedback about their own abilities, find a pleasure-oriented approach to (physical) culture and thereby experience a feeling of initiative and causation through play. Second, the *openness and uncertainty* of the outcome is a further characteristic of play. Particularly for children and adolescents, the uncertainty—which is often difficult to bear—and the associated risk of failure seem to be dimensions of play that promote individual development and growth. Playing confronts children and adolescents with multiple challenges and it supports to establish a relational relationship between someone's world of experience and the person's relevant environment. While playing, children exhibit a multitude of social behaviors and interactions, and take up various social status roles (46). These roles mirror to a certain extent the life-worlds, in which the children are growing up. Third, play is *a separate activity* that takes place in a special world that is clearly distinguishable from the world of day-to-day life. Play takes place in its own time and space. Ideally, nothing is created through playful activity that is of significance outside that activity. In this sense, play is, fourth, an *unproductive activity* that is sufficient in itself but in contrast to the ordinary day-to-day life. Fifth, since cultural ideas and conventions have an effect on how to play, play appears to be a *regulated activity*, but its rules may well conflict with the legal or day-to-day regulations of the living environment. Due to the conscious "as-if" character of the activity, play is, sixth, also a *fictional activity* whose "unreality" stimulates dedicated playing and the experience of joy both during as well as after play.

In principle, children's play can contribute to the development of intrinsic motivation and competence, decision-making and problem-solving skills, self-control and emotional regulations, friendship skills and social capital (3). Children's free play also embodies the dynamic of the dramatic increase and decrease of tension. Hence, play allows to practice the drama of interpersonal relationships in a protected environment in a casual way (47). As such, play plays an important role in Piaget's process of accommodation and assimilation and also serves for empowerment.

The fact that children's play particularly contributes to the experience of joy makes it such a valuable tool for public health programs. From the perspective of critical sociology, however, it is questionable, whether activities like "energetic play" (36), "free active play" (36), "active play" (38, 41) or "active outdoor play" (39, 48), which are implemented as parts of public health programs, are indeed fun for the children. The use of these terms in the context of public health is not neutral. Rather, it can be regarded as a sign of objectification and functionalisation in the current discourse on play in public health and physical activity promotion (26). Making "active play" or "active free play" a research object and promoting it as part of public health concerns may (re-)define the way play is understood and experienced. From the perspective of a sociology of the child, Alexander et al., among others, have already hinted at the underlying paradox in this discourse: advocating, promoting and discussing children's play might reshape it into a new form that is purpose-driven and thus no longer free and intrinsically motivated (6). In this sense, a highly pre-structured, functionalised playing activity bears the risk that it no longer primarily aims at what Sutton-Smith identifies as the main function of free play of children: that it simply "makes them happier" (7).

From the perspective of critical sport sociology, a more reflective discussion of functionalized play is needed that pays attention to the current "reframing of children's leisure lives" (6). Such a critical reflection should particularly focus on the potential harmful consequences of transforming a leisure activity that allows risk-taking and provides fun (which is what childhood should be about in the first place) into a much more constrained, managed, and supervised intervention.

The functionalisation of play in the field of health promotion has a particularly interesting dynamic in the form of so-called "serious games." Marsh (49) defines serious games as follows: *"Serious games are digital games, simulations, virtual environments and mixed reality/media that provide opportunities to engage in activities through responsive narrative/story, gameplay or encoun- ters to inform, influence, for well-being, and/ or experience to convey meaning. (. . .) Serious games are identified along a continuum from games for purpose at one end, through to experiential environments with minimal or no gaming characteristics for experience at the other end."* These games are developed, designed, marketed and distributed by companies. Within the framework of the serious games, health-related content is taken up and integrated into an exciting story, which should ensure a sustainable motivation for healthy behavior. At the same time, the companies are oriented toward selling the games and thus primarily follow a market logic. To the extent that business enterprises, due to their market interest, integrate algorithms into the games that create dependency on playing or even play addiction, the health promotion intention is thwarted. Thus, e-games may deviate from the idea of free children's games in two respects: On the one hand, the games are pre-programmed, methodised and internationalized to a large extent.

In this regard, one can also expect effects of social inequality. In milieus, in which physical activity is considered a relevant instrument to foster the development of children, functionalised e-games will probably be given to children, while milieus that are far away from movement will become impoverished in terms of physical activity. On the other hand, the attempt to encourage children to consume these games in a sustainable way and—linked to this—to buy updates or new versions, prevent adolescents from freely deciding for or against the game. Given that the particularly motivating health-promoting e-games for children are most at risk to cause dependency, guidance of children becomes of central importance.

Current statistics on the media behavior of children during the COVID-19-pandemic show how important supervision of children's use of digital technologies is. According to a recent German FORSA survey with 500 children on behalf of a large German health insurance, 95 percent of all parents report that their children spent significantly m ore t ime i n f ront o f PCs and smartphones during time of school lockdowns (50). In this regard, it is not only the use of communication technologies, social media, streaming services or e-games, but also the massive upswing of digital learning that leads to an increase of time spent sedentarily. Only in a small percentage of the children, this behavioral change is compensated by physical activity, for example by more outdoor activities in gardens or parks (38 percent).

A Facebook Messenger survey on behalf of ParentsTogether with over 3,000 parents came to a similar conclusion in the USA (51). The average time spent online has doubled for kids during the crisis. Almost half of the children spent more than 6 h online per day (compared to only 8.29% before), 26% of kids even spent more than 8 h online (compared to 4% previously) during the lockdown. The most prominent platforms and apps used by children whose parents completed the survey were mostly non-educational: YouTube (78.21%), Netflix (49.64%), and TikTok (33.41%) (51).

CONCLUSIONS

The functionalisation of play in the context of health promotion basically attempts to resolve a paradox: to integrate the motivational characteristics of free play into an actually unfree setting. This idea is well-intentioned and principally aimed at promoting the best interests of children. However, so far there has been no empirical evidence on its actual outcome. In a highly digitalized social world characterized by functionalization, isolation, and commercialization, there are hardly any spaces left in which children can have development-promoting experience without adult guidance. Serious games that are designed to promote a healthier behavior in children are therefore not necessarily the best answer on global health challenges. This is even more true when considering the potential opposite effects to those intended, namely if serious games increase the children's sedentary time. From a critical-sociological perspective, there is another interesting dynamic in the functionalization of play in form of e-games. Implicitly, this dynamic means that public health authorities delegate some of their responsibility for the promotion of citizens' health (comparable with similar tendencies in the field of education) to commercial enterprises whose interests by no means fully coincide with the tasks of public institutions. One could therefore say that governments do not fulfill their obligation to secure collective goods for society but that they leave gaps to be filled by commercial enterprises.

The question remains what public health strategies can be recommended to promote "healthy and development-promoting" play? Instead of pre-structured games, some of which take place on the computer, public health should rather aim to create stimulating movement environments in which children can act freely, invent their own rules, test these rules, measure each other, learn to cooperate, i.e., to make use of the socialization potential of sport and movement, which is neglected in guided, controlled worlds. This includes, firstly, the appropriation and questioning of norms and, secondly, the ability to develop design possibilities where social norms are lacking. Secondly, this includes learning the ability to act autonomously and to apply social norms in a reflective and flexible manner, both of which are a prerequisite for the development of an "ego-strength." Thirdly, this also includes developing the competence to weigh self-interest against group interests in less pre-structured game worlds and to be able to make decisions that meet social obligations without neglecting one's own goals. PA-promoting free play areas should ideally be linked locally to schools and kindergartens to ensure that all children are reached. These areas should not be supervised and it should be left to the children themselves how and what they play. If one considers the socially contagious effects of free play, then it is to be expected that children will get moving.

Monitoring children's play then could focus on the infrastructures of settings in which free play should take place. Thereby, the design for the settings should also make sure to differentiate target groups in alignment with how they are affected from the decline of PA and to which degrees.

Parents who are involved in children's life, public health professionals, and researchers who are interested in understanding and monitoring children's play can bring back happiness to children's play. In this regard, children's play need to be contextualized in a holistic way. Parents, professionals, and researchers need to put children's perspectives and experience at center. From this perspective, the monitoring of play environments for children should primarily focus on whether play can "simply make children happy" (45). If this works, one can ultimately also expect benefits with regard to the children's physical, mental, and social health.

AUTHOR CONTRIBUTIONS

AF had the idea for the paper. AF and AT wrote and edited the draft article. All authors contributed to the article and approved the submitted version.

REFERENCES

United Nations. *Convention on the Rights of the Child.* New York, NY: United Nations (1990).

Holloway SL, Pimlott-Wilson H. Enriching children, institutionalizing childhood? Geographies of play, extracurricular activities, and parenting in England. *Ann Assoc Am Geogr.* (2014) 104:613– 27. doi: 10.1080/00045608.2013.846167

Gray P. The decline of play and the rise of psychopathology in children and adolescents. *Am J Play.* (2011) 3:443–63.

Chudacoff HP. *Children at Play: An American History.* New York, NY: New York University Press (2007).

Foyster E, Marten J. Introduction. In: Foyster E, Marten J, editors. *A Cultural History of Childhood and Family in the Age of Enlightenment.* New York, NY: Berg Publishers (2010). p. 1–13. doi: 10.5040/9781350049635-005

Alexander SA, Frohlich K, Fusco C. *Play, Physical Activity and Public Health: The Reframing of Children's Leisure Lives.* London: Routledge (2018).

Sutton-Smith B. *Emotional Breaches in Play and Narrative. Children in Play, Story, and School.* New York, NY: Guilford Press (2001). p. 161–76.

Beck U, Beck-Gernsheim E. *Individualization: Institutionalized Individualism and Its Social and Political Consequences.* London: SAGE Publications Ltd. (2001).

Thiel A, Gropper H. Sport in an individualized and digitalized society: more important than ever? *Eur J Sport Soc.* (2017) 14:287–90. doi: 10.1080/16138171.2017.1421298

Thiel F. *Ökologie als Thema: Überlegungen zur Pädagogisierung Einer Gesellschaftlichen Krisenerfahrung.* Weinheim: Deutscher Studien Verlag (1996).

Kelly L, Duran RL, Miller-Ott AL. Helicopter parenting and cell-phone contact between parents and children in college. *South Commun J.* (2017) 82:102–14. doi: 10.1080/1041794X.2017.1310286

Odenweller KG, Booth-Butterfield M, Weber K. Investigating helicopter parenting, family environments, and relational outcomes for millennials. *Commun Stud.* (2014) 65:407–25. doi: 10.1080/10510974.2013.811434

Frost JL. *A History of Children's Play and Play Environments: Toward a Contemporary Child-Saving Movement.* New York, NY: Routledge (2010).

Burdette HL, Whitaker RC. A national study of neighborhood safety, outdoor play, television viewing, and obesity in preschool children. *Pediatrics.* (2005) 116:657–62. doi: 10.1542/peds.2004-2443

Zeiher H. Kindheitsträume: Zwischen Eigenständigkeit und Abhängigkeit. In: Beck U, Beck-Gernsheim E, editors. *Riskante Freiheiten: Individualisierung in modernen Gesellschaften.* Frankfurt: Suhrkamp (1994). p. 353–75.

Valentine G, McKendrck J. Children's outdoor play: exploring parental concerns about children's safety and the changing nature of childhood. *Geoforum.* (1997) 28:219–35. doi: 10.1016/S0016-7185(97) 00010-9

Valentine G. "Oh yes i can." "oh no you can't": children and parents' understandings of kids' competence to negotiate public space safely. *Antipode.* (1997) 29:65–89. doi: 10.1111/1467-8330.00035

Janssen I. Hyper-parenting is negatively associated with physical activity among 7–12year olds. *Prev Med.* (2015) 73:55–9. doi: 10.1016/j.ypmed.2015.01.015

Cline FW, Fay J. *Parenting With Love and Logic: Teaching Children Responsibility.* Colorada Springs, CO: Pinon (1990).

Hunt J. Make room for daddy ... and mommy: helicopter parents are here. *J Acad Administr Higher Educ.* (2008) 4:9–12.

Carver A, Timperio AF, Crawford D. Playing it safe: the influence of neighbourhood safety on children's physical activity - a review. *Health Place.* (2008) 14:217–27. doi: 10.1016/j.healthplace.2007.06.004

Timperio AF, Crawford D, Telford A, Salmon J. Perceptions about the local neighborhood and walking and cycling among children. *Prev Med.* (2004) 38:39–47. doi: 10.1016/j.ypmed.2003.09.026

Powell EC, Ambardekar EJ, Sheehan KM. Poor neighborhoods: safe playgrounds. *J Urban Health.* (2005) 82:403–10. doi: 10.1093/jurban/jti099

Veitch J, Bagley S, Ball K, Salmon J. Where do children usually play? A qualitative study of parents' perceptions of influences on children's active free-play. *Health Place.* (2006) 12:383–93. doi: 10.1016/j.healthplace.2005.02.009

Farley TA, Meriwether RA, Baker ET, Watkins LT, Johnson CC, Webber LS. Safe play spaces to promote physical activity in inner-city children: results from a pilot study of an environmental intervention. *Am J Public Health.* (2007) 97:1625–31. doi: 10.2105/AJPH.2006.092692

Frohlich KL, Alexander SAC, Fusco C. All work and no play? The nascent discourse on play in health research. *Soc Theory Health.* (2013) 11:1– 18. doi: 10.1057/sth.2012.18

Kepper MM, Staiano AE, Katzmarzyk PT, Reis RS, Eyler AA, Griffith DM, et al. Using mixed methods to understand women's parenting practices related to their child's outdoor play and physical activity among families living in diverse neighborhood environments. *Health Place.* (2020) 62:102292. doi: 10.1016/j.healthplace.2020.102292

Kantrowitz B, Tyre P. *The Fine Art of Letting Go.* Newsweek (2006).

Statista. *Umfrage Handybesitz (Survey on Cellphone Ownership).* (2020). Available online at: https://de.statista.com/statistik/daten/studie/1106/ umfrage/handybesitz-bei-jugendlichen-nach-altersgruppen (accessed June 09, 2020).

Liepelt R, Dolk T, Hommel B. Self-perception beyond the body: the role of past agency. *Psychol Rev.* (2017) 81:549–59. doi: 10.1007/s00426-016-0766-1

Holdampf-Wendel A, Shahd M, Hampe K. *Jung und Vernetzt: Kinder und Jugendliche in der Digitalen Gesellschaft.* Berlin: Bitkom (2014).

Konrath S, O'Brien EH, Hsing C. Changes in dispositional empathy in American college students over time: a meta-analysis. *Personal Soc Psychol Rev.* (2011) 15:180–98. doi: 10.1177/1088868310377395

Ackermann J. Playing computer games as social interaction – an analysis of LAN-Parties. In: Fromme J, Unger A, editors. *Computer Games and New Media Cultures A Handbook of Digital Games Studies.* Dordrecht: Springer (2012).

Tillmann A, Hugger K-U. Mediatisierte Kindheit: Aufwachsen in mediatisierten Lebenswelten. In: Tillmann A, Fleischer S, Hugger K-U, editors. *Handbuch Kinder und Medien.* Wiesbaden: Springer (2014). p. 31–46. doi: 10.1007/978-3-531-18997-0_2

Cole H, Griffiths MD. Social interactions in massively multiplayer online role-playing gamers. *Cyberpsychol Behav.* (2007) 10:575– 83. doi: 10.1089/cpb.2007.9988

World Health Organization. *Guidelines on Physical Activity, Sedentary Behaviour and Sleep for Children Under 5 Years of Age.* Geneva: WHO (2019).

Yogman M, Garner A, Hutchinson J, Hirsh-Pasek K, Golinkoff RM. The power of play: a pediatric role in enhancing development in young children. *Pediatrics.* (2018) 142:e20182058. doi: 10.1542/peds.2018-2058

Demetriou Y, Bucksch J, Hebestreit A, Schlund A, Niessner C, Schmidt SCE, et al. Germany's 2018 report card on physical activity for children and youth. *German J Exerc Sport Res.* (2019) 49:113–126. doi: 10.1007/s12662-019-00578-1

Tremblay MS, Gray C, Babcock S, Barnes J, Bradstreet CC, Carr D, et al. Position statement on active outdoor play. *Int J Environ Res Public Health.* (2015) 12:6475–505. doi: 10.3390/ijerph120606475

Australian Government Department of Health. *Move and Play Every Day: National Physical Activity Recommendations for Children 0–5 Years.* Canberra: DoH (2014).

Tremblay MS, Barnes JD, González SA, Katzmarzyk PT, Onywera VO, Reilly JJ, et al. Global matrix 2.0: report card grades on the physical activity of children and youth comparing 38 countries. *J Phys Act Health.* (2016) 13(11 Suppl. 2):S343–66. doi: 10.1123/jpah.2016-0594

Alexander SA, Frohlich KL, Fusco C. 'Active play may be lots of fun, but it's certainly not frivolous': the emergence of active play as a health practice in Canadian public health. *Sociol Health Illness.* (2014) 36:1188– 204. doi: 10.1111/1467-9566.12158

Gill T. *No Fear: Growing Up in a Risk-Averse Society.* London: Calouste Gulbenkian Foundation (2007).

Brown S. *Play: How it Shapes the Brain, Opens the Imagination, and Invigorates the Soul.* Toronto: Penguin Group (2009).

Callois R. *Man, Play and Games.* Champaign, IL: University of Illoins Press (1961).

Arnott L. An ecological exploration of young children's digital play: Framing children's social experiences with technologies in early childhood. *Early Yeaes.* (2016) 36:271–88. doi: 10.1080/09575146.2016.1 181049

Grupe O. *Bewegung, Spiel und Leistung im Sport: Grundthemen der Sportanthropologie.* Schorndorf: Hofmann (1982).

Boxberger K, Reimers AK. Parental correlates of outdoor play in boys and girls aged 0 to 12-a systematic review. *Int J Environ Res Public Health.* (2019) 16:190. doi: 10.3390/ijerph16020190

Marsh T. Serious games continuum: between games for purpose and experiential environments for purpose. *Entertainment Comp.* (2011) 2:61– 8. doi:10.1016/j.entcom.2010.12.004

Krankenkasse K. *Corona-Ferien: Computer & Handy Ziehen Kinder Magisch an.* (2020). Available online at: https://www.kkh.de/presse/fokusthemen/ corona-ferien?_ga=2.243483525.1021165674.1589528859-1005594104. 1589528859 (accessed June 09, 2020).

Parentstogether Foundation. *Survey Shows Parents Alarmed as Kids' Screen Time Skyrockets During COVID-19 Crisis* [Press release]. Available online at: https://parents-together.org/survey-shows-parents-alarmed-as-kids- screen-time-skyrockets-during-covid-19-crisis/ (accessed June 09, 2020)

6

Diverse Effects of Thermal Conditions on Performance of Marathon Runners

Thadeu Gasparetto[1†] and Cornel Nesseler[2†]*

[1] Department of Management, National Research University Higher School of Economics, Saint Petersburg, Russia,
[2] Business School, Norwegian University of Science and Technology, Trondheim, Norway

***Correspondence:**
Cornel Nesseler
cornel.m.nesseler@ntnu.no

† These authors have contributed equally to this work*

Heat exposure affects human performance in many ways. Both physiological (i.e., glycogen sparing, oxygen uptake, thermoregulation) and biomechanical mechanisms (i.e., contact time, knee flexion, muscle activity) are affected, hence reducing performance. However, the exposure affects persons differently. Not all athletes necessarily experience an identical thermal condition similarly, and this point has been overlooked to date. We analyzed endurance performances of the top 1000 runners for every year during the last 12 New York City Marathons. Thermal conditions were estimated with wet-bulb globe temperature (WBGT) and universal thermal climate index (UTCI). Under identical thermal exposure, the fastest runners experienced a larger decline in performance than the slower ones. The empirical evidence offered here not only shows that thermal conditions affect runners differently, but also that some groups might consistently suffer more than others. Further research may inspect other factors that could be affected by thermal conditions, as pacing and race strategy.

Keywords: performance, marathon, heat stress, wet-bulb globe temperature, universal thermal climate index

INTRODUCTION

The negative effects of heat exposure are widely known. Labor productivity is negatively impacted by heat exposure in the workplace (Dunne et al., 2013; Cheung et al., 2016; Chavaillaz et al., 2019). Previous research regarding heat exposure focuses on the effects between low- and high-risk labor (Hsiang et al., 2017), the amount of time individuals are exposed (Hancock et al., 2007), and degrees of work stress (Kjellstrom et al., 2018). A point that has been overlooked is that groups of workers within the same labor activity might experience the impacts of identical heat exposure differently (Dear, 2018).

Heat exposure and global warming have many socioeconomic impacts (Watts et al., 2018), including increased death rates (Hsiang et al., 2017; Mora et al., 2017), occupational injuries (Spector et al., 2016; Varghese et al., 2018), reduced economic production (Burke et al., 2015; Fishman et al., 2019; Martinich and Crimmins, 2019), and loss of labor productivity (Dunne et al., 2013; Zare et al., 2015; Chavaillaz et al., 2019). A broad literature exists discussing the negative impacts on labor productivity (Flouris et al., 2018). Physiological effects (Ladell, 1955; Hellon et al., 1956; Liu et al., 2017) are mainly associated with declines in productivity as a consequence of heat stress, but external elements such as clothing (Kampmann et al., 2012), work patterns (Yi and Chan, 2015; Takakura et al., 2017), leisure (Dyble et al., 2019), cooling systems (Tanabe et al., 2015), lifestyle (Trezza et al., 2015), and physical activity (Zander et al., 2015) can also restrain these effects.

Research has examined the impacts of global warming and heat exposure on labor productivity at different geographic levels: global (Ely et al., 2007; Dell et al., 2012; Dunne et al., 2013; Burke et al., 2015; Chavaillaz et al., 2019), national (Cheung et al., 2016; Hsiang et al., 2017; Fishman et al., 2019; Martinich and Crimmins, 2019), and regional (Barreca et al., 2016). Additionally, authors have examined these effects between gender groups (Witterseh et al., 2004), industries, income classes (Zander et al., 2015), indoor vs. outdoor conditions (Cheung et al., 2016), work risk groups (Hsiang et al., 2017), and degrees of heat stress (Kjellstrom et al., 2018). Contemporary research offers adaptation options (Day et al., 2019), limits (Sherwood and Huber, 2010), and recommendations (Watts et al., 2018) on how to cope with global warming and heat exposure.

The negative effects of heat exposure have been extensively researched in sports settings as well. Coris et al. (2004) emphasize heat and humidity as significant risk factors for human exercise. Armstrong et al. (2007) find that heat stress causing organ system dysfunction and failure is a relevant cause for athletes to withdraw from their activities. Tyler et al. (2016) find that heat adaptation is beneficial, however, they state that it depends on the duration of the training (in days). Périard et al. (2015) find, in addition to Tyler et al. (2016), that heat adaptation depends on the kind of heat (e.g., dry or humid hear) and several other factors, such as intensity or frequency. Brotherhood (2008) broadly examines the impacts of heat stress in exercise and sports. Such negative impacts are reported in such diverse sports as cycling (Tatterson et al., 2000), triathlon (Massimino, 1988; Gosling et al., 2008), baseball (Kurakake et al., 1988), and football (Mohr et al., 2012).

Being an outdoor endurance event, marathon running is a sport that researchers have examined carefully for the impacts of heat exposure. Indeed, there is robust evidence of negative effects of weather on performance of marathon runners. Numerous researchers (e.g., Trapasso and Cooper, 1989; Suping et al., 1992; Ely et al., 2007; Montain et al., 2007; Maughan, 2010; Roberts, 2010; Vihma, 2010; Miller-Rushing et al., 2012; Del Coso et al., 2013; Maffetone et al., 2017; Knechtle et al., 2018, 2019; and Nikolaidis et al., 2019b) have found that higher temperatures result in slower finishing times for both elite and amateur runners.

Although the negative impact of heat exposure is well known, it is plausible to assume that not all individuals react similarly to heat. Indeed, Dear (2018) indicates that heterogeneity among workers may result in diverse productivity under similar heat exposure. Although sport is a plausible setting in which heat exposure could have diverse effects, this important element has not been extensively studied in the previous literature. In the context of marathon running, the topic has been discussed by Ely et al. (2007), Montain et al. (2007), and Vihma (2010). They emphasize that slower runners experience larger reductions in performance than elite runners. However, their main argument is that slower runners experience more heat stress because they run for longer periods than faster runners. Our hypothesis, on the other hand, is that even though top runners run for shorter periods, they perform the task (the race) more intensely than slower runners. Hence, they could suffer more from a performance penalty than slower runners.

MATERIALS AND METHODS

We analyze runner performance in the same, constant setting (New York City Marathon) over twelve events (from 2006 to 2018 – the marathon was canceled in 2012). The New York City Marathon takes place at the first Sunday of November. All information regarding race course, rules, and results can be found at https://www.nyrr.org/tcsnycmarathon. Marathon runners are especially prone to heat stress (Roberts, 2010; Smith et al., 2016) as a consequence of the particular characteristics of a marathon, a highly physiologically demanding activity (Ely et al., 2007).

The present setting allows for an appropriate identification of impacts from thermal conditions for the following reasons: (1) goals and outputs are clear: runners seek to be as fast as they can and are ranked according to their performance; (2) similar circumstances: (2.1) all competitors run the same distance and course: 42.195 km (26.219 miles) in New York City over a period of 12 years; (2.2) all athletes are under identical thermal conditions at the same event; (2.3) no seasonal bias – every event happens on the first Sunday of November; and (2.4) no dressing bias – all runners wear similar uniforms. Previous works inspecting the impact of weather on runners analyzed different events at the same time, which undermines the identification of heat exposure effects (Ely et al., 2007; Montain et al., 2007), used air temperature and precipitation as weather conditions (Roberts, 2010; Vihma, 2010), or examined smaller samples each season (Trapasso and Cooper, 1989; Suping et al., 1992; Maffetone et al., 2017; Knechtle et al., 2018) than the current work.

Model and Variables

We examine the impact of heat exposure on performance (p) by multiple linear modeling as follows:

$$p_{it} = \beta_0 + \beta_1 C_{jt} w_t + \beta_2 C_{jt} w_t^2 + \upsilon W_{it} + \varepsilon_i$$

where p is performance, measured by the finishing time in seconds; i is an individual runner; t is a year; C is a matrix of clusters $j = 1, 2, 3,$ or 4; w is thermal condition, measured by WBGT or UTCI, both in Celsius scale (°C), at the beginning of each marathon; $\boldsymbol{W}$ is a vector of control variables. The control variables are age, gender, nationality, number of previous participations, the defined clusters, and start corral dummy (since 2008). An alternative model inspecting a quadratic age effect (cf., Lara et al., 2014; Nikolaidis et al., 2019a) is also carried out but both terms – first and second order – shows insignificant effect and does not influence the results. Start corral was established in the New York Marathon in 2008 with the aim to offer safer conditions for runners by an ordered and smooth flow. It is currently the standard start approach in most major marathon events worldwide. The variables of interest are two interaction terms in each equation: interactions between a heat exposure index (WBGT or UTCI) and its squared term and the defined clusters. It aims to capture the nonlinear impact that heat exposure might have on productivity, as observed by Burke et al. (2015). We use temperature in Celsius degrees throughout the paper. Fahrenheit degrees are related as follows: F =°C * 1.8000+ 32.00.

Thermal condition is calculated by the WBGT and the UTCI at the start time of each marathon. WBGT is the most popular measure of heat exposure (Epstein and Moran, 2006; Kjellstrom et al., 2009; Lemke and Kjellstrom, 2012) and is currently an ISO standard (ISO, 2017). UTCI is a more recent index that affords a slightly different measure of thermal perception (Zare et al., 2018). Brocherie and Millet (2015) discuss some potential limitations regarding WBGT by measuring the severity of the thermal conditions on sport practice. They indicate that UTCI is more appropriate for sport heat stress modeling. However, most of the recent literature still uses WBGT as a bioclimatic index. Therefore, we decided to include both. Both indexes incorporate temperature, solar radiation, wind speed, and humidity, but differ in their calculations. Specifically, WBGT is calculated as follows:

$$WBGT = 0.7 * T_w + 0.2 * T_b + 0.1 * T_d$$

where T_w is wet-bulb temperature; T_b is black globe temperature; and T_d ambient temperature (Epstein and Moran, 2006). UCTI is calculated as follows:

$$UTCI = f\,(T_a;\, T_{mrt};\, va;\, RH) = T_a + Offset(T_a;\, T_{mrt};\, va;\, RH)$$

where T_a is air temperature; T_{mrt} is air mean radiant temperature; *va* is wind speed; and *RH* is relative humidity (Błażejczyk et al., 2013). Air temperature, solar radiation, wind speed, and humidity are the inputs in our calculations. Brocherie and Millet (2015) suggest these basic weather elements for WBGT calculation. Both indexes were automatically calculated using the heat stress calculator available at http://www.climatechip.org.

The data comprises the top-1000 overall runners for each event. This sample represents about 2% of total participants for each year. Of these, 89.70% completed the race in less than 3 h – the slowest runner in the sample finished in 3:04:43. Previous work habitually uses subjective criteria to separate runners into groups (e.g., top-3, top-10, top-50, and top-100). Nevertheless, such an arbitrary definition is bound to lead to misspecifications. For instance, the 11th place in a year might be more similar to the runners of the top-10 *group* than compared to the top-50 group. Therefore, to appropriately examine whether groups experience thermal conditions differently, runners were clustered by their performance on each event. The hierarchical clustering through the average linkage method was used to establish the clusters. This method is chosen because of the hierarchical, top-down distribution of runners according to finishing times. The method clusters the data by considering the distance between two clusters as equal to the average distance from any members of both clusters (Ward, 1963; Rokach and Maimon, 2005). There are 222 observations (1.85%) in Cluster 1; 600 observations (5.00%) in Cluster 2; 2192 observations (18.27%) in Cluster 3; and 8985 observations (74.88%) in Cluster 4. **Figure 1** shows the percentage of runners for every cluster for every year. Reasons for changes could be, e.g., the (non-)participation of some runners in specific years, the increase (decrease) in their performances, injuries prior or during the events, or several other external elements that we cannot capture with our data.

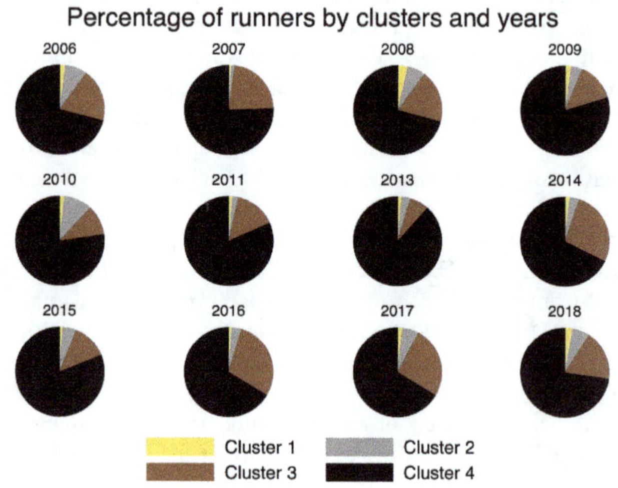

FIGURE 1 | Percentage of runners by clusters and years.

RESULTS AND DISCUSSION

The output of the regressions is given in **Table 1**. All control variables show the expected coefficients. The results also confirm the nonlinear effects of thermal conditions on performance (Burke et al., 2015). In line with previous findings, higher temperatures reduced the performance of runners. However, the results show that each cluster reacts to identical thermal conditions differently. **Figures 2, 3** show the predictive marginal effects of WBGT (°C) and UCTI (°C) by each cluster. We choose the range of values of temperature (*x*-axis) from the minimum valid value of WBGT and UTCI in our sample (+3°C and −5°C, respectively) up to the maximum "Do not start" (DNS) temperature for a marathon (+20°C WBGT) (Roberts, 2010).

The general result is that higher temperatures reduce performance in marathons, corroborating previous findings (Ely et al., 2007; Roberts, 2010; El Helou et al., 2012; Miller-Rushing et al., 2012; Del Coso et al., 2013; Cheung et al., 2016; Maffetone et al., 2017; Knechtle et al., 2018). The tipping point of productivity (about +8°C WBGT) is similar to what has been found before. Montain et al. (2007) showed a progressive decrease in performance in temperatures above 5–10°C WBGT, while Knechtle et al. (2018) observed reduced performances of runners under air temperatures higher than +8°C.

However, the current work refutes earlier research that suggests that faster runners suffer less than slower runners (Ely et al., 2007, Montain et al., 2007; Vihma, 2010). In earlier research, the argument was made that slower runners are exposed to heat stress for longer periods and hence suffer more. However, we assume that when analyzing all participants in a marathon, the slower runners (mainly amateurs) tend to have lower performances under higher temperatures not only because of the time exposed, but also due to their inferior level of training and weaker physiological adaptations and metabolic rates than elite runners. Therefore, a comparison among a relatively more homogeneous group of runners, as performed in the current

TABLE 1 | Effects of WBGT and UTCI on performance by clusters of runners.

Variables	Dependent variable: Performance	
	(*w* = WBGT)	**(*w* = UTCI)**
Cluster 1*Heat Index	−141.7***	−19.58***
	(40.83)	(7.60)
Cluster 2*Heat Index	−202.9***	−12.89**
	(23.54)	(5.24)
Cluster 3*Heat Index	−138.3***	−22.56***
	(12.63)	(2.06)
Cluster 4*Heat Index	−58.75***	−21.82***
	(6.55)	(1.22)
Cluster 1*Heat Index^2	9.16***	1.23*
	(2.74)	(0.73)
Cluster 2*Heat Index^2	13.03***	0.48
	(1.58)	(0.51)
Cluster 3*Heat Index^2	9.25***	1.50***
	(0.84)	(0.22)
Cluster 4*Heat Index^2	3.79***	1.10***
	(0.44)	(0.12)
Cluster 2	967.1***	794.7***
	(148.3)	(33.13)
Cluster 3	1,457***	1,486***
	(136.0)	(30.74)
Cluster 4	2,007***	2,298***
	(131.4)	(29.73)
Previous Participations	−23.47***	−23.36***
	(1.66)	(1.63)
Age	5.27***	5.02***
	(0.35)	(0.34)
Gender	51.61***	47.17***
	(10.16)	(10.01)
Start Corral	−77.97***	−90.81***
	(7.15)	(6.77)
Constant	8,893***	8,539***
	(294.6)	(261.8)
Nationality	Yes	Yes
Observations	11,999	11,999
Adjusted R-squared	0.80	0.81

*Standard errors in parentheses. ***$p < 0.01$, **$p < 0.05$, *$p < 0.1$.*

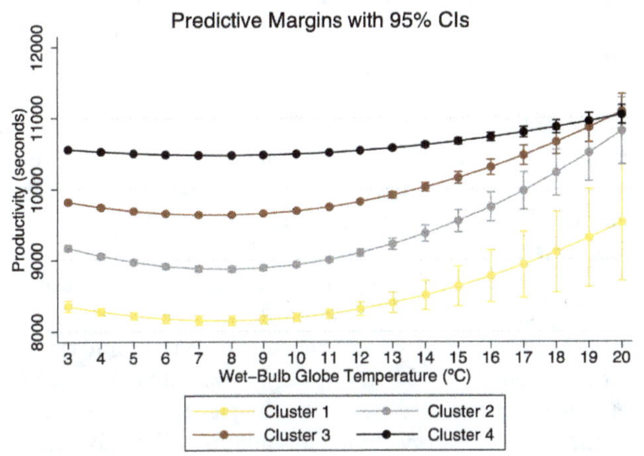

FIGURE 2 | Marginal Impact of WBGT on performance by clusters.

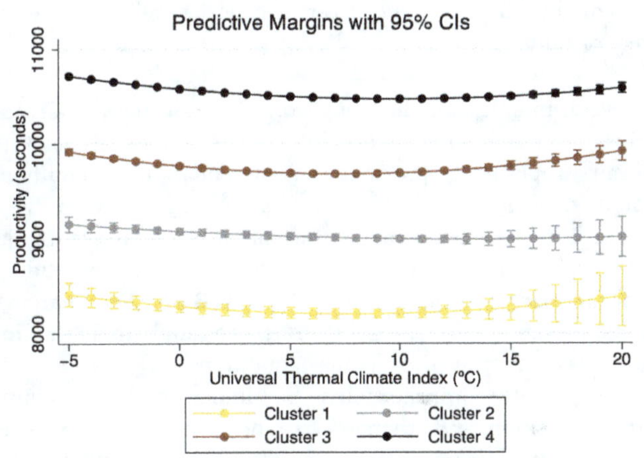

FIGURE 3 | Marginal Impact of UTCI on performance by clusters.

work, is needed to understand whether thermal conditions impact them differently as well.

Our results indicate that top runners suffer higher decreases in performances than slower ones. As shown in **Figures 2, 3**, when comparing finishing times under optimal (+8°C WBGT) and DNT temperatures (+20°C WBGT), the present results indicate an average decrease of about 1,376 s (16.89%), 1,942 s (21.89%), 1,149 s (15.04%), and 569 s (5.44%) for groups 1, 2, 3, and 4, respectively. Faster runners perform the same task at a higher intensity than slower ones, and therefore thermal conditions affect their performance more than the slower groups. Del Coso et al. (2013) previously suggested that runners with higher levels of fatigue could not sustain their habitual pace, and accordingly their performance deteriorates. Therefore, although less skilled runners spend longer periods under heat exposure, their relatively less intense activity explains, to some extent, the reduced negative impact from higher temperatures when compared to top runners.

Psychological elements would also be associated with such performance penalties for faster runners. World-class and elite runners – the fastest in a major marathon – are in a highly competitive situation: pressure to win, earning places in other major events, or achieving certain results because of financial incentives from sponsors. These performance pressures in sports usually result in injuries (Strauss and Curry, 1983) and in some cases may drive top athletes to behave unethically (Volkwein, 1995; Barroso et al., 2008). Donahue et al. (2006) shows that intrinsic and extrinsic motivations are appropriate to prevent elite athletes from unethical behaviors, but they do not eliminate the pressure for good results. Therefore, top-level runners would try to surpass their physiological limits to cope with the negative effects of heat stress, and hence may suffer a bigger performance penalty than slower runners under identical conditions. Unfortunately, our data does not allow us to investigate this matter further, but additional studies are encouraged that focus on these types of questions.

Further research could also exploit the limitations of this paper. Doherty et al. (2020) assess the effect of many training elements on marathon performance but, because of a lack of data availability, they were not included in the present research. Indeed, certain training patterns might help coping with negative effects of heat stress. Pacing and other race strategies are also important elements in marathoners' performance, but were not available for the current research. Further research could examine how heat exposure influences pacing for different groups of athletes as well as analyze optimal strategies that handle certain environmental conditions during marathons. Studies focusing on thermal impacts on gender and age groups are also encouraged. Finally, the variation of thermal conditions during a marathon is an interesting factor that certainly impacts race performance and that should be examined as well. Understanding these elements is essential to maximize sports performance as well as assure the safety of runners.

Several practical implications from this research are already reported in the literature. However, our output is very relevant supporting previous recommendations. Marathons should happen under temperatures around +8°C WBGT, assuring higher levels of performance and safety for all participants. Additionally, organizers should avoid competitions with thermal conditions over +20°C WBGT. The marginal effects presented here can help runners to adjust their training sessions considering the thermal conditions. We may assume that the negative impacts might be similar for both training and competition and, therefore, runners should be aware of these performance penalties not only on the race day, but also during their whole preparation. Finally, the evidence that faster runners suffer from a greater performance penalty than slower ones under identical thermal conditions suggests an opportunity for performance' optimization for top-runners. Researchers and athletes together have to search for ways to maximize performance under such conditions.

The results here are important for future research regarding the impact of thermal conditions on performance. We demonstrate that marathon runners suffer from thermal conditions in different ways: under identical thermal conditions, top runners experience a substantially greater performance decrement than slower runners. This finding, which contradicts previous research, is the key contribution of the present research. Marathon is a genuine competitive sport, which makes these results relevant for other sport settings (e.g., triathlon, cross-country skiing, cycling) (Orr, 2020). However, the results are not exclusively valid for the sport sphere since heterogeneous performance levels can be found in numerous settings where individual-, group-, and firm-variation is regularly observed. For instance, further research is encouraged that investigates the physiological responses of different groups of professional workers – both athletes and non-athletes – based on their skill level. Researchers should be aware of these elements and examine as precisely as possible each specific case prior to performing estimations for future scenarios. Understanding why groups experience heat stress differently under identical circumstances is crucial for relevant scientific and policy recommendations.

AUTHOR CONTRIBUTIONS

All authors listed have made a substantial, direct and intellectual contribution to the work, and approved it for publication.

REFERENCES

Armstrong, L. E., Casa, D. J., Millard-Stafford, M., Moran, D. S., Pyne, S. W., and Roberts, W. O. (2007). Exertional heat illness during training and competition. *Med. Sci. Sports Exerc.* 39, 556–572.

Barreca, A., Clay, K., Deschenes, O., Greenstone, M., and Shapiro, J. S. (2016). Adapting to climate change: the remarkable decline in the US temperature-mortality relationship over the twentieth century. *J. Polit. Econ.* 124, 105–159. doi: 10.1086/684582

Barroso, O., Mazzoni, I., and Rabin, O. (2008). Hormone abuse in sports: the antidoping perspective. *Asian J. Androl.* 10, 391–402. doi: 10.1111/j.1745-7262.2008.00402.x

Błażejczyk, K., Jendritzky, G., Bröde, P., Fiala, D., Havenith, G., Epstein, Y., et al. (2013). An introduction to the universal thermal climate index (UTCI). *Geogr. Pol.* 86, 5–10. doi: 10.7163/gpol.2013.1

Brocherie, F., and Millet, G. P. (2015). Is the wet-bulb globe temperature (WBGT) index relevant for exercise in the heat? *Sports Med.* 45, 1619–1621. doi: 10.1007/s40279-015-0386-8

Brotherhood, J. R. (2008). Heat stress and strain in exercise and sport. *J. Sci. Med. Sport* 11, 6–19. doi: 10.1016/j.jsams.2007.08.017

Burke, M., Hsiang, S. M., and Miguel, E. (2015). Global non-linear effect of temperature on economic production. *Nature* 527, 235–239. doi: 10.1038/nature15725

Chavaillaz, Y., Roy, P., Partanen, A. I., Da Silva, L., Bresson, É, Mengis, N., et al. (2019). Exposure to excessive heat and impacts on labour productivity liked to cumulative CO emissions. *Sci. Rep.* 9:13711.

Cheung, S. S., Lee, J. K. W., and Oksa, J. (2016). Thermal stress, human performance, and physical employment standards. *Appl. Physiol. Nutr. Metab.* 41, S148–S164.

Coris, E. E., Ramirez, A. M., and Van Durme, D. J. (2004). Heat illness in athletes: the dangerous combination of heat, humidity and exercise. *Sports Med.* 34, 9–16. doi: 10.2165/00007256-200434010-00002

Day, E., Fankhauser, S., Kingsmill, N., Costa, H., and Mavrogianni, A. (2019). Upholding labour productivity under climate change: an assessment of adaptation options. *Clim. Policy* 19, 367–385. doi: 10.1080/14693062.2018.1517640

Dear, K. (2018). Modelling productivity loss from heat stress. *Atmosphere* 9, 1–9.

Del Coso, J., Fernández, D., Abián-Vicen, J., Salinero, J. J., González-Millán, C., Areces, F., et al. (2013). Running pace decrease during a marathon is positively related to blood markers of muscle damage. *PLoS One* 8:e57602. doi: 10.1371/journal.pone.0057602

Dell, M., Jones, B. F., and Olken, B. A. (2012). Climate change and economic growth: evidence from the last half century. *Am. Econ. J. Macroecon.* 4, 66–95. doi: 10.1257/mac.4.3.66

Doherty, C., Keogh, A., Davenport, J., Lawlor, A., Smyth, B., and Caulfield, B. (2020). An evaluation of the training determinants of marathon performance: a meta-analysis with meta-regression. *J. Sci. Med. Sport* 23, 182–188. doi: 10.1016/j.jsams.2019.09.013

Donahue, E. G., Miquelon, P., Valois, P., Goulet, C., Buist, A., and Vallerand, R. J. (2006). A motivational model of performance-enhancing substance use in elite athletes. *J. Sport Exerc. Psychol.* 28, 511–520. doi: 10.1123/jsep.28.4.511

Dunne, J. P., Stouffer, R. J., and John, J. G. (2013). Reductions in labour capacity from heat stress under climate warming. *Nat. Clim. Change* 3, 563–566. doi: 10.1038/nclimate1827

Dyble, M., Thorley, J., Page, A. E., Smith, D., and Migliano, A. B. (2019). Engagement in agricultural work is associated with reduced leisure time among Agta hunter-gatherers. *Nat. Hum. Behav.* 3, 792–796. doi: 10.1038/s41562-019-0614-6

Epstein, Y., and Moran, D. S. (2006). Thermal comfort and the heal stress indices. *Industrial Health* 44, 388–398. doi: 10.2486/indhealth.44.388

El Helou, N., Tafflet, M., Berthelot, G., Tolaini, J., Marc, A., Guillaume, M., et al. (2012). Impact of environmental parameters on marathon running performance. *PLoS One* 7:e37407. doi: 10.1371/journal.pone.0037407

Ely, M. R., Cheuvront, S. N., Roberts, W. O., and Montain, S. J. (2007). Impact of weather on marathon-running performance. *Med. Sci. Sports Exerc.* 39, 487–493. doi: 10.1249/mss.0b013e31802d3aba

Fishman, R., Carillo, P., and Russ, J. (2019). Long-term impacts of exposure to high temperatures on human capital and economic productivity. *J. Environ. Econ. Manage.* 93, 221–238. doi: 10.1016/j.jeem.2018.10.001

Flouris, A. D., Dinas, P. C., Ioannou, L. G., Nybo, L., Havenith, G., Kenny, G. P., et al. (2018). Workers' health and productivity under occupational heat strain: a systematic review and meta-analysis. *Lancet Planet Health* 2, e521–e531. doi: 10.1016/s2542-5196(18)30237-7

Gosling, C. M., Gabbe, B. J., McGivern, J., and Forbes, A. B. (2008). The incidence of heat casualties in sprint triathlon: the tale of two Melbourne race events. *J. Sci. Med. Sport* 11, 52–57. doi: 10.1016/j.jsams.2007.08.010

Hancock, P. A., Ross, J. M., and Szalma, J. L. (2007). A meta-analysis of performance response under thermal stressors. *Human Factors* 49, 851–877. doi: 10.1518/001872007x230226

Hellon, R. F., Lind, A. R., and Weiner, J. S. (1956). The physiological reactions of men of two age groups to a hot environment. *J. Physiol.* 133, 118–131. doi: 10.1113/jphysiol.1956.sp005570

Hsiang, S., Kopp, R., Jina, A., Rising, J., Delgado, M., Mohan, S., et al. (2017). Estimation economic damage from climate change in the United States. *Science* 356, 1362–1369.

ISO (2017). *ISO 7243:2017. Ergonomics of the Thermal Environment – Assessment of Heat Stress using the WBGT (wet bulb globe temperature) Index.* Geneva: ISO.

Kampmann, B., Bröde, P., and Fiala, D. (2012). Physiological responses to temperature and humidity compared to the assessment by UTCI, WGBT and PHS. *Int. J. Biometeorol.* 56, 505–513. doi: 10.1007/s00484-011-0410-0

Kjellstrom, T., Holmer, I., and Lemke, B. (2009). Workplace heat stress, health and productivity – an increasing challenge for low and middle-income countries during climate change. *Global Health Action* 2:10.3402/gha.v2i0.2047. doi: 10.3402/gha.v2i0.2047

Kjellstrom, T., Freyberg, C., Lemke, B., Otto, M., and Briggs, D. (2018). Estimating population heat exposure and impacts on working people in conjunction with climate change. *Int. J. Biometeorol.* 62, 291–306. doi: 10.1007/s00484-017-1407-0

Knechtle, B., Di Gangi, S., Rüst, C. A., Rosemann, T., and Nikolaidis, P. T. (2018). Men's participation and performance in the Boston Marathon from 1897 to 2007. *Int. J. Sports Med.* 39, 1018–1027. doi: 10.1055/a-0660-0061

Knechtle, B., Di Gangi, S., Rüst, C. A., Villiger, E., Rosemann, T., and Nikolaidis, P. T. (2019). The role of weather conditions on running performance in the Boston Marathon from 1972 to 2018. *PLoS One* 14:e0212797. doi: 10.1371/journal.pone.0212797

Kurakake, S., Sugawara, K., Kumae, T., Shimaoka, A., Mathida, K., and Okamura, N. (1988). A study on the effect of physical load of baseball umpire, during a baseball game in the summer. *Japanese J. Hygiene* 42, 1013–1022. doi: 10.1265/jjh.42.1013

Ladell, W. S. S. (1955). The effects of water and salt intake upon the performance of men working in hot and humid environments. *J. Physiol.* 127, 11–46. doi: 10.1113/jphysiol.1955.sp005235

Lara, B., Salinero, J. J., and Del Coso, J. (2014). The relationship between age and running time in elite marathoners is U-shaped. *Age* 36, 1003–1008. doi: 10.1007/s11357-013-9614-z

Lemke, B., and Kjellstrom, T. (2012). Calculating workplace WBGT from meteorological data: a tool for climate change assessment. *Industrial Health* 50, 267–278. doi: 10.2486/indhealth.ms1352

Liu, W., Zhong, W., and Wargocki, P. (2017). Performance, acute health symptoms and physiological responses during exposure to high air temperature and carbon dioxide concentration. *Build. Environ.* 114, 96–105. doi: 10.1016/j.buildenv.2016.12.020

Maffetone, P. B., Malcata, R., Rivera, I., and Laursen, P. B. (2017). The Boston marathon versus the world marathon majors. *PLoS One* 12:e0184024. doi: 10.1371/journal.pone.0184024

Martinich, J., and Crimmins, A. (2019). Climate damages and adaptation potential across diverse sectors of the United States. *Nat. Clim. Change* 9, 397–404. doi: 10.1038/s41558-019-0444-6

Massimino, F. A. (1988). Common triathlon injuries: special considerations for multisport training. *Ann. Sports Med.* 4, 82–86.

Miller-Rushing, A. J., Primack, R. B., Phillips, N., and Kaufmann, R. K. (2012). Effects of warming temperatures on winning times in the Boston Marathon. *PLoS One* 7:e43579. doi: 10.1371/journal.pone.0043579

Mohr, M., Nybo, L., Grantham, J., and Racinais, S. (2012). Physiological responses and physical performance during football in the heat. *PLoS One* 7:e39202. doi: 10.1371/journal.pone.0039202

Montain, S. K., Ely, M. R., and Cheuvront, S. N. (2007). Marathon performance in thermally stressing conditions. *Sports Med.* 37, 320–323. doi: 10.2165/00007256-200737040-00012

Mora, C., Dousset, B., Caldwell, I. R., Powell, F. E., Geronimo, R. C., Bielecki, C. R., et al. (2017). Global risk of deadly heat. *Nat. Clim. Change* 7, 501–506.

Maughan, R. J. (2010). Distance running in hot environments: a thermal challenge to the elite runner. *Scand. J. Med. Sci. Sports* 20, 95–102. doi: 10.1111/j.1600-0838.2010.01214.x

Nikolaidis, P. T., Di Gangi, S., Chtourou, H., Rüst, C. A., Rosemann, T., and Knechtle, B. (2019b). The role of environmental conditions on marathon running performance in men competing in Boston marathon from 1897 to 2018. *Int. J. Environ. Res. Public Health* 16:614. doi: 10.3390/ijerph16040614

Nikolaidis, P. T., Alvero-Cruz, J. R., Villiger, E., Rosemann, T., and Knechtle, B. (2019a). The age-related performance decline in marathon running: the paradigm of the Berlin marathon. *Int. J. Environ. Res. Public Health* 16, 1–12.

Orr, M. (2020). On the potential impacts of climate change on baseball and cross-country skiing. *Managing Sport Leisure* 25, 307–320. doi: 10.1080/23750472.2020.1723436

Périard, J. D., Racinais, S., and Sawka, M. N. (2015). Adaptations and mechanisms of human heat acclimation: applications for competitive athletes and sports. *Scand. J. Med. Sci. Sports* 25, 20–38. doi: 10.1111/sms.12408

Roberts, W. O. (2010). Determining a "Do not start" temperature for a marathon on the basis of adverse outcomes. *Med. Sci. Sports Exerc.* 42, 226–232. doi: 10.1249/mss.0b013e3181b1cdcf

Rokach, L., and Maimon, O. (2005). "Clustering methods," in *Data Mining and Knowledge Discovery Handbook*, eds O. Maimon, and L. Rokach (Berlin: Springer), 321–352.

Sherwood, S. C., and Huber, M. (2010). An adaptability limit to climate change due to heat stress. *Proc. Natl. Acad. Sci. U.S.A.* 107, 9552–9555. doi: 10.1073/pnas.0913352107

Smith, K. R., Woodward, A., Lemke, B., Otto, M., Chang, C. J., Mance, A. A., et al. (2016). The last summer olympics? Climate change, health, and work outdoors. *Lancet* 388, 642–644. doi: 10.1016/s0140-6736(16)31335-6

Spector, J. T., Bonauto, D. K., Sheppard, L., Busch-Isaksen, T., Calkins, M., Adams, D., et al. (2016). A case-crossover study of heat exposure and injury risk in outdoor agricultural workers. *PLoS One* 11:e0164498. doi: 10.1371/journal.pone.0164498

Strauss, R. H., and Curry, T. J. (1983). Social factors in wrestlers' health problems. *Phys. Sportsmed.* 11, 86–99. doi: 10.1080/00913847.1983.11708685

Suping, Z., Guanglin, M., Yanwen, W., and Ji, L. (1992). Study of the relationships between weather conditions and the marathon race, and of meteorotropic effects on distance runners. *Int. J. Biometeorol.* 36, 63–68. doi: 10.1007/BF01208915

Takakura, J. Y., Fujimori, S., Takahashi, K., Hijioka, Y., Hasegawa, T., Honda, Y., et al. (2017). Cost of preventing work place heat-related illness through worker breaks and the benefit of climate-change mitigation. *Environ. Res. Lett.* 12, 1–12.

Tanabe, S., Haneda, M., and Nishihara, N. (2015). Workplace productivity and individual thermal satisfaction. *Build. Environ.* 91, 42–50. doi: 10.1016/j.buildenv.2015.02.032

Tatterson, A. J., Hahn, A. G., Martini, D. T., and Febbraio, M. A. (2000). Effects of heat stress on physiological responses and exercise performance in elite cyclists. *J. Sci. Med. Sport* 3, 186–193. doi: 10.1016/s1440-2440(00)80080-8

Trapasso, L. M., and Cooper, J. D. (1989). Record performances at the Boston marathon: biometeorological factors. *Int. J. Biometeorol.* 33, 233–237. doi: 10.1007/bf01051083

Trezza, B. M., Apolinario, D., de Oliveira, R. S., Busse, A. L., Gonçalves, F. L. T., Saldiva, P. H. N., et al. (2015). Environmental heat exposure and cognitive performance in older adults: a controlled trial. *Age* 37, 1–10.

Tyler, C. J., Reeve, T., Hodges, G. J., and Cheung, S. S. (2016). The effects of heat adaptation on physiology, perception and exercise performance in the heat: a meta-analysis. *Sports Med.* 46, 1699–1724. doi: 10.1007/s40279-016-0538-5

Varghese, B. M., Hansen, A., Bi, P., and Pisaniello, D. (2018). Are workers at risk occupational injuries due to heat exposure? A comprehensive literature review. *Safety Sci.* 110, 380–392. doi: 10.1016/j.ssci.2018.04.027

Vihma, T. (2010). Effects of weather on the performance of marathon runners. *Int. J. Biometeorol.* 54, 297–306. doi: 10.1007/s00484-009-0280-x

Volkwein, K. A. E. (1995). Ethics and top-level sport - a paradox? *Int. Rev. Sociol. Sport* 30, 311–320. doi: 10.1177/101269029503000305

Ward, J. H. (1963). Hiearchical grouping to optimize an objective function. *J. Am. Stat. Assoc.* 58, 236–244. doi: 10.1080/01621459.1963.10500845

Watts, N., Amann, M., Arnell, N., Ayeb-Karlsson, S., Belesova, K., Berry, H., et al. (2018). The 2018 report of the Lancet countdown on health and climate change: shaping the health of nations for centuries to come. *Lancet* 392, 2479–2514.

Witterseh, T., Wyon, D. P., and Clausen, G. (2004). The effects of moderate heat stress and open-plan office noise distraction on SBS symptoms and of the performance of office work. *Indoor Air* 14, 30–40. doi: 10.1111/j.1600-0668.2004.00305.x

Yi, W., and Chan, A. P. C. (2015). Optimal work pattern for construction workers in hot weather: a case study in Hong Kong. *J. Comput. Civil Eng.* 29, 1–11.

Zander, K., Botzen, W., Oppermann, E., Kjellstrom, T., and Garnett, S. T. (2015). Heat stress causes substantial labour productivity loss in Australia. *Nature Clim. Change* 5, 647–651. doi: 10.1038/nclimate2623

Zare, S., Hasheminejad, N., Shirvan, H. E., Hemmatjo, R., Sarebanzadeh, K., and Ahmadi, S. (2015). Heat stress causes substantial labour productivity loss in Australia. *Nat. Clim. Change* 5, 647–651. doi: 10.1038/nclimate2623

Zare, S., Hasheminejad, N., Shirvan, H. E., Hemmatjo, R., Sarebanzade, K., and Ahmadi, S. (2018). Comparing universal thermal climate index (UTCI) with selected thermal indices/environmental parameters during 12 months of the year. *Weather Clim. Extrem.* 19, 49–57. doi: 10.1016/j.wace.2018.01.004

7

Representative Percentile Curves of Physical Fitness from Early Childhood to Early Adulthood

Claudia Niessner [1], Till Utesch [2], Doris Oriwol [1,3], Anke Hanssen-Doose [3], Steffen C. E. Schmidt [1], Alexander Woll [1], Klaus Bös [1] and Annette Worth [3]*

[1] Institute of Sport and Sport Science, Karlsruhe Institute of Technology, Karlsruhe, Germany, [2] Department of Pedagogical Assessment and Potential Development, Institute of Educational Sciences, University of Münster, Münster, Germany, [3] Institute of Movement and Sport, University of Education, Karlsruhe, Germany

***Correspondence:**
Claudia Niessner
claudia.niessner@kit.edu

Introduction: Monitoring of physical fitness in youth is important because physical fitness is a summative indicator of health. From a developmental and preventive perspective, physical fitness levels are relatively stable from childhood to early adulthood. Thus, it is important to monitor physical fitness on a population based level being able to intervene at early stages (1). In order to reliably assess and evaluate the physical fitness of youth, a reliable system of standard values based on representative data is required. The aim of this analysis is to report sex- and age-specific physical fitness percentile curves from childhood to early adulthood in a nationwide sample in Germany.

Methods: We use data from the nationwide representative Motorik Modul (MoMo) Study in Germany (data collection wave 1: 2009–2012; age: 4–23 years; n = 3,742; 50.1% female). Physical fitness was assessed by means of the MoMo test profile covering four dimensions of physical fitness (strength, endurance, coordination, and flexibility) and including eight physical fitness items. Percentile curves were fitted using the LMS transformation method of Cole and Green.

Results: Standardized age- and sex-specific physical fitness percentiles were calculated for eight items: ergometric endurance testing, standing long jump, push-ups, sit-ups, jumping side-ways, balancing backwards, static stand, and stand and reach test. The physical fitness curves differ according to gender and the fitness dimension. Physical fitness improvements with age are linear (e.g., max. strength) or curvilinear (e.g., coordination) and have their stagnation points at different times over the course of adolescence.

Discussion: Our results provide for the first time sex- and age-specific physical fitness percentile curves for Germany from 4 to 17 years. Differences in curve-shapes indicating a timed and capacity-specific physical fitness development. Nationwide German physical fitness percentiles can be useful in comparing different populations (e.g., cross-country), reporting secular trends, comparing special groups, and to evaluate physical fitness interventions.

Keywords: health-related, performance, skill-related, LMS, reference, monitoring, Germany, youth

INTRODUCTION

Physical fitness levels play a major role in overall healthy child and youth development (2). Representing powerful biomarkers of health status already in early childhood, especially the maintenance of satisfactory fitness levels is highly connected with current public health issues as physical development (3), the prevention of diabetes, obesity (4), cardiovascular disease risk factors (5), cancer and mental health (2, 6). Therefore, it is important to monitor population fitness levels longitudinally to being able to intervene at an early stage (7, 8). The importance of such monitoring has also been shown by critical decreases in physical fitness levels in a large world-wide sample (9).

The specific selection of appropriate definitions, assessments and subsequent test interpretations are important in the scientific as well as practical fields of human health and sports sciences. The construct of physical fitness consists of two components (10): on the one hand, health-related fitness includes cardiovascular endurance, strength endurance, explosive muscular strength, body composition as well as flexibility (10). On the other hand, skill-related fitness is defined as agility, balance, coordination, speed, power and reaction time (10). Physical fitness can be accessed via laboratory as well as field tests. Although laboratory tests using sophisticated material are capable of providing very objective and detailed outcomes, these tests are not suitable for comprehensive monitoring of physical fitness levels in large scale studies across cities, states or countries. Here, single field tests assessing specific fitness domains are often utilized and gathered in standardized test batteries to comprehensively cover physical fitness [e.g., FitnessGram (11), Eurofit (12), German Motor Performance Test 6–18 (13)]. Among various widely known and broadly used single test items, the MoMo Motor Performance Test (14) was compiled using the most widely used single item tests in Europe in order to broadly and longitudinally assess physical fitness from early childhood to early adulthood.

In Germany, it has been shown that certain physical fitness components are relatively stable between cohorts from childhood to early adulthood while others increase or decrease (3, 15). In order to successfully monitor physical fitness levels over time in a representative manner, it is necessary to provide up-to-date normative data of the specific test items. Many researchers, but also physical education teachers or sport coaches assess physical fitness from their students and need valid and simple possibilities judging their physical fitness performance (16). Therefore, this study aims to provide up-to-date age- and sex-related percentile curves of persons aged four to 17 years for frequently used test items:

(1) Ergometric endurance testing, (2) standing long jump, (3) push-ups, (4) sit-ups, (5) jumping side-ways, (6) balancing backwards (7) static stand, and (8) stand and reach test.

METHODS

The study was conducted according to the Declaration of Helsinki. Ethics approval was obtained by the University of Konstanz (Wave 1). The Federal Commissioner for the "data protection" and "freedom of information" was informed about the study and approved it.

Participants

Data were obtained from the nationwide German Motorik-Modul study (MoMo). The MoMo study is an in-depth module study of the German Health Interview and Examination Survey for Children and Adolescents which was conducted by The Robert Koch-Institute (RKI, Berlin) since 2003 (17, 18). The MoMo study provides nationwide representative data on the physical fitness and physical activity status (19). The study was set up in 2003 (2003–2006 MoMo Baseline). Two consecutive survey waves were conducted until now: MoMo Wave 1 (2009–2012) and MoMo Wave 2 (2014–2017). Children and adolescents were invited to the physical fitness tests at central locations within close proximity to their homes in the 167 cities and municipalities.

The data of 3,284 children and adolescents (1,644 female, 1,646 male) aged 4–17 years were reported in figures below while LMS curve modeling used data of persons till 23 years ($N = 3{,}742$; male 49.9% $N = 1{,}868$; female 50.1% $N = 1{,}874$) from the MoMo Wave 1 survey (2009–2012) was used to model physical fitness percentiles of children and adolescents. We have modeled the percentile curves up to 23 years, as the model fit for the percentile curves become better and more accurate with more data and thus over a larger age range. From the age of 17 years on, however, our sample is no longer representative for Germany, so we report only the data up to 17 years. Characteristics of the whole sample including individual level of socioeconomic status (SES) (20), BMI (21), and type of residential area (22) differentiated by age group and sex are shown in **Supplement Table 1** in the Supplement Material.

Detail information about mean values of all physical fitness tests for age groups and gender can be found here (23).

Sampling

To ensure a diverse sample of German children and adolescents, a nationwide, stratified, multi-stage sample with two evaluation levels was drawn (24).

First, a systematic sample of 167 primary sampling units was selected from an inventory of German communities that were stratified according to the BIK classification system that measures the level of urbanization and the geographic distribution (17). The probability of any community being picked was proportional to the number of inhabitants younger than 18 years in that community. Second, an age stratified sample of randomly selected children and adolescents was drawn from the official registers of local residents. At the second measurement point (KiGGS Wave 1 study), 12,368 children and adolescents participated (18). This sample built the population for the MoMo Wave 1 subsample. 6,076 from KiGGS Wave 1 were randomly assigned to MoMo Wave 1. From those, 3,994 participated in MoMo (65.7%). After excluding participants without a valid physical fitness test (one test item was sufficient), a total of 3,742 children and adolescents 4–23 years remained for this analysis.

Representativeness

Weighting procedure was used to account for potential bias in outcome variables caused by selective unit nonresponse (24). In the first step, inverse probability weights were applied via logistic regression to eliminate differences in outcome variables between the MoMo subsample and the weighted representative KiGGS sample. In the second step, the MoMo subsample was stratified using data of the German Micro Census 2010 to ensure representativeness of the target population (German children and adolescents aged 4–17 years) regarding sex, age, region, migration background, and education level (25).

Material

The MoMo Motor Performance Test (14) was developed in order to broadly cover the construct of physical fitness. The physical fitness tests were carried out in the time frame from 8 a.m. to 6 p.m. Trained testing stuff conducted the tests with the children and adolescents in a one-to-one supervision. Testing always start with the coordination tasks followed by the strength tasks and at the end the endurance test on the bike ergometer was carried out. The duration of the test is about 60 min. The test items originated from common validated test profiles and were pretested, optimized, discussed with experts, and documented in a comprehensive test manual (14). The overall reliability was calculated using the standardized total value and results in a correlation of $r = 0.97$ ($p = 0.00$) and no significant difference in mean value. The objectivity (tested using different test directors) is very good ($r = 0.98$ to 0.99), the percentage difference is less than one percentage point for all test items (26). It consists of eight items covering health-related (i.e., endurance, strength endurance, lower body explosive muscular strength, and flexibility) and skill-related fitness domains (i.e., balance, coordination), which are covered by the following test items:

Cardiovascular endurance was assessed using a static bicycle ergometer test. It measures the aerobic endurance capacity of participants using a sequential step test design. The test is started at a calculated input load of 0.5 watt/kg body weight and a cadence of 70 revolutions per minute (rpm). Each load level is held for two minutes. Then the load is increased by 0.5 watts per kilogram of body weight. Each level is shown on a digital display. For the assessment of the performance the power at a heart rate of 170 bpm (Physical Working Capacity [PWC170]) were used. The test stops at three occasions: (1) if there is a pulse of above 190 (participants up to 10 years) or above 180 (participants from 11 years), respectively, (2) if the cadence falls below 50 rpm for more than 20 s, or (3) if participants want to stop due to subjective exhaustion. Children aged 4–5 years did not participate in the test.

Strength endurance is assessed for upper extremities as well as body core via sit-ups and push-ups. Firstly, participants perform sit-ups to cover body core strength endurance in a lying position with bent legs. The test instructor fixes the feet on the ground. The fingertips touch the temples in order to avoid pulling the neck. At each sit-up, participants need to touch the knees with their elbows without lifting the basin. Subjects repeat as many correct sit-ups as possible in 40 s. Secondly, push-ups were performed in order to cover upper extremities strength endurance starting with hands together at the lower back. In a first step, participants push their body up with a plank body angle. When the arms are straight, subjects touch one hand with the other hand and return the starting position with constant body control. The resulting variable is the number of repeated correct push-ups in 40 s. Children aged 4–5 years did not partake in these two tests.

Explosive muscular strength of the lower extremities is assessed via standing long jump. Participants start at a line, which is marked on a tartan mat. It is important that subjects jump using both legs together and do not fall backwards after landing the jump. Otherwise, the jump has to be repeated. Two jumps were performed while the maximum jump is counted.

Coordination including Balance is assessed via jumping sideways, static stand and balancing backwards. For the jumping sideways task the test instructor creates two adjacent 50 cm squares with 5 cm lines. Participants have to jump from one to the other square like a pendulum jumping with both legs without touching the boundaries. After a 1-min pause, subjects have a second trial. The test instructor counts the number of correct jumps in 15 s.

Balance is assessed via static stand and more dynamic balancing backwards. Firstly, static jump measures sensomotoric regulation of precision tasks on a 3 cm broad beam. Participants have to balance on the beam without touching the own leg, the beam or the ground. Test instructor counts the number of mistakes in one minute. Secondly, balancing backwards assesses dynamic whole-body balance on three differently broad. Subjects have two trials each on a 6 cm, on a 4.5 cm, and on a 3 cm beam. Test instructor counts the number of steps from each participant before touching the ground while reaching a maximum of eight steps per beam (total max. 48 steps).

Flexibility of the lower extremities is assessed via stand and reach. Stand and reach specifically measures the flexibility of the lower back and hamstring muscles. Test instructors measure the level of the fingers with the feet recording to zero. Negative values are associated with not being able to reach one's own toes while positive values are related to reaching further than the toes. Participants have to stay in the final position for two seconds in order to avoid swinging execution of the task. Subjects have two trials for this test.

Data Analysis: LMS Curves

Age- and sex-specific percentile values (P5, P10, P15, P30, P50, P70, P85, P90, and P95) were calculated and percentile curves were fitted using the LMS transformation method of Cole and Green (27). The LMS method summarizes the changing distribution by three curves representing the median (M), coefficient of variation (L), and skewness (S) (expressed as a Box-Cox power). Using penalized likelihood the three curves can be fitted as cubic splines by non-linear regression, and the extent of smoothing required can be expressed in terms of smoothing parameters or equivalent degrees of freedom (27). The values of L, M and S were constrained to change smoothly with age, and the fitted values can be used to construct any required percentile curves (28). All analyses were performed with LMS chartmaker pro (V. 2.3). When modeling some extreme values resulted

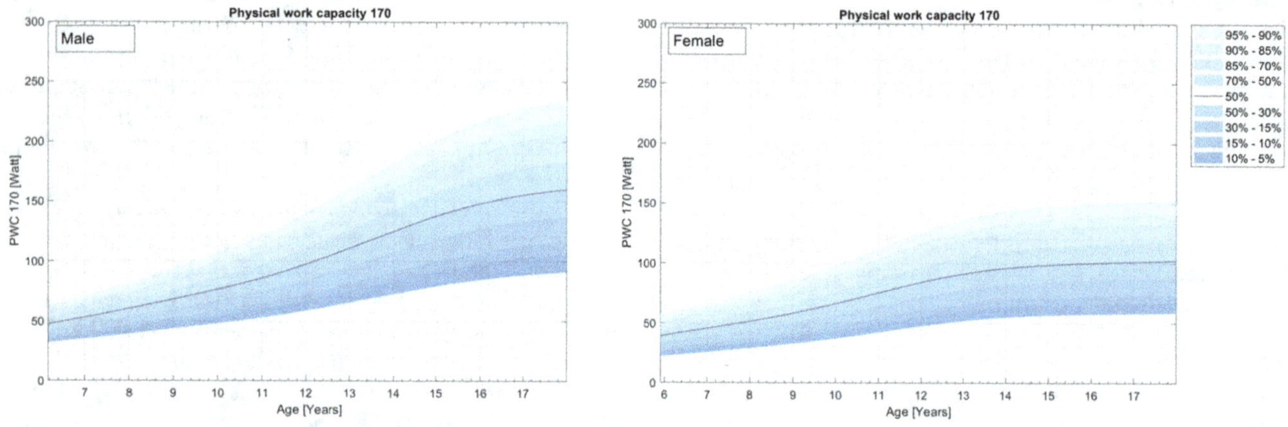

FIGURE 1 | Cardiovascular endurance curves (Physical Work Capacity 170, ergometric bicycle test) for the representative sample of German boys and girls aged 4–17 years.

in the sample of computational instabilities in the application of the method. For this reason, values were excluded which exceeded plus and minus three standard deviations. The number of degrees of freedom for the splines is considered optimal, following a recommendation by Cole (29), if the model's deviance (P Deviance and SBC Black Bayesian Criterion) with a further increase of 1° of freedom does not improve by more than 8. In addition, a visual quality control was conducted: Empirical and fitted centiles plotted on top of each other. This is an accurate technique in which the observations are divided into age groups (half-yearly). Empirical centiles are computed for each group, and these are plotted together with the fitted curves. If everything is right, the fitted curves should be close to the point estimates (that is, within sampling error). Quantile-quantile plot (Q–Q plot) of the z-scores were also applied. The display plots the quantiles of the theoretical distribution (on the horizontal axis) against those of the empirical distribution (on the vertical axis).

RESULTS

Physical fitness indicators for 3,742 children and adolescents from a representative (for 2010) nationwide German sample were used to develop percentile curves for male (49.9%) and female (50.1%) students aged 4–23 years. **Supplement Table 1** and **Figures 1–4** demonstrate the distributions and corresponding standardized age-based percentiles of all items separated for male and female subjects. We present figures to reproduce the shape of the percentile curves but at the same time provide the data basis for concrete physical fitness comparisons using the data in the tables for practical use.

Cardiovascular Endurance

The results for cardiovascular endurance can be found in **Figure 1** and **Supplement Table 2.**

Although the lowest percentile curves for fitness are relatively flat, a steady increase in mean aerobic performance is seen as children enter adolescence. On average, girls had a maximum fitness between ages 14 and 15 years, while boys, on average, had a maximum fitness between 15 and 16 years. Both sexes demonstrated a slight decrease after these peaks.

Strength

Sit-Ups

Results for strength are represented in **Figure 2** and **Supplement Tables 3–5.**

There is a steady increase in mean strength performance from childhood to adolescence. On average, girls had a maximum fitness between ages 11 and 12 years, while boys, on average, reach their maximum performance probably at the 17–18 years. The girls demonstrated a slight decrease after the peak.

Push-Ups

For females, the lowest percentile curves for fitness are relatively flat. On average, girls had a maximum strength performance at the age of 11 years (3). Boys also demonstrate a steady increase in mean strength performance over childhood and adolescence for all percentile curves except for the highest percentiles. The female percentile curve demonstrates a slight decrease after the peak for the highest percentiles or a stabilization for the other percentile curves.

Standing Long Jump

There is a steady increase in mean strength performance of the standing long jump from childhood to adolescence for both sexes. On average, standing long jump performance in girls stabilizes at the age of 11 years, while boys, demonstrate a steady increase. Both sexes demonstrated no decrease in this timespan.

Coordination Including Balance

Figure 3 and **Supplement Tables 6–8** show the results for coordination including jumping sideways, static stand, and balancing backwards.

Jumping Side-Ways

There is a steady increase in mean jumping sideways performance from childhood to adolescence for both sexes. On average, performance stabilizes

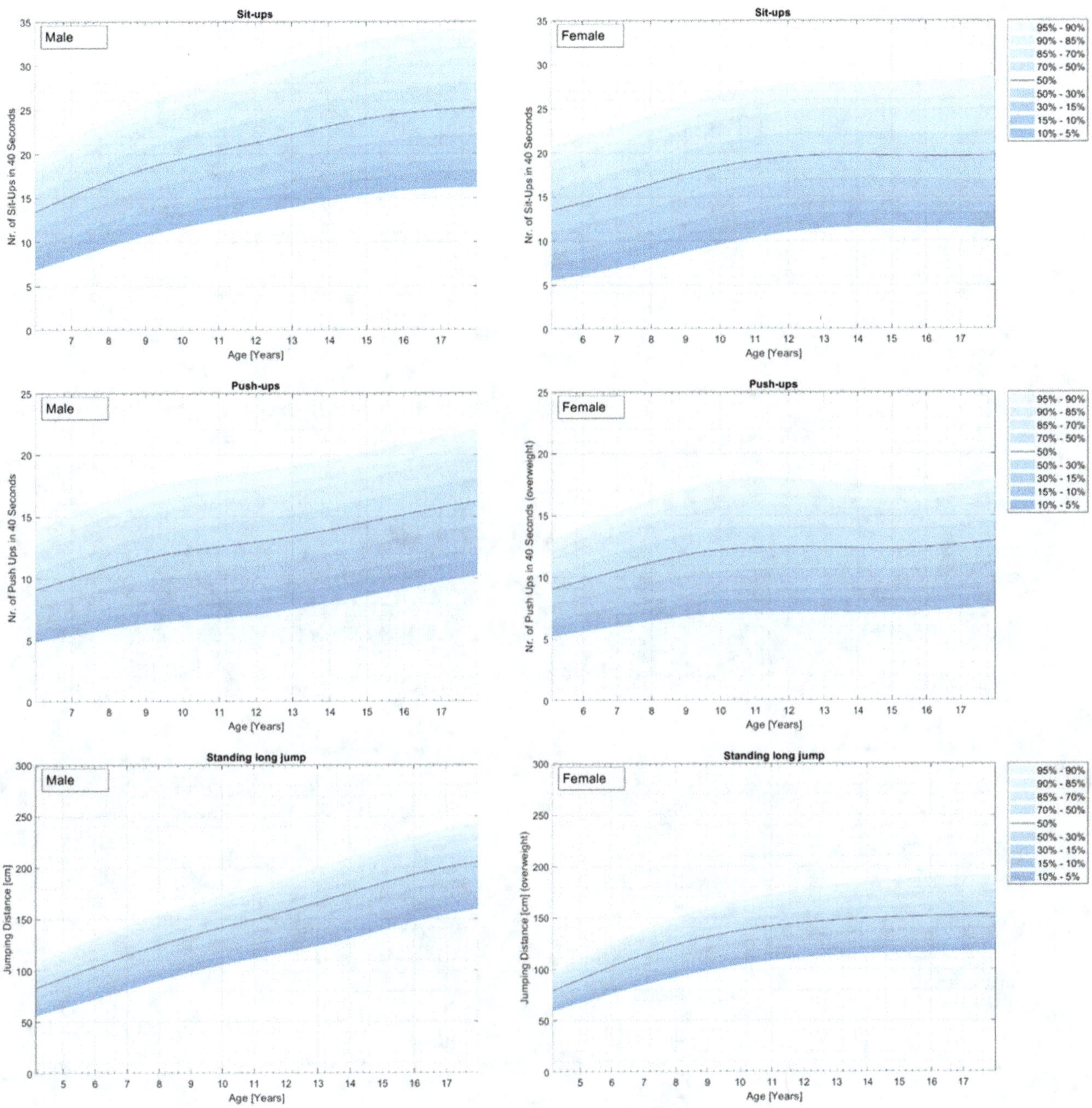

FIGURE 2 | Strength curves for the representative sample of German boys and girls aged 4–17 years for the testitems Sit-ups (top), Push-ups (middle), and Standing long jump (bottom).

for both sexes at the age between 12 and 14 years. Both sexes demonstrated no decrease in this timespan.

Static Stand

There is a steady decrease in mean ground contact from childhood to adolescence for both sexes up to 10–12 years. After that, performance stabilizes. There is a ceiling effect for the high percentiles.

Balancing Backwards

There is a steady increase in mean balancing performance from childhood to adolescence for both sexes. On average, performance stabilizes for both sexes at an age of 9 years. Both sexes demonstrated no decrease in this timespan.

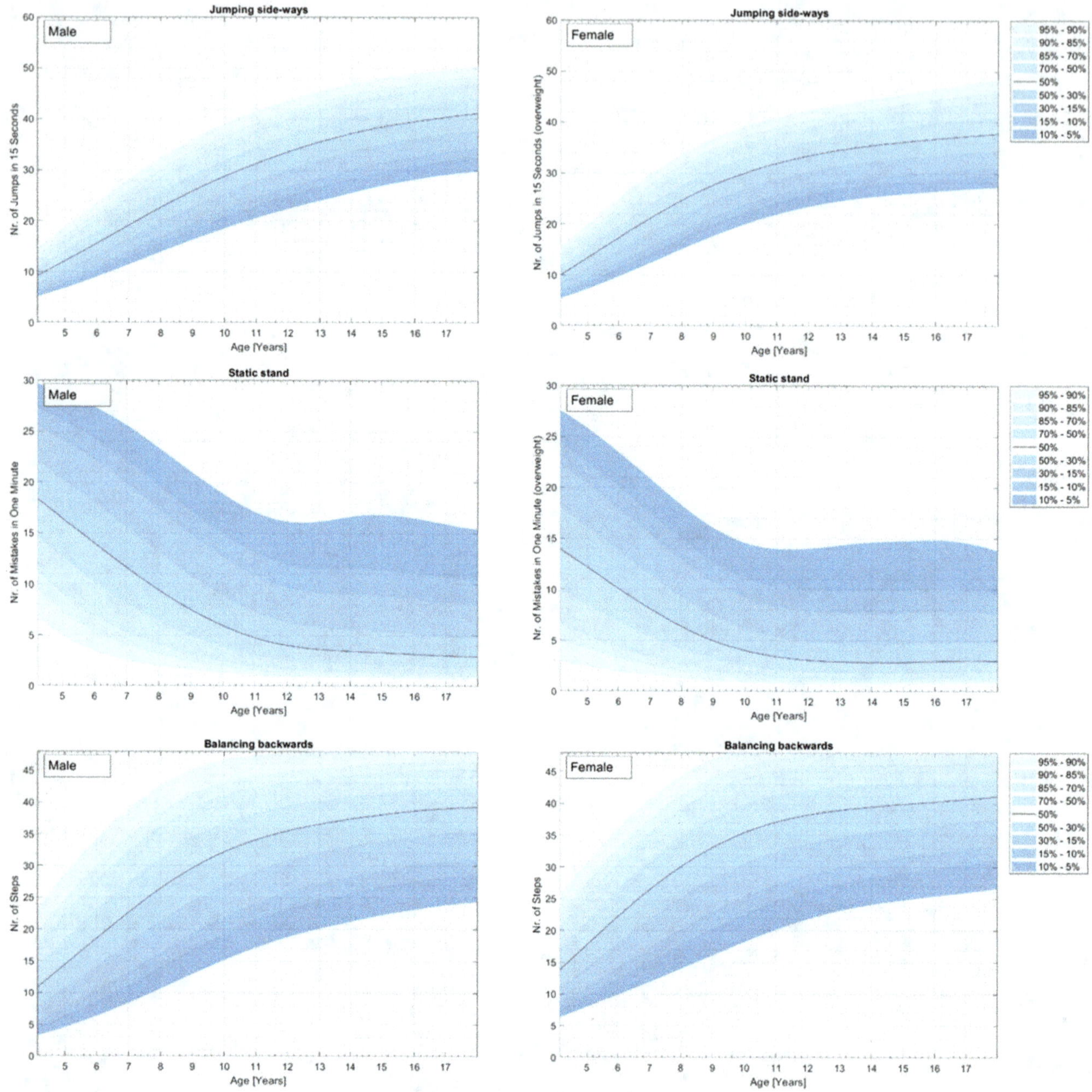

FIGURE 3 | Coordination curves for the representative sample of German boys and girls aged 4–23 years for the test items jumping side-ways (top), static stand (middle), and balancing backwards (bottom).

Flexibility

Results for flexibility are represented in **Figure 4** and **Supplement Table 9**.

Stand and Reach

In mean, both sexes demonstrate relatively flat percentile curves. Percentiles show a siccors effect with increasing age between the low and the high percentile curves. The low percentile curves decrease steady whereas high percentile curves increase steady from childhood to adolescence.

DISCUSSION

Poor physical fitness levels are associated with negative health trajectories from early childhood to adulthood e.g., (2, 4, 6). Therefore, it is an important public health goal to improve

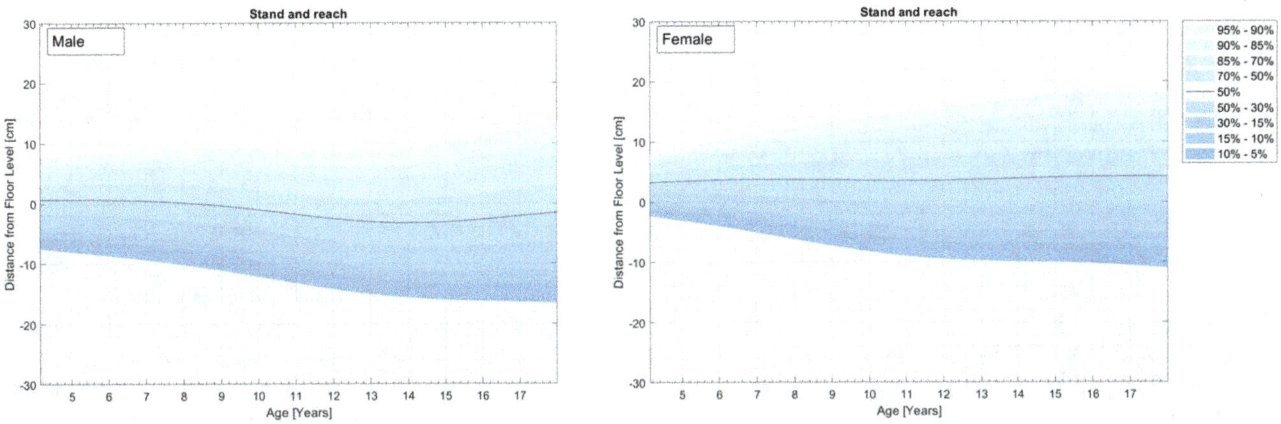

FIGURE 4 | Flexibility curves (Stand and reach) for the representative sample of German boys and girls aged 4–23 years.

and maintain physical (i.e., skill-related and especially health-related) fitness levels of children and adolescents as well as their physical self-concepts in order to foster physical activity behavior, e.g., (30, 31). In this regard, public health as well as politics need reliable and valid assessments and representative normative data in order to validly classify people's current fitness level according to their sex and current age. Unfortunately, these normative data did not exist for all fitness assessments and representative samples so far. Therefore, the aim of this study was to provide normative LMS percentile curves for several physical fitness parameters for typical developed German children and adolescents. Using LMS curves provides several advantages for representative normative data. Firstly, the sample size of each age group can be relatively small as the age and sex dependent groups were in the current study, because each age group benefits from adjacent age groups which increases overall accuracy and power of the normative data. Secondly, these adjacent age groups increase the developmental character of the normative data for longitudinal analyses purposes as it has been established for BMI (32) and Bioelectrical Impedance percentiles (33). This is clearly a benefit but also a limitation of this study, because smoothing algorithms might damage the validity of the data under specific circumstances. Therefore, the LMS curves were examined in-depth theory-driven.

Fitting MLS percentile curves for Germany (MoMo Wave 1, 2009–2012) enables us to compare the physical fitness in Germany with other nations which have percentile curves and using same test items. As an example for using our percentile curves we conducted a comparison for the test item standing long jump, as a highly standardized test item, with current European standard values of Tomkinson et al. (34). Boys (9–17 years) in Germany perform worse than their European peers in almost all age groups (e.g., boys 17 year. German P50 = 200,00 cm, European P50 = 205.8 cm). The standing long jump performance of German girls (9–17), on the other hand, is comparable to the European peer group (1). There are some other countries presenting physical fitness percentile curves [Australia: (35), Spain: (36), US Wisconsin: (37), Europe: (34)]. These percentile curves partly allow comparisons between countries, but these comparisons must be interpreted with caution, since the test items, the survey periods, and the samples differ. At first sight, physical fitness levels of populations have a continuous character rather than dichotomous (strict criterion-based "healthy" or "non-healthy"). Hence, it is intuitive to expect most information about children within very detailed percentiles and such population-based percentile distribution curves (and values) can be seen as very useful for public health cross-sectional assessment and prospective evaluation of interventions. However, from a test theoretical point of view (i.e., considering measurement error, test instructor effects, etc.), motor test performance should be interpreted in validated categorization system (or in percentile ranges) instead of single percentile values, because development is rarely truly (38–41). In this regard, percentile curves were provided based on internationally comparable values (i.e., percentiles 5, 10, 20, 30, 50, 70, 80, 90, and 95 as well as interim curves) which have successfully been shown for the measurement of physical fitness across childhood (32, 34, 42).

How "high" the level of physical fitness should be has not been sufficiently researched so far, but it is assumed that certain threshold values of physical fitness should be reached by every child to ensure growing up healthy. Some authors give a fitness level of less than percentile 5 as an indicator of health risks and thus define this value as the boundary between "healthy" and "increased risk for diseases" e.g., (33, 43). The problem with this definition might be that it is based on standard values and do not provide information regarding how the values relates to health (44). The only health-related fitness test that tries to circumvent this problem is the FitnessGram test battery (11) and the VO_2max test (45). However, the test items used at Fitnessgram correspond to the type of test used in the MoMo study (e.g., push-up, sit-up, etc.), but they differ in terms of their execution and/or duration. As a result, the health-related fitness cut-off points defined in the FitnessGram cannot be transferred to the MoMo study. However, the determination of cut-off points and so define thresholds on the basis of the MoMo study is in progress, e.g., we are working on the conversion of the PWC 170 values of our study into VO2max values via ergonizer software for sports medical performance diagnostics. The aim is to use the thresholds identified by Ruiz et al. (45) in their systematic literature search for studies that determined a cardiorespiratory fitness cut point that predicted cardiovascular disease risk in children and adolescents.

In Conclusion, we present LMS coefficient relating to representative physical fitness p ercentile r anges i n o rder to provide cut-offs for children with positive but also negative fitness values.

The new LMS curves are available by year from age 4 to 17 years. These LMS coefficient make it easy to compare children's physical fitness levels within one age branch, but also between age brands and longitudinally. We recommend to use these new, rather than old, LMS curves to transform children's raw performances into standard values that enable (the) identification of children especially in the peripheral areas 16. Finally, we emphasize that the presented normative data should be regularly updated and put in to context with older data to monitor trends in physical fitness performance.

ETHICS STATEMENT

The studies involving human participants were reviewed and approved by Karlsruhe Institute of Technology. Written informed consent to participate in this study was provided by the participants' legal guardian/next of kin.

AUTHOR CONTRIBUTIONS

CN and TU drafted the initial manuscript and reviewed and revised the manuscript. CN and DO coordinated and supervised data collection. CN, DO, and SS modeling the percentile curves. AWol, AWor, and KB conceptualized and designed the study. AH-D supervised data collection and critically reviewed the manuscript for important intellectual content. All authors have read and approved the submitted manuscript.

ACKNOWLEDGMENTS

The MoMo-Study is a national representative study carried out in collaboration with the Robert Koch-Institute in Berlin. A complete list of the participating researchers of the MoMo-Study group can be found on the MoMo website (www.sport.kit.edu/MoMo/). Thank you to Human Kinetics, Inc., for the permission to reuse parts of the abstract (1).

REFERENCES

Albrecht C, Oriwol D, Hanssen-Doose A, Woll A, Worth A. German percentile curves of physical fitness from childhood to early adulthood-the MoMo-Study. *J Phys Act Health.* (2018) 15:50. doi: 10.1123/jpah.2018-0535

Ortega FB, Ruiz JR, Castillo M, Sjöström M. Physical fitness in childhood and adolescence: a powerful marker of health. *Int J Obes.* (2008) 32:1- 11. doi: 10.1038/sj.ijo.0803774

Albrecht C. *Entwicklung und Einflussfaktoren der Entwicklung der motorischen Leistungsfähigkeit im Kindes- und Jugendalter. Befunde der MoMo-Längsschnittstudie.* Karlsruhe: KIT Scientific Publishing (2016).

Dwyer T, Magnussen CG, Schmidt MD, Ukoumunne OC, Ponsonby A-L, Raitakari OT, et al. Decline in physical fitness from childhood to adulthood associated with increased obesity and insulin resistance in adults. *Diabetes Care.* (2009) 32:683–7. doi: 10.2337/dc08-1638

Hamer M, O'Donovan G, Batty D, Stamatakis E. Estimated cardiorespiratory fitness in childhood and cardiometabolic health in adulthood: 1970 British Cohort Study. *Scand J Med Sci Sports.* (2020) 30:932–8. doi: 10.1111/sms.13637

Ruiz JR, Castro-Piñero J, Artero EG, Ortega FB, Sjöström M, Suni J, et al. Predictive validity of health-related fitness in youth: a systematic review. *Br J Sports Med.* (2009) 43:909–23. doi: 10.1136/bjsm.2008.0 56499

Cleland VJ, Ball K, Magnussen C, Dwyer T, Venn A. Socioeconomic position and the tracking of physical activity and cardiorespiratory fitness from childhood to adulthood. *Am J Epidemiol.* (2009) 170:1069– 77. doi: 10.1093/aje/kwp271

Minatto G, Barbosa Filho VC, Berria J, Petroski EL. School- based interventions to improve cardiorespiratory fitness in adolescents: systematic review with meta-analysis. *Sports Med.* (2016) 46:1273–92. doi: 10.1007/s40279-016-0480-6

Tomkinson GR, Lang JJ, Tremblay MS. Temporal trends in the cardiorespiratory fitness of children and adolescents representing 19 high-income and upper middle-income countries between 1981 and 2014. *Br J Sports Med.* (2019) 53:478–86. doi: 10.1136/bjsports-2017-097982

Caspersen CJ, Powell KE, Christenson GM. Physical activity, exercise, and physical fitness: definitions and distinctions for health-related research. *Public Health Rep.* (1985) 100:126–31.

The Copper Institute. *Fitnessgram and Activitygram Test Administration Manual, 4th ed.* Dallas, TX: Human Kinetics (2010).

Kemper HCG, Van Mechelen W. Physical fitness testing of children: a European perspective. *Pediatr Exer Sci.* (1996) 8:201–14. doi: 10.1123/pes.8.3.201

Bös K, Schlenker L, Albrecht C, Büsch D, Lämmle L, Müller H, et al. *Deutscher Motorik Test 6-18 (DMT 6-18). Manual und Internetbasierte Auswertungssoftware.* Hamburg: Czwalina (2016).

Worth A, Woll A, Albrecht C, Karger C, Mewes N, Oberger J, et al. . *MoMo-Laengsschnittstudie "Physical Fitness and Physical Activity as Determinants of Health Development in Children and Adolescents" Testmanual zu den Motorischen Tests und den Anthropometrischen Messungen (KIT Scientific Reports; 7700).* Karlsruhe: KIT Scientific Publishing (2015).

Utesch T, Zinner J, Büsch D. Stabilität der physischen Fitness im Kindesalter. *Ger J Exerc Sport Res.* (2018) 48:404–14. doi: 10.1007/s12662-018-0500-9

Utesch T, Dreiskämper D, Strauss B, Naul R. The development of the physical fitness construct across childhood. *Scand J Med Sci Sports.* (2018) 28:212– 9. doi: 10.1111/sms.12889

Kurth B-M, Kamtsiuris P, Hölling H, Schlaud M, Dölle R, Ellert U, et al. The challenge of comprehensively mapping children's health in a nation- wide health survey: Design of the German KiGGS-Study. *BMC Public Health.* (2008) 8:1–8. doi: 10.1186/1471-2458-8-196

Lange M, Butschalowsky HG, Jentsch F, Kuhnert R, Schaffrath AR, Schlaud M, et al. The first KiGGS follow-up (KiGGS Wave 1): study conduct, sample design, and response. *Bundesgesundheitsblatt, Gesundheitsforschung, Gesundheitsschutz.* (2014) 57:747–61. doi: 10.1007/s00103-014-1973-9

Woll A, Albrecht C, Worth A. *Motorik-Module (MoMo) - the KiGGS Wave 2 Module to Survey Motor Performance and Physical Activity.* Robert Koch-Institut, Epidemiologie und Gesundheitsberichterstattung. (2017).

Lampert T, Muters S, Stolzenberg H, Kroll LE, KiGGSSG. Measurement of socioeconomic status in the KiGGS study: first follow-up (KiGGS Wave 1). *Bundesgesundheitsblatt Gesundheitsforschung Gesundheitsschutz.* (2014) 57:762–70. doi: 10.1007/s00103-014-1974-8

Cole TJ, Lobstein T. Extended international (IOTF) body mass index cut- offs for thinness, overweight and obesity. *Pediatr Obes.* (2012) 7:284– 94. doi: 10.1111/j.2047-6310.2012.00064.x

Hoffmeyer-Zlotnik JHP, editor. *Instrument der Wohnquartiersbeschreibung [Tools to Describe Residential Areas]*. Mannheim: Informationszentrum Sozialwissenschaften der Arbeitsgemeinschaft Sozialwissenschaftlicher Institute e.V., Bonn (2005).

Albrecht C, Hanssen-Doose A, Bös K, Schlenker L, Schmidt S, Wagner M, et al. Motorische Leistungsfähigkeit von Kindern und Jugendlichen in Deutschland. *Sportwiss.* (2016) 46:294–304. doi: 10.1007/s12662-016-0421-4

Kamtsiuris P, Lange M, Schaffrath AR. The German Health Interview and Examination Survey for Children and Adolescents (KiGGS): sample design, response and nonresponse analysis. *Bundesgesundheitsblatt Gesundheitsforschung Gesundheitsschutz.* (2007) 50:547–56. doi: 10.1007/s00103-007-0215-9

Schmidt SC, Henn A, Albrecht C, Woll A. Physical activity of German children and adolescents 2003-2012: the MoMo-study. *Int J Environ Res Public Health.* (2017) 14:1375. doi: 10.3390/ijerph14111375

Oberger J, Romahn N, Opper E, Tittlbach S, Wank V, Woll, et al., editors. *Untersuchungen zur Motorischen Leistungsfähigkeit und Körperlich- Sportlichen Aktivität im Rahmen des Kinder-und Jugendgesundheitssurveys des Robert-Koch-Institutes Berlin. [Examination of motor performance and physical activity in the KiGGS-Study]*. Hamburg: Czwalina (2006).

Cole TJ, Green PJ. Smoothing reference centile curves: the lms method and penalized likelihood. *Stat Med.* (1992) 11:1305– 19. doi: 10.1002/sim.4780111005

Castro-Piñero J, Ortega FB, Keating X, González-Montesinos JL, Sjöstrom M, Ruíz, JR. Percentile values for aerobic performance running/walking field tests in children aged 6 to 17 years; influence of weight status. *Nutrición hospitalaria.* (2011) 26:572–8. doi: 10.1590/S0212-16112011000300021

Pan H, Cole TJ. A comparison of goodness of fit tests for age-related reference ranges. *Stat Med.* (2004) 23:1749–65. doi: 10.1002/sim.1692

Stodden DF, Goodway J, Langendorfer SJ, Roberton MA, Rudisill M, Garcia C, et al. A developmental perspective on the role of motor skill competence in physical activity: an emergent relationship. *Quest.* (2008) 60:290–306. doi: 10.1080/00336297.2008.10483582

Utesch T, Dreiskämper D, Naul, Roland, Geukes K. Understanding physical (in-) activity, overweight, and obesity in childhood: effects of congruence between physical self-concept and motor competence. *Sci Rep.* (2018) 8:1– 10. doi: 10.1038/s41598-018-24139-y

Schmidt SC, Bosy-Westphal A, Niessner C, Woll A. Representative body composition percentiles from bioelectrical impedance analyses among children and adolescents. The MoMo study. *Clin Nutr.* (2019) 38:2712– 20. doi: 10.1016/j.clnu.2018.11.026

Miguel-Etayo P de, Gracia-Marco L, Ortega FB, Intemann T, Foraita R, Lissner L, et al. Physical fitness reference standards in European children: the IDEFICS study. *Int J Obes.* (2014) 38:S57–S66. doi: 10.1038/ijo.2014.136

Tomkinson G, Carver K, Atkinson F, Daniell N, Lewis L, Fitzgerald J, et al. European normative values for physical fitness in children and adolescents aged 9-17 years: results from 2 779 165 Eurofit performances representing 30 countries. *Br J Sports Med.* (2018) 52:1445– 56. doi: 10.1136/bjsports-2017-098253

Catley M, Tomkinson G. Normative health-related fitness values for children: analysis of 85347 test results on 9-17-year-old Australians since 1985. *Br J Sports Med.* (2013) 47:98–108. doi: 10.1136/bjsports-2011-0 90218

Castro-Piñero J, Ortega FB, Keating X, González-Montesinos JL, Sjöstrom M, Ruíz, et al. Percentile values for aerobic performance running/walking field tests in children aged 6 to 17 years; influence of weight status. *Nutr Hosp.* (2011) 26:572–8. doi: 10.5641/027013610X13088554297035

Carrel AL, Bowser J, White D, Moberg DP, Weaver B, Hisgen J, et al. Standardized childhood fitness percentiles derived from school-based testing. *J Pediatr.* (2012) 161:120–4. doi: 10.1016/j.jpeds.2012.01.036

Linacre JM. New approaches to determining reliability and validity. *Res Q Exer Sport.* (2000) 71:129–36. doi: 10.1080/02701367.2000.11082796

Strauss B, Büsch D, Tenenbaum G, editors. *New Developments in Measurement and Testing.* Boston, MA: Wiley (2007).

Utesch T, Bardid F, Huyben F, Strauss B, Tietjens M, Martelaer K de, et al. Using Rasch modeling to investigate the construct of motor competence in early childhood. *Psychol Sport Exer.* (2016) 24:179– 87. doi: 10.1016/j.psychsport.2016.03.001

Utesch T, Strauß B, Tietjens M, Büsch D, Ghanbari M-C, Seidel I. Die Überprüfung der Konstruktvalidität des Deutschen Motorik-Tests 6-18 für 9-bis 10-Jährige. *Z Sportpsychol.* (2015) 22:77–90. doi: 10.1026/1612-5010/a000143

Cole TJ, Bellizzi MC, Flegal KM, Dietz WH. Establishing a standard definition for child overweight and obesity worldwide: international survey. *BMJ.* (2000) 320:1240. doi: 10.1136/bmj.320.7244.1240

Ortega FB, Artero EG, Ruiz JR, España-Romero V, Jiménez- Pavón D, Vicente-Rodriguez G, et al. Physical fitness levels among European adolescents: the HELENA study. *Br J Sports Med.* (2011) 45:20–9. doi: 10.1136/bjsm.2009.062679

Adegboye A, Anderssen S, Froberg K, Sardinha L, Heitmann B, Steene-Johannessen J, et al. Recommended aerobic fitness level for metabolic health in children and adolescents: a study of diagnostic accuracy. *Br J Sports Med.* (2011) 45:722–8. doi: 10.1136/bjsm.2009. 068346

Ruiz JR, Cavero-Redondo I, Ortega FB, Welk GJ, Andersen LB, Martinez-Vizcaino V. Cardiorespiratory fitness cut points to avoid cardiovascular disease risk in children and adolescents; what level of fitness should raise a red flag? A systematic review and meta- analysis. *Br J Sports Med.* (2016) 50:1451–8. doi: 10.1136/bjsports-2015-0 95903

8

Validity and Reliability of a Commercially Available Indoor Tracking System to Assess Distance and Time in Court-Based Sports

*Enrique Colino[1], Jorge Garcia-Unanue[1], Javier Sanchez-Sanchez[2], Javier Calvo-Monera[3], Manuel Leon[1], María Jose Carvalho[4], Leonor Gallardo[1], Jose Luis Felipe[2] and Archit Navandar[2]**

[1] IGOID Research Group, University of Castilla–La Mancha, Toledo, Spain, [2] Faculty of Sport Sciences, Universidad Europea de Madrid, Madrid, Spain, [3] Nothingbutnet S.L., Valencia, Spain, [4] Faculdade de Desporto da Universidade do Porto, Porto, Portugal

***Correspondence:**
Archit Navandar
archit.navandar@universidadeuropea.es;
archit89@gmail.com

The aim of this study was to evaluate the validity and reliability of a commercially available local position measurement (LPM) tracking system when assessing distance and running time at different speeds. Fifteen male healthy athletes performed 15 m displacements at walking, running and sprinting speed. Data recorded by the LPM system were compared to those from the reference equipment, consisting of measuring tape and electronic timing gates placed at 0, 5, 10, and 15 m. Mean error, mean absolute error (MAE), standard deviation (SD) of the measurement error, maximum measurement error and root mean square error (RMSE) were calculated to determine the validity for distance and the running time variables. Product-moment correlation and intraclass correlation coefficient (ICC) were also used for the running time. Finally, the reliability of the distance was carried out comparing data from the three repetitions with the standard tape measure using a linear mixed model and the typical error as mean coefficient of variation (CV) (%). MAE shows errors under 0.18 m for the distance variable at all speeds and under 0.08 s for the running time variable at all speeds, except from 15 m at walking. Product-moment correlations were high to nearly perfect for running time (range: 0.60–0.99), ICC varied between high (0.75–0.90) and extremely high (>0.99) for most measures, and coefficients of variation remained almost invariable as speed increased (walking: 2.16; running: 2.52; sprinting: 2.20). The tested LPM system represents a valid and reliable method for monitoring distance during different constant speeds over a straight line, as long as there is no signal loss. However, the running time errors could be too large for performance tests that require acute precision.

Keywords: team sports, player tracking, indoor tracking, training load, match analysis

INTRODUCTION

Accurate assessment of athletes' movement profile during training and match play in team sports presents useful information that could assist coaches and trainers in the development of specific conditioning activities and recovery strategies (Duffield et al., 2010). Initially, computer-based tracking systems were used for assessing players at constant running speeds such as distance covered and time spent during sports-specific tasks (Edgecomb and Norton, 2006). However, this analysis technique required large amounts of time and was overall difficult to implement when simultaneously assessing large groups of athletes or entire teams. In the last few years, advancements in technology have led to the introduction and rapid proliferation of sophisticated systems such as multiple camera semi-automatic systems, global positioning systems (GPS) and local position measurement (LPM) systems. These technologies are capable of quickly recording and processing the players' physical exertions throughout an entire match or training session (Carling et al., 2008).

The development of these technologies has mostly been linked with outdoor sports such as football which has seen the rapid evolution of multiple camera and GPS systems, bringing forth a significant improvement in sport performance and player management, thereby contributing to the emergence of a whole new industry. The main contribution of these technologies is that they allow the concurrent analysis of running speeds of numerous players to be completed on a routine basis with affordable expenses (Buchheit et al., 2014).

Computerized analysis using multiple camera, semi-automatic, video match-analysis systems has proved to be a valid and reliable tool to measure player movements and actions, and to classify the game events in professional competitions (Di Salvo et al., 2007, 2008; Carling et al., 2008). However, installing and using this technology generally requires a large investment in economic terms that represents a limitation in most sports.

Global positioning systems devices have also been widely assessed for their validity and reliability in measuring distance, time, speed and acceleration during different sporting actions over the last decade (Edgecomb and Norton, 2006; Barbero-Alvarez et al., 2010; Coutts and Duffield, 2010; Coutts and Duffield, 2010; Gray et al., 2010; Jennings et al., 2010; Waldron et al., 2011; Varley et al., 2012; Vickery et al., 2014), and it has led to GPS being the preferred technology used in player tracking. However, the main limitation of GPS technology is that it requires an "open" sky without obstructions above athletes that ensures clear space for positional data acquisition from satellites. This constraint prevents GPS devices from being used in indoor sports such as basketball or handball. Thus, other technologies such as LPM have been used for the assessment of athletes' movement profile indoors.

The LPM technology has seen moderate improvements over the last few years, resulting in better stability and precision. The declared relative position measurement accuracy of some of these systems is around 3 cm which can be measured up to 1 kHz (Buchheit et al., 2014). This technology consists of radio systems based on a Bluetooth Low Energy (BLE) radio signals which provide location information through a network of antennas (base stations) and transponders. These base stations are positioned around the playing area to be measured while the transponders are worn by the athletes.

There is limited information regarding the validity and reliability of commercially available indoor tracking systems using LPM technology for assessing constant running speeds during indoor team sports (Frencken et al., 2010; Siegle et al., 2013; Link et al., 2018; Linke et al., 2018). Although LPM systems have been reported to offer higher validity for measuring athletes' position compared to video and GPS technology (Linke et al., 2018), they still have the highest deviations when measuring distance, which might also cause relevant limitations for the assessment of sprint performance especially over short distances (Link et al., 2018). In the past few years, this type of positioning system has experienced an increasing commercialization, and some of them are currently being used by different basketball teams of the highest category in Spain. The present work aims to assess the validity and reliability of distance and running time measured by means of an LPM system at different speeds, providing an initial contribution for the assessment of this technology.

MATERIALS AND METHODS

Experimental Approach to the Problem

Participants performed repeated straight-line displacements at different speeds while distance and time were assessed using the LPM system and compared to the reference values. Actual distance was measured using a calibrated tape measure and time was measured using four pairs of dual-beam photocells (Witty, Microgate, Bolzano, Italy) placed at the starting line and every 5 m. This technology has been previously considered as a reference tool in the measurement of distances and time (Buchheit et al., 2014) and is the recommended technology to register accurate and reliable short sprint results in scientific research (Haugen and Buchheit, 2016). The tests were conducted in an indoor sport facility with parquet surface, normally used by a basketball team of the ACB (first division of Spanish basketball).

Subjects

Fifteen trained male athletes (age: 26 ± 3 years; height: 1.85 ± 0.06 m; weight: 79 ± 3 kg) were randomly chosen from a population of basketball players that volunteered to participate in the study. Participants were informed about the experimental procedures and the potential risks and benefits resulting from participating in the study, and they all signed an institutionally approved informed consent document, as outlined in the Declaration of Helsinki. The study protocol was approved by the Local Ethics Committee.

Procedures

Each participant completed nine 15-m displacements on a straight line separated by 1 min of passive recovery, following procedures mentioned previously (Jennings et al., 2010). The first three displacements were made at a comfortable walking speed; displacements 4 to 6 were performed running at gentle pace; and the last three displacements were performed sprinting at maximum speed. To expand the scope of the study at different speeds and distances, timing gates were placed at 0, 5, 10, and 15 m. Total time (0–15 m) and times of each of the three 5-m splits (0–5, 5–10, and 10–15 m) were recorded.

For the calculation of the distances traveled in a specific time, the LPM system considered the start time of each displacement as that when the first movement occurred (i.e., the first increase on the velocity curve above zero (Petersen et al., 2009; Jennings et al., 2010). This starting time was associated with the moment that the athlete went through the timing gate placed at 0 m mark. Then, the time from the timing gates was used to indicate the end of the movement for each known distance. Thus, for a time interval determined by two successive cuts of timing gates, distance measured with the LPM system was compared to the current distance between both timing gates.

In addition, the time taken to complete the distance of 15 m (according to the LPM system) was recorded. This data was compared to the time recorded by the timing gates for the same distance. Therefore, distances and times recorded by the LPM system in each test were compared to the taped distances and the times obtained from the timing gates, respectively. Only trials where an accurate measurement was made by both the timing gates (trials discarded for timing gate measurement error: walking = 2, jogging = 4, sprinting = 19) and the LPM system (trials discarded due to momentary drop in signal: walking = 5, jogging = 3, and sprinting = 12) were considered for analysis.

LPM System

The system used in this study is commercially known as NBN23 (Nothing But Net, Valencia, Spain) and is composed of two different elements. First, the system hardware was created by the Finnish company Quuppa (Nokia Corporation, 2014). This technology consists of locators and the devices that the players carry (tags) which were placed on the waist, at the back of the trousers at the height of the sacrum. This position represents the approximate position of the center of mass of the subject and avoids a possible shielding of the signal with the participant's own body. Tags are emission devices, and the system works by triangulating the signal they emit. The frequency at which they send information can be varied between 9, 17, 33, and 50 Hz. The frequency band is 2.4 GHz, the system delay is 100 ms with a capacity of 400 information packets per second. In this study, eight locators (firmware v9.047) placed in two groups of four at a height of 13.51 m (**Figure 1**) were used along with eight different tags at a frequency of 17 Hz (Nokia Technologies Oy, 2014).

Secondly, the specific software for the LPM system was used (Nothingbutnet v1.1.3, Spain, 2016). This software adds a Kalman filter to the position coordinates (given in terms of *X* and *Y*) provided by Quuppa to reduce noise and measurement error with a cut-off frequency of 3 Hz. The distance traveled was calculated through the position changes on the *X* and *Y* axes. To carry out the tests, the participant started from a static position on the free throw line.

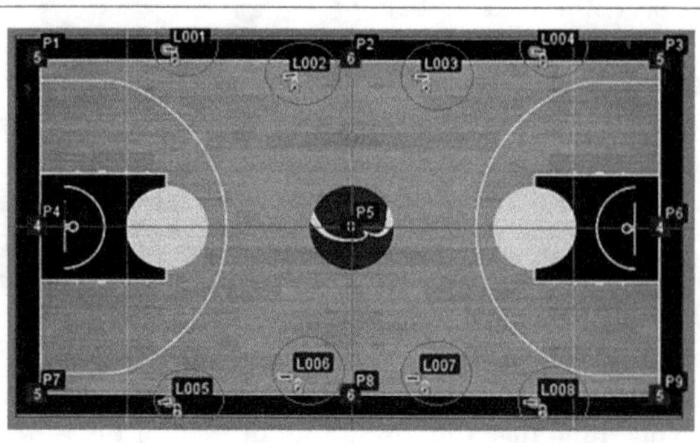

FIGURE 1 | The positioning of the locaters (L) and reference points (P) of the NBN system.

Statistical Analyses

Mean error, mean absolute error (MAE), standard deviation (SD) of the measurement error, maximum measurement error and root mean square error (RMSE) were determined for assessing validity of the distance variable, considering the tape measurement as the standard. A plot with the difference between criterion and LPM distance in each speed and 5-m split (0–5, 5–10, and 10–15 m) was also added.

Validity of the running time variable was performed between the times recorded using the LPM system and the interval times recorded by the timing gates for equal distances. Product-moment correlation (r), intraclass correlation coefficient (ICC), absolute agreement with 95% confidence intervals (Field, 2013) and Bland–Altman plots were used. Moreover, similar to the distance measures, MAE, SD of the measurement error, maximum measurement error and RMSE were determined taking the timing gates data as the standard. Product-moment correlation results were evaluated as trivial (<0.10), small (0.10–0.30), moderate (0.30–0.50), large (0.50–0.70), very large (0.70–0.90), nearly perfect (0.90–1.00) scores (Johnston et al., 2014). ICC were evaluated as very low (<0.20), low (0.20–0.50), moderate (0.50–0.75), high (0.75–0.90), very high (0.90–0.99), and extremely high (>0.99) scores (Buchheit et al., 2014).

The reliability of the distance was carried out comparing data from the three repetitions with the standard tape measure using a linear mixed model. For this model, the repetition was considered as the fixed factor, and the participant was the random factor. Furthermore, typical error as mean coefficient of variation (CV) (%) was calculated by the Hopkins reliability spreadsheet (Hopkins, 2015), and used among the three trials for each velocity (walking, running, and sprinting). Once CV was established, it was divided into criterion categories, being rated as good (CV < 5%), moderate (CV 5 to 10%) or poor (CV > 10%) (Atkinson and Nevill, 1998; Duthie et al., 2003; Johnston et al., 2014).

Normality and homogeneity of the variance were previously tested and assumed by the Kolmogorov Smirnov test and the Levene's statistical analysis. The level of significance was established at $p < 0.05$. Data were analyzed using SPSS version 21.0 (SPSS Inc., Chicago, IL, United States) and SAS University Edition (SAS Institute Inc., 2015, Cary, NC, United States).

RESULTS

Tables 1, 2 show the errors measured between the LPS system and the gold standard measurement: the fixed taped distance and the timing gates. The mean error, and the MAE show values under 0.18 m for the distance variable at all speeds, which is lower than 5% of the actual measured value (**Figures 2, 3**). In case of the time

TABLE 1 | Validity and agreement of the distance variable.

	N	Mean error (m)	MAE (m)	SD of measurement error (m)	Max error (m)	RMSE (m)
Walking						
0–5 m	38	0.08	0.13	0.20	0.76	0.22
5–10 m	38	−0.08	0.10	0.11	0.37	0.14
10–15 m	38	0.03	0.11	0.15	0.34	0.15
0–10 m	38	0.01	0.13	0.19	0.70	0.19
0–15 m	38	0.03	0.12	0.16	0.45	0.16
Jogging						
0–5 m	38	0.05	0.13	0.18	0.52	0.19
5–10 m	38	−0.06	0.12	0.18	0.49	0.19
10–15 m	38	−0.02	0.13	0.19	0.56	0.19
0–10 m	38	0.01	0.16	0.21	0.54	0.19
0–15 m	38	−0.01	0.12	0.15	0.34	0.15
Running						
0–5 m	14	0.08	0.12	0.14	0.29	0.15
5–10 m	14	0.05	0.15	0.23	0.73	0.23
10–15 m	14	−0.13	0.18	0.24	0.68	0.26
0–10 m	14	0.13	0.15	0.25	0.91	0.27
0–15 m	14	0.00	0.17	0.26	0.70	0.26

N, number of trials; MAE, mean absolute error; SD, standard deviation; RMSE, root mean square error; Max error, maximum error; MAE and RMSE were determined with respect to the measured distance.

TABLE 2 | Validity and agreement of the time variable.

Variables	*N*	Mean error (s)	MAE (s)	SD of measured error (s)	Max error (s)	RMSE (s)	*r*	ICC
Walking								
0–5 m	38	−0.04	0.05	0.08	0.36	0.09	0.96	0.97
5–10 m	38	−0.02	0.03	0.02	0.10	0.04	0.99	0.99
10–15 m	38	−0.03	0.07	0.14	0.83	0.16	0.80	0.87
0–10 m	38	−0.06	0.07	0.07	0.38	0.10	0.99	0.99
0–15 m	38	−0.08	0.12	0.14	0.85	0.18	0.97	0.98
Running								
0–5 m	38	−0.02	0.03	0.02	0.08	0.03	0.99	0.99
5–10 m	38	−0.03	0.03	0.03	0.10	0.04	0.99	0.99
10–15 m	38	−0.00	0.05	0.07	0.29	0.09	0.88	0.94
0–10 m	38	−0.05	0.05	0.04	0.14	0.06	0.99	0.99
0–15 m	38	−0.05	0.08	0.06	0.29	0.10	0.98	0.99
Sprinting								
0–5 m	14	−0.02	0.02	0.02	0.05	0.03	0.97	0.96
5–10 m	14	−0.02	0.04	0.04	0.13	0.50	0.60	0.71
10–15 m	14	−0.03	0.04	0.03	0.11	0.06	0.64	0.59
0–10 m	14	−0.04	0.05	0.04	0.18	0.07	0.77	0.79
0–15 m	14	−0.07	0.08	0.04	0.15	0.09	0.89	0.83

MAE, mean absolute error; SD, standard deviation; Max error, maximum error; RMSE, root mean square error; r, product-moment correlation; ICC, intraclass correlation coefficient.

variable a slightly higher value of MAE was recorded at the longer distances. In this case, the ICC went from high to extremely high values at walking and running speeds, while at sprinting speed it presents moderate to very high correlation values. In spite of the lower coefficients at sprinting speed, correlations values are still above the threshold of moderate magnitude.

Table 3 shows the reliability results of distance data. In this case, all the values fit within the best criterion category (good). Unlike the previous cases, results show a great consistency in all speeds and distances, with mean CVs remaining below 3% for all speeds (walking: 2.16; running: 2.52; sprinting: 2.20).

Finally, **Table 4** shows the reliability of the differences in distances between the LPM system measurement and the taped measurement. The results show that the differences between the trials only varied for the 0–15 m distance at a walking speed, and inter-participant differences were observed for the 0–10 m walking distance.

DISCUSSION

This paper presents the validity and reliability of an LPM measuring system for distance and running time during different constant speeds over a straight line. The validity of the system, which consisted of a set of tags placed at the sacrum of the player, was measured against taped distances and timing gates.

When assessing distance validity, results show that the LPM system either over or underestimates the actual distance, but the MAE are well under 0.18 m (percentage of differences is less than 2%). The magnitude of this difference were over those declared by Frencken et al. (2010) when assessing accuracy and validity of an equivalent LPM device in smaller, straight line distances (0.2%), but under that declared for GPS devices when assessing distance at different speeds over a 200 m on a straight line (0.8–2.8%) (Gray et al., 2010). It is important to consider that some noise-inducing variables such as a slightly forward position of the device at the beginning or end of the trial, can cause these differences. Furthermore, the SD of measurement error varied from 0.11 to 0.26 m, but this issue was not discussed in these previous studies.

On the other hand, the results of the present study show that the LPM system offers a higher accuracy than that shown by GPS in other studies such as Coutts and Duffield (2010) (3.6–7.1%), Gray et al. (2010) (0.5–9.8%), Duffield et al. (2010) (4.0–30.0%) or Jennings et al. (2010) (9.0–32.4%), although some of those studies consisted of more complex validation protocols including turns and curved movement paths.

Possibly, one of the most frequent uses in these monitoring systems is the quantification of the load as accumulated distance at different speeds, as previous studies refer to these individual movements in team sports (Gray et al., 2010). Therefore, the LPM system analyzed can be used to quantify distances in simple movements with the same or greater precision than those obtained through a system like the GPS. However, more research is needed involving complex circuits and routes that mimic the movement patterns of sports such as basketball, handball or futsal.

When assessing running time spent to cover a certain distance, validity correlation ranged from very large to nearly perfect in walking and running speeds (0.80–0.99), in agreement to those described by Frencken et al. (2010). When assessing running

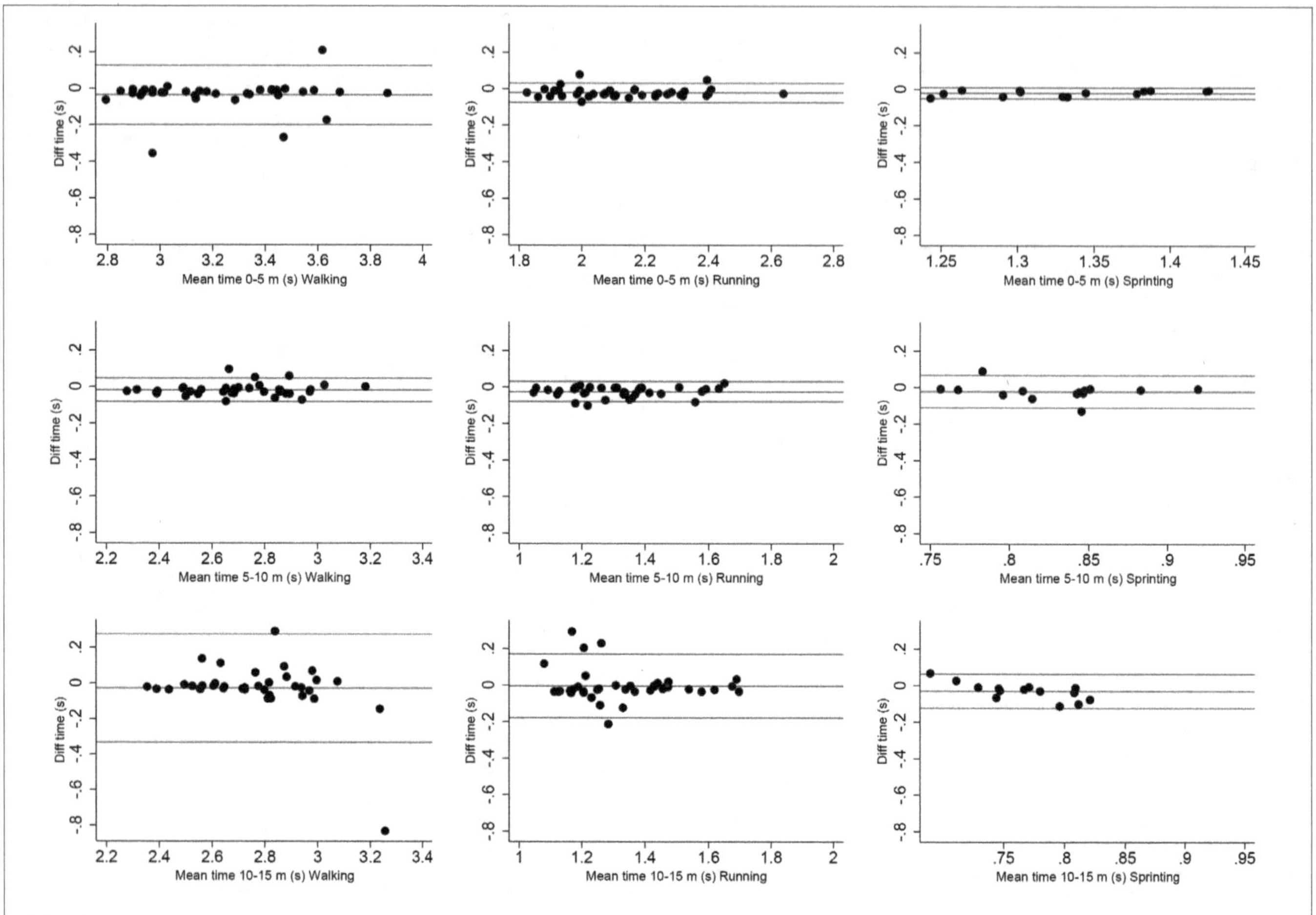

FIGURE 2 | Bland-Altman plots representing the differences between the time measured by the NBN system and the standard timing gates.

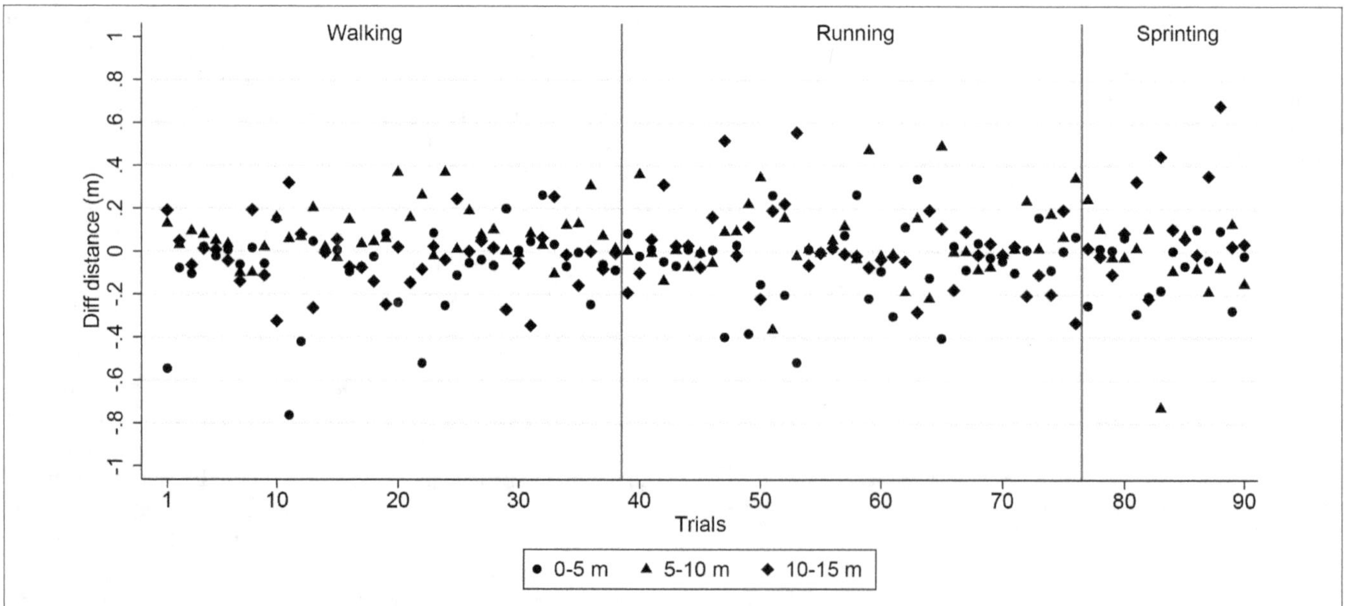

FIGURE 3 | Bland-Altman plots representing the differences between the distance measured by the NBN system and the taped distances.

TABLE 3 | Reliability of the distance variable (typical error presented as the mean CV).

Distance interval	CV walking (%)	CV running (%)	CV sprinting (%)
0–5 m	3.0	2.4	2.3
5–10 m	2.6	4.1	2.3
10–15 m	2.8	3.2	4.3
0–10 m	1.3	2.0	0.6
0–15 m	1.1	0.9	1.5

CV, coefficient of variation.

TABLE 4 | Reliability of the differences in distances between the taped distance and the distance measured by the local position measurement (LPM) system.

	Fixed effects				Random effects	
	F	df1	df2	*p*	Wald *Z*	*p*
Walking						
0–5 m	3.15	2	22.92	0.062	1.90	0.06
5–10 m	1.04	2	35.00	0.366	−1.46	0.14
10–15 m	0.05	2	23.53	0.952	0.57	0.57
0–10 m	2.61	2	22.65	0.096	2.03	0.04†
0–15 m	3.51	2	35.00	0.041*	−0.42	0.67
Jogging						
0–5 m	0.22	2	21.65	0.803	1.83	0.07
5–10 m	0.12	2	35.00	0.889	−1.88	0.06
10–15 m	0.78	2	35.00	0.468	−0.33	0.74
0–10 m	0.27	2	35.00	0.767	0.17	0.87
0–15 m	1.12	2	22.71	0.344	1.25	0.21
Running						
0–5 m	1.13	2	6.67	0.378	1.04	0.30
5–10 m	0.50	2	4.18	0.639	1.26	0.21
10–15 m	0.49	2	11.00	0.625	−0.18	0.86
0–10 m	0.38	2	4.89	0.701	1.65	0.10
0–15 m	0.98	2	6.98	0.422	0.44	0.66

*A linear mixed model was used with the repetition being the fixed effect and the athlete being the random effect. *Indicates a significant difference between the difference of the measures in the different repetitions. †Indicates a significant difference between participants in different repetitions. All tests were carried out with α = 0.05.*

time at sprinting speed the correlation values down to large (0.60–0.97). In relative terms, the percentage of difference varied between 0 and 2.48% at walking and running speeds and between 4.35 and 6.68% at sprinting speed. In addition, the ICC varied between a high (0.75–0.90) and extremely high (>0.99) except in two time-variables at sprinting speed, where it is still moderate (0.50–0.75). However, MAE remain similar in all speeds, which varied between 0.02 and 0.12. In agreement with previous research validating GPS devices, the accuracy of the LPM system decreased slightly as speed increased (Edgecomb and Norton, 2006; Coutts and Duffield, 2010; Duffield et al., 2010; Jennings et al., 2010; Vickery et al., 2014). These differences are once more in line with those described by Frencken et al. (2010) (1.3–3.9%) and are lower than those generally described for speed in GPS devices as in Duffield et al. (2010) (10–30%). Furthermore, the LPM system provides better level of accuracy for measures of running time compared with other tracking devices such as GPS where ICC has been reported to vary from 0.10 to 0.70 (Duffield et al., 2010) or from 0.50 to 0.86 (Vickery et al., 2014).

The reliability of the LPM system when measuring distance traveled during each bout was good (CV < 5%), being this consistent as speed increases from walking to maximal sprint, and this was confirmed by the linear mixed model. The overall reliability of the LPM system data across all trials remains within the ranges that have been described for other LPM systems (0.4–2.0%) (Frencken et al., 2010) or other tracking devices. For example, regarding GPS systems, Barbero-Alvarez et al. (2010) reported CVs of between 1.2 and 1.7% for summated maximal speed and peak speed expressed during 15 and 30-m repeated sprint tests over seven trials. Others such as Coutts and Duffield (2010) reported good-to-moderate CVs for total distance (3.6–7.1%) and peak speed (2.3–5.8%) when assessing validity and reliability of different GPS devices. However, studies assessing reliability of other tracking devices generally report that the higher the speed, the greater the measurement error (Duffield et al., 2010; Gray et al., 2010; Vickery et al., 2014). Contrarily, in the present study better reliability was observed as intensity increases, with the lowest CVs corresponding to the highest speed.

The measurement can be considered as useful for precise measurements when the noise is at least equal to or lower than the smallest worthwhile change (SWC) (Haugen and Buchheit, 2016). The SWC could be defined as 0.2 multiplied by the between-subject SD (Hopkins et al., 2009; Ferioli et al., 2018). In this study the SWC is between 0.01 and 0.06 s in 5 m splits for the time measurement (between 0.8 and 2.75%). The SD of measurement errors were between 0.02 and 0.14 s in the 5 m splits, which could make the random error higher than the differences in performance between players, presenting a limitation of its use in performance tests carried out over short distances. Nevertheless, it can be a useful device in determining accumulated loads in training and games.

Another limitation of this study was that time and distance were only assessed over standard straight-line 15-m displacements and that true peak speed was not measured directly. Quite often, short sprints, changes of direction and brief maximal accelerations of >1 s are completed in team sports. Although previous methodologies were followed to match the start of timing gates and LPM measurement, there are still possible errors because the LPM system may start recording a few ms before the first timing light cut. There is also a spatial limitation since it was possible that in some specific points of the field (bands or corners) the LPM system could measure differently depending on the distance to the system receivers. Finally, this study also has its own measurement error associated with timing gates. Among them, the possible swinging of arms and legs, an error that can reach 0.02 s (Haugen et al., 2014) and errors associated with the height or distance of the photocells (Cronin and Templeton, 2008). Therefore, the scope of this work is limited, and it is possible that important data may be missed due to the protocol design. Future research should examine the efficacy of this system when assessing more complex protocols.

CONCLUSION

The tested LPM system represents a valid and reliable method for monitoring distance and running time during constant speeds over a straight line as long as there is no signal loss. Intensity appears to affect the LPM system running time accuracy, being this lower as speed increases. The typical error measured with CV (%) shows a great consistency regardless of speed and distance, with good reliability results. This implies that the LPM system provides similar consistency than other tracking devices such as GPS system and could be useful for training purposes and determinate external workload. However, the random part of measurement error is higher than the SWC, so the LPM could not be a good system to evaluate performance tests carried out at high speeds in short distances.

ETHICS STATEMENT

This study was carried out in accordance with the recommendations of the Institutional Research Board of the Universidad de Castilla-La Mancha, Toledo, Spain with written informed consent from all subjects. All subjects gave written informed consent in accordance with the Declaration of Helsinki. The protocol was approved by the Ethics Committee of the Universidad de Castilla-La Mancha, Toledo, Spain.

AUTHOR CONTRIBUTIONS

EC coordinated the research, drafted the initial manuscript, and carried out the statistical analyses. JG-U, JF, and AN substantially contributed to the analysis and interpretation of the data. JS-S helped on the conceptualization and design of the study. JC-M, MC, and ML coordinated the data collection process. All authors contributed to the manuscript revision, read, and approved the submitted version.

ACKNOWLEDGMENTS

All authors would like to thank Diego Galdón Tébar for his collaboration, and the 15 volunteers who participated in the study during the data collection process.

REFERENCES

Atkinson, G., and Nevill, A. M. (1998). Statistical methods for assessing measurement error (reliability) in variables relevant to sports medicine. *Sports Med.* 26, 217–238. doi: 10.2165/00007256-199826040-00002

Barbero-Alvarez, J. C., Coutts, A., Granda, J., Barbero-Alvarez, V., and Castagna, C. (2010). The validity and reliability of a global positioning satellite system device to assess speed and repeated sprint ability (RSA) in athletes. *J. Sci. Med. Sport* 13, 232–235. doi: 10.1016/j.jsams.2009.02.005

Buchheit, M., Allen, A., Poon, T. K., Modonutti, M., Gregson, W., and Di Salvo, V. (2014). Integrating different tracking systems in football: multiple camera semi-automatic system, local position measurement and GPS technologies. *J. Sports Sci.* 32, 1844–1857. doi: 10.1080/02640414.2014.942687

Carling, C., Bloomfield, J., Nelsen, L., and Reilly, T. (2008). The role of motion analysis in elite soccer: contemporary performance measurement techniques and work rate data. *Sports Med.* 38, 839–862. doi: 10.2165/00007256-200838100-00004

Coutts, A. J., and Duffield, R. (2010). Validity and reliability of GPS devices for measuring movement demands of team sports. *J. Sci. Med. Sport* 13, 133–135. doi: 10.1016/j.jsams.2008.09.015

Cronin, J. B., and Templeton, R. L. (2008). Timing light height affects sprint times. *J. Strength Cond. Res.* 22, 318–320. doi: 10.1519/JSC.0b013e31815fa3d3

Di Salvo, V., Baron, R., Tschan, H., Calderon Montero, F. J., Bachl, N., and Pigozzi, F. (2007). Performance characteristics according to playing position in elite soccer. *Int. J. Sports Med.* 28, 222–227. doi: 10.1055/s-2006-924294

Di Salvo, V., Benito, P. J., Calderon, F. J., Di Salvo, M., and Pigozzi, F. (2008). Activity profile of elite goalkeepers during football match-play. *J. Sports Med. Phys. Fitness* 48, 443–446.

Duffield, R., Reid, M., Baker, J., and Spratford, W. (2010). Accuracy and reliability of GPS devices for measurement of movement patterns in confined spaces for court-based sports. *J. Sci. Med. Sport* 13, 523–525. doi: 10.1016/j.jsams.2009.07.003

Duthie, G., Pyne, D., and Hooper, S. (2003). The reliability of video based time motion analysis. *J. Hum. Mov. Stud.* 44, 259–271.

Edgecomb, S. J., and Norton, K. I. (2006). Comparison of global positioning and computer-based tracking systems for measuring player movement distance during Australian football. *J. Sci. Med. Sport* 9, 25–32. doi: 10.1016/j.jsams.2006.01.003

Ferioli, D., Bosio, A., Bilsborough, J. C., La Torre, A., Tornaghi, M., and Rampinini, E. (2018). The preparation period in basketball: training load and neuromuscular adaptations. *Int. J. Sports Physiol. Perform.* 13, 991–999. doi: 10.1123/ijspp.2017-0434

Field, A. (2013). *Discovering Statistics Using IBM SPSS Statistics*, 3rd Edn. London: Sage.

Frencken, W. G., Lemmink, K. A., and Delleman, N. J. (2010). Soccer-specific accuracy and validity of the local position measurement (LPM) system. *J. Sci. Med. Sport* 13, 641–645. doi: 10.1016/j.jsams.2010.04.003

Gray, A. J., Jenkins, D., Andrews, M. H., Taaffe, D. R., and Glover, M. L. (2010). Validity and reliability of GPS for measuring distance travelled in field-based team sports. *J. Sports Sci.* 28, 1319–1325. doi: 10.1080/02640414.2010.504783

Haugen, T., and Buchheit, M. (2016). Sprint running performance monitoring: methodological and practical considerations. *Sports Med.* 46, 641–656. doi: 10.1007/s40279-015-0446-0

Haugen, T. A., Tønnessen, E., Svendsen, I. S., and Seiler, S. (2014). Sprint time differences between single-and dual-beam timing systems. *J. Strength Cond. Res.* 28, 2376–2379. doi: 10.1519/JSC.0000000000000415

Hopkins, W. G. (2015). Spreadsheets for analysis of validity and reliability. *Sportscience* 19, 36–42.

Hopkins, W. G., Marshall, S. W., Batterham, A. M., and Hanin, J. (2009). Progressive statistics for studies in sports medicine and exercise science. *Med. Sci. Sports Exerc.* 41, 3–13. doi: 10.1249/MSS.0b013e31818cb278

Jennings, D., Cormack, S., Coutts, A. J., Boyd, L., and Aughey, R. J. (2010). The validity and reliability of GPS units for measuring distance in team sport specific running patterns. *Int. J. Sports Physiol. Perform.* 5, 328–341. doi: 10.1123/ijspp.5.3.328

Johnston, R. J., Watsford, M. L., Kelly, S. J., Pine, M. J., and Spurrs, R. W. (2014). Validity and interunit reliability of 10 Hz and 15 Hz GPS units for assessing athlete movement demands. *J. Strength Cond. Res.* 28, 1649–1655. doi: 10.1519/JSC.0000000000000323

Link, D., Weber, M., Linke, D., and Lames, M. (2018). Can positioning systems replace timing gates for measuring sprint time in ice hockey? *Front. Physiol.* 9:1882. doi: 10.3389/fphys.2018.01882

Linke, D., Link, D., and Lames, M. (2018). Validation of electronic performance and tracking systems EPTS under field conditions. *PLoS One* 13:e0199519. doi: 10.1371/journal.pone.0199519

Petersen, C., Pyne, D., Portus, M., and Dawson, B. (2009). Validity and reliability of GPS units to monitor cricket-specific movement patterns. *Int. J. Sports Physiol. Perform.* 4, 381–393. doi: 10.1123/ijspp.4.3.381

Siegle, M., Stevens, T., and Lames, M. (2013). Design of an accuracy study for position detection in football. *J. Sports Sci.* 31, 166–172. doi: 10.1080/02640414.2012.723131

Varley, M. C., Fairweather, I. H., and Aughey, R. J. (2012). Validity and reliability of GPS for measuring instantaneous velocity during acceleration, deceleration, and constant motion. *J. Sports Sci.* 30, 121–127. doi: 10.1080/02640414.2011.627941

Vickery, W. M., Dascombe, B. J., Baker, J. D., Higham, D. G., Spratford, W. A., and Duffield, R. (2014). Accuracy and reliability of GPS devices for measurement of sports-specific movement patterns related to cricket, tennis, and field-based team sports. *J. Strength Cond. Res.* 28, 1697–1705. doi: 10.1519/JSC.0000000000000285

Waldron, M., Worsfold, P., Twist, C., and Lamb, K. (2011). Concurrent validity and test-retest reliability of a global positioning system (GPS) and timing gates to assess sprint performance variables. *J. Sports Sci.* 29, 1613–1619. doi: 10.1080/02640414.2011.608703

9

Can School-Based Physical Activity Projects such as Skipping Hearts have a Long-Term Impact on Health and Health Behavior?

Lisa Baumgartner[1]*, Tanja Postler[1], Christine Graf[2], Nina Ferrari[2], Bernhard Haller[3], Renate Oberhoffer-Fritz[1] and Thorsten Schulz[1]

[1] TUM Department of Sport and Health Sciences, Institute of Preventive Pediatrics, Technical University of Munich, Munich, Germany, [2] Institute of Movement and Neurosciences, German Sport University Cologne, Cologne, Germany, [3] Institute of Medical Informatics, Statistics and Epidemiology, Technical University of Munich, Munich, Germany

***Correspondence:**
Lisa Baumgartner
lisa.baumgartner@tum.de

Low physical activity, limited motor skills, and an increased number of overweight or obese children are major public health problems. Numerous school-based programs try to improve physical activity and health behavior in children but investigations on sustainable effects of these programs are rare. Therefore, we examined the long-term effects of the *Skipping Hearts* health promotion project. 486 children (57.7% female, 9.0 ± 0.6 years at baseline) participated in this non-randomized controlled longitudinal trial within a follow-up period of 3.5 years. Of these, 286 subjects received a one-time 90-min workshop in rope skipping (Basic-Workshop) and 140 additionally received 10 lessons in rope skipping (Champion-Program), 78 students served as controls. Anthropometrics, blood pressure, motor skills, screen-based media use, self-assessment of physical fitness, and physical activity were collected at both measurement points; endurance capacity and health-related quality of life only at follow-up. Standard deviation scores of body-mass-index ($\eta^2 = 0.005$) and systolic blood pressure ($\eta^2 = 0.006$) decreased, while diastolic blood pressure ($\eta^2 = 0.004$), motor performance ($\eta^2 < 0.001$), physical fitness, subjective physical activity ($\eta^2 = 0.008$), and screen-based media use ($\eta^2 = 0.001$) increased without significant difference in development between groups (all $p > 0.05$). At follow-up, groups did not differ in endurance capacity ($\eta^2 = 0.010$) and health-related quality of life ($\eta^2 < 0.001$). *Skipping Hearts* does not affect the long-term improvement of health status, motor performance, or health behavior. To improve the effects, the project should be implemented as a daily routine in schools to force the transfer of health behavior-related knowledge. Nevertheless, the project offers a physical activity that can be performed in children's everyday life without high costs.

Keywords: physical activity, health behavior, accelerometry, body composition, long-term evaluation, children, adolescents

INTRODUCTION

Poor physical activity in childhood and adolescence is associated with a higher risk for cardiovascular and chronic diseases and is, therefore, a major public health problem (1, 2). Several studies have found an adverse correlation between regular physical activity in childhood and adolescence and body mass index (BMI), waist circumference, and blood pressure (3–6). Having these risk factors at an early age leads to higher mortality and morbidity in adulthood (7). Ward et al. (8) report a 1 in 10 probability that 5-year-old obese children will not be obese by the age of 35 years.

Although countless projects promoting physical activity in this span of life exist, only 26% of German children and adolescents meet the recommendation of at least 60 min of moderate-to-vigorous physical activity (MVPA) per day (9, 10). It is of great significance that the physical activity level declines with increasing age during childhood and adolescence. Jekauc et al. (11) found an age-related continuous decrease in physical activity, especially in girls. The probability of meeting the World Health Organization's physical activity recommendations decreases every year by 17% in childhood and by 19% in adolescence (11).

The maturation of distinct motor skills is of crucial importance for early childhood development. Several studies have shown a positive correlation between motor skills and total, light-to-moderate, and MVPA in childhood and adolescence (12–14). Regular physical activity is not only important for physical health, but it is also associated with psychical well-being at an early age (15). Finne et al. (16) have shown a positive relationship between physical activity and health-related quality of life (HRQoL) and a negative association between HRQoL and screen-based media use (SBM), respectively. Therefore, the need for programs promoting health behavior, health status, and physical performance in childhood is particularly high.

Numerous projects and intervention studies, both national and international, promote physical activity in this age group with the main goal of changing their behavior towards a healthier lifestyle. The conceptions of these projects range from one-time offers to regular interventions lasting several hours and weeks, from projects limited to physical activity promotion to multimodal projects including nutrition or stress management, and from the integration only of children to the additional inclusion of parents (17). School seems to be particularly suitable as a setting for such projects since nowhere else can so many different children and adolescents be reached at the same time (18). Furthermore, Pate et al. (19) point out that it is an important task for schools to promote health behavior because of the increasing number of overweight children and adolescents.

Previous school-based programs in primary schools in Germany showed only a limited impact on children's health and health behavior. The URMEL-ICE study found no short-term effect on BMI but on waist circumference and subscapular skinfold thickness (20). The program "Join the Healthy Boat" resulted in a short-term reduction in cardiovascular disease risk and SBM, improvements in motor skills and a tendency of higher physical activity pattern (21–23). Graf et al. (24) conducted the CHILT Project which aimed to promote a healthy lifestyle in primary schools and consisted of health education lessons, physical activity breaks, and games for leisure. After 4 years, they observed higher improvements in lateral jumping and balancing backwards in the intervention group (25). Concerning the measured endpoints, Dobbins et al. (17) conclude in their systematic review that school-based interventions to promote physical activity and fitness have little or no effect on television viewing behavior, physical activity, blood pressure, and BMI. In addition, the authors suggest that significant changes in physical activity were observed in programs with longer duration and that interventions with significant effects included changes in school curricula and printed teaching materials. The recent review by Love et al. (26) also concludes that school-based intervention programs do not lead to a change in physical activity and that there are no differences between girls and boys and between children from different socioeconomic backgrounds. Changing health and health behavior through school-based programs is a necessary task from the point of view of public health, but also a challenging one in order to achieve the required effects in the short and long-term.

Of particular note is the fact that a long-term evaluation of such projects and interventions over the years is rather rare: only 2 out of 23 school-based intervention studies that measured the impact on physical activity duration had a follow-up of 12 months or more (17).

In 2006, the German Heart Foundation initiated the *Skipping Hearts* project, which aims to promoting physical activity and an active lifestyle through rope skipping during childhood. Skipping rope is the modern form of jumping rope and strengthens physical fitness, complex movement patterns, and social skills in girls and boys (27). The project is free of charge for schools and contains a two-staged concept: a one-time 90-min Basic-Workshop (supervision of a trainer of the German Heart Foundation) and the subsequent Champion-Program with 10 45-min rope skipping lessons (standardized curricula, implementation by the teacher). All participating schools and classes receive a package of materials, including a teacher's handbook. Up until August 2017, 12,487 school classes had completed the Basic-Workshop and 2,924 school classes had received the Champion-Program. In total, more than 500,000 children participated in *Skipping Hearts*. Therefore, *Skipping Hearts* is one of the largest projects promoting physical activity in Germany. It is well-described in a short-term evaluation with a 5-month follow-up, where the positive effects of both project parts on physical activity, body composition, and motor skills were determined (28).

This study aimed to investigate the long-term effect of the established *Skipping Hearts* project on anthropometric and cardiovascular parameters, motor performance, self-assessed physical fitness level, physical activity, SBM, and HRQoL in

Abbreviations: BMI, body mass index; DBP, diastolic blood pressure; HRQoL, health-related quality of life; MVPA, moderate-to-vigorous physical activity; SBM, screen-based media use; SBP, systolic blood pressure; SDS, standard deviation score; SH-B, skipping hearts basic group; SH-CH, skipping hearts champion group.

children. Therefore, an additional follow-up examination 3 years later was conducted. The effect sizes of the short-term evaluation were small and it was therefore of interest whether the Basic-Workshop and Champion-Program led to the effects being maintained or strengthened in the long term or whether the effects disappeared. We hypothesized that only the Champion-Program leads to long-term improvements in the mentioned parameters and that the Basic Workshop shows no long-term effects.

MATERIALS AND METHODS

Study Design

Skipping Hearts was evaluated in a non-randomized controlled longitudinal design between 2011 and 2016. The study included a fitness test (anthropometrics, health parameters, and motor skills), a health behavior questionnaire, and an accelerometer-based assessment of children (baseline: 10/2011-03/2012, follow-up: 03/2015-07/2015). Moreover, children's exercise capacity and HRQoL were evaluated in cross-section with a self-assessment and external assessment (parents). Informed consent was obtained from all children and parents.

Sampling Procedures

The sample consisted of the same subjects as the short-term evaluation study—pupils in the 3rd and 4th grade of primary school in Upper Bavaria (28). Children who only received the 90-min Basic-Workshop comprised group SH-B. Group SH-CH consisted of pupils who received the Champion-Program in addition to the Basic-Workshop. The schools registered with the German Heart Foundation for the *Skipping Hearts* project. It was up to the schools to decide whether a class would be involved in the Basic-Workshop only (42 classes) or also in the Champion-Program (26 classes). The control group (18 classes) consisted of children from schools that had neither the Basic-Workshop nor the Champion-Program. Between baseline and follow-up, the former primary school children moved to secondary school and were invited individually to join in the follow-up examination at a sports hall near their former primary school. Of 1,662 children with baseline data (838 SH-B, 480 SH-CH, 344 control group), 1,124 children (67.62%) were invited during the recruiting process and 538 (32.37%) were lost to follow-up. The main reason for loss to follow-up was inaccessibility at their secondary schools due to missing contact data.

An a priori power analysis with a small effect size ($f = 0.1$) and a power of 80% revealed a required total sample of $n = 246$ and thus $n = 82$ per group. A total of 486 students out of 1,124 (43.2%) joined in the follow-up examination. Of these, 286 only participated in the Skipping Hearts Basic-Workshop (SH-B), 140 additionally received the Skipping Hearts Champion-Program (SH-CH), and 78 served as controls. The required sample size from the power analysis was achieved in SH-B and SH-CH, in the control group it was only slightly below. A total of 307 parents of the 486 children with longitudinal data answered a questionnaire at follow-up.

Of 105 children with baseline data for short-term accelerometer-based assessment, 43 (41.0%) again took part in the accelerometer-based measurement at follow-up, 27 (25.7%) could not be contacted and 35 (33.3%) refused to participate in the long-term assessment. Seven of 43 subjects did not provide any data and 16 did not meet the inclusion criteria. Due to the small sample size of 20 subjects with baseline and follow-up data, the accelerometer-based assessment was supplemented by a cross-sectional survey at follow-up: 6 children with non-usable baseline data and 102 children without prior activity measurement, who volunteered for accelerometer measurement, were included. In total, of 151 subjects with follow-up examination, 90 completed the activity measurement, 41 did not provide any data, and 20 did not meet the inclusion criteria.

Follow-up examination was voluntary, and the fitness test took place in the afternoon during the children's leisure time. For renewed participation in the study, all children got a gym bag and took part in a lottery game with 1 × 2 concert tickets or 1 × 2 tickets for a German professional soccer league match as the main prize.

Materials

Blood pressure was measured using Mobil-O-Graph ambulatory blood pressure monitoring system (IEM Healthcare, Stolberg, Germany). After a rest period of at least 5 minutes, the measurement was taken on the left upper arm in a sitting position with the blood pressure cuff at heart level. Individual cuff size was determined by upper arm circumference (29). Based on German reference data, BMI was transformed into standard deviation scores (SDS), according to Kromeyer-Hauschild et al. (30) and systolic (SBP) and diastolic blood pressure (DBP) according to Neuhauser et al. (31).

Body fat was measured using the near-infrared technique (Futrex Advanced Body Fat Analyzer 6100 A/ZL, Futrex, Inc, Maryland, USA) on the right and left upper arm in the middle of the biceps brachii muscle (32). This method has high reliability and can be used in pediatric longitudinal studies to monitor changes in body fat over time (33). The mean of both measurements was used for further analyses.

Standing long jump, jumping sideways, 20-m sprint, and 6-min run were performed to conduct motor performance (34). The 6-min run was only performed in the follow-up examination. The measurement procedure is described in Postler et al. (28) and Graf et al. (24). SDS of these motor tests were calculated according to Bös et al. (34). To make a statement about general motor performance, a motor score was calculated from the three tests that were performed at all times (standing long jump, jumping sideways and 20-m sprint). This was composed of the mean value of the SDS values of the measured parameters and thus forms a single, meaningful parameter for motor performance. The test-retest reliability of the individual tests used ranges from $\alpha = 0.89$ to $\alpha = 0.92$ and the tests show a good overall validity (34). In our study, the reliability of the motor score was $\alpha = 0.71$ for the baseline and $\alpha = 0.77$ for the follow-up measurement.

Activity levels were recorded using the MoMo activity questionnaire (35). The physical activity score was calculated according to Prochaska et al. (36) as the mean value of the questions "How many of the last 7 days have you been physically active for at least 60 min a day?" and "How many days in a normal week are you physically active for at least 60 min a day?" The physical activity score has acceptable reliability and validity in comparison to accelerometer measurements (36). The Cronbach's alpha of the physical activity score was $\alpha = 0.76$ for the baseline and $\alpha = 0.84$ for the follow-up measurement. To assess SBM, children were asked about their daily consumption of TV/video, computer/Internet, gaming consoles, and mobile phone according to Lampert et al. (37) and estimation of their fitness level (How well do you think your physical performance is [=fitness]?) was collected in five categories from "very well" to "not at all well." An SBM index (h/day) was built according to Finne et al. (16). Although the SBM index was used in the reported study, it has not yet been checked for reliability and validity. The reliability of SBM in our study was $\alpha = 0.49$ for the baseline and $\alpha = 0.51$ for the follow-up measurement.

A subsample performed an accelerometer-based measurement using Actigraph GT3X+ to assess objective physical activity, particularly the time spent in MVPA. Study participants should wear the accelerometer for 1 week all day on the right hip. Inclusion criteria were wearing the accelerometer at least 7 h daily on at least 3 workdays and 1 weekend day (38, 39). The cut-points of Freedson et al. (40) were used to determine activity intensity levels. An activity of fewer than 100 counts/min was generally defined as sedentary activity (41). Epoch length was 60 s. Data were classified as wear time and non-wear time according to the algorithm of Choi et al. (42). Besides, children recorded their daily physical activity and wear time in an activity protocol.

The KINDL-R questionnaire was used to assess the HRQoL of children through self-report and parent-report (43). The questionnaire was only used in the follow-up examination. It contains 24 items in 6 subscales (physical well-being, emotional well-being, self-esteem, family, friends, and school), whereby four items make up one subscale. Subscale scores and the total score are transformed from 0 to 100 with a higher score expressing a better HRQoL. In addition to HRQoL, parents were asked about their child's physical activity according to Prochaska et al. (36) (no personal data available). The psychometric characteristics of the KINDL-R revealed a reliability of $\alpha = 0.54$ to $\alpha = 0.73$ for the subscales and $\alpha = 0.82$ for the total score (44). Satisfactory convergent validity is generally attributed to the subscales and the total score (45). The reliability of the scores in our study ranged from $\alpha = 0.43$ (friends) to $\alpha = 0.74$ (family) in the self-report and from $\alpha = 0.66$ (friends) to $\alpha = 0.83$ (physical well-being) in the parent-report. The overall HRQoL score reliability was $\alpha = 0.83$ and $\alpha = 0.87$ in the self-report and the parent-report, respectively.

Standard operation procedure for follow-up was identical to the standard operation procedure for baseline examination. All measurements were performed by previously trained staff.

Statistical Analysis

Mean and standard deviations are reported for continuous data, median for non-normally distributed continuous data. Absolute and relative frequencies are shown for categorical data.

A comparison of baseline data of originally included participants who were willing to take part in the long-term assessments and those who refused to perform (children who could not be contacted were not considered). Welch two-sample t-tests were used to examine differences between children with follow-up and children without follow-up in anthropometrics, cardiovascular parameters, motor performance, physical activity, and SBM at baseline. Fisher's exact test was used for the categorical variable physical fitness in this analysis.

One-way analysis of variance for metric variables and Kruskal–Wallis tests for categorical variables were used for group comparisons at baseline.

Analysis of variance for repeated measures considering time as within-subjects variable and group as between-subjects variable for anthropometrics, cardiovascular parameters, motor performance, physical activity score, and SBM were used to examine changes between baseline and follow-up in total and between SH-B, SH-CH, and the control group over time for all 486 participants with baseline and follow-up data. For the categorical variable physical fitness, we used Wilcoxon signed rank test and Pearson's Chi-squared test in this analysis.

Due to the small sample size in the accelerometer-based assessment, Wilcoxon signed rank test was used to analyze the change between follow-up and baseline data in accelerometer data in total. We further calculated the differences between follow-up and baseline data and used Kruskal Wallis test to analyze the changes between groups, respectively.

Changes over time within groups were examined using paired t-tests for anthropometrics, cardiovascular parameters, motor performance, physical activity score, and SBM, and Wilcoxon signed rank tests for accelerometer data and assessment of physical fitness (Bonferroni correction $p < 0.0167$).

One-way analysis of variance was used to analyze only cross-sectional data of follow-up measurement: accelerometer ($n = 90$), 6-min run ($n = 477$), physical activity score (parental report), and HRQoL for both parental report ($n = 307$) and self-report ($n = 455$).

Statistical data analysis was performed using SPSS Statistics 23.0 (IBM Corp., Armonk, NY, USA) and R 3.3.3 (R Foundation for Statistical Computing, Vienna, Austria). The level of significance was set at $p < 0.05$ and $p < 0.1$ was set as the tendency of significance. Effect size is reported for all analyses of variance.

RESULTS

Dropout-Analysis: Differences in Subjects With or Without Participation in Long-Term Assessment at Baseline

Children who participated in follow-up had better baseline values in BMI (16.7 ± 2.36 vs. 17.5 ± 2.99, $p < 0.001$), BMI-SDS (0.07 ± 0.96 vs. 0.20 ± 1.07, $p < 0.001$), body fat (15.3 ± 3.14 vs. 15.7 ± 3.63, $p = 0.040$), SBP (113.5 ± 10.9 vs. 115.1 ± 12.0, $p = 0.022$), SBP-SDS (1.34 ± 1.28 vs. 1.52 ± 1.37, $p = 0.027$) and motor performance (0.34 ± 0.73 vs. 0.08 ± 0.72, $p < 0.001$) than children who didn't participate in the follow-up (**Table 1**). No significant differences were found in

TABLE 1 | Dropout-analysis: differences in subjects with or without participation in long-term assessment at baseline.

	Participation in long-term assessment			No participation in long-term assessment			*p*-value
Welch two-sample *t*-tests	***n***	**Mean (SD)**	**95% CI**	***n***	**Mean (SD)**	**95% CI**	
Age (years)	486	8.98 (0.60)	[8.93, 9.04]	638	9.09 (0.65)	[9.04, 9.14]	**0.005**
Height (cm)	478	135.1 (6.71)	[134.5, 135.7]	631	135.6 (6.87)	[135.0, 136.1]	0.260
Weight (kg)	478	30.7 (6.32)	[30.1, 31.3]	631	32.5 (7.78)	[31.8, 33.1]	**<0.001**
BMI (kg/m^2)	478	16.7 (2.36)	[16.5, 16.9]	631	17.5 (2.99)	[17.3, 17.7]	**<0.001**
BMI-SDS	478	0.07 (0.96)	[−0.15, 0.02]	631	0.20 (1.07)	[0.11, 0.28]	**<0.001**
Body fat (%)	476	15.3 (3.14)	[15.0, 15.6]	626	15.7 (3.63)	[15.4, 16.0]	**0.040**
SBP (mmHg)	460	113.5 (10.9)	[112.5, 114.4]	618	115.1 (12.0)	[114.1, 116.0]	**0.022**
SBP-SDS	460	1.34 (1.28)	[1.22, 1.46]	618	1.52 (1.37)	[1.42, 1.63]	**0.027**
DBP (mmHg)	460	70.3 (9.08)	[69.4, 71.1]	618	71.0 (9.61)	[70.3, 71.8]	0.191
DBP-SDS	460	1.18 (1.39)	[1.06, 1.31]	614	1.28 (1.46)	[1.17, 1.40]	0.268
Motor performance	464	0.34 (0.73)	[0.28, 0.41]	608	0.08 (0.72)	[0.03, 0.14]	**<0.001**
Physical activity score (days/week)	405	4.06 (1.82)	[3.88, 4.24]	567	3.87 (1.82)	[3.72, 4.02]	0.108
MVPA relative (% of wear time)	20	22.5 (3.73)	[20.7, 24.23]	59	22.8 (6.61)	[21.1, 24.5]	0.837
MVPA absolute (minutes/day)	20	170.3 (30.3)	[156.1, 184.4]	59	168.2 (51.0)	[154.9, 181.5]	0.866
SBM (h/day)	365	1.79 (1.99)	[1.58, 1.99]	496	2.09 (2.74)	[1.85, 2.33]	0.075
Fisher's exact test		***n* (%)**			***n* (%)**		***p*-value**
Physical fitness		454 (100)			614 (100)		0.169
Very well		197 (43.4)			230 (37.5)		
Well		191 (42.1)			271 (44.1)		
Medium		61 (13.4)			105 (17.1)		
Not as well		3 (0.7)			7 (1.1)		
Not at all well		2 (0.4)			1 (0.2)		

Significant results marked in bold types. BMI, body mass index; SBP, systolic blood pressure; DBP, diastolic blood pressure; SDS, standard deviation score; MVPA, moderate-to-vigorous physical activity; SBM, screen-based media use.

the number of days/week with daily at least 60 min of physical activity (4.06 ± 1.82 vs. 3.87 ± 1.82, $p = 0.108$) and relative (22.5 ± 3.73 vs. 22.8 ± 6.61, $p = 0.837$), absolute minutes in MVPA per day (170.3 ± 30.3 vs. 168.2 ± 51.0, $p = 0.866$) and self-assessment of own physical fitness at baseline. Children with participation in long-term assessment showed a tendency of lower SBM (1.79 ± 1.99 vs. 2.09 ± 2.74, $p = 0.075$) at baseline.

Baseline Characteristics

Four hundred and eighty six children (256 female) had baseline and follow-up data with a mean age at baseline of 8.98 ± 0.60 years (**Table 2**). 10.0% were classified as underweight, 9.6% as overweight, and 2.5% as obese. Mean age in SH-B (9.06 ± 0.64) was ~2 months higher than in SH-CH (8.89 ± 0.59, $p = 0.019$) and in the control group (8.87 ± 0.46, $p = 0.038$). SH-B (4.13 ± 1.77, $p = 0.033$) and SH-CH (4.20 ± 1.87, $p = 0.038$) reported higher physical activity compared to controls (3.53 ± 1.82). Groups did not significantly differ in BMI, body fat, blood pressure, motor performance, objectively measured physical activity, and SBM (*p*-values not shown). At baseline, 85.4% of the participating children (SH-B: 87.9%, SH-CH: 83.6%, control group: 80.6%, $p = 0.582$) reported a good or very good own physical fitness.

Changes Between Baseline and Follow-Up in Total

Height (Δ 21.2 ± 3.53, $p < 0.001$), weight (Δ 15.0 ± 5.08 $p < 0.001$), BMI (Δ 1.86 ± 1.47, $p < 0.001$), body fat (Δ 6.41 ± 3.39, $p < 0.001$), SBP (Δ 5.74 ± 13.1, $p < 0.001$), DBP (Δ 4.27 ± 10.3, $p < 0.001$), DBP-SDS (Δ0.14 ± 1.57, $p = 0.027$) and motor performance (Δ0.16 ± 0.57, $p < 0.001$) increased from baseline to follow-up (**Table 2**). Age- and sex-independent BMI-SDS (Δ −0.06 ± 0.52, $p = 0.025$) and SBP-SDS (Δ −0.24 ± 1.48, $p = 0.014$) decreased over time and prevalence of overweight and obesity remained constant ($\chi^2 = 3.98, p = 0.409$). Subjective physical activity score (Δ0.58± 2.22, $p < 0.001$) and daily SBM (Δ 1.61 ± 2.56, $p < 0.001$) increased between baseline and follow-up. A decline of MVPA-minutes ($z = -3.92$, $p < 0.001$) and percentage of MVPA-minutes of daily wear time ($z = -3.92$, $p < 0.001$) was observed. The assessment of own physical fitness declined between baseline and follow-up ($z = -10.0, p < 0.001$).

Changes Between Baseline and Follow-Up Within Groups

Height, weight, BMI, SBP, DBP, and SBM increased between baseline and follow-up in all groups (**Table 3**). BMI-SDS only decreased in SH-CH (Δ −0.11 ± 0.49, $p = 0.006$). SH-B (Δ −0.34 ± 1.52, $p < 0.001$) and not SH-CH decreased in SBP-SDS. DBP-SDS did not change over time within all groups. Motor

TABLE 2 | Descriptive statistics of baseline and follow-up data.

	Baseline		Follow-Up		*p*-value	η^2
Paired *t*-tests from ANOVA for repeated measures	**Mean (SD)**	**95% CI**	**Mean (SD)**	**95% CI**		
Age (years)	8.98 (.60)	[8.93, 9.04]	12.4 (0.60)	[12.3, 12.4]	**<0.001**	1.00
Height (cm)	135.1 (6.71)	[134.5, 135.7]	156.3 (8.22)	[155.6, 157.0]	**<0.001**	0.996
Weight (kg)	30.7 (6.32)	[30.7, 31.3]	45.6 (9.91)	[44.8, 46.5]	**<0.001**	0.873
BMI (kg/m^2)	16.7 (2.36)	[16.5, 16.9]	18.5 (2.95)	[18.3, 18.8]	**<0.001**	0.557
BMI-SDS	−0.07 (0.96)	[−0.15, 0.02]	−0.13 (1.07)	[−0.22, −0.03]	**0.025**	0.010
Body fat (%)	15.3 (3.14)	[15.0, 15.6]	21.70 (5.34)	[21.2, 22.2]	**<0.001**	0.739
SBP (mmHg)	113.4 (10.8)	[112.2, 114.4]	119.2 (12.0)	[118.0, 120.3]	**<0.001**	0.153
SBP-SDS	1.34 (1.27)	[1.22, 1.46]	1.10 (1.26)	[0.98, 1.22]	**0.014**	0.013
DBP (mmHg)	70.2 (9.04)	[69.4, 71.1]	74.5 (8.19)	[73.8, 75.3]	**<0.001**	0.136
DBP-SDS	1.18 (1.38)	[1.06, 1.31]	1.33 (1.21)	[1.21, 1.44]	**0.027**	0.011
Motor performance	0.35 (0.73)	[0.28, 0.42]	0.51 (0.74)	[0.45, 0.58]	**<0.001**	0.057
Physical activity score (days/week)	4.06 (1.82)	[3.88, 4.24]	4.64 (1.69)	[4.47, 4.81]	**<0.001**	0.064
SBM (h/day)	1.77 (1.92)	[1.56, 1.97]	3.38 (2.38)	[3.12, 3.63]	**<0.001**	0.242
Wilcoxon signed rank tests	**Median**		**Median**			
MVPA relative (% of wear time)	22.6		8.7		**<0.001**	
MVPA absolute (minutes/day)	170.8		74.6		**<0.001**	
Wilcoxon signed rank tests	***n* (%)**		***n* (%)**			
Physical fitness	439 (100)		439 (100)		**<0.001**	
Very well	190 (43.3)		75 (17.1)			
Well	185 (42.1)		227 (51.7)			
Medium	59 (13.4)		123 (28.0)			
Not as well	3 (0.07)		14 (3.2)			
Not at all well	2 (0.05)		0 (0.0)			

Significant results marked in bold types. BMI, body mass index; SBP, systolic blood pressure; DBP, diastolic blood pressure; SDS, standard deviation score; MVPA, moderate-to-vigorous physical activity; SBM, screen-based media use.

performance significantly increased over time in both project groups (SH-B: Δ0.17± 0.57, SH-CH: Δ0.16 ± 0.54, $p < 0.001$ for both). Between baseline and follow-up, self-reported physical activity score increased in SH-B (Δ0.53 ± 2.20, $p = 0.001$) and the control group (Δ 1.02 ± 2.04, $p < 0.001$), but not in SH-CH. Absolute and relative MVPA ($z = -2.52, p = 0.012$) significantly decreased over time in SH-CH. Between baseline and follow-up, all groups significantly decreased in their assessment of own physical fitness (SH-B: $z = -7.48$, SH-CH: $z = -5.26$, control group: $z = -4.09, p < 0.001$ for all).

Changes Between Baseline and Follow-Up Between Groups: Long-Term Effect of *Skipping Hearts*

Mean changes in all anthropometric and cardiovascular parameters over time did not differ between groups (**Table 4**). In subjective physical activity, no change over time was observed in SH-B and SH-CH compared to controls ($p = 0.243$). A tendency of lower decline of MVPA-minutes in SH-B and SH-CH compared to controls ($\chi^2 = 5.09, p = 0.078$) but not in percentage of MVPA-minutes of daily wear time ($\chi^2 = 2.92, p = 0.232$) was found. Mean changes in SBM over time did not differ between groups. Self-reported physical fitness showed no interaction between group and time ($\chi^2 = 0.30, p = 0.990$).

Additional Analyzes at Follow-Up

Due to the little number of subjects with accelerometer data at both times of measurement, additionally data derived at the long-term assessment were analyzed without consideration of baseline data to estimate possible outlasting effects of SH. Groups did not differ in the daily MVPA-minutes ($p = 0.568$), percentage of MVPA-minutes of daily wear time ($p = 0.488$) and endurance capacity ($p = 0.098$, **Table 5**). In parental report, no significant group differences were determined in the physical activity score of the children (SH-B: 4.07 ± 1.73, SH-CH: 4.23 ± 1.74, control group: 3.91 ± 1.61, $p = 0.605$, $\eta^2 = 0.003$). In self-assessment of children and parent-report, no significant group differences in total score and all subscales of KINDL-R were observed.

DISCUSSION

This study aimed to evaluate the long-term effects of the *Skipping Hearts* health promotion project, a donation-funded project of the German Heart Foundation. A positive effect

TABLE 3 | Descriptive statistics of baseline and follow-up data (SH-B, SH-CH, control group) and intra-group development over time.

	SH-B						SH-CH						Control group					
		Baseline		Follow-Up		*p*-value*		Baseline		Follow-Up		*p*-value*		Baseline		Follow-Up		*p*-value*
Paired *t*-tests	*n*	Mean (SD)	95% CI	Mean (SD)	95% CI		*n*	Mean (SD)	95% CI	Mean (SD)	95% CI		*n*	Mean (SD)	95% CI	Mean (SD)	95% CI	
Age (years)	268	9.06 (0.64)	[8.99, 9.14]	12.4 (0.64)	[12.4, 12.5]	**<0.001**	140	8.89 (0.59)	[8.79, 8.99]	12.3 (0.58)	[12.2, 12.4]	**<0.001**	78	8.87 (0.46)	[8.77, 8.97]	12.2 (0.47)	[12.1, 12.3]	**<0.001**
Height (cm)	260	135.3 (6.56)	[134.5, 136.0]	156.5 (7.71)	[155.6, 157.4]	**<0.001**	140	135.3 (7.07)	[134.1, 136.4]	156.5 (8.98)	[155.0, 158.0]	**<0.001**	78	134.2 (6.55)	[132.7, 135.7]	155.1 (8.46)	[153.2, 157.0]	**<0.001**
Weight (kg)	260	30.5 (6.19)	[29.8, 31.3]	45.5 (9.16)	[44.4, 46.6]	**<0.001**	140	30.9 (6.04)	[29.9, 32.0]	45.9 (10.24)	[44.2, 47.7]	**<0.001**	78	30.7 (7.27)	[29.1, 32.3]	45.6 (11.7)	[43.0, 48.3]	**<0.001**
BMI (kg/m^2)	260	16.6 (2.26)	[16.3, 16.8]	18.5 (2.75)	[18.1, 18.8]	**<0.001**	140	16.8 (2.23)	[16.4, 17.2]	18.6 (3.03)	[18.1, 19.1]	**<0.001**	78	16.9 (2.88)	[16.2, 17.5]	18.8 (3.46)	[18.0, 19.5]	**<0.001**
BMI-SDS	260	−0.13 (0.92)	[−0.24, −0.01]	−0.17 (1.04)	[−0.30, −0.04]	0.209	140	0.03 (0.92)	[−0.13, 0.18]	−0.09 (1.06)	[−0.26, 0.09]	**0.006**	78	−0.03 (1.14)	[−0.29, 0.22]	−0.06 (1.20)	[−0.33, 0.21]	0.687
Body fat (%)	258	15.4 (3.18)	[15.0, 15.8]	21.9 (5.13)	[21.2, 22.5]	**<0.001**	139	15.3 (3.16)	[14.8, 15.8]	21.7 (5.42)	[20.7, 22.6]	**<0.001**	78	14.8 (2.97)	[14.2, 15.5]	21.3 (5.88)	[19.9, 22.6]	**<0.001**
SBP (mmHg)	246	113.7 (10.7)	[112.3, 115.0]	118.6 (12.4)	[117.0, 120.1]	**<0.001**	134	112.7 (10.7)	[110.9, 114.5]	119.1 (11.2)	[117.2, 121.0]	**<0.001**	77	113.8 (11.4)	[111.2, 116.4]	121.1 (12.2)	[118.3, 123.9]	**<0.001**
SBP-SDS	246	1.35 (1.27)	[1.19, 1.51]	1.01 (1.30)	[0.85, 1.18]	**0.001**	134	1.26 (1.29)	[1.04, 1.48]	1.11 (1.17)	[0.91, 1.31]	0.196	77	1.44 (1.25)	[1.15, 1.72]	1.36 (1.24)	[1.08, 1.64]	0.662
DBP (mmHg)	246	70.5 (9.00)	[69.3, 71.6]	74.1 (7.99)	[73.1, 75.1]	**<0.001**	134	69.6 (9.06)	[68.1, 71.2]	74.6 (7.55)	[73.3, 75.8]	**<0.001**	77	70.6 (9.21)	[68.5, 72.7]	75.6 (9.76)	[73.4, 77.8]	**<0.001**
DBP-SDS	246	1.21 (1.38)	[1.03, 1.38]	1.26 (1.19)	[1.11, 1.41]	0.571	134	1.09 (1.38)	[0.86, 1.33]	1.34 (1.10)	[1.15, 1.52]	0.075	77	1.26 (1.39)	[0.94, 1.57]	1.51 (1.44)	[1.18, 1.83]	0.202
Motor performance	260	0.37 (0.74)	[0.28, 0.46]	0.53 (0.71)	[0.45, 0.62]	**<0.001**	136	0.30 (0.69)	[0.18, 0.42]	0.46 (0.79)	[0.32, 0.59]	**0.001**	60	0.39 (0.81)	[0.19, 0.60]	0.57 (0.74)	[0.38, 0.76]	0.040
Physical activity score (days/week)	207	4.13 (1.77)	[3.89, 4.37]	4.66 (1.64)	[4.44, 4.89]	**0.001**	113	4.20 (1.87)	[3.85, 4.55]	4.63 (1.78)	[4.30, 4.96]	0.050	58	3.53 (1.82)	[3.06, 4.01]	4.55 (1.57)	[4.14, 4.97]	**<0.001**
SBM (h/day)	182	1.77 (2.00)	[1.48, 2.06]	3.32 (2.14)	[3.01, 3.64]	**<0.001**	97	1.78 (2.07)	[1.37, 2.20]	3.54 (2.99)	[2.94, 4.14]	**<0.001**	56	1.73 (1.31)	[1.38, 2.08]	3.26 (1.88)	[2.75, 3.76]	**<0.001**
Wilcoxon tests		**Median**		**Median**				**Median**		**Median**				**Median**		**Median**		
MVPA relative (% of wear time)	5	22.9		7.80		0.043	8	21.9		8.90		**0.012**	7	22.6		7.90		0.018
MVPA absolute (minutes/day)	5	171.0		67.0		0.043	8	164.5		76.6		**0.012**	7	188.6		67.9		0.018
Wilcoxon tests		***n* (%)**		***n* (%)**				***n* (%)**		***n* (%)**				***n* (%)**		***n* (%)**		
Physical fitness	289					**<0.001**	128					**<0.001**	72					**<0.001**
Very well		103 (43.1)		37 (15.5)				57 (44.5)		25 (19.5)				30 (41.7)		13 (18.1)		
Well		107 (44.8)		130 (54.4)				50 (39.1)		62 (48.4)				28 (38.9)		35 (48.6)		
Medium		25 (10.5)		66 (27.6)				20 (15.6)		37 (28.9)				14 (19.4)		20 (27.8)		
Not as well		2 (0.8)		6 (2.5)				1 (0.8)		4 (3.1)				0 (0.0)		4 (5.6)		
Not at all well		2 (0.8)		0 (0.0)				0 (0.0)		0 (0.0)				0 (0.0)		0 (0.0)		
Not at all well																		

Corrected according to Bonferroni (significant when $p < 0.0167$). Significant results marked in bold types. SH-B, skipping hearts basic; SH-CH, skipping hearts champion; BMI, body mass index; SBP, systolic blood pressure; DBP, diastolic blood pressure; SDS, standard deviation score; MVPA, moderate-to-vigorous physical activity; SBM, screen-based media use.

TABLE 4 | Δ (follow-up−baseline) and group/time-interaction effect in anthropometric and cardiovascular parameters, motor performance, physical activity score and screen-based media use.

	SH-B			SH-CH			Control group				η^2
	Δ (follow-up−baseline)			Δ (follow-up−baseline)			Δ (follow-up−baseline)			*p*-value	
ANOVA for repeated measures	*n*	**Mean (SD)**	**95% CI**	*n*	**Mean (SD)**	**95% CI**	*n*	**Mean (SD)**	**95% CI**	**time*goup**	
Age (years)	268	3.37 (0.04)	[3.37, 3.38]	140	3.37 (0.04)	[3.36, 3.37]	78	3.36 (0.07)	[3.35, 3.38]	0.100	0.009
Height (cm)	260	21.2 (3.39)	[20.8, 21.6]	140	21.3 (3.76)	[20.7, 21.9]	78	20.9 (3.60)	[20.1, 21.8]	0.791	0.001
Weight (kg)	260	14.9 (4.71)	[14.4, 15.5]	140	15.0 (5.44)	[14.1, 15.9]	78	15.0 (5.63)	[13.7, 16.2]	0.990	<0.001
BMI (kg/m^2)	260	1.88 (1.40)	[1.71, 2.05]	140	1.80 (1.59)	[1.54, 2.07]	78	1.88 (1.49)	[1.54, 2.21]	0.873	0.001
BMI-SDS	260	−0.04 (0.53)	[−0.11, 0.02]	140	−0.11 (0.49)	[−0.20, −0.03]	78	−0.03 (0.55)	[−0.15, 0.10]	0.338	0.005
Body fat (%)	258	6.43 (3.24)	[6.03, 6.83]	139	6.37 (3.33)	[5.81, 6.93]	78	6.43 (3.99)	[5.53, 7.33]	0.986	<0.001
SBP (mmHg)	246	4.89 (13.5)	[3.20, 6.59]	134	6.41 (12.0)	[4.36, 8.46]	77	7.26 (13.5)	[4.19, 10.3]	0.299	0.005
SBP-SDS	246	−0.34 (1.52)	[−0.53, −0.15]	134	−0.15 (1.37)	[−0.39, 0.08]	77	−0.08 (1.52)	[−0.42, 0.27]	0.281	0.006
DBP (mmHg)	246	3.66 (10.0)	[2.40, 4.92]	134	4.92 (10.3)	[3.15, 6.68]	77	5.05 (11.1)	[2.54, 7.57]	0.399	0.004
DBP-SDS	246	0.06 (1.53)	[−0.14, 0.25]	134	0.24 (1.57)	[−0.02, 0.51]	77	0.25 (1.69)	[−0.14, 0.63]	0.438	0.004
Motor performance	260	0.17 (0.57)	[0.10, 0.24]	136	0.16 (0.54)	[0.07, 0.25]	60	0.17 (0.64)	[0.01, 0.34]	0.976	<0.001
Physical activity score (days/week)	207	0.53 (2.20)	[0.23, 0.83]	113	0.43 (2.33)	[0.00, 0.87]	58	1.02 (2.04)	[0.48, 1.55]	0.243	0.008
SBM (h/day)	182	1.55 (2.36)	[1.21, 1.90]	97	1.78 (3.10)	[1.21, 1.90]	56	1.53 (2.12)	[0.96, 2.09]	0.789	0.001

SH-B, skipping hearts basic; SH-CH, skipping hearts champion; BMI, body mass index; SBP, systolic blood pressure; DBP, diastolic blood pressure; SDS, standard deviation score; SBM, screen-based media use.

TABLE 5 | Group comparison in 6-min run, MVPA, and HRQoL at long-term assessment.

	SH-B			SH-CH			Control group			*p*-value	η^2
One-way ANOVA	*n*	**Mean (SD)**	**95% CI**	*n*	**Mean (SD)**	**95% CI**	*n*	**Mean (SD)**	**95% CI**		
6-min run (meter)	262	1,076.6 (120.1)	[1,062.0, 1,091.2]	137	1,075.7 (122.5)	[1,055.0, 1,096.4]	78	1,043.8 (124.8)	[1,015.7, 1,072.0]	0.098	0.010
MVPA relative (% of wear time)	35	9.07 (3.70)	[7.80, 10.34]	27	9.99 (3.92)	[8.44, 11.5]	28	10.2 (4.03)	[8.58, 11.7]	0.488	0.016
MVPA absolute (minutes/day)	35	74.1 (29.9)	[63.8, 84.3]	27	80.8 (29.4)	[69.1, 92.4]	28	81.3 (31.6)	[69.0, 93.6]	0.568	0.013
KINDL-R self-report											
Total	261	74.0 (11.1)	[72.6, 75.3]	131	74.4 (12.2)	[72.3, 76.5]	63	73.7 (12.1)	[70.6, 76.7]	0.911	<0.001
Physical well-being	261	75.7 (16.9)	[73.6, 77.2]	130	75.4 (18.8)	[72.1, 78.6]	63	77.4 (17.1)	[73.1, 81.7]	0.739	0.001
Emotional well-being	259	82.0 (14.6)	[80.1, 83.7]	129	83.1 (14.9)	[80.6, 85.7]	62	82.3 (12.8)	[79.0, 85.5]	0.725	0.001
Self-esteem	259	55.7 (20.5)	[53.2, 58.2]	128	56.2 (22.8)	[52.2, 60.2]	61	56.0 (20.4)	[50.8, 61.2]	0.971	<0.001
Family	261	85.7 (16.3)	[83.7, 87.7]	131	84.8 (16.1)	[82.0, 87.6]	63	83.1 (17.3)	[78.8, 87.5]	0.534	0.003
Friends	258	78.0 (14.7)	[76.2, 79.8]	131	78.6 (15.9)	[75.8, 81.3]	63	76.1 (16.8)	[71.8, 80.3]	0.555	0.003
School	261	66.7 (17.9)	[64.5, 68.9]	131	68.0 (19.3)	[64.7, 71.4]	63	67.0 (20.2)	[62.0, 72.1]	0.807	0.001
KINDL-R parent-report											
Total	177	78.6 (8.7)	[77.3, 79.9]	88	76.7 (10.2)	[74.5, 78.8]	40	75.4 (11.2)	[71.8, 79.0]	0.082	0.016
Physical well-being	177	81.3 (14.9)	[79.1, 83.6]	88	77.3 (17.9)	[73.5, 81.1]	40	75.9 (16.2)	[73.5, 81.1]	0.050	0.020
Emotional well-being	177	84.0 (11.1)	[82.3, 85.6]	87	82.1 (12.7)	[79.4, 84.8]	40	81.4 (14.1)	[76.9, 85.9]	0.303	0.008
Self-esteem	177	70.9 (13.8)	[68.9, 73.0]	88	69.5 (13.5)	[66.7, 72.4]	40	67.2 (14.8)	[62.5, 71.9]	0.288	0.008
Family	177	79.5 (15.0)	[77.3, 81.7]	89	79.4 (14.2)	[76.4, 82.4]	40	79.2 (12.0)	[75.4, 83.1]	0.991	<0.001
Friends	177	77.6 (12.7)	[75.7, 79.5]	88	76.5 (13.9)	[73.5, 79.4]	40	73.4 (15.3)	[68.6, 78.3]	0.210	0.010
School	175	78.3 (14.3)	[76.2, 80.5]	87	75.3 (17.2)	[71.6, 78.9]	40	75.2 (14.1)	[70.7, 79.7]	0.219	0.010

SH-B, skipping hearts basic; SH-CH, skipping hearts champion; MVPA, moderate-to-vigorous physical activity.

of the *Skipping Hearts* Basic-Workshop and Champion-Program regarding the long-term improvement of health and health behavior could not be determined, but a tendency towards a less pronounced decrease of physical activity was observed.

While Postler et al. (28) found significant short-term improvements in motor performance and body fat (SH-B and SH-CH compared to controls) as well as activity level (SH-CH compared to controls), the long-term evaluation could not confirm the positive short-term results. SH-B and SH-CH did not show diverging development in anthropometrics, cardiovascular parameters, motor performance, SBM, and HRQoL compared to the control group between baseline and follow-up. Despite the tendency for *Skipping Hearts* to prevent an age-related decrease of physical activity, this result might be influenced by the high dropout rate of 44.9% in accelerometer measurement.

A decline in BMI-SDS and SBP-SDS was found in all groups. This indicates an age- and sex-independent improvement in these parameters. Furthermore, children in all groups improved their motor performance and physical activity score but the results of objective accelerometer data do not confirm this improvement. The decline within the 3.5 years from baseline to follow-up is in line with the literature: Physical activity decreases between childhood and adolescence (46–49). Even though a direct effect of *Skipping Hearts* was not found, participation in a study-related fitness test can be a motivational factor for children to increase their health status and fitness level. However, comparison of baseline data between children willing to participate in the long-term assessment and those who refused revealed that the healthier children participated again at follow-up. This indicates that the follow-up examination was not attended by those children who were the main target group of the project. Therefore, the current study population was more likely to stay in their initial healthy state.

A review of the relevant literature reveals that there are no consistent findings regarding the long-term effectiveness of prevention and health promotion projects at school. After a 1-year school-based physical activity intervention and a follow-up of 3 years, Meyer et al. (50) found a long-term increase in aerobic fitness compared to controls, but no sustainable effects on physical activity, cardiovascular parameter, and quality of life. Kobel et al. (22) also reported no significant increase in physical activity but a significant decrease in SBM in girls in a 1-year follow-up of the cluster-randomized longitudinal study "Join the Healthy Boat." Anderson et al. (51) conducted a school-based cluster-randomized controlled trial including lessons-plans, teaching materials, parental-child homework activities, training for teachers, and health promotion strategies for parents; but they observed no effect on MVPA and sedentary behavior. In contrast, Lahti et al. (52) reported higher levels of physical activity compared to controls 4 years after ending a 7-year intervention at school. Furthermore, Vander Ploeg et al. (53) observed a greater increase in activity on school days and on weekends in the intervention group 2 years after the implementation of a comprehensive school health program.

In a Cochrane Review of 2013, Dobbins et al. (17) suggest that school-based interventions only have limited effects regarding BMI, blood pressure, pulse rate, and physical activity level. This is interesting insofar as only one out of 44 had a follow-up measurement at 4 years after intervention and the majority of studies had the point of measurement directly post-intervention. Because the findings of every new intervention study are consistent with those from other studies, the probability of improving the tested parameters in a short-term intervention study is high. However, statements regarding the effectiveness of an intervention should be treated with caution because they do not reveal anything about a long-term effect. A long-lasting increase in activity levels and motor performance should be the main goal of every project related to prevention and health promotion research. Therefore, it is not surprising that *Skipping Hearts* is not able to sustainably enable children to do more physical activity. Indeed, the short-term effectiveness of *Skipping Hearts*—both the Basic-Workshop and the Champion-Program—has to be viewed as an unexpected success.

Skipping Hearts is not a controlled and scientifically supported intervention, but a donation-funded project of a foundation. The Champion-Program of *Skipping Hearts* is planned as a continuous implementation of 10 45-min prepared lessons. The responsibility of implementation lies within the school administration because there is no supervisor. To a certain extent, the implementation of the Champion-Program is therefore entirely up to the teachers themselves. It may well be that this individual responsibility for the implementation process is the most crucial point for its effectiveness. It can be assumed that teachers implemented the lessons during and not in addition to sports education. On measurement days at school, teachers gave this verbal feedback and mentioned that they did not meet the given guidelines—the large majority did not conduct all 10 lessons and reduced the physical activity duration. To get a detailed insight into the assessment of the project and its conception and implementation into the daily routine of schools, qualitative interviews were conducted with the teachers and headmasters of 64 participating schools. Furthermore, a nationwide survey of all teachers and headmasters ($n = 1474$) who participated in *Skipping Hearts* since its beginning in 2006 was performed. These data are currently being analyzed and will be published elsewhere.

To achieve a long-term effect of the Champion-Program, it may be therefore necessary to instruct trained supervisors at school who serve as contact persons for all teachers. The fact that this concept can be successful is shown by Vander Ploeg et al. (53) in the evaluation of a comprehensive school health approach. A key component of the intervention was the placement of a full-time school health facilitator at each school, who was dedicated to promoting healthy living. Furthermore, Lahti et al. (52) postulate that education for a sustainable active way of living is possible when interventions are implemented in the daily routine of schools. It therefore may be necessary to strive for sustainable implementation of rope skipping in the daily routine of schools. Offering lessons in shorter bouts must not necessarily harm the effectiveness of the Champion-Program. In their systematic review, Barr-Anderson et al. (54) highlight that short, 10–15-min, bouts daily can increase physical activity—if these bouts are implemented in the daily routine of schools.

Taken these findings together, several points impair the proposed project goal, specifically the sustainable motivation of children to be physically active all their lives. Therefore, we recommend considering the following suggestions in the future program planning of *Skipping Hearts*: The Champion-Program should be conducted according to the guidelines of the German Heart Foundation and should be implemented in the daily routine of schools after the end of the project to obtain sustained rope skipping. The project should also force the transfer of knowledge about health behavior, and all involved teachers should undergo specific training. Furthermore, a supervisor should be provided for all schools, who serves as a contact person if problems occur while implementing the project. Teachers should directly motivate pupils to practice rope skipping as part of their school routine (e.g., during their school break) and should integrate parents further into the project (e.g., practicing together at home). Nevertheless, the easy and uncomplicated character of the *Skipping Hearts* project should remain unchanged. With rope skipping, the project offers a physical activity that can be performed in children's everyday life without high costs.

The results are limited due to the non-randomized design of the study, specified by Postler et al. (28). *Skipping Hearts* is not a scientifically supported and controlled intervention but a school project that was carried out under everyday conditions. In addition, the long-term evaluation of *Skipping Hearts* was added subsequently to the short-term evaluation. Therefore, the recruitment of the "original" sample turned out to be very time-consuming and difficult. Since the previous evaluation was not designed for the long-term, there were no contact details for the participants. Children could no longer be reached via the former elementary schools, as they had meanwhile moved on to a secondary school. Therefore, intensive research was carried out in all secondary schools in the catchment area of the former primary schools, and a variety of measures were undertaken to provide information about the continuation of this short-term evaluation. Nevertheless, the missing data could have biased the results. Given that the follow-up examination was voluntary and took place in the afternoon, compounded with the problem that many children could not even be invited due to missing personal data, the participation rate of 43.3% is quite successful. Furthermore, baseline differences between children with and without follow-up of the anthropometric parameter and motor skills could have led to biased results. It should be noted that children answered the questionnaire on their own without the control of teachers or parents. Restrictions regarding the project itself are described in Postler et al. (28). Although good reliability is reported for near-infrared technology in children and adolescents, body fat measured with near-infrared technology is overestimated compared to densitometry by hydrostatic weighing (33). However, the same measurement methodology was applied at all measurement points, as the NIR is suitable for longitudinal studies. The socio-economic status of the parents, the migration background, and the nutritional behavior of the children were not sufficiently investigated in this study. These confounding factors could influence both the collected parameters and the effectiveness of *Skipping Hearts*, which we did not record within this study.

In summary, the observed short-term effects of *Skipping Hearts* could not be confirmed after 3 years. We did not observe long-term effects on children's cardiovascular health, motor skills, physical activity, or quality of life. Nevertheless, *Skipping Hearts* can certainly be used as an initial impulse, but for a long-term effect, the project needs to be revised and schools should be more proactive regarding the promotion of students' health. In addition, every program promoting physical activity and motor skills in youth should strive for the long-term, and intervention studies should test a sustainable effect.

ETHICS STATEMENT

The studies involving human participants were reviewed and approved by German Sport University Cologne (project number 113/2014). Written informed consent to participate in this study was provided by the participants' legal guardian/next of kin.

AUTHOR CONTRIBUTIONS

TP, CG, NF, RO-F, and TS designed the study. LB, TP, and TS performed the data collection. BH performed the data analysis. LB and TP assisted in data analysis and drafted the manuscript. All authors reviewed, edited, and approved the manuscript.

ACKNOWLEDGMENTS

We thank all students and colleagues, especially Tobias Engl and Michael Meyer (Institute of Preventive Pediatrics, Technical University of Munich), for their tireless engagement during data collection and processing. Furthermore, we thank all the children, parents, teachers, and headmasters who participated in this study.

REFERENCES

Andersen LB, Riddoch C, Kriemler S, Hills AP. Physical activity and cardiovascular risk factors in children. *Br J Sports Med.* (2011) 45:871– 6. doi: 10.1136/bjsports-2011-090333

Jimenez-Pavon D, Konstabel K, Bergman P, Ahrens W, Pohlabeln H, Hadjigeorgiou C, et al. Physical activity and clustered cardiovascular disease risk factors in young children: a cross-sectional study (the IDEFICS study). *BMC Med.* (2013) 11:172. doi: 10.1186/1741-7015-11-172

Dalene KE, Anderssen SA, Andersen LB, Steene-Johannessen J, Ekelund U, Hansen BH, et al. Cross-sectional and prospective associations between physical activity, body mass index and waist circumference in children and adolescents. *Obes Sci Pract.* (2017) 3:249–57. doi: 10.1002/osp4.114

Janssen I, Leblanc AG. Systematic review of the health benefits of physical activity and fitness in school-aged children and youth. *Int J Behav Nutr Phy.* (2010) 7:40. doi: 10.1186/1479-5868-7-40

Knowles G, Pallan M, Thomas GN, Ekelund U, Cheng KK, Barrett T, et al. Physical activity and blood pressure in primary school children: a longitudinal study. *Hypertension.* (2013) 61:70–5. doi: 10.1161/HYPERTENSIONAHA.112.201277

Tremblay MS, LeBlanc AG, Kho ME, Saunders TJ, Larouche R, Colley RC, et al. Systematic review of sedentary behaviour and health indicators in school-aged children and youth. *Int J Behav Nutr Phys Act.* (2011) 8:98. doi: 10.1186/1479-5868-8-98

Weihrauch-Bluher S, Schwarz P, Klusmann JH. Childhood obesity: increased risk for cardiometabolic disease and cancer in adulthood. *Metabolis.* (2019) 92:147–52. doi: 10.1016/j.metabol.2018.12.001

Ward ZJ, Long MW, Resch SC, Giles CM, Cradock AL, Gortmaker SL. Simulation of growth trajectories of childhood obesity into Adulthood. *New Engl J Med.* (2017) 377:2145–53. doi: 10.1056/NEJMoa1703860

World Health Organization. *Global Recommendations on Physical Activity for Health.* Geneva: World Health Organization (2010).

Finger JD, Varnaccia G, Borrmann A, Lange C, Mensink G. Körperliche Aktivität von Kindern und Jugendlichen in Deutschland - Querschnittsergebnisse aus KiGGS Welle 2 und Trends. *J Health Monitor.* (2018) 3.:24–31. doi: 10.17886/RKI-GBE-2018-006.2

Jekauc D, Reimers AK, Wagner MO, Woll A. Prevalence and socio- demographic correlates of the compliance with the physical activity guidelines in children and adolescents in Germany. *BMC Public Health.* (2012) 12:714. doi: 10.1186/1471-2458-12-714

Fisher A, Reilly JJ, Kelly LA, Montgomery C, Williamson A, Paton JY, et al. Fundamental movement skills and habitual physical activity in young children. *Med Sci Sports Exer.* (2005) 37:684–8. doi:10.1249/01.MSS.0000159138.48107.7D

Iivonen KS, Saakslahti AK, Mehtala A, Villberg JJ, Tammelin TH, Kulmala JS, et al. Relationship between fundamental motor skills and physical activity in 4-year-old preschool children. *Percept Mot Skills.* (2013) 117:627– 46. doi: 10.2466/10.06.PMS.117x22z7

Larouche R, Boyer C, Tremblay MS, Longmuir P. Physical fitness, motor skill, and physical activity relationships in grade 4 to 6 children. *Appl Physiol Nutr Metab.* (2014) 39:553–9. doi: 10.1139/apnm-2013-0371

Wu XY, Han LH, Zhang JH, Luo S, Hu JW, Sun K. The influence of physical activity, sedentary behavior on health-related quality of life among the general population of children and adolescents: a systematic review. *PLoS ONE.* (2017) 12:e0187668. doi: 10.1371/journal.pone.0187668

Finne E, Bucksch J, Lampert T, Kolip P. Physical activity and screen- based media use: cross-sectional associations with health-related quality of life and the role of body satisfaction in a representative sample of German adolescents. *Health Psychol Behav Med.* (2013) 1:15–30. doi: 10.1080/21642850.2013.809313

Dobbins M, Husson H, DeCorby K, LaRocca RL. School-based physical activity programs for promoting physical activity and fitness in children and adolescents aged 6 to 18. *Cochrane DB Syst Rev.* (2013) 2013:Cd007651. doi: 10.1002/14651858.CD007651.pub2

Story M, Nanney MS, Schwartz MB. Schools and obesity prevention: creating school environments and policies to promote healthy eating and physical activity. *Milbank Q.* (2009) 87:71–100. doi: 10.1111/j.1468-0009.2009.00548.x

Pate RR, Davis MG, Robinson TN, Stone EJ, McKenzie TL, Young JC. Promoting physical activity in children and youth: a leadership role for schools: a scientific statement from the American Heart Association Council on nutrition, physical activity, and metabolism (Physical Activity Committee) in collaboration with the councils on cardiovascular disease in the Young and Cardiovascular Nursing. *Circulation.* (2006) 114:1214– 24. doi: 10.1161/CIRCULATIONAHA.106.177052

Brandstetter S, Klenk J, Berg S, Galm C, Fritz M, Peter R, et al. Overweight prevention implemented by primary school teachers: a randomised controlled trial. *Obes Facts.* (2012) 5:1–11. doi: 10.1159/000336255

Lämmle C, Kobel S, Wartha O, Wirt T, Steinacker JM. Intervention effects of a school-based health promotion program on children's motor skills. *Z Gesundh Wiss.* (2016) 24:185–92. doi: 10.1007/s10389-016-0715-x

Kobel S, Wirt T, Schreiber A, Kesztyus D, Kettner S, Erkelenz N, et al. Intervention effects of a school-based health promotion programme on obesity related behavioural outcomes. *J Obes.* (2014) 2014:476230. doi: 10.1155/2014/476230

Drenowatz C, Wartha O, Brandstetter S, Steinacker JM. Effects of a teacher-centred, school-based intervention program on health behavior and cardiovascular disease risk in elementary school children. *ISRN Public Health.* (2013) 2013:513183. doi: 10.1155/2013/513183

Graf C, Koch B, Falkowski G, Jouck S, Christ H, Stauenmaier K, et al. Effects of a school-based intervention on bmi and motor abilities in childhood. *J Sport Sci Med.* (2005) 4:291–9.

Graf C, Koch B, Falkowski G, Jouck S, Christ H, Staudenmaier K, et al. School- based prevention: effects on obesity and physical performance after 4 years. *J Sports Sci.* (2008) 26:987–94. doi: 10.1080/02640410801930176

Love R, Adams J, van Sluijs EMF. Are school-based physical activity interventions effective and equitable? A meta-analysis of cluster randomized controlled trials with accelerometer-assessed activity. *Obes Rev.* (2019) 20:859–70. doi: 10.1111/obr.12823

Pfister G. Traditional games as "Sport for All" - from traditional rope jumping to modern rope skipping. *TAFISA Magazine.* (2008) 10–6.

Postler T, Schulz T, Oberhoffer R. Skipping hearts goes to school: short-term effects. *Dtsch Z Sportmed.* (2017) 68:148–56. doi: 10.5960/dzsm.2017.288

Neuhauser H, Thamm M. Blutdruckmessung im Kinder- und Jugendgesundheitssurvey (KiGGS). *Bundesgesundheitsblatt Gesundheitsforschung Gesundheitsschutz.* (2007) 50:728. doi: 10.1007/s00103-007-0234-6

Kromeyer-Hauschild K, Wabitsch M, Kunze D, Geller F, Geiß HC, Hesse V, et al. Perzentile für den Body-mass-Index für das Kindes- und Jugendalter unter Heranziehung verschiedener deutscher Stichproben. *Monatsschrift Kinderheilkunde.* (2001) 149:807–18. doi: 10.1007/s001120 170107

Neuhauser H, Schienkiewitz A, Rosario AS, Dortschy R, Kurth BM. *Referenzperzentile für Anthropometrische Maßzahlen und Blutdruck aus der Studie zur Gesundheit von Kindern und Jugendlichen in Deutschland (KiGGS).* Berlin: Robert Koch-Institut (2013).

Fthenakis ZG, Balaska D, Zafiropulos V. Uncovering the FUTREX-6100XL prediction equation for the percentage body fat. *J Med Eng Technol.* (2012) 36:351–7. doi: 10.3109/03091902.2012.708382

Cassady SL, Nielsen DH, Janz KF, Wu YT, Cook JS, Hansen JR. Validity of near infrared body composition analysis in children and adolescents. *Med Sci Sports Exerc.* (1993) 25:1185–91. doi: 10.1249/00005768-199310000-00016

Bös K, Schlenker L, Büsch D, Lämmle L, Müller H, Oberger J, et al. *Deutscher Motorik-Test 6–18 (DMT 6–18).* 2nd ed. Hamburg: Czwalina (2016).

Schmidt S, Will N, Henn A, Reimers AK, Woll A. *Der Motorik-Modul Aktivitätsfragebogen MoMo-AFB: Leitfaden zur Anwendung und Auswertung.* Karlsruhe: KIT (2016).

Prochaska JJ, Sallis JF, Long B. A physical activity screening measure for use with adolescents in primary care. *Arch Pediatr Adolesc Med.* (2001) 155:554–9. doi: 10.1001/archpedi.155.5.554

Lampert T, Sygusch R, Schlack R. Nutzung elektronischer medien im jugendalter. *Bundesgesundheitsblatt Gesundheitsforschung Gesundheitsschutz.* (2007) 50:643–52. doi: 10.1007/s00103-007-0225-7

Stone MR, Rowlands AV, Eston RG. Relationships between accelerometer-assessed physical activity and health in children: impact of the activity- intensity classification method. *J Sport Sci Med.* (2009) 8:136–43.

Robertson W, Stewart-Brown S, Wilcock E, Oldfield M, Thorogood M. Utility of accelerometers to measure physical activity in children attending an obesity treatment intervention. *J Obes.* (2011) 2011:398918. doi: 10.1155/2011/398918

Freedson P, Pober D, Janz KF. Calibration of accelerometer output for children. *Med Sci Sports Exer.* (2005) 37:523– 30. doi: 10.1249/01.mss.0000185658.28284.ba

Trost SG, Loprinzi PD, Moore R, Pfeiffer KA. Comparison of accelerometer cut points for predicting activity intensity in youth. *Med Sci Sports Exer.* (2011) 43:1360–8. doi: 10.1249/MSS.0b013e318206476e

Choi L, Liu Z, Matthews CE, Buchowski MS. Validation of accelerometer wear and nonwear time classification algorithm. *Med Sci Sports Exer.* (2011) 43:357–64. doi: 10.1249/MSS.0b013e3181ed61a3

Ravens-Sieberer U, Bullinger M. Assessing health-related quality of life in chronically ill children with the German KINDL: first psychometric and content analytical results. *Qual Life Res.* (1998) 7:399–407. doi: 10.1023/A:1008853819715

Bullinger M, Brütt AL, Erhart M, Ravens-Sieberer U, the BSG. Psychometric properties of the KINDL-R questionnaire: results of the BELLA study. *Eur Child Adolesc Psychiatry.* (2008) 17:125–32. doi: 10.1007/s00787-008-1014-z

Ravens-Sieberer U, Ellert U, Erhart M. *Gesundheitsbezogene Lebensqualität von Kindern und Jugendlichen in Deutschland: Eine Normstichprobe für Deutschland aus dem Kinder- und Jugendgesundheitssurvey (KIGGS).* Berlin: Robert Koch-Institut; Epidemiologie und Gesundheitsberichterstattung (2007). doi: 10.1007/s00103-007-0244-4

Farooq MA, Parkinson KN, Adamson AJ, Pearce MS, Reilly JK, Hughes AR, et al. Timing of the decline in physical activity in childhood and adolescence: gateshead millennium cohort study. *Brit J Sport Med.* (2017) 52:1002–6. doi: 10.1136/bjsports-2016-096933

Dumith SC, Gigante DP, Domingues MR, Kohl HW. Physical activity change during adolescence: a systematic review and a pooled analysis. *Int J Epidemiol.* (2011) 40:685–98. doi: 10.1093/ije/dyq272

Martins J, Marques A, Loureiro N, da Costa FC, Diniz J, de Matos MG. Trends and age-related changes of physical activity among portuguese adolescent girls from 2002-2014: highlights from the health behavior in school-aged children study. *J Phys Act Health.* (2019) 16:281–7. doi: 10.1123/jpah.2018-0092

Rutten C, Boen F, Seghers J. Changes in physical activity and sedentary behavior during the transition from elementary to secondary school. *J Phys Act Health.* (2014) 11:1607–13. doi: 10.1123/jpah.2012-0465

Meyer U, Schindler C, Zahner L, Ernst D, Hebestreit H, van Mechelen W, et al. Long-term effect of a school-based physical activity program (KISS) on fitness and adiposity in children: a cluster-randomized controlled trial. *PLoS ONE.* (2014) 9:e87929. doi: 10.1371/journal.pone. 0087929

Anderson EL, Howe LD, Kipping RR, Campbell R, Jago R, Noble SM, et al. Long-term effects of the Active for Life Year 5 (AFLY5) school-based cluster-randomised controlled trial. *BMJ Open.* (2016) 6:e010957. doi: 10.1136/bmjopen-2015-010957

Lahti A, Rosengren BE, Nilsson JA, Karlsson C, Karlsson MK. Long- term effects of daily physical education throughout compulsory school on duration of physical activity in young adulthood: an 11- year prospective controlled study. *BMJ Open Sport Exerc Med.* (2018) 4:e000360. doi: 10.1136/bmjsem-2018-000360

Vander Ploeg KA, McGavock J, Maximova K, Veugelers PJ. School-based health promotion and physical activity during and after school hours. *Pediatrics.* (2014) 133:e371–8. doi: 10.1542/peds.2013-2383

Barr-Anderson DJ, AuYoung M, Whitt-Glover MC, Glenn BA, Yancey AK. Integration of short bouts of physical activity into organizational routine a systematic review of the literature. *Am J Prev Med.* (2011) 40:76– 93. doi: 10.1016/j.amepre.2010.09.033

10

Longitudinal Study of Individual Exercises in Elite Rhythmic Gymnastics

Elena Sierra-Palmeiro[1], Marta Bobo-Arce[1], Alexandra Pérez-Ferreirós[2] and María A. Fernández-Villarino[2]*

[1] *Department of Physical Education and Sports, Faculty of Sports Science and Physical Education, University of A Coruña, A Coruña, Spain,* [2] *Department of Especial Teaching, Faculty of Education and Sports Sciences, University of Vigo, Pontevedra, Spain*

***Correspondence:**
Elena Sierra-Palmeiro
elena.sierra@udc.es

The performance evolution in rhythmic gymnastics depends on changes in code of points. At the beginning of each Olympic cycle the code of points changes and therefore, the content of the competition exercises, as well. This study aimed to analyze – for each apparatus – the evolution of number of technical elements and final score over the last two decades (last 13 world championships), how they have been affected by changed code of points, and how the final score relates to the number of technical elements performed. The sample consisted of 416 exercises in five apparatus: ball (96), rope (40), hoop (96), ribbon (88), and clubs (96). The following variables were gathered: code of points, apparatus, technical group, total number of elements, final classification, and final score. Linear mixed-effects models were used to examine the effects on the number of elements and final score in each apparatus. The number of technical elements increased in all apparatus, between 7.4 and 20% over a 10-year period. There were mixed evolutions of final score between the different apparatus, between −6.3 and 14% over a 10-year period. There is small increase in number of elements in hoop and a small decrease in rope after a code change. There was a small decrease in final score in championships after a code change in hoop, moderate in clubs and ribbon, and large in rope. There was a negative relationship between number of elements performed and final score in clubs. In conclusion, the code change generally effects the final score negatively, but there were apparatus specific effects of code change on number of elements and relationship between number of elements and final score.

Keywords: code of points, apparatus, technical elements, performance analysis, rule change, world championship

INTRODUCTION

Rhythmic gymnastics is a sport that combines technical, aesthetic, and artistic parameters with the aim of reproducing an optimal execution model, both in matter of form and execution (Díaz-Pereira et al., 2014). When a gymnast performs her competition routine, she coordinates her body movements with handling of an apparatus (ball, clubs, tape, hoop or rope) in a choreographic composition accompanied by music.

The optimal execution model that the gymnast strive for is determined by both quantitative and qualitative criteria specified in the code of points. The code of points is set by the International Gymnastics Federation and are updated each Olympic cycle. It is therefore, considered the basis for the internal logic of the sport or strategy (the possibilities of interaction of gymnast with space, time, apparatus, with other gymnast, and with the criteria of success or failure), as well as a key factor when composing the competition routines and practice planning (Ávila-Carvalho et al., 2012a; Massidda and Calò, 2012; Leandro et al., 2017).

In the last 20 years, the International Gymnastics Federation has made numerous changes to the code of points aiming to increase the objectivity of the judges scoring, and to stimulate the development of the sport. These code changes have resulted in structural changes to the competition routines. For example, Ávila-Carvalho et al. (2011) have shown that the compositions of the routines have evolved toward increasing the difficulty and variety in body movements, and toward a higher technical mastery and enrichment in the apparatus handling.

In an attempt to understand the competitive model and performance in the rhythmic gymnastics, several studies have analyzed the composition of competition routines, both in group and individual events (Ávila-Carvalho et al., 2011, 2012a; Trifunov and Slovodanka, 2013; Agopyan, 2014). However, most have analyzed a single competition, and none have considered the changes in the code of points over time. Moreover, they have focused solely on the artistic content or on the difficulty of the body movements. Further, the results of these studies have highlighted the constant and rapid evolution of the sport, stressing the need to continuously perform these kind of studies (Čuk et al., 2012; Hökelmann et al., 2012; Massidda and Calò, 2012; Bučar et al., 2013; Pelin, 2013).

Given the limitations in earlier studies, there is a need for longitudinal studies analyzing the evolution of competition routine compositions and performance over time, which would provide valuable new information on the factors affecting the performance in rhythmic gymnastics (Ávila-Carvalho et al., 2012b; Leandro et al., 2017). Further, it could provide new insight into the effects of changes to the code of points on the performance. Finally, it would provide valuable insights for rhythmic gymnastics coaches, enabling them to make more informed decisions when planning practices and learning activities to improve the skills in each apparatus. This study aims to analyze – for each apparatus – the evolution of number of technical elements and final score over the last two decades (last 13 world championships), how they have been affected by changed code of points, and how the final score relates to the number of technical elements performed.

MATERIALS AND METHODS

Sample

The sample consisted of 416 individual rhythmic gymnastics routines performed in the final round of each apparatus in the last 13 rhythmic gymnastics world championships (1997–2018). The total sample comprised 96 ball, 96 clubs, 96 hoop, 88 ribbon, and 40 rope routines. Only four of the apparatus are used in each competition, with the International Gymnastics Federation choosing which are to be included before each championship. Which apparatus were used in each championship is presented in **Table 1**. Eight routines were performed in all final rounds for each apparatus and championship. The study was conducted in accordance with the ethical standards of sports science (Harris and Atkinson, 2009). The study did not require an ethical committee approval, as only publicly available data was used.

Procedure and Variables

Video recordings of all routines were obtained from the International Gymnastics Federation website[1]. All recordings were checked to ensure that the entire surface of the floor and the gymnast's performance were visible throughout the routine. Two international rhythmic gymnastics judges (Ph.D. in sports science and rhythmic gymnastics) with at least of 15 years of international judging experience observed the recordings and counted the number of elements performed in each routine. The final score was taken from the official records on the International Gymnastics Federation website. The year, apparatus, code of points used, number of elements, and final score was registered for each routine.

Each apparatus has a number of technical groups determined by the code of points (**Table 2**). The judges recorded the elements performed within each technical group of the apparatus used for the routine. The sum of elements in all technical groups was then considered as the total number of elements in the routine. To assess the reliability, 10 randomly chosen routines (two for each apparatus) were observed by both judges. After a period of 2 weeks, the routines were re-observed. The inter-rater reliability was, for ball ICC(2,1) = 1, clubs ICC(2,1) = 0.98, hoop ICC(2,1) = 1, ribbon ICC(2,1) = 0.96, rope = 0.87. The intra-rater reliability was, for ball ICC(2,1) = 0.96, clubs ICC(2,1) = 1, hoop ICC(2,1) = 1, ribbon ICC(2,1) = 0.96, rope = 0.87.

The code of points was transformed into a dichotomous variable (code change), indicating whether the code of points used was the same as in the previous championship or had changed. No change of code of points was considered as reference in all analyses. As the maximal obtainable score varied between the different code of points, all scores were rescaled to a maximum of 20 points, which is the maximum score. To measure the evolution over time, a continuous variable indicating the year of the championship was used. The maximum point and whether the code of points changed for each championship is presented in **Table 1**.

Statistical Analysis

All statistical analyses and graphics were produced using R 3.5.1. The mean and standard deviation (SD) for each apparatus and championship are presented graphically together with the occurrence of code change.

[1] www.gymnastics.sport

TABLE 1 | Code change, maximum score, and apparatus used in each championship.

Championship	Code change	Maximum score	Ball	Clubs	Hoop	Ribbon	Rope
Berlin 1997	Change	10	✓	–	✓	✓	✓
Madrid 2001	Change	30	✓	✓	✓	–	✓
Budapest 2003	Stable	30	✓	✓	✓	✓	–
Baku 2005	Change	20	✓	✓	✓	✓	–
Patras 2007	Stable	20	–	✓	✓	✓	✓
Mie 2009	Change	30	✓	✓	–	✓	✓
Moscow 2010	Stable	30	✓	✓	✓	–	✓
Montpelier 2011	Stable	30	✓	✓	✓	✓	–
Kiev 2013	Change	20	✓	✓	✓	✓	–
Izmir 2014	Stable	20	✓	✓	✓	✓	–
Stuttgart 2015	Stable	20	✓	✓	✓	✓	–
Pesaro 2017	Change	20	✓	✓	✓	✓	–
Sofia 2018	Stable	20	✓	✓	✓	✓	–

Linear mixed-effects models were used to assess the evolution over time and the effects of code change on the number of elements performed. A linear model was fitted to predict the number of elements for each apparatus, including year as continuous, and code change as dichotomous fixed effects. The models included random intercepts for the individual gymnasts, as well as for each competition. Further, linear mixed-effects models were also used to assess the evolution over time, effect of code change and of number of elements on the final score. A linear model was fitted to predict the final score for each apparatus, including year as continuous, code change as dichotomous, and number of elements as continuous fixed effects. The models included random intercepts for the individual gymnasts, as well as for each competition.

By using regression modeling, it is possible to assess the specific effects of each variable, accounting for the influence of the other ones. As each apparatus comprise its own independent competition, a model was fitted to each of them in both cases. To account for repeated measures of the same gymnast in several championships, gymnast was included as a random factor in the model. To account for the potential influence of different maximum scores in the championships on final score and number of elements, it was included as a fixed factor.

Initially, all two-way interactions were included in the model. However, the interaction between year and number of elements had no effect on the final score and was therefore excluded from the final models. The assumptions of normality and homoscedasticity of residuals were checked by inspecting qq-plots, plots of residual vs. predicted values, residuals vs. predictors and SDs for the different levels of the predictors. The inspection did not reveal violations of the assumptions.

The difference in number of elements and final score between championships with and without code change are presented using estimated marginal means, with 95% confidence intervals (CI). The evolution of number of elements and final score over a 10-year time period is presented by multiplying the simple effect of year by 10 and are also expressed as percentages of the grand mean. This is done both overall for the full sample and comparing between championships with and without code change. Finally, the relationship between final score and number of elements are presented as standardized effect sizes by multiplying the simple effects of number of elements by two SD of the number of elements in the original sample. Standardized effect sizes were also calculated by dividing the difference by the SD derived from all random variance components of the models (Westfall et al., 2014). The standardized effect sized for the number of elements are interpreted as small (≥0.2), moderate (≥0.6), large (≥1.2), very large (≥2.0) and extremely large (≥4.0) (Hopkins et al., 2009). For final score, the standardized effect sizes are interpreted as small (≥0.3), moderate (≥0.9), large (≥1.6), very large (≥2.5) and extremely large (≥4.0) (Malcata and Hopkins, 2014).

RESULTS

The mean and SD of number of elements and final score for each championship and apparatus are presented in **Figures 1, 2**. The evolution over time, together with indications of when

TABLE 2 | Technical groups in each apparatus.

Apparatus	Technical groups
Ball	Throws and catches, bounces, roll on the floor, roll over body segments, unstable balance, and handling.
Clubs	Small circles, mills, throws and catches, tappings, asymmetric movements, unstable balance, and handling.
Hoop	Roll on the floor, roll over body segments, rotations, throws and catches, passing through, passing over, unstable balance, and handling.
Ribbon	Spirals, snakes, throws and catches, boomerang throw, releases, passing through, passing over, and handling.
Rope	Passing through with jump, passing through with a part of body, throws and catches, releases and catches, rotations, unstable balance, and handling.

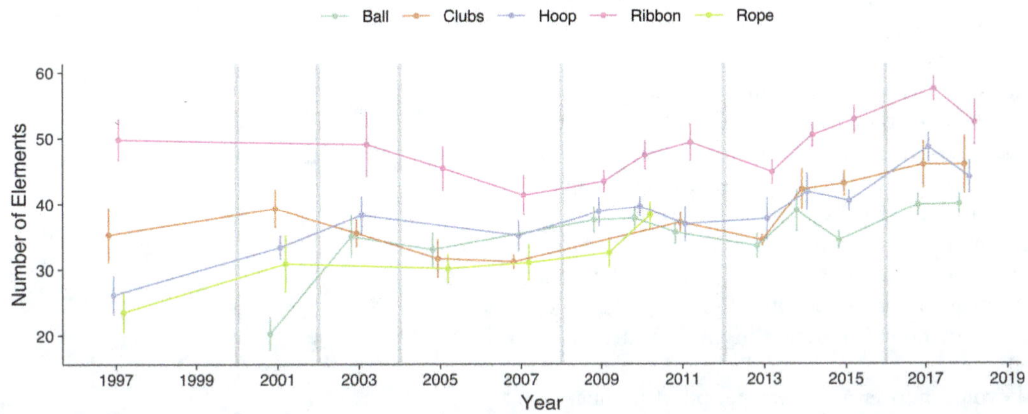

FIGURE 1 | Evolution of average number of elements with standard deviation for each apparatus. Vertical lines indicate code change.

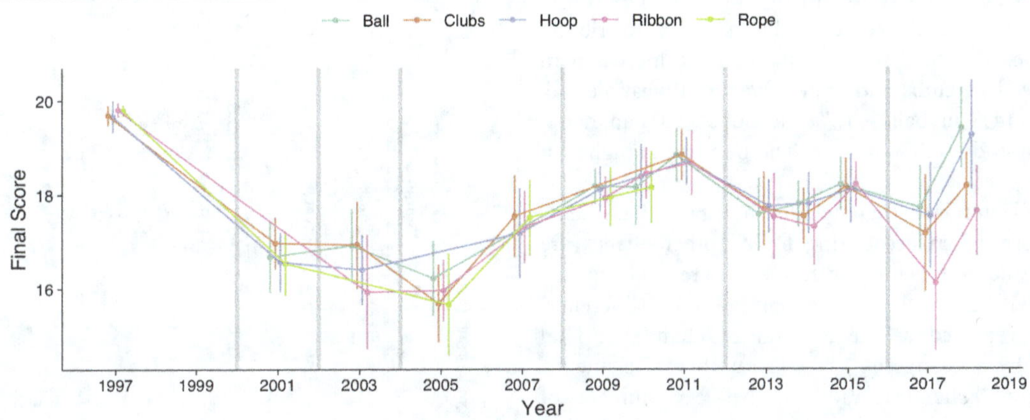

FIGURE 2 | Evolution of average final score with standard deviation for each apparatus. Vertical lines indicate code change.

TABLE 3 | Estimated means with and without code change for number of elements and final score.

	No code change			Code change								
		95% CI			95% CI			95% CI			95% CI	
	Estimate	**Lower**	**Upper**	**Estimate**	**Lower**	**Upper**	**Difference**	**Lower**	**Upper**	**ES**	**Lower**	**Upper**
Number of elements												
Ball	35.8	27.0	44.5	35.3	30.1	40.6	−0.4	−11.1	10.2	−0.1	−1.6	1.4
Clubs	38.3	32.8	43.8	37.9	32.2	43.6	−0.4	−8.7	7.8	0.0	−1.0	0.9
Hoop	37.4	34.9	39.9	39.7	36.8	42.6	2.3	−1.7	6.4	0.4	−0.3	1.1
Ribbon	48.7	44.3	53.0	48.4	43.3	53.6	−0.3	−7.1	6.6	0.0	−0.9	0.9
Rope	32.0	16.2	47.7	30.1	14.8	45.4	−1.9	−28.1	24.4	−0.3	−5.0	4.3
Final score												
Ball	17.5	17.0	18.1	17.5	17.2	17.9	0.0	−0.7	0.7	0.0	−0.5	0.6
Clubs	18.6	17.7	19.4	16.9	16.0	17.8	−1.7	−3.0	−0.4	−0.9	−1.7	−0.2
Hoop	18.3	17.5	19.2	17.4	16.5	18.4	−0.9	−2.2	0.4	−0.5	−1.2	0.2
Ribbon	18.2	17.8	18.6	16.6	16.1	17.0	−1.6	−2.2	−1.0	−1.1	−1.5	−0.7
Rope	19.0	16.1	21.8	16.1	13.6	18.6	−2.9	−9.0	3.2	−2.1	−6.6	2.4

CI, confidence interval; ES, effect size.

code changes occurred are presented graphically for number of elements (**Figure 1**) and final score (**Figure 2**).

The estimated means of number of elements and final score for championships with and without code change, when accounting for change over time and number of elements, are presented in **Table 3** together with the raw and standardized difference. There is no clear general difference in number of elements between championships with and without code change. There is small increase in number of elements in hoop and a small decrease in rope after a code change. The final score is generally lower in championships after a code change, with small difference in hoop, moderate in clubs and ribbon, and large in rope.

The estimated evolution over a 10-year period of number of elements and final score, when accounting for all other effects, are presented in **Table 4**. Moreover, the estimated evolution for championships with and without code change, as well as difference are also presented in **Table 4**. The number of elements has increased for all apparatus. Over a 10-year period, it increased 20% in ball, 12% in clubs, 20% in hoop, 7.4% in ribbon and 13% in rope. The final score seems to have increased in ball and decreased in clubs and rope. Over a 10-year period, the change was 14% in ball, −1.7% in clubs, 2.8% in hoop, −0.6% in ribbon and −6.3% in rope. The increase is higher in ribbon and rope.

The estimated standardized effect of number of elements on the final score, when accounting for all other effects, are presented in **Table 5** together with the separate effects for championships with and without code change and the difference. The effects are reported as the amount of change in final score produced by a change of 2 SD in number of elements. There is no clear general relationship between number of elements performed and final score. The only clear relationship is a negative one in clubs. In ball there is a small difference, with a negative relationship in championships without rule change, and a positive relationship in championships with code change. In rope, there is also a small difference, with a positive relationship in championships without rule change, and a negative relationship in championships with code change.

DISCUSSION

The aims of this study were to analyze the evolution of the performance in rhythmic gymnastics in the last two decades and describe how the number of technical elements performed with the apparatus are related to the performance of the gymnasts. In general, the changes to the code of points have affected the number of technical elements performed and the final score differently for the different apparatus. The relationship between number of technical elements and final score were also apparatus specific. According to Ávila-Carvalho et al. (2012b), the technical apparatus elements used in the routine composition varies according to the type of apparatus, stressing the importance of studying each apparatus separately. If the

TABLE 4 | Estimated 10-year evolution overall, with and without code change for number of elements and final score.

				No code change			Code change								
		95% CI			95% CI			95% CI			95% CI			95% CI	
	Estimate	Lower	Upper	Estimate	Lower	Upper	Estimate	Lower	Upper	Difference	Lower	Upper	ES	Lower	Upper
Number of elements															
Ball	7.1	−7.9	22.1	5.4	−18.8	29.6	8.8	−1.6	19.3	3.4	−18.8	25.6	0.5	−2.7	3.6
Clubs	4.7	−1.0	10.5	5.9	−2.6	14.4	3.5	−6.9	14.0	−2.4	−17.6	12.9	−0.3	−2.0	1.5
Hoop	7.6	4.6	10.6	7.8	3.7	12.0	7.3	1.9	12.8	−0.5	−8.0	7.1	−0.1	−1.4	1.2
Ribbon	3.6	−2.3	9.6	3.1	−4.3	10.5	4.2	−6.3	14.6	1.0	−12.6	14.6	0.1	−1.7	1.9
Rope	4.1	−27.7	35.8	6.3	−39.5	52.2	1.8	−42.2	45.7	−4.6	−68.2	59.0	−0.8	−12.1	10.4
Final score															
Ball	2.5	1.6	3.5	3.2	1.7	4.7	1.9	1.1	2.6	−1.4	−2.8	0.1	−0.2	−0.4	0.0
Clubs	−0.3	−1.2	0.7	−1.2	−2.6	0.2	0.7	−1.0	2.4	1.8	−0.7	4.3	0.2	−0.1	0.5
Hoop	0.5	−0.6	1.5	−0.2	−1.6	1.2	1.1	−0.7	3.0	1.3	−1.2	3.9	0.2	−0.2	0.7
Ribbon	−0.1	−0.7	0.5	−1.4	−2.1	−0.7	1.2	0.3	2.2	2.7	1.4	4.0	0.4	0.2	0.5
Rope	−1.1	−6.1	4.0	−3.5	−8.8	1.7	1.4	−10.4	13.3	5.0	−4.5	14.5	0.9	−0.8	2.6

CI, confidence interval; ES, effect size.

TABLE 5 | Estimated effect of two standard deviation change in number of elements on final score overall, with and without rule change.

					No code change			Code change							
		95% CI			95% CI			95% CI			95% CI			95% CI	
	Estimate	Lower	Upper	Estimate	Lower	Upper	Estimate	Lower	Upper	Estimate	Lower	Upper	ES	Lower	Upper
Ball	0.3	−0.4	1.1	−0.4	−1.6	0.8	1.1	0.1	2.0	1.5	0.0	3.0	0.3	0.0	0.5
Clubs	−0.6	−1.2	0.1	−0.3	−1.1	0.6	−0.9	−1.8	0.1	−0.6	−1.8	0.6	−0.1	−0.3	0.1
Hoop	0.0	−0.5	0.6	0.3	−0.7	1.3	−0.2	−0.8	0.4	−0.5	−1.7	0.6	−0.1	−0.2	0.1
Ribbon	0.2	−0.4	0.8	0.2	−0.6	1.0	0.2	−0.7	1.1	0.0	−1.1	1.2	0.0	−0.1	0.1
Rope	−0.1	−0.6	0.3	1.0	0.4	1.7	−1.3	−2.0	−0.7	−2.3	−3.2	−1.4	−0.3	−0.4	−0.2

CI, confidence interval; ES, effect size.

work with an apparatus implies a technique and a specific coordination with the body, it also implies specific motor and physical performance (Botti and Nascimento, 2011). However, care should be taken when interpreting the results for rope, as it has not been present in any world championship since 2010.

During the two decades observed, the number of technical elements has increased for all apparatus. This suggests that the impact of apparatus skills on the final score has increased, as well as the coordination between the movement of the apparatus and body (Tsopani et al., 2012). In the same way, this increase has meant that each modification to the code of points have sought an increased precision in the performance evaluation criteria. There was no clear effect of code change on the number of elements or its evolution over time, which might mean that the code changes had not substantial effect on the number of elements. It might also mean that the different code changes affected the number of elements differently. Leandro et al. (2015) points out that the updates to the code of points are directed toward increasing the complexity of the interaction between the gymnast and the apparatus in the routines, either through an increase in number of elements or the degree of coordination difficulty. The characteristics of the specific apparatus might affect the amount of possible ways for the gymnasts to interact with the apparatus.

In championships with a new code of points, the final score decreased. That is, a code change significantly affects the performance of the gymnasts, who must modify their workouts and learn new possible technical elements. Aspects such as the variety and diversity of the compositions can be compromised, and until a stabilization of the score code occurs, the richness and spectacularity of the compositions diminish. Similarly, a code change means both new evaluation criteria and implementations, as well as the fact that new technical elements are introduced. All this contributes to the quality of the artistic composition of a routine and to the development of the sport (Levre, 2011). Leandro et al. (2017) point out the difficulty of making an accurate judgment in the elements of the apparatus. Particularly, the technical elements of the apparatus, such as masters, are considered by the judges to be less objective to evaluate. The work with the apparatus sometimes demands an extraordinary coordination, perfect technical control and specificity that hinder the work of the judge. Each new code change requires a search by the coaches for skilful interaction (gymnast-apparatus) and the increase of technical elements of the apparatus in the compositions, with the aim of improving the performance in competition. In the same way, for the judges it requires the definition of new objective criteria that allows a correct and precise evaluation of the performance.

As for the relationship between number of elements and final score, the only clear findings were that higher number of elements relates to lower final score in clubs. As pointed out above, the specific characteristics of each apparatus affects the relationship between number of elements and final score. There seem to be a more positive relationship between number of elements and final score in competitions with rule change in ball and a negative one in rope. Probably, as with the hoop and clubs, the characteristics of the ball and the rope would allow us to understand this relationship. However, the lack of data related to rope does not allow us to have an objective assessment (it has not been in competition for the last 8 years).

The present study has some limitations that should be considered. The analysis of competition routines should also focus on qualitative aspects of the technical elements of each apparatus, such as variety and diversity. These aspects are determining factors in the quality and richness of the compositions and they contribute to the development and evolution of the sport, and therefore its modernization. Therefore, an evaluation of judges and coaches on the changes that the code of points makes, both in the training models and in the evaluation criteria, would increase the perspective of analysis of the presented data.

CONCLUSION

Throughout the evaluated period, the number of technical elements of the apparatus that the gymnasts perform in their competition routines has increased, although each time the code of points change the performance of the gymnasts decreases. With each Olympic cycle new forms of coordination between gymnast and apparatus must be developed, which has increased the repercussion of the technical elements of the apparatus in the score of the competition routines and the complexity of the compositions.

This type of analysis provides information about the performance indicators as well as knowing how they are affected by the changes in the code of points. This information can be used by coaches to improve the composition strategies of the exercises, both increasing the complexity of the technical elements and the interaction between gymnast and apparatus. It also provides information to the judges for the definition of new evaluation criteria that allows a better adjustment of the evaluation in competition.

AUTHOR CONTRIBUTIONS

All authors participated in the study design, documentation, development, and writing of the manuscript.

REFERENCES

Agopyan, A. (2014). Analysis of the body movement difficulties of individual elite rhythmic gymnastics at London 2012 Olympic games finals. *J. Sci. Res.* 19, 1554–1565.

Ávila-Carvalho, L., Klentrou, P., and Levre, E. (2012a). Handling, throws, catches and collaborations in elite group rhythmic gymnastics. *Sci. Gymnastics J.* 4, 37–47.

Ávila-Carvalho, L., Klentrou, P., Palomero, M., and Levre, E. (2012b). Analysis of the technical content of elite rhythmic gymnastics group routines. *Open Sports Sci. J.* 5, 146–153. doi: 10.2174/1875399x01205010146

Ávila-Carvalho, L., Palomero, M., and Levre, E. (2011). Estudio del valor artístico de los ejercicios de conjunto de Gimnasia Rítmica de la Copa del Mundo de Portimao 2017 y 2008. *Apunts Educ. Física y Deporte* 103, 68–75.

Botti, M., and Nascimento, J. V. (2011). The teaching-learning-training process in rhythmic gymnastics supported by the ecological theory. *Sci. Gymnastics J.* 3, 35–48.

Bučar, M., Čuk, I., Pajek, J., Kovac, M., and Leskosek, B. (2013). Is the quality of judging in women artistic gymnastics equivalent at major competitions of different levels? *J. Hum. Kinet.* 37, 173–181. doi: 10.2478/hukin-2013-0038

Čuk, I., Fink, H., and Leskošek, B. (2012). Modeling the final score in artistic gymnastics by different weights of difficulty and execution. *Sci. Gymnastics J.* 4, 73–82.

Díaz- Pereira, M. P., Gómez-Conde, I., Escalona, M., and Olivieri, D. M. (2014). Automatic recognition and scoring of olympic rythmic gymnastic movements. *Hum. Mov. Sci.* 34, 63–80. doi: 10.1016/j.humov.2014.01.001

Harris, D. J., and Atkinson, G. (2009). Ethical standards in sport and exercise science research. *Int. J. Sport Med.* 30, 701–702. doi: 10.1055/s-0029-1237378

Hökelmann, A., Breitkreutz, T., and Livioty, G. (2012). "Changes in performance structure during group competitions in rhythmic gymnastics," in *Book of Abstracts of the World Congress of the Performance Analysis of Sport IX*, eds M. Peters and P. O. Ďonoghue (Worcester: University of Worcester).

Hopkins, W. G., Marshall, S. W., Batterham, A. M., and Hanin, J. (2009). Progressive statistics for studies in sports medicine and exercise science. *Med. Sci. Sports Exerc.* 41, 3–12. doi: 10.1249/MSS.0b013e31818cb278

Leandro, C., Ávila-Carvalho, L., Sierra-Palmeiro, E., and Bobo Arce, M. (2015). Accuracyin judgment the difficulty score in elite rhythmic gymnastics individual routines. *Sci. Gymnastics J.* 7, 81–93.

Leandro, C., Ávila-Carvalho, L., Sierra-Palmeiro, E., and Bobo Arce, M. (2017). Judging in rhythmic gymnastics at diferente levels of performance. *J. Hum. Kinet.* 60, 159–165. doi: 10.1515/hukin-2017-0099

Levre, E. (2011). *Technical principles for the new framework. Crossroads to the future.* Switzerland: International Federation of Gymnastics Scientific Commission, 1–8.

Malcata, R. M., and Hopkins, W. G. (2014). Variability of competitive performance of elite athletes: a systematic review. *Sports Med.* 44, 1763–1774. doi: 10.1007/s40279-014-0239-x

Massidda, M., and Calò, M. C. (2012). Performance scores and standings during the 43rd artistic gymnastics world championships, 2011. *J. Sports Sci.* 30, 1415–1420. doi: 10.1080/02640414.2012.710759

Pelin, R. A. (2013). Studies regarding the rhythmic gymnastics from the olympic games. *Sport Soc.* 13:61. doi: 10.1136/bjsports-2017-09 7972

Trifunov, T., and Slovodanka, D. (2013). The structure of difficulties in the routines of the best world and serbian rhythmic gymnastics. *Fizička Kultura* 67, 120–129. doi: 10.5937/fizkul1302120t

Tsopani, D., Dallas, G., Tasika, N., and Tinto, A. (2012). The effect of different teaching system in learning rhythmic gymnastics apparatus motor skills. *Sci. Gymnastics J.* 4, 55–62.

Westfall, J., Kenny, D. A., and Judd, C. M. (2014). Statistical power and optimal design in experiments in which samples of participants respond to samples of stimuli. *J. Exp. Psychol. Gen.* 143, 2020–2045. doi: 10.1037/xge000 0014

11

Intervention Effects of a Kindergarten-Based Health Promotion Programme on Motor Abilities in Early Childhood

Susanne Kobel[1], Lea Henle[2], Christine Laemmle[1], Olivia Wartha[1], Bertram Szagun[2] and Juergen Michael Steinacker[1]*

[1] Division of Sports and Rehabilitation Medicine, Department of Internal Medicine, University Hospital Ulm, Ulm, Germany,
[2] Faculty Social Work, Health & Nursing, University of Applied Sciences Ravensburg-Weingarten, Weingarten, Germany

***Correspondence:**
Susanne Kobel
susanne.kobel@uni-ulm.de

Background: Physical activity is positively related to motor abilities. Especially in childhood, an active lifestyle is important to support healthy motor development. The low-threshold health promotion programme "Join the Healthy Boat" in kindergartens promotes physical activity in order to also improve motor abilities. Here, effects of the programme on children's motor abilities after 1 year were investigated.

Materials and Methods: The longitudinal study included 419 children (3.7 ± 0.6 years) from 58 kindergartens throughout south-west Germany (intervention: 254, control: 165). Children in the intervention group received physical activity promotion with a focus on motor ability development, led by teachers, through one kindergarten year; children in the control group followed the normal kindergarten routine. At baseline and follow-up, motor tests (3-min-run, one-leg-stand, standing long jump, sit-and-reach-test) were performed, anthropometric measures (body weight and height) were taken and a parental questionnaire was issued. Intervention effects were assessed using differential measures (follow-up – baseline) adjusted for gender, age, socioeconomic status (SES) and baseline values, with covariance analyses.

Results: Children in the intervention group showed a significant improvement in endurance performance ($F(1.329) = 20.95,\ p < 0.000,\ \eta_p^2 = 0.060$), which applies to boys $\left(F(1,172) = 13,66,\ p \leq 0.000,\ \eta_p^2 = 0,074\right)$ and girls $\left(F(1,152) = 7,48,\ p \leq 0.007, \eta_p^2 = 0,047\right)$. No significant intervention effects on endurance performance were found for children with low baseline values, children with a low SES, and children aged 5 years, nor for any other assessed motor ability.

Conclusions: The theory-based, teacher-centered intervention promoting physical activity in order to also improve motor abilities has shown a positive effect on endurance performance in kindergarten children, but no other motor ability. Future interventions should therefore be either longer, more intense and take into account children's age, initial level of performance and their SES. In addition, the influence of teachers should be considered more closely in future research.

Keywords: physical activity, children, preschool, endurance performance, socio-economic status

INTRODUCTION

From an early age, physical activity supports a healthy growing-up as well-children's development of their motor abilities (1, 2). However, research shows that physical activity levels of children have declined in recent years, and that only half of kindergarten-aged children are sufficiently physically active (3–5). In Germany, 43% of 3–6-year-old girls and 49% of the boys are moderately to vigorously physically active for at least 1 h per day (4). These global recommendations [moderate to vigorous physical activity for at least 1 h per day (6)] can only be seen as a minimum of daily physical activity (6). Children between the ages of three and four (6) and 4 and 6 years of age (7) are encouraged to engage in a minimum of 180 min of physical activity per day, respectively, which includes structured and unstructured activities (7). In general, it is advised to reduce periods of inactivity and increased levels of physical activity have shown to result in greater health benefits such as prevention of obesity, developing an active lifestyle throughout childhood, adolescence and into adulthood, as well as greater cognitive and academic achievements (4, 8).

It is undisputed that physical activity and motor abilities are interrelated (9). Developing adequate motor abilities is considered as one of the key developmental tasks in early childhood (10), for health-related fitness, the promotion of physical activity as well as the prevention of overweight and sedentary behavior (11–13). In addition, studies were able to show that the level of motor abilities during childhood is positively associated with later physical activity behavior (14). Furthermore, a positive correlation between motor abilities and various developmental areas, such as cognitive abilities and language acquisition have been suggested (15–17).

Along with the decline in physical activity in recent decades, various studies also indicate a change in motor abilities in childhood and adolescence (12, 18, 19). For children at kindergarten age, there are only very few evidence-based studies that have addressed changes in motor abilities over recent years. Overall, the results available to date do not show a uniform picture; compared to previous generations, significant changes can only be seen in individual motor abilities, especially in the energetic-conditional area and flexibility (10, 20, 21).

The positive impact of physical activity on children's motor abilities, health and health behaviors is subject of ongoing health research. Findings of various evaluation studies of physical activity promotion measures suggest that targeted promotion of physical activity can positively support the development of motor abilities even at kindergarten age (22–27). Therefore, it is recommended to integrate physical activity promotion into children's everyday lives from an early age on in order to promote a physically active lifestyle and encourage more movement experiences so motor abilities can be developed (4, 28–31).

Since it is one of the first educational institutions children enter, kindergarten is ideally suited for early support of health resources, as it is possible to realize behavior as well as environmental change. In Germany, visiting a kindergarten is voluntary, still, almost all children – independent of their social background – between the ages of three and six can be reached here (32, 33). It is primarily used as a child care offer, not comparable with school, i.e., without fixed curriculum but some recommendations of promoting certain developmental areas during the time children are at kindergarten (e.g., knowledge, creativity, motor skills etc.). The theory-guided health promotion programme "Join in the Healthy Boat" aims to intervene in that setting and offers kindergarten teachers materials to realize bespoke recommendations in health-related areas. The intention of this low-threshold behavioral and preventive intervention is to promote children's health behaviors in kindergartens (34) with the focus on physical activity, nutrition and leisure time activities in order to inter alia improve children's motor abilities. Without adding extra lessons or interfering too much, the teacher-based programme supports and structures already present elements of the daily kindergarten routine such as educational lessons, physical activity sessions, and trips into more health promoting ones. Against the background of the already identified need for early promotion of physical activity and motor abilities, this study investigated intervention effects of the health promotion programme on kindergarten children's motor abilities.

MATERIALS AND METHODS

Study Design

For this cluster randomized longitudinal study, nearly 8,000 kindergartens in south-west Germany were contacted by mail. 398 kindergarten teachers of 66 kindergartens provided written, informed consent for participation in the study. After that, a three-stage randomization on the basis of kindergarten size [see (34)] was performed to assign kindergarten children to intervention or control group, which resulted in a drop-out of 22 kindergarten teachers and therefore eight kindergartens. More detailed information can be found elsewhere (34).

The framework-guided (35) study was conducted in kindergartens throughout south-west Germany. Before and after the intervention period of 1 year, age-appropriate tests and measurements were carried out in the kindergartens of all participating children whose parents had given their written informed consent and children their assent. After those examinations, a parental questionnaire was issued. After baseline measurements were completed, the kindergartens were divided into intervention and control group. Kindergartens in the intervention group implemented the "Healthy Boat" programme during one kindergarten year; the control group carried on with their normal kindergarten routine (starting with the programme after follow-up measurements were completed). However, it has to be assumed that children in the control group also received some kind of health-promotion since the Ministry of Culture, Youth and Sport recommends health promotion at kindergartens, however does not give any guidance on how to implement it (32).

The theory-based intervention (36, 37) consists of weekly exercises and games lessons with the focus to improve children's motor abilities, also includes ready-to-use ideas, action alternatives, and instructions to get children to be more physically active and gain knowledge about their body and health, as well as eat more healthily (38). Additionally, ideas on how to re-arrange rooms and outdoor spaces for more opportunities to be physically active as well as helpful structures and norms were presented to enable the development of healthy eating habits. Further, short activity games (5–7 min each) designed to promote children's physical activity and motor abilities were incorporated into the daily kindergarten routine and delivered by the kindergarten teachers (more details: 34).

The here reported results were assessed as a secondary outcome of the programme. Primary outcomes as well as other secondary aspects of the programme are reported elsewhere (39–42).

Instruments

Children's flexibility (sit-and-reach), balance (one-legged stand), and speed strength (standing long jump) were assessed using the KiMo-Test (43), children's endurance performance was assessed during a 3-min run (44). Skilled examiners carried out the tests on a one-to-one basis, including trained students who recorded the results.

During a kindergarten visit, children's height (m) and body weight (kg) were measured to ISAK standards (45) by trained staffed using a stadiometer and calibrated electronic scales (Seca 213 and Seca 826, respectively, Seca Weighing and Measuring Systems, Hamburg, Germany). Based on height and weight, children's body mass index (BMI; kg/m^2) was calculated and subsequently converted to BMI percentiles based on German reference data (46). Children thereafter were classified into under-/normal weight (percentiles < 90), overweight (percentiles ≥ 90) and obese (percentiles ≥ 97).

Socio-demographic information as well as children's and parental health behaviors were collected via parental questionnaire. For the present study, data on children's physical activity behavior {"On how many days of a normal week is your child physically active for a total of at least 60 min a day?" [WHO guideline (6)]} was derived from bespoke questionnaire, as well as their leisure time activities ("Is your child physically active in/out of a sports club?"). In order to calculate children's socioeconomic status (SES), based on the so-called Winkler index (47), highest parental education level, their occupation and the household income were used. This was followed by a division into a low, medium and high SES.

Statistical Analyses

For the performed analyses, a significance level of $\alpha \leq 5\%$ was defined; data were calculated using SPSS Statistics 25 (SPSS Inc., Chicago, IL, US). Effect strength was evaluated using the partial eta square (η_p^2) $\geq$ 0.059. To check randomization, the two groups were screened for possible differences based on various characteristics. For nominally scaled variables chi-square tests; for ordinal scaled variables, Mann-Whitney U-tests, and for metric variables, t-tests for independent samples were used. In addition, t-tests for dependent samples were used to analyse within group effects. The differential measures (follow-up - baseline) of all dependent variables (motor tests) were checked for existing differences and analyzed by covariance analyses (ANCOVA). Based on the current state of research, the factors intervention/control group, gender, age, and SES were included in the statistical model in order to examine intervention effects; participation in organized sports was originally planned to be included as well but showed no effect in any models, so it was disregarded. In the case of intervention effects, the results were stratified for different characteristics.

RESULTS

Sample Descriptives

After plausibility checks, the valid sample included 558 children from 58 kindergartens. Since only children who had completed the full motor test battery at baseline and follow-up were included, 139 children were excluded from the dataset and the thereafter analyzed sample consists of 419 children (254 in the intervention group, 165 in the control group) from 53 kindergartens (ranging from 3 to 30 children per kindergarten).

Table 1 shows the sample's baseline characteristics; the two groups differ significantly in their composition in terms of gender ($\chi^2 = 9.95$; $p = 0.002$). For their motor abilities, at baseline, the children in both groups achieved similar levels of endurance performance (3-min run) as well as flexibility (sit-and-reach) and lower limb strength (long jump). For balance (one-legged stand) however, there was a significant difference at baseline with children in the intervention group performing significantly better than those in the control group [$t_{(417)} = 3.19, p = 0.002$].

Association of Physical Activity and Organized Sports

At baseline, there was a significant difference for meters run during 3 min between those children who were physically active for a minimum of 60 min per day on at least 4 days per week and those who are not [$t_{(334)} = -2.29, p = 0.02$]. Children who are physically active on most days per week for 1 h achieved 13.5 m more than those who are less physically active (266.7 (± 47.7) m vs. 253.3 (± 46.3) m, respectively). This effect however, could not be observed for any other motor ability, nor for children's organized sports participation on any of the tested motor variables or at follow-up.

Intervention Effects

After 1 year, both groups improved their endurance performance significantly as well as their balance and lower limb strength. A decrease in trunk flexibility was evident in both groups, however only significant in the intervention group.

As shown in **Figure 1**, at follow-up, the children in the intervention group ran on average 55.3 m more in 3 min than at baseline; children in the control group improved their endurance performance with 31.6 m more than the previous year significantly less, even if adjusted for gender, age, SES and baseline values ($F\,(1.329) = 20.95$, $p < 0.000$, $\eta_p^2 = 0.060$). The overall model explains 37.5% of the variance (*adjusted* $R^2 = 0.375$, $F\,(6.329) = 34.49$, $p < 0.000$, $\eta_p^2 = 0.386$).

The intervention effect remains for both genders; boys $\left(F\,(1.172) = 13.66,\ p \leq 0.000,\ \eta_p^2 = 0.074\right)$ and girls $\left(F\,(1.152) = 7.48,\ p \leq 0.007, \eta_p^2 = 0.047\right)$, adjusted for age, SES and baseline values. The model for the boys explains 36.7% of the variance (*adjusted* $R^2 = 0.367$, $F\,(5.172)$ 21.49, $p <$ 0.000, $\eta_p^2 = 0.384$), the model for the girls explains 36.6% of

TABLE 1 | Baseline characteristics of the total sample, intervention and control group.

	Missing values	Intervention group	Control group	Total sample
Number (n; %)		254 (60.6)	165 (39.4)	419 (100)
Gender [boys] (n; %)[a]		140 (55.1)	74 (44.8)	214 (51.1)
Age [years] (m; sd)		3.7 (0.6)	3.7 (0.5)	3.7 (0.6)
Body weight [kg] (m; sd)	7	17.4 (2.4)	17.4 (2.8)	17.4 (2.6)
Height [cm] (m; sd)	6	105.6 (5.8)	105.8 (5.4)	105.0 (5.6)
BMI percentiles (m; sd)	7	51.1 (25.6)	47.9 (26.2)	49.8 (25.9)
Overweight/obese (n; %)	7	14 (5.6)	9 (5.5)	23 (5.6)
Socio-economic status (n; %)	83			
Low		19 (9.4)	13 (9.8)	32 (9.5)
Medium		67 (33.0)	46 (34.6)	113 (33.6)
High		117 (57.6)	74 (55.6)	191 (56.8)
Physical activity				
Physically active during leisure time (organized and unorganized) (n; %)	67	175 (82.5)	105 (75.0)	280 (79.5)
Participation in organized sports (n; %)	19	121 (51.1)	83 (50.9)	204 (51.0)
MVPA for at least 1 h/day [n days] (m; sd)	83	2.7 (2.0)	2.3 (1.8)	2.5 (2.0)
MVPA for at least 1 h/day on most (i.e., 4 or more) days/week (n; %)	83	57 (27.5)	27 (20.9)	84 (25.0)
Motor abilities at baseline (m; sd)				
3-min run [m]		253.8 (48.6)	257.8 (43.9)	255,3 (46.8)
One-legged stand [n floor contacts][b]		18.4 (8.6)	21.2 (9.0)	19.5 (8.8)
Sit-and-reach [cm]		2.7 (4.7)	2.3 (6.0)	2.5 (5.2)
Standing long jump [cm]		67.6 (20.0)	63.6 (21.2)	66.0 (20.5)

[a]*significant difference between both groups (p = 0.04);* [b]*significant difference between both groups (p = 0.002).*
n, number; m, mean; sd, standard deviation; overweight/obese, BMI percentiles ≥ 90; MVPA, moderate to vigorous physical activity.

the variance ($adjusted\ R^2 = 0.366$, $F(5.152)\ 17.11$, $p < 0.000, \eta_P^2 = 0.386$).

For the remaining three motor tests, no intervention effects were found (**Table 2**). Further, no gender differences in motor abilities could be seen within the study year; which applies to intervention and control group.

Stratified Intervention Effects on Endurance Performance

For the intervention effect on endurance performance, it became apparent that the initial performance level ($F(1.329) = 1661.01$, $p < 0.000$, $\eta_P^2 = 0.329$), children's gender $\left(F(1.329) = 4.89,\ p < 0.028,\ \eta_P^2 = 0.015\right)$, age $\left(F(1.329) = 4.25,\ p < 0.040,\ \eta_P^2 = 0.013\right)$ and SES $\left(F(2.329) = 3.82,\ p < 0.023,\ \eta_P^2 = 0.023\right)$ are significantly associated with endurance performance.

Initial Performance

Children with low initial performance showed the greatest increase in endurance performance in control and intervention group. Yet, only children with average and high baseline performance in the 3-min run benefited from the intervention, controlled for group factor, age, gender, and SES ($intervention: \bar{x}_{average} = 56.92;\ \bar{x}_{high} = 23.76;\ control : \bar{x}_{average} = 28.91;\ \bar{x}_{high} = -3.4$). In both performance groups (high and average), the development of endurance performance was significantly higher than that of children in the control group with the same initial level ($average: F(1.160) = 15.07,\ p \leq 0.000,\ \eta_P^2 = 0.09;\ high: F(1.78) = 5.54, p = 0.02;\ \eta_P^2 = 0.07$). In children with low motor abilities at baseline, no intervention effect was seen ($low: intervention: \bar{x}_{low} = 87.51;\ control: \bar{x}_{low.} = 78.10;\ F(1,80) = 0.94,\ p = 0.336,\ \eta_P^2 = 0.01$).

Socio-Economic Status

Intervention effects are also seen in children with medium ($medium\ SES: \bar{x}_{IG} = 61.46;\ \bar{x}_{CG} = 25.37;\ F = (1.108)\ 11.74,\ p \leq 0.001, \eta_P^2 = 0.10$) and high SES ($high\ SES: \bar{x}_{IG} = 56.44;\ \bar{x}_{CG} = 39.32;\ F = (1.186)\ 8.14,\ p \leq 0.005, \eta_P^2 = 0.04$). Children with low SES in the intervention group did not significantly increase their endurance performance in comparison to those in the control group ($low\ SES: \bar{x}_{IG} = 41.37;\ \bar{x}_{CG} = 17.31;\ F(1.27) = 2.26,\ p = 0.144,\ \eta_P^2 = 0.08$).

Age

Three- and four-year-old children benefited from the intervention ($3\ years: \bar{x}_{IG} = 63.88;\ \bar{x}_{CG} = 48.98;\ F(1.106) = 5.60,\ p \leq 0.02, \eta_P^2 = 0.05$) ($4\ years: \bar{x}_{IG} = 54.25;\ \bar{x}_{CG} = 24.94;\ F(1.200) = 12.01,\ p \leq 0.001, \eta_P^2 = 0.06$), whereas, 5-year-old children in the intervention group performed no differently than those in the control group ($5\ years: \bar{x}_{IG} = 43.63;\ \bar{x}_{CG} = 0.5;\ F(1.12) = 3.69,\ p \leq 0.08, \eta_P^2 = 0.24$).

DISCUSSION

This study investigated intervention effects of the health promotion programme "Join the Healthy Boat" on motor abilities through kindergarten-based physical activity promotion.

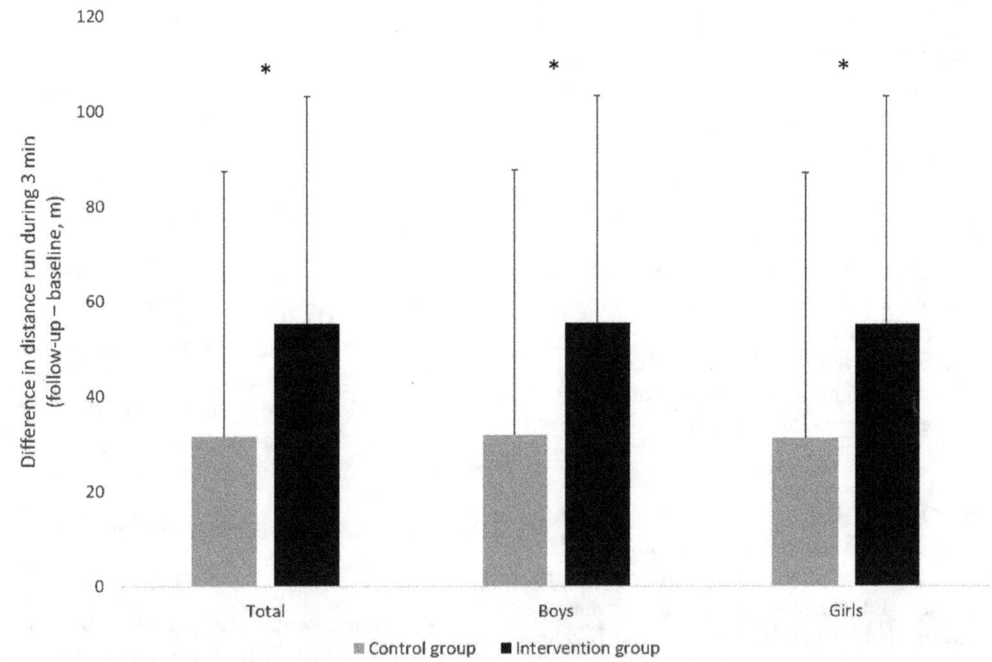

FIGURE 1 | Development of endurance performance (3 min run; difference follow-up – baseline) for total sample, boys and girls as well as intervention and control group. Values are displayed as means and standard deviation, *significant difference ($p < 0.05$).

TABLE 2 | Intervention effects for motor abilities of intervention and control group, for total sample, boys and girls [difference follow-up – baseline; values are displayed as m (sd)].

	Intervention group			Control group		
	Boys (n = 149)	**Girls (n = 114)**	**Total (n = 254)**	**Boys (n = 74)**	**Girls (n = 91)**	**Total (n = 165)**
3-min run [m][a,b,c]	55.4 (48.5)	55.2 (47.2)	55.3 (47.9)	32.0 (49.0)	31.3 (55.8)	31.6 (52.7)
One-legged stand [n floor contacts][b]	−6.4 (8.7)	−5.9 (8.1)	−6.2 (8.4)	−9.7 (8.7)	−8.8 (9.4)	−9.2 (9.1)
Sit-and-reach [cm]	−1.6 (5.5)	−0.8 (4.3)	−1.3 (5.0)	−1.1 (4.9)	−0.1 (5.6)	−0.5 (5.3)
Standing long jump [cm]	20.9 (20.0)	17.0 (20.4)	19.2 (20.2)	21.3 (21.2)	20.4 (19.8)	20.8 (20.3)

[a] significant difference between intervention and control group ($p < 0.001$), adjusted for baseline values, age, gender and SES; [b] significant difference for boys between intervention and control group ($p < 0.001$), adjusted for baseline values, age and SES; [c] significant difference for girls between intervention and control group ($p \leq 0.007$), adjusted for baseline values, age, and SES.

n, number; m, mean; sd, standard deviation, SES, socio-economic status.

Within the 1-year study period, children in both groups (control and intervention) have improved their endurance, strength and balance; and decreased their trunk flexibility. Since early childhood is considered to be a phase of rapid motor development (48, 49), it is not surprising that the entire sample has improved in three out of four motor abilities. Physiological and physical changes support that development process (49), but during those years at kindergarten, motor abilities are practiced and completed mainly through the children's urge to play and move.

This is where the here investigated programme tries to intervene. During the intervention period, the teachers were asked to implement 20 exercise and games lessons as well as 30 ready-to-use action alternatives and ideas in order to get children to be more physically active and gain knowledge about their body and health as well as eat more healthily. In order to incorporate additional physical activity into the daily kindergarten routine, short activity games of 5–7 min each were introduced and performed twice a day. This was as much as the pedagogical advisory board, which was consulted during intervention planning, considered as possibly feasible to incorporate into a normal kindergarten routine if high and lasting implementation of the intervention was sought.

Bounce, Flexibility, and Balance

Various kindergarten-based health promotion programmes have shown to have significant effects on bounce, balance and motor coordination in early childhood (22, 24, 26, 27). While there is a tendency for an increased development of bounce (standing long jump) in the intervention group, none of the above mentioned results can be confirmed by the here available results of "Join the Healthy Boat."

The result of flexibility and balance (sit-and-reach and one-legged stand) indicate that children in the control group tended to perform slightly better than their counterparts in the intervention group and even showed a decrease in trunk flexibility in both groups after 1 year. The latter maybe age-related but one can only speculate to why this showed statistical significance in the intervention group. Similarly, to why - although no significant differences were found - balance tended to be slightly more pronounced in children in the control group, although they started off with worse values at baseline. Especially the short activity games of the intervention, which were implemented twice a day, have plenty of exercises to use and practice balance, as well as flexibility. According to teachers' information on implementation rates (not shown), those activities were used very regularly and children enjoyed performing those exercises.

Endurance Performance

Further, this low-threshold intervention, mainly promoting daily physical activity in order to inter alia increase children's motor abilities found significant intervention effects for endurance performance, when controlled for gender, age, SES and baseline values; this applies to boys as well as girls, although there were more boys in the intervention group, compared to the control group. Since aerobic endurance is considered a positive predictor of well-developed health-related fitness (50), which again is positively associated with various health aspects such as cardiovascular health and weight status (51), endurance performance is looked at in most interventions assessing children's motor abilities. Like Latorre-Román et al. (25) who were able to show similar effects using a shorter (10 weeks) but much more intense programme including 3 weekly exercise lessons á 30 min focussing on the promotion of physical fitness through aerobic exercise games. Correspondingly, the health promotion programme "Ballabeina" was able to demonstrate positive intervention effects on endurance performance in kindergartens with a high proportion of children with migration background (26). This has also been confirmed for slightly older children (first and second grade of primary school) where children in the intervention group but especially boys with migration background benefited from a low-threshold school-based health and physical activity promotion and showed significantly improved endurance performance after 1 year (40, 41).

Age Differences in Endurance Performance

Then again, looking at the significant intervention effects (for endurance performance) in more detail, it becomes apparent that children's initial motor abilities, SES, and age are significantly associated to their development of endurance performance. Three-year-olds in intervention and control group were the most likely to improve their endurance performance. Yet, significant intervention effects were found for children aged three and four, but not five. Reasons for this are unclear, especially since the materials provided for the intervention include actual activity games and exercises but also lessons for children to gain knowledge, which should theoretically address the older children more but maybe there was already a limit reached. It is difficult to valuate these findings, since only one study in kindergarten children known to date has differentiated their results according to age. In contrast to the results reported here, Birnbaum et al. (22) found intervention effects only for 4.3–5 year old children on bounce and coordination during jumping. Yet, their results and these can only be compared with each other to a limited extent, since different motor abilities were assessed.

Differences in Endurance Performance on the Basis of Initial Performance Level

With regards to different levels of motor abilities, it was repeatedly reported that children who have particularly weak motor abilities benefit most from interventions at an early age (16, 24). Although here, the largest increase in endurance performance in both groups was seen in children with low abilities, intervention effects were only visible in children with moderate and high endurance performance at baseline. This is contraire to another German study examining effects of a physical activity promotion measure in kindergarten children, where children with low and moderate motor abilities were more likely to benefit from the intervention (24). However, the performance groups of that study (24) refer to an entire motor abilities test and have been determined on the basis of the standard values. Endurance performance levels of children in the present study were determined by quartiles of the sample distribution. In order to judge why the here assessed measure has shown effects only in children with moderate and high initial endurance performance, further qualitative details should have been collected. Whether it was that children with little interest in physical activity and possibly thus low motor ability levels were not reached because of reasons on their side, such as lack of motivation; or even on the teacher's side, e.g., excluding those children from some exercises because they know they cannot do them well so they want to spare them the disappointment. Further, maybe some of the children with low motor abilities have a pathological condition, that was not considered here.

Differences in Endurance Performance on the Basis of Socio-Economic Background

In addition to age and initial endurance performance, children's SES was also associated to their motor abilities during the intervention period. Stratified analyses for SES showed that intervention effects on endurance performance were only significant in children from a middle and high socio-economic background; even though there was a tendency for children with low SES in the intervention group to show better results in the 3-min run. Children with low SES also showed less change in performance levels compared to those with medium and high SES; this applies to children in the intervention as well as the control group. It is already known that children with a lower SES are less physically active (4) and display worse motor abilities than children with a high SES (52, 53). Based on the present findings however, it should be considered to not only work holistically and preventive in the kindergarten setting but to try and reach those children from a socio-economically disadvantaged background as well as their parents especially with an intervention and a more specific and intense health promotion measure. "Join the Healthy Boat" already tries to reach parents with regular information about health promoting content, including letters in different languages, but possibly those letters and information do not reach parents of children from a socio-economically disadvantaged background and more joint activities, including exercises or hands-on information are needed.

While findings show that some motor abilities can be influenced by targeted promotion in early life already, and that for endurance performance "Join the Healthy Boat" can be applied in that area, there are also several limitations to be considered when interpreting the here presented results. In contrast to other physical activity promotion interventions, the duration of the individual exercise sessions (two short exercises per day and on average one game, lesson or activity per week) is below average (24–27), which may have resulted in the low intervention effects. Yet, it should be noted (as mentioned above) that this intervention was designed as a low-threshold measure so it would not interfere with the daily kindergarten routine in order to ensure high implementation rates. This however, is in conflict with a longer duration of individual physical activity sessions, as recommended by Jaščenoka and Petermann (54). On the positive side, because of the little interference of this health-promotion programme in the day-to-day routine, this intervention can be carried out from the first year at nursery, throughout kindergarten to the end of primary school, and thus support a healthy lifestyle including physical activity and well-developed motor abilities over nearly 10 years during a formative phase in children's lives. Nonetheless, this study only lasted 1year and follow-up assessments were carried out straight after a 6-week summer break with no intervention, so it can be surmised that a follow-up before the holidays (55), a shorter more intense or a multi-year low-level implementation would have had stronger effects. Further, the often discussed influence of teachers on children's development but also on the quality of health promotion measures in kindergartens (54) was not taken into consideration. On a further limiting note, only four motor tests were used in this study (speed was ignored). Motor abilities, however, are understood as the sum of all control and function processes that underlie posture and movement (56) and therefore all dimensions (endurance, strength, coordination, speed and flexibility) should be taken into account (57); again, this was owed to feasibility. Additionally, there were significantly more boys in the intervention group, compared to the control group, which might have led to a distortion of the results, at least in some aspects. Also, since "Join the Healthy Boat" encompasses physical activity promotion in order to promote motor abilities as well as nutrition advice and a reduction of screen media use in order to achieve a holistic change in health behavior, the intervention effects can probably not solely be attributed to the physical activity module of the programme, but rather that the intervention in its entirety could have led to the results. Moreover, data on physical activity, leisure time behavior and SES were taken from a parental questionnaire, which leads to the possibility of a systematic bias due to recall and social desirability bias. Finally, although the sample was large, its representativeness and transferability to other regions are limited since only children from kindergartens in south-west Germany were included and participation was voluntary. Yet, the cluster-randomized longitudinal design of the intervention study with an intervention and control group is a strength of this study.

CONCLUSION

To summarize, the relationship between physical activity and motor abilities and their positive relationship to health and development of children is well-established. For kindergartens, there are only few studies examining the influence of health promotion measures on motor abilities. The present study contributes to new findings in the bespoke research gap. The kindergarten-based health promotion programme "Join the Healthy Boat" has shown positive effects on aerobic endurance, and thus on a health-related measure, in both boys and girls after a 1-year intervention. This could be achieved by a low-threshold intervention with a comparatively short duration of exercise sessions. There was no evidence of intervention effects for children with a low initial endurance performance, for children from a low socio-economical background, and for older children. In order to achieve development in terms of coordination, bounce and flexibility (which were also assessed but showed no increases), it may be necessary to have a longer lasting and/or more specific and intense intervention. This and some qualitative data on why those groups could not be reached should be investigated in future studies. The results of existing intervention studies suggest that measures with the aim to promote physical activity of kindergarten children have positive effects on endurance performance. Structured and evidence-based physical activity promotion measures should be used to support motor abilities from an early age on and across all social groups in different settings. In future interventions, motor-impaired children and children from socially disadvantaged families should be given special attention and materials should also be designed on a target-group-specific basis.

ETHICS STATEMENT

The studies involving human participants were reviewed and approved by The Ministry of Education, as well as Ulm University's ethics committee (https://www.uni-ulm.de/einrichtungen/ethikkommission-der-universitaet-ulm/) have approved the study. Written informed consent to participate in this study was provided by the participants' legal guardian/next of kind; participants' verbal assent was also given. Written informed consent to participate in this study was provided by the participants' legal guardian/next of kin.

AUTHOR CONTRIBUTIONS

SK, OW, CL, and JS designed the study. SK, OW, and CL carried out the study. SK, LH, and BS performed the statistical analyses. SK and LH drafted the manuscript. OW, CL, BS, and JS revised the manuscript. All author contributed to the article and approved the submitted version.

financed by the Baden-Württemberg Foundation, which had no influence on the content of this paper.

ACKNOWLEDGMENTS

The authors would like to thank all members of the programme Join the Healthy Boat for their input, as well as all student assistants who were involved in the performance of measurements, and especially all teachers and families for their participation.

REFERENCES

Strong WB, Malina RM, Blimkie CJ, Daniels SR, Dishman RK, Gutin B, et al. Evidence based physical activity for school-age youth. *J Pediatr.* (2005) 146:732–7. doi: 10.1016/j.jpeds.2005.01.055

Andersen LB, Harro M, Sardinha LB, Froberg K, Ekelund U, Brage S, et al. Physical activity and clustered cardiovascular risk in children: a cross- sectional study (The European Youth Heart Study). *Lancet.* (2006) 368:299– 304. doi: 10.1016/ S0140-6736(06)69075-2

Andersen E, Borch-Jenssen J, Øvreås S, Ellingsen H, Jørgensen KA, Moser T. Objectively measured physical activity level and sedentary behavior in Norwegian children during a week in preschool. *Prev Med Rep.* (2017) 7:130–5. doi: 10.1016/j.pmedr.2017.06.003

Finger JD, Varnaccia G, Borrmann A, Lange C, Mensink G. Physical activity among children and adolescents in Germany. Results of the cross- sectional KiGGS Wave 2 study and trends. *J Health Monitor.* (2018) 3:24– 31. doi: 10.17886/RKI-GBE-2018-0232

Kyhälä AL, Reunamo J, Ruismäki H. Preschool children are more physically active and less sedentary on weekdays compared with weekends. *J Early Childh Educ Res.* (2018) 7:100–26.

World Health Organization. *Guidelines on Physical Activity, Sedentary Behaviour and Sleep for Children Under 5 Years of Age.* Geneva: World Health Organization. (2019). Available online at: https://apps.who.int/iris/handle/ 10665/311664 (accessed April 7, 2020).

Pfeifer K, Banzer W, Ferrari N, Füzéki E, Geidle W, Graf C, et. al. "Empfehlungen für bewegung *[Recommendations for physical activity]*," In: Rütten A, Pfeifer K, editors. *Nationale Empfehlungen für Bewegung und Bewegungsförderung [National Recommendations for Physical Activity and Physical Activity Promotion].* Erlangen-Nürnberg: FAU (2016). p. 17–64.

Kwon S, Janz KF, Letuchy EM, Burns TL, Levy SM. Active lifestyle in childhood and adolescence prevents obesity development in young adulthood. *Obesity* (2015) 23:2462–9. doi: 10.1002/oby.21262

Laukkaneen A, Pesola A, Havu M, Sääkslahti A, Finni T. Relationship between habitual physical activity and gross motor skills is multifaceted in 5- to 8-year-old children. *Scand J Med Sci Sports.* (2014) 24:e102– 10. doi: 10.1111/sms.12116

Bös K, Ulmer J. Motorische entwicklung im kindesalter *[Motor development during childhood]. Monatsschr Kinderheilk.* (2003) 151:14–21. doi: 10.1007/s00112-002-0623-8

Holfelder B, Schott N. Relationship of fundamental movement skills and physical activity in children and adolescents: a systematic review. *Psychol Sport Exerc.* (2014) 15:382–91. doi: 10.1016/j.psychsport.2014.03.005

Lopes L, Santos R, Pereira B, Lopes VP. Associations between sedentary behavior and motor coordination in children. *Am J Hum Biol.* (2012) 24:746– 52. doi: 10.1002/ajhb.22310

Luz C, Rodrigues LP, Meester AD, Cordovil R. The relationship between motor competence and health-related fitness in children and adolescents. *PLoS ONE.* (2017) 12:e0179993. doi: 10.1371/journal.pone.01 79993

Lubans DR, Morgan PJ, Cliff DP, Barnett LM, Okely AD. Fundamental movement skills in children and adolescents. *Sports Med.* (2010) 40:1019– 35. doi: 10.2165/11536850-000000000-00000

Jaščenoka J, Walter F, Petermann F, Korsch F, Fiedler S, Daseking M. Zum zusammenhang von motorischer und kognitiver entwicklung im vorschulalter *[The relationship between motor and cognitive development in early childhood]. Kindh Entwickl.* (2018) 27:142–52. doi: 10.1026/0942-5403/a000254

Rethorst S, Fleig P, Willimczik K. "Effekte motorischer förderung im kindergartenalter *[Effects of motor promotion in early childhood]*," In: Schmidt W, editor. *Zweiter Deutscher Kinder- und Jugendsportbericht: Schwerpunkt: Kindheit [Second German children's and youth sports report: Focus: Childhood].* Schorndorf: Hofmann (2009). p. 237–54.

Voelcker-Rehage C. Der zusammenhang zwischen motorischer und kognitiver entwicklung im frühen kindesalter – ein teilergebnis der MODALIS-studie *[The relationship between motor and cognitive development in early childhood]. Dtsch Z Sportmed.* (2005) 56:358–63. doi: 10.1016/j.jsams.2014.09.007

Bös K. Motorische leistungsfähigkeit von kindern und jugendlichen *[Motor performance of children and adolescents]*," In: Schmidt W, Hartmann-Tews I, Brettschneider WD, editors. *Erster Deutscher Kinder- und Jugendsportbericht: Schwerpunkt: Kindheit [First German children's and youth sports report: Focus: Childhood].* Schorndorf: Hofmann (2003). p. 85–107.

Fransen J, Pion J, Vandendriessche J, Vandorpe B, Vaeyens R, Lenoir R, et al. Differences in physical fitness and gross motor coordination in boys aged 6–12 years specializing in one versus sampling more than one sport. *J Sport Sci.* (2012) 30:379–86. doi: 10.1080/02640414.2011.642808

Spengler S, Rabel M, Kuritz AM, Mess F. Trends in motor performance of first graders: a comparison of cohorts from 2006 to 2015. *Front Pediatr.* (2017) 5:206. doi: 10.3389/fped.2017.00206

Tomkinson GR, Olds TS. Secular changes in pediatric aerobic fitness test performance: the global picture. *Pediatr Fitness.* (2007) 50:46– 66. doi: 10.1159/000101075

Birnbaum J, Geyer C, Kirchberg F, Manios Y, Koletzko B. Effects of a kindergarten-based, family-involved intervention on motor performance ability in 3- to 6-year-old children: the ToyBox-study. *J Sports Sci.* (2017) 35:377–84. doi: 10.1080/02640414.2016.1166390

Kambas A, Antoniou P, Xanthi G, Heikenfeld R, Taxildaris K, Godolias G. Unfallverhütung durch schulung der bewegungskoordination bei kindergartenkindern *[Accident prevention through development of coordination in kindergarten children]. Dtsch Z Sportmed.* (2004) 55:44–7.

Krombholz H. Untersuchung der entwicklung und förderung von kindern mit unterschiedlichem motorischem leistungsstand im vorschulalter *[Investigation on the development and support of preschool children with different motor abilities]. Z Sportpsychol.* (2015) 22:63–76. doi: 10.1026/1612-5010/a000142

Latorre-Román PA, Mora-López D, García-Pinillos F. Effects of a physical activity programme in the school setting on physical fitness in preschool children. *Child Care Health Dev.* (2018) 44:427–32. doi: 10.1111/cch.12550

Puder JJ, Marques-Vidal P, Schindler C, Zahner L, Niederer I, Bürgi F, et al. Effect of multidimensional lifestyle intervention on fitness and adiposity in predominantly migrant preschool children (Ballabeina): cluster randomised controlled trial. *BMJ.* (2011) 343:d6195. doi: 10.1136/bmj.d6195

Roth K, Kriemler S, Lehmacher W, Ruf KC, Graf C, Hebestreit H. Effects of a physical activity intervention in preschool children. *Med Sci Sports Exerc.* (2015) 47:2542–51. doi: 10.1249/MSS.00000000000 00703

Albrecht C, Hanssen-Doose A, Bös K, Schlenker L, Schmidt S, Wagner M, et al. Motorische leistungsfähigkeit von kindern und jugendlichen in deutschland *[Motor performance of children and adolescents in Germany]. Sportwiss.* (2016) 46:294–304. doi: 10.1007/s12662-016- 0421-4

Ketelhut K, Stang H, Holzweg M. Einfluss des sozialen einzugsgebietes auf die motorische leistungsfähigkeit und das aktivitätsverhalten im kindergartenalter *[Influence of the social environment in motor performance and physical activity at preschool-age]. Dtsch Z Sportmed.* (2011) 62:47–51.

Morgan PJ, Barnett LM, Cliff DP, Okely AD, Scott HA, Cohen KE, et al. Fundamental movement skill interventions in youth: a systematic review and meta-analysis. *Pediatr.* (2013) 132:e1361–83. doi: 10.1542/peds.2013- 1167

Zimmer R. *Handbuch Bewegungserziehung: Grundlagen für Ausbildung und Pädagogische Praxis [Handbook movement education: Basics for training and pedagogical practice].* Freiburg: Verlag Herder GmbH (2013).

Ministry of Culture, Youth and Sport of the State Baden-Württemberg (2011). *Orientierungsplan für Bildung und Erziehung in Baden-Württembergischen Kindergärten und Weiteren Kindertageseinrichtungen [Orientation plan for education and upbringing in kindergartens and other day care centres of Baden-Wuerttemberg]*. Available online at: http://kindergaerten-bw.de/ Lde/Startseite/ Fruehe+Bildung/Material_Orientierungsplan (accessed April 7, 2020).

Federal Statistical Office (2018). *Staat & Gesellschaft - Kinder- & Jugendhilfe Betreuungsquote - Statistisches Bundesamt [State & society - child and youth welfare - childcare quota - federal statistical office]*. Available online at: https://www.destatis.de/DE/Themen/Gesellschaft-Umwelt/Soziales/ Kindertagesbetreuung/_inhalt.html (accessed June 3, 2020).

Kobel S, Wartha O, Wirt T, Dreyhaupt J, Lämmle C, Friedemann EM, et al. Design, implementation, and study protocol of a kindergarten- based health promotion intervention. *BioMed Res Internat.* (2017) 2017:4347675. doi: 10.1155/2017/4347675

Glasgow RE, Vogt TM, Boles SM. Evaluating the public health impact on health promotion interventions: The RE-AIM framework. *Am J Pub Health.* (1999) 89:1322–7. doi: 10.2105/ajph.89.9.1322

Bandura A. Social cognitive theory: an agentic perspective. *Ann Rev Psychol* (2001) 52:1–26. doi: 10.1146/annurev.psych.52.1.1

Bronfenbrenner U. "Ökologische sozialisationsforschung. ein bezugsrahmen *[Ecological socialisation research. A frame of reference]*," In: Bauer U, Bittlingmayer U, Scherr A, editors. *Handbuch Bildungs- und Erziehungssoziologie [Handbook of education's sociology]*. Wiesbaden: VS Verlag für Sozialwissenschaften (2012). p. 167–76.

Wartha O, Lämmle C, Kobel S, Wirt T, Steinacker JM. Aufbau des bewegungsmoduls des schulbasierten gesundheitsförderprogramms "komm mit in das gesunde boot" *[Development of the activity module of the school-based health promotion programme "Join the Healthy Boat"]. Dtsch Z Sportmed* (2017) 68:20–6. doi: 10.5960/dzsm.2016.265

Kobel S, Wartha O, Lämmle C, Dreyhaupt J, Steinacker JM. Intervention effects of a kindergarten-based health promotion programme on obesity related behavioural outcomes and BMI percentiles. *Prev Med Rep.* (2019) 15:100931. doi: 10.1016/j.pmedr.2019. 100931

Lämmle C, Kobel S, Wartha O, Wirt T, Steinacker JM. Intervention effects of a school-based health promotion program on children's motor skills. *J Pub Health.* (2016) 24:185–92. doi: 10.1007/s10389-016- 0715-x

Lämmle C, Wartha O, Kobel S, Wirt T, Kelso A, Kutzner C, et al. Intervention effects of the school-based health promotion program "join the healthy boat" on motor abilities of children with migration background. *Health.* (2017) 9:520–33. doi: 10.4236/health.2017.93037

Kobel S, Wartha O, Steinacker JM. Correlates of active transport to school in German primary school children. *Dtsch Z Sportmed.* (2019) 70:67– 74. doi: 10.5960/dzsm.2019.369

Dordel S, Koch B, Klein D. *Der KiMo (Kindergarten Mobil)-Test: Motorikscreening für Kinder im Alter von 3-6 Jahren [The KiMo (kindergarten mobile) -test: motor screening for children aged 3-6 years]*. Testmanual. Available online at: https://fitnessolympiade.de/pdfs/Testmanual_KiMo.pdf (accessed June 3, 2020).

Oja L, Jürimäe T. Assessment of motor ability of 4- and 5-year-old children. *Am J Hum Biol.* (1997) 9:659–64. doi: 10.1002/(SICI)1520- 6300(1997)9:5<659::AID-AJHB12>3.0.CO;2-L

Stewart A, Marfell-Jones M, Olds T, de Ridder H. *International Standards for Anthropometric Assessment.* Lower Hutt: ISAK (2011).

Kromeyer-Hauschild K, Wabitsch M, Kunze D, Geller F, Geiß HC, Hesse V, et al. Perzentile für den body-mass-index für das kindes- und jugendalter unter heranziehung verschiedener deutscher stichproben *[Percentiles of body mass index in children and adolescents evaluated form different regional German studies]. Monatsschr Kinderheilk.* (2001) 149:807– 18. doi: 10.1007/ s001120170107

Lampert T, Kroll LE. "Messung des sozioökonomischen status in sozialepidemiologischen Studien *[Assessment of socio-economic status in social epidemiological studies]*," In: Richter M, Hurrelmann K, editors. *Gesundheitliche Ungleichheit: Grundlagen, Probleme, Konzepte [Health inequality: basics, problems, concepts]*. Wiesbaden: VS Verlag für Sozialwissenschaften (2006). p. 297–319.

Hardy LL, King L, Farrell L, Macniven R, Howlett S. Fundamental movement skills among Australian preschool children. *J Sci Med Sport.* (2010) 13:503– 8. doi: 10.1016/j.jsams.2009.05.010

Winter R, Hartmann C. "Die motorische entwicklung des menschen von der geburt bis ins hohe alter (Überblick) *[Human motor development from birth to old age (overview)]*," In: Meinel K, Schnabel G, editors. *Bewegungslehre. Sportmotorik. Abriss Einer Theorie der Sportlichen Motorik Unter Pädagogischem Aspekt [Movement theory. Sports motor skills. Outline of a theory of motor skills from an educational point of view]*. Aachen: Meyer & Meyer Verlag (2015). p. 243–373.

Vlahov E, Baghurst TM, Mwavita M. Preschool motor development predicting high school health-related physical fitness: a prospective study. *Percept Motor Skills.* (2014) 119:279–91. doi: 10.2466/10.25.PMS.119c16z8

Ortega FB, Ruiz JR, Castillo MJ, Sjöström M. Physical fitness in childhood and adolescence: a powerful marker of health. *Int J Obes.* (2008) 32:1– 11. doi: 10.1038/sj.ijo.0803774

Klein M, Fröhlich M, Pieter A, Emrich E. Socio-economic status and motor performance of children and adolescents. *Eur J Sport Sci.* (2016) 16:229– 36. doi: 10.1080/17461391.2014.1001876

Morley D, Till K, Ogilvie P, Turner G. Influences of gender and socioeconomic status on the motor proficiency of children in the UK. *Hum Move Sci.* (2015) 44:150–6. doi: 10.1016/j.humov.2015.08.022

Jaščenoka J, Petermann F. Bewegungsförderung im kindergarten – was ist notwendig, was ist überflüssig? *[Physical activity promotion in kindergartens – what is necessary, what is unnecessary?] Frühe Bildung.* (2018) 7:231– 4. doi: 10.1026/2191-9186/a000403

Carrel AL, Clark RR, Peterson S, Eickhoff J, Allen DB. School-based fitness changes are lost during the summer vacation. *Arch Pediatr Adolesc Med.* (2007) 161:561–4.

Bös K, Mechling H. "Motorik *[Motor skills]*," In: Röthig P, Becker H, Carl HK, Kayser D, Prohl R, editors. *Sportwissenschaftliches Lexikon [Lexicon of sport science]* Schorndorf: Hofmann (1992). p. 319–22.

Lämmle L, Tittlbach S, Oberger J, Worth A, Bös K. A two-level model of motor performance ability. *J Exerc Sci Fitness.* (2010) 8:41– 49. doi: 10.1016/S1728-869X(10)60006-8

12

The Beginning of Senior Career in Team Sport is Affected by Relative Age Effect

*Corrado Lupo[1], Gennaro Boccia[1], Alexandru Nicolae Ungureanu[1], Riccardo Frati[2], Roberto Marocco[2] and Paolo Riccardo Brustio[1]**

[1] NeuroMuscularFunction Research Group, School of Exercise & Sport Sciences, Department of Medical Sciences, University of Turin, Turin, Italy, [2] School of Exercise & Sport Sciences, SUISM, University of Turin, Turin, Italy

***Correspondence:**
Paolo Riccardo Brustio
paoloriccardo.brustio@unito.it

Many previous studies in national team sports did not report evidence about relative age effect (RAE) in senior categories. This study aimed for the first time to determine if the RAE may specifically affect the early, but not the late, phase of senior career in elite team sports. A total of 3,319 birthdates (basketball: n = 642; rugby: n = 572; soccer: n = 1318; volleyball: n = 337; water polo: n = 450) of elite senior players were analyzed. Senior players with an age lower or equal to the 25° percentile of age were considered as *early phase* players while the others as *late phase* players. Separate Poisson regression models were applied to investigate the RAE in each sport (overall, and for *early phase* and *late phase* subgroups). Considering the overall sample, players born close to the beginning of the year were 1.57, 1.34, 2.69, 1.48, and 1.45 times more likely to reach first and second Italian division of basketball, rugby, soccer, volleyball, and water polo respectively, than those born in the last part of the year. RAE was present in all *early phase* subgroups. Differently, in the *late phase* subgroups the RAE was present only in soccer. Data highlighted a bias in the selection of senior teams, which may limit the chance to identify talented players born late in the second part of the year. Italian sport federations should promote the talent development of relatively younger players by equally promoting the joining of young players to senior teams.

Keywords: talent identification, biological age, team sports, physical maturation, RAE

INTRODUCTION

In sport context, birthdates are usually chosen to gather sport categories of adolescents and young athletes. Literature reported that in youth teams' relatively older players (i.e., athletes born close to cut-off date of selection) and relatively younger players (i.e., athletes born far away to cut-off date of selection) may present large differences in physical and psychological maturation (Cobley et al., 2009; Lovell et al., 2015). As consequence, relatively older players are advantaged in sport performance if compared with relatively younger players (Cobley et al., 2009) and have more probabilities to be selected by coaches and talent scouts (Lovell et al., 2015; Furley and Memmert, 2016; Sarmento et al., 2018). This leads to an over-representation of athletes born close to selection date. This phenomenon is recognized with the name of Relative Age Effect (RAE) (Barnsley et al., 1985; Musch and Grondin, 2001; Boccia et al., 2017).

The RAE has been successively observed in several individual (Cobley et al., 2018; Kearney et al., 2018; Brustio et al., 2019) and team sports. In the latter sport area, this phenomenon has been especially investigated in soccer (Fumarco and Rossi, 2015; Gonzalez-Villora et al., 2015; Sierra-Diaz et al., 2017; Brustio et al., 2018; Rađa et al., 2018), basketball (Arrieta et al., 2016;

Rubajczyk et al., 2017; Steingrover et al., 2017; Ibanez et al., 2018), and rugby union (Till et al., 2010; McCarthy et al., 2016; Jones et al., 2018), but also in other team sports such as volleyball (Campos et al., 2016) and water polo (Barrenetxea-Garcia et al., 2018). Despite the pervasiveness of RAE in youth sport teams, controversial results were found at senior professional level (Delorme et al., 2009; Romann et al., 2018). For example, large RAE was found in soccer (Gonzalez-Villora et al., 2015; Brustio et al., 2018), while small or negligible RAE was observed in other sport teams such rugby league (Delorme et al., 2009; Till et al., 2010; Jones et al., 2018), basketball (Delorme et al., 2009; Werneck et al., 2016; López de Subijana and Lorenzo, 2018), volleyball (Campos et al., 2016) and water polo (Barrenetxea-Garcia et al., 2018). A discrepancy in RAE at senior professional level may also emerge in relation to the countrywide. For example, in a nationwide analysis of most popular sports in Switzerland (Romann et al., 2018), despite authors found an overall RAE in male athletes, RAE associated to single sports reported substantial differences. Similarly, Delorme et al. (2009) showed in French male professional players a different pattern in RAE according to the sport teams considered. Specifically, a significant RAE was observed only in ice-hockey while only a trend was detected in handball and rugby union but not in basketball, soccer or volleyball. Interesting, a different trend was observed in female professional players, where RAE was found to be small or not present at all (for an extensive review and meta-analysis see Smith et al., 2018). Indeed, the social context, the level of competition, the popularity, and number of active participants may affect the presence of RAE (Musch and Grondin, 2001). The paucity of studies focused on RAE of different team sports in the same countrywide is evident, and further studies are strongly needed.

New evidences underlined a reversal RAE at senior professional level, where relative younger players may have the greatest potentiality for a later success (McCarthy et al., 2016; Till et al., 2016). In other words, it is possible that relative younger players may have the chance to be identified and selected at senior professional level at late stage of their career. Accordingly, as previously suggested, it is possible that RAE magnitude may differ in the early and late phase of professional senior career (Brustio et al., 2018). Indeed, it is likely to hypothesize that only the first years of senior career may be affected by the RAE. This would mean that the relatively older athletes (i.e., those born close to the selection date) may be advantaged in entering the senior teams. Despite this sensible hypothesis, previous studies, focusing on RAE at senior level, investigated the senior teams without differentiating between the athletes in the first years of senior career and the others (Delorme et al., 2009; Till et al., 2010; Werneck et al., 2016; Jones et al., 2018; López de Subijana and Lorenzo, 2018).

Thus, the aim of this study was to quantify the prevalence and magnitude of RAE in male Italian context at professional senior level (i.e., first and second division), focusing on basketball, rugby (i.e., rugby union, 15 players each team), soccer, volleyball, and water polo, which are the most popular team sports in Italy[1]. In addition, RAE was separately quantified for players competing in the early (*early phase* players) and later (*late phase* players) stage of their senior career in order to determine if the RAE in senior team may be influenced over time.

MATERIALS AND METHODS

Design

Birthdates of 3,319 male athletes were collected from the first and second Italian division of basketball, rugby, soccer, volleyball and water polo for the 2017–2018 seasons. Date of birth was obtained from different sources such as TransferMarkt database for soccer players and web sites of clubs for the other sports. Data collection has been performed at the end of the season, when the teams' rosters are consolidated after eventual players moving among different clubs. All players included in the rosters of senior teams were considered in this analysis regardless of the age.

Procedure

A total of 642 (mean age = 25.6 ± 5.6 years), 572 (mean age = 24.2 ± 4.5 years), 1318 (mean age = 25.0 ± 5.0 years), 337 (mean age = 25.6 ± 5.5 years), and 450 (mean age = 25.6 ± 6.3 years) male elite players were analyzed in basketball, rugby, soccer, volleyball, and water polo, respectively. The 18, 7, 9 4, and 24 % of the subjects in basketball, rugby, soccer, volleyball, and water polo, respectively aged less than 18 years. Players' names were removed from the data set. Since our data are based on anonymous resources, no informed consent was requested. This study was approved by the local ethics committee of the University of Turin (Italy) and conducted in accordance with the declaration of Helsinki.

Statistical Analyses

To explore the possible differences in RAE between *early phase* and *late phase* players, the whole sample of each sport was split in two subgroups on the basis of their age. Those senior players with an age lower or equal to the 25° percentile of age of the considered sport (i.e., the first quartile of players in terms of age) were considered as *early phase* players; the rest of sample was considered as *late phase* players. It is likely that *early phase* players (i.e., the younger players in the senior sample) were those in their first years of their adult career. In absence of the actual year of entering the senior team, the age of the player has been considered as the most sensible index to determine if a player is in the early or late phase of his adult career.

In Italy, the youth categories are based on calendar years, for which all young players born from 1st January to 31st December of a calendar year are grouped together. Thus, the birth week (W_B) and the time of birth (T_B) of each player were computed according to previous studies (Brustio et al., 2018, 2019; Doyle and Bottomley, 2018, 2019). W_B indicates the week of the year of player's birth while T_B indicates how far from the beginning of the year a player was born (range score between 0 and 1).

In line with recent studies on RAE (Brustio et al., 2018, 2019; Doyle and Bottomley, 2018, 2019; Rađa et al., 2018), a separate Poisson regression was applied to investigate the RAE in each

[1] https://www.coni.it

team sport following the formula $y = e^{(b0 + b1x)}$. Specifically, y represents the frequency of birth in a given week while x represents the T_B. Moreover, the Index of Discrimination (ID), which provided the relative odds of being selected for a player born in the first versus last week of the competition year (Doyle and Bottomley, 2018, 2019), was calculated as e^{-b1}. Finally, likelihood ratio R^2 was computed (Cohen et al., 2013). All data were analyzed in MATLAB R2017b (Mathworks, Natick, MA, United States).

RESULTS

Figure 1 reports the scatter-plots of relative birth frequency by week, the red line in the **Figure 1** represents the best fit of the Poisson regression modeling the frequency of birth in a given week the T_B. **Table 1** shows the descriptive statistic of W_B and T_B, and the output of Poisson regression for each subgroup and sport. The **Table 1** shows that the players of each considered sport were born at beginning of the year (mean T_B range: 0.42–0.48). Moreover, players born close to the beginning of the year (i.e., in the first week of the year) were 1.57, 1.34, 2.69, 1.48, and 1.45 times more likely to reach first and second Italian division of basketball, rugby, soccer, volleyball, and water polo than those born in the last part (i.e., last week) of the year (see ID values).

The cut-off ages for discriminating *early phase* and *late phase* subgroups were: 19 years, for basketball and water polo; 21 years, for rugby and soccer; and 22 years, for volleyball. According to these scenarios, the results suggested that the amount of RAE was greater in the *early phase* than *late phase* subgroup of players in each sport. In fact, the Poisson regressions were significant for *early phase* players in basketball ($p < 0.0001$; $R^2 = 0.19$), rugby ($p = 0.01$; $R^2 = 0.14$), soccer ($p < 0.0001$; $R^2 = 0.47$), volleyball ($p < 0.03$; $R^2 = 0.16$), and water polo ($p < 0.04$; $R^2 = 0.12$). Differently, Poisson regression was significant for *late phase* subgroups, only in soccer ($p < 0.0001$; $R^2 = 0.47$), but not in the other sports. The T_B indexes in all sports were lower in *early phase* compared to *late phase* subgroups (see **Figure 1**). In addition, coherently to the above-mentioned results, IDs indexes in all sports were greater in *early phase* compared to *late phase* subgroups (see **Table 1**).

DISCUSSION

The aim of this study was to examine the prevalence and magnitude of RAE at senior professional level in Italian team sports, discriminating male players in relation to *early* or *late phase* of career. For this purpose, the birthdates distribution of basketball, rugby, soccer, volleyball, and water polo players competing in the first and second Italian Championships was recorded. The main finding consisted of a large over-representation of players born close to the beginning of the calendar year in early, but not in late, phase of senior career. Soccer was an exception, showing that even *late phase* players presented evidence of RAE, despite smaller than *early phase*.

Considering the overall sample, evidence of RAE was found in each considered team sport. To quantify the RAE, we adopted the ID which consists in the relative odds of being selected

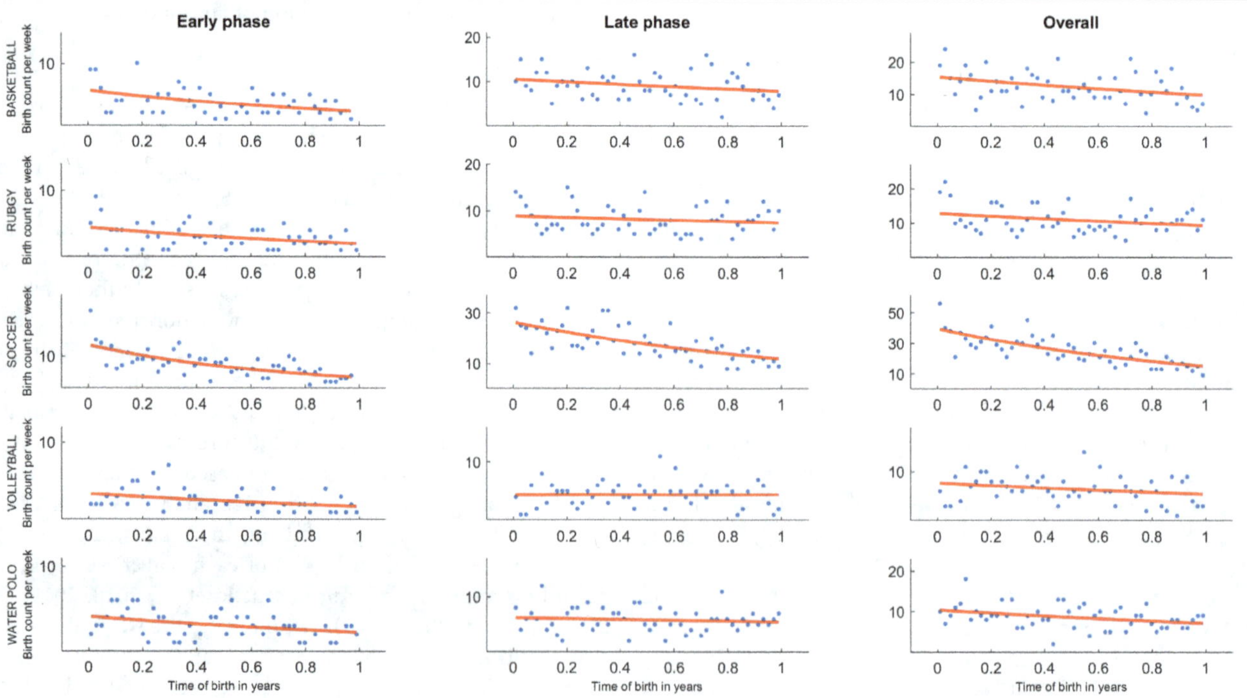

FIGURE 1 | Scatter-plots of birthdates reported for each team sport (i.e., basketball, rugby, soccer, volleyball, and water polo) in relation to the entire samples, and to the *early phase* and *late phase* career subgroups. The red line represents the best fit of the Poisson regression.

TABLE 1 | Poisson regression results in basketball, rugby, soccer, volleyball, and water polo.

		Basketball	Rugby	Soccer	Volleyball	Water polo
Overall	N	642	572	1318	337	450
	W_B	25 ± 15	25 ± 16	22 ± 14	25 ± 14	25 ± 15
	T_B	0.46 ± 0.29	0.48 ± 0.3	0.42 ± 0.28	0.47 ± 0.27	0.45 ± 0.29
	b_0	2.732	2.541	3.687	2.058	2.337
	b_1	−0.454	−0.294	−1.000	−0.392	−0.370
	ID	**1.57**	**1.34**	**2.69**	**1.48**	**1.45**
	R^2	0.12	0.07	0.6	0.07	0.11
	p value	<0.0001	0.04	<0.0001	0.04	0.02
Early phase	N	168	149	376	115	147
	W_B	23 ± 15	24 ± 16	21 ± 14	23 ± 15	23 ± 15
	T_B	0.42 ± 0.28	0.44 ± 0.30	0.39 ± 0.27	0.42 ± 0.28	0.43 ± 0.28
	b_0	1.714	1.457	2.581	1.243	1.415
	b_1	−0.866	−0.729	−1.333	−0.716	−0.611
	ID	**2.38**	**2.07**	**3.79**	**2.05**	**1.84**
	R^2	0.19	0.14	0.47	0.16	0.12
	p value	<0.0001	0.01	<0.0001	0.03	0.04
Late phase	N	474	423	942	222	303
	W_B	25 ± 15	26 ± 16	23 ± 14	26 ± 14	26 ± 15
	T_B	0.48 ± 0.29	0.49 ± 0.3	0.43 ± 0.28	0.49 ± 0.27	0.49 ± 0.29
	b_0	2.351	2.171	3.283	1.472	1.820
	b_1	−0.288	−0.152	−0.829	0.037	−0.145
	ID	**1.33**	**1.16**	**2.29**	**0.96**	**1.12**
	R^2	0.06	0.02	0.47	0	0.01
	p value	0.07	0.37	<0.0001	0.87	0.56

W_B, week in which players born; T_B, time of birth; ID, Index of Discrimination.

for an athlete born in the first versus the last week of the calendar year (Doyle and Bottomley, 2018, 2019). In this study, the IDs ranged from 1.34 to 2.69 underlined the presence of RAE in all considered team sports. Thus, the present results showed a different pattern in senior Italian context compared to International ones, where RAE was small or negligible as observed in basketball (Delorme et al., 2009; Werneck et al., 2016; López de Subijana and Lorenzo, 2018), rugby league (Till et al., 2010), volleyball (Campos et al., 2016) and water polo at senior level (Barrenetxea-Garcia et al., 2018). On the other hand, it possible that the proportion of players with less than 18 years (overall mean = 12%) in analyzed teams may partially influence the results contradicting previous results in senior teams and in accordance with other studies which describe RAE in European National Teams (Arrieta et al., 2016). However, as outlined before, controversial results may arise in relation to the countrywide, because the social context, the level of competitiveness, the popularity, and number of active participants affect the magnitude of RAE (Musch and Grondin, 2001; Cobley et al., 2009; Wattie et al., 2015). Thus, this finding should be considered specific to Italian context and cannot be generalized to other countries. Some speculations could be provided to more deeply interpret the results of the present study. The team sports of our study may be considered as highly physical demanding sports, where strength and power represent a substantial role. Since physical maturation is related to muscular strength, endurance, and speed, and is important to obtain successful performances (Musch and Grondin, 2001; Cobley et al., 2009), relatively older players could be more favored than younger counterparts. Moreover, soccer, basket, rugby, and water polo are invasion sports and characterized by physical contacts, where higher muscular strength and body dimensions are directly favorable. Differently, despite volleyball is not an invasion sport, greater body dimension and physical capabilities can be favorable as well. This can explain the fact that also volleyball presented RAE values in line with the other sports, even if it is not an invasion sport. Beyond the physical aspect, the influence of social agents such as parents, coaches or the athletes themselves, especially at the beginning of the careers, may amplify RAE (e.g., best coaches, facilities, equipment, higher self-expectations) (Hancock et al., 2013). Furthermore, also environmental factors, such as birthplace, may positively impact on athletes' development and increase the opportunity to obtain success in sport (Côté et al., 2006).

Soccer is the sport more affected by RAE (**Table 1**). Players born near the cut-off date of selection are nearly three times more likely to play in the first or second division. The larger RAE in soccer may be related to the fact that soccer is the most popular sport in Italy. In fact, the high professionalism of the first and second division can be associated to a more severe player selection in comparison with other team sports. Moreover, the greater attractiveness of soccer compared to other sports in term of media presence and higher funding (Romann et al., 2018) might explain the larger RAE in soccer. In other words, we may speculate that the relative inferior popularity and number of active participants of basketball, rugby, volleyball, and water polo in Italy, and consequent more opportunities to be selected in elite teams may have minimized the RAE. As consequence, even though soccer can benefit from a huge number of players, its talent selection seems to risk more than other team sports to lose valuable elite players only because of a late physical maturation occurring during the youth phase of career. Therefore, it could be hypothesized a paradoxical phenomenon, where an effective and trivial talent selection is developed in minor team sports and soccer, respectively.

The most interesting result of this study was that in basketball, rugby, volleyball, and water polo, the RAE was present only in *early phase* subgroup (IDs ranged = 1.84–2.38) but not in the *late phase* subgroup (IDs ranged = 0.96–1.33). This finding highlights that, in these sports, relatively younger players may still suffer the initial disadvantage undergone in youth career (Cobley et al., 2009) during their *early phase* of adult career (McCarthy et al., 2016; Till et al., 2016). In soccer, the results presented the same trend but with even more pronounced RAE. Indeed, the ID was extraordinarily large in *early phase* subgroup (ID = 3.8) and lower, but still large, in *late phase* subgroup (ID = 2.3). Taken together, the present findings show that the relatively older soccer players (i.e., those born close the beginning of the year) are facilitated in entering the senior professional teams. Moving from youth to senior team is a delicate passage in players' careers. However, it seems that the relatively older players have early chances to join the senior teams compared to the relatively younger players. Anyway, for relatively younger players, further opportunities to play with senior team should be offered to optimize the process of talent development. However, it is known that the excessive research of immediate successes in youth categories could prevent the promotion of long-term talent development, leading coaches to select youth players with more mature physical characteristics (Lovell et al., 2015; Furley and Memmert, 2016; Sarmento et al., 2018).

This study presents some limitations. The study considered the whole roster of the selected teams. Hence, it included also foreign players as well as players with less than 18 years. These aspects could potentially influence the observed RAE and the cut-off age used to categorize *early phase* and *late phase* players. Moreover, the present study did not investigate the possible causal factors of RAE, such individual performance during a season (e.g., total minutes and number of the match played) or individual characteristics (e.g., physical fitness performance, physical maturation, and anthropometrical measures) which may better describe the phenomenon. Additionally, the present study focused on male competitions only. Due to the possible small effect of RAE in female sport contexts (Smith et al., 2018), future studies are needed to investigate this phenomenon in the *early* and *late* phase of female players' career. Finally, the present study considered only one year of completion (e.g., 2017–2018 season). Furthermore, studies are needed to investigate the RAE considering the starting age of the players in elite teams as well as the phenomenon longitudinally.

CONCLUSION

At senior professional level, a large over-representation of players born close to the beginning of the year is evident in all popular Italian team sports. However, this trend significantly emerged for the *early phase* of players' career, whereas it was weaker for the *late phase*, which was significant only in soccer. Therefore, these data suggested that relatively older players have more chances to join senior teams especially at the beginning of their adult career.

To limit the negative RAE consequence, Italian sport federations should provide different solutions to advantage all athletes with different time points of development (Hurley et al., 2001; Romann and Cobley, 2015; Mann and van Ginneken, 2017; Haycraft et al., 2018). Since results of present study showed that the RAE is more evident in the early phase of players' career, practitioners should try to find solutions to support athletes in the transition from youth to senior teams. Taking in mind that even relatively younger players can reach top-level senior competition, team sports coaches should consider the later development trajectories of youth athletes. Thus, they should promote the talent development of the relatively younger players by equally promoting the joining of young players to senior teams.

AUTHOR CONTRIBUTIONS

CL, GB, and PRB conceptualized and supervised the study and wrote the original draft of the manuscript. All authors investigated the study, wrote, reviewed, and edited the manuscript. PRB carried out the formal analysis. CL acquired the funding.

REFERENCES

Arrieta, H., Torres-Unda, J., Gil, S. M., and Irazusta, J. (2016). Relative age effect and performance in the U16, U18 and U20 european basketball championships. *J. Sports Sci.* 34, 1530–1534. doi: 10.1080/02640414.2015.1122204

Barnsley, R. H., Thompson, A. H., and Barnsley, P. E. (1985). Birthdate and performance: the relative age effect. *Can. J. Hist. Sport Phys. Educ.* 51, 23–28.

Barrenetxea-Garcia, J., Torres-Unda, J., Esain, I., and Gil, S. M. (2018). Relative age effect and left-handedness in world class water polo male and female players. *Laterality* 24, 259–273. doi: 10.1080/1357650X.2018.1482906

Boccia, G., Rainoldi, A., and Brustio, P. R. (2017). Relative age effect in males, but not females, undergraduate students of sport science. *Sport Sci. Health* 13, 349–353. doi: 10.1007/s11332-017-0364-7

Brustio, P. R., Kearney, P. E., Lupo, C., Ungureanu, A. N., Mulasso, A., Rainoldi, A., et al. (2019). Relative age influences performance of world-class track and field athletes even in the adulthood. *Front. Psychol.* 10:1395. doi: 10.3389/fpsyg.2019.01395

Brustio, P. R., Lupo, C., Ungureanu, A. N., Frati, R., Rainoldi, A., and Boccia, G. (2018). The relative age effect is larger in Italian soccer top-level youth categories and smaller in Serie A. *PLoS One* 13:e0196253. doi: 10.1371/journal.pone.0196253

Campos, F. A. D., Stanganelli, L. C. R., Rabelo, F. N., Campos, L. C. B., and Pellegrinotti, Í. L. (2016). The relative age effect in male volleyball championships. *Int. J. Sports Sci.* 6, 116–120.

Cobley, S., Abbott, S., Dogramaci, S., Kable, A., Salter, J., Hintermann, M., et al. (2018). Transient relative age effects across annual age groups in national level australian swimming. *J. Sci. Med. Sport* 21, 839–845. doi: 10.1016/j.jsams.2017.12.008

Cobley, S., Baker, J., Wattie, N., and McKenna, J. (2009). Annual age-grouping and athlete development: a meta-analytical review of relative age effects in sport. *Sports Med.* 39, 235–256. doi: 10.2165/00007256-200939030-00005

Cohen, J., Cohen, P., West, S. G., and Aiken, L. S. (2013). *Applied Multiple Regression/Correlation Analysis for the Behavioral Sciences.* New York, NY: Routledge.

Côté, J., Macdonald, D. J., Baker, J., and Abernethy, B. (2006). When "where" is more important than "when": birthplace and birthdate effects on the achievement of sporting expertise. *J. Sports Sci.* 24, 1065–1073. doi: 10.1080/02640410500432490

Delorme, N., Boiche, J., and Raspaud, M. (2009). The relative age effect in elite sport: the French case. *Res. Q. Exerc. Sport* 80, 336–344. doi: 10.1080/02701367.2009.10599568

Doyle, J. R., and Bottomley, P. A. (2018). Relative age effect in elite soccer: more early-born players, but no better valued, and no paragon clubs or countries. *PLoS One* 13:e0192209. doi: 10.1371/journal.pone.0192209

Doyle, J. R., and Bottomley, P. A. (2019). The relative age effect in european elite soccer: a practical guide to poisson regression modelling. *PLoS One* 14:e0213988. doi: 10.1371/journal.pone.0213988

Fumarco, L., and Rossi, G. (2015). *Relative Age Effect on Labor Market Outcomes for High Skilled Workers–Evidence from Soccer.* Available at: http://www.bbk.ac.uk/management/docs/workingpapers/WP9.pdf (accessed January 18, 2019).

Furley, P., and Memmert, D. (2016). Coaches' implicit associations between size and giftedness: implications for the relative age effect. *J. Sports Sci.* 34, 459–466. doi: 10.1080/02640414.2015.1061198

Gonzalez-Villora, S., Pastor-Vicedo, J. C., and Cordente, D. (2015). Relative age effect in UEFA championship soccer players. *J. Hum. Kinet.* 47, 237–248. doi: 10.1515/hukin-2015-0079

Hancock, D. J., Adler, A. L., and Cote, J. (2013). A proposed theoretical model to explain relative age effects in sport. *Eur. J. Sport Sci.* 13, 630–637. doi: 10.1080/17461391.2013.775352

Haycraft, J. A. Z., Kovalchik, S., Pyne, D. B., Larkin, P., and Robertson, S. (2018). The influence of age-policy changes on the relative age effect across the Australian rules football talent pathway. *J. Sci. Med. Sport* 21, 1106–1111. doi: 10.1016/j.jsams.2018.03.008

Hurley, W., Lior, D., and Tracze, S. (2001). A proposal to reduce the age discrimination in Canadian minor hockey. *Can. Public Policy* 27, 65–75.

Ibanez, S. J., Mazo, A., Nascimento, J., and Garcia-Rubio, J. (2018). The relative age effect in under-18 basketball: effects on performance according to playing position. *PLoS One* 13:e0200408. doi: 10.1371/journal.pone.0200408

Jones, B. D., Lawrence, G. P., and Hardy, L. (2018). New evidence of relative age effects in "super-elite" sportsmen: a case for the survival and evolution of the fittest. *J. Sports Sci.* 36, 697–703. doi: 10.1080/02640414.2017.1332420

Kearney, P. E., Hayes, P. R., and Nevill, A. (2018). Faster, higher, stronger, older: relative age effects are most influential during the youngest age grade of track and field athletics in the United Kingdom. *J. Sports Sci.* 36, 2282–2288. doi: 10.1080/02640414.2018.1449093

López de Subijana, C., and Lorenzo, J. (2018). Relative age effect and long-term success in the Spanish soccer and basketball national teams. *J. Hum. Kinet.* 65, 197–204. doi: 10.2478/hukin-2018-0027

Lovell, R., Towlson, C., Parkin, G., Portas, M., Vaeyens, R., and Cobley, S. (2015). Soccer player characteristics in english lower-league development programmes: the relationships between relative age, maturation, anthropometry and physical fitness. *PLoS One* 10:e0137238. doi: 10.1371/journal.pone.0137238

Mann, D. L., and van Ginneken, P. J. (2017). Age-ordered shirt numbering reduces the selection bias associated with the relative age effect. *J. Sports Sci.* 35, 784–790. doi: 10.1080/02640414.2016.1189588

McCarthy, N., Collins, D., and Court, D. (2016). Start hard, finish better: further evidence for the reversal of the RAE advantage. *J. Sports Sci.* 34, 1461–1465. doi: 10.1080/02640414.2015.1119297

Musch, J., and Grondin, S. (2001). Unequal competition as an impediment to personal development: a review of the relative age effect in sport. *Dev. Rev.* 21, 147–167. doi: 10.1006/drev.2000.0516

Rađa, A., Padulo, J., Jelaska, I., Ardigò, L. P., and Fumarco, L. (2018). Relative age effect and second-tiers: no second chance for later-born players. *PLoS One* 13:e0201795. doi: 10.1371/journal.pone.0201795

Romann, M., and Cobley, S. (2015). Relative age effects in athletic sprinting and corrective adjustments as a solution for their removal. *PLoS One* 10:e0122988. doi: 10.1371/journal.pone.0122988

Romann, M., Rossler, R., Javet, M., and Faude, O. (2018). Relative age effects in Swiss talent development - a nationwide analysis of all sports. *J. Sports Sci.* 36, 2025–2031. doi: 10.1080/02640414.2018.1432964

Rubajczyk, K., Swierzko, K., and Rokita, A. (2017). Doubly disadvantaged? The relative age effect in poland's basketball players. *J. Sports Sci. Med.* 16, 280–285.

Sarmento, H., Anguera, M. T., Pereira, A., and Araujo, D. (2018). Talent identification and development in male football: a systematic review. *Sports Med.* 48, 907–931. doi: 10.1007/s40279-017-0851-7

Sierra-Diaz, M. J., Gonzalez-Villora, S., Pastor-Vicedo, J. C., and Serra-Olivares, J. (2017). Soccer and relative age effect: a walk among elite players and young players. *Sports* 5:E5. doi: 10.3390/sports5010005

Smith, K. L., Weir, P. L., Till, K., Romann, M., and Cobley, S. (2018). Relative age effects across and within female sport contexts: a systematic review and meta-analysis. *Sports Med.* 48, 1451–1478. doi: 10.1007/s40279-018-0890-8

Steingrover, C., Wattie, N., Baker, J., Helsen, W. F., and Schorer, J. (2017). The interaction between constituent year and within-1-year effects in elite German youth basketball. *Scand. J. Med. Sci. Sports* 27, 627–633. doi: 10.1111/sms.12672

Till, K., Cobley, S., Morley, D., O'Hara, J., Chapman, C., and Cooke, C. (2016). The influence of age, playing position, anthropometry and fitness on career attainment outcomes in rugby league. *J. Sports Sci.* 34, 1240–1245. doi: 10.1080/02640414.2015.1105380

Till, K., Cobley, S., Wattie, N., O'Hara, J., Cooke, C., and Chapman, C. (2010). The prevalence, influential factors and mechanisms of relative age effects in UK Rugby League. *Scand. J. Med. Sci. Sports* 20, 320–329. doi: 10.1111/j.1600-0838.2009.00884.x

Wattie, N., Schorer, J., and Baker, J. (2015). The relative age effect in sport: a developmental systems model. *Sports Med.* 45, 83–94. doi: 10.1007/s40279-014-0248-9

Werneck, F., Coelho, E., de Oliveira, H., Júnior, D. R., Almas, S., de Lima, J., et al. (2016). Relative age effect in olympic basketball athletes. *Sci. Sports* 31, 158–161. doi: 10.1016/j.scispo.2015.08.004

13

Children's Physical Activity, Academic Performance and Cognitive Functioning

Vedrana Sember*, Gregor Jurak, Marjeta Kovač, Shawnda A. Morrison and Gregor Starc

Laboratory for the Diagnostics of Somatic and Motor Development, Faculty of Sport, University of Ljubljana, Ljubljana, Slovenia

****Correspondence:***
Vedrana Sember
vedrana.sember@fsp.uni-lj.si

Researching the relationship between physical activity and academic performance is becoming an important research topic due to increasing evidence about the positive effect of physical activity on cognitive functioning. The present systematic review and meta-analysis (PROSPERO registration number: CDR132118) is a unique contribution to the recently published reviews since it only includes interventions longer than 6 weeks and acknowledges the influence of the qualifications of practitioners who deliver interventions. After identifying 14,245 records in five databases and selecting 247 full-text articles assessed for eligibility, 44 interventions passed all eligibility criteria. This meta-analysis uses validity generalization in a random effects model, which shows that academic performance itself is not solely caused by increased physical activity. The weighted mean population effect of all included interventions was $r_W = 0.181$. Most of the studies had serious limitations since they did not report physical activity intensity, which is an essential component to achieving positive exercise effects on cognition. In addition, the qualifications of the staff who administer the interventions were largely ignored in existing literature. It was found that 13 out of 20 physical activity interventions with significant positive effects on academic performance were performed by practitioners who held higher qualifications in the field of physical education and exercise science, who could mediate higher physical activity intensities of the given interventions. The population effect in studies where interventions were administered by practitioners with lower qualifications in the field ($r_W = 0.14$) was lower compared to interventions performed by staff with higher qualifications ($r_W = 0.22$). There was also a significant difference in academic performance with regard to staff qualification level ($\chi = 4.464$; $p = 0.035$). In addition to activity duration, future physical activity intervention studies including those investigating academic performance should focus on the importance of physical activity intensity and include measures of physical fitness as objective indicators to enable more reliable analyses to establish physical activity influence on academic performance.

Keywords: physical activity, academic performance, teaching qualifications, children, adolescents, intervention

INTRODUCTION

Regular physical activity (PA) at an adequate intensity and duration is indispensable for maintaining a healthy lifestyle due to its continued positive impact on skeletal (1), metabolic (2), cardiovascular (3) and psychosocial functioning of the human body (4). Low levels of PA, on the other hand, lead to low cardiorespiratory fitness and are associated with a decline in academic performance (AP) (5), possibly due to the deterioration of brain structure, and thus, cognitive abilities and brain function (6–8). PA increases oxygen saturation (9) and angiogenesis (10) in brain areas responsible for task performance. The positive effects of PA on the prefrontal cortex and the hippocampus have been emphasized in many studies (11–13). Furthermore, the molecular architecture and behavior of the basal ganglia may also be directly influenced by PA (8).

Some studies have found positive results between PA and academic performance (AP) (14–17), whereas other studies have found no difference, or even negative correlations between the two factors (18, 19). Review articles using effect size (ES) suggest that PA itself has positive effects on AP (6). For example, one of the earliest meta-analyses in which 1,260 ES were calculated, reported an overall ES of 0.25 and suggested that PA has a small, yet positive effect on cognition (20). ES has been shown to be the largest in studies investigating cognition as a function of fitness level (ES = 0.53). For example, Sibley and Etnier (6) calculated ES for each study that met their study eligibility criteria. They concluded that there is a statistically-significant positive effect of PA on cognition in children, reporting an overall ES of 0.32.

Contemporary children often experience a lack of physical exercise and an abundance of sedentariness in their school and domestic environments, which inevitably leads to deterioration of PA. School-based PA as a part of the normal physical education classes (PE) and extracurricular activities are often the only stable access to PA for many children, and have shown to provide a significant impact on classroom behavior (21), self-esteem (4), self-image (22), and cognitive function (5–7). This is why the competencies of PE teachers and other specialists who deliver school-based PA programmes are so critical, and can affect student outcomes considerably. Formally gained knowledge and professional experiences that assure the professional competencies of the practitioners are key elements for the safe and effective implementation of any PA-enhancing intervention (23, 24). However, the professional competencies of the practitioners who deliver such interventions (and really, any school-based PA programme), are often ignored or not represented in the literature. This meta-analysis does differentiates professional qualifications of staff who perform interventions and measurements in the physical activity classes.

In this regard, our meta-analysis provides a unique contribution to the recently published reviews (25–29), since it exclusively includes interventions longer than 6 weeks (30) and also considers the influence of the qualifications of the PE teachers and practitioners administering the interventions.

Thus, the main purpose of this review is to examine whether primary and secondary school children who were involved in PA-enhancing school-based interventions demonstrated higher AP than their peers who were not involved in regular PA, and whether the improvements observed in AP were influenced by practitioners with higher professional competencies compared to less qualified practitioners. This review examines only those interventions completed in studies with an experimental design, and which reportclear and reliable measures and indicators of both PA and AP. The studies also had to be implemented in school settings.

METHODS

The meta-analysis was performed and reported in accordance with the Preferred Reporting Items for Systematic Reviews and Meta-Analysis (PRISMA) guidelines (31, 32). The present work was registered at the International Prospective Register for Systematic Reviews, identification code CDR132118.

Literature Search

Two review authors (VS and GS) independently searched literature from databases PubMed, Scopus and ScienceDirect, which were accessed between January 2017 and July 2017 and searches were re-run from February 2019 and June 2019. Gray literature of published interventions and systematic reviews was searched through Google Scholar and Dart electronic databases from February 2019 to June 2019. Unpublished studies won't be sought. The international prospective register of systematic reviews (PROSPERO database) was also searched to identify any unpublished and/or important ongoing meta-analyses. Titles and abstracts of studies retrieved using search string and those from additional sources were screened independently by two review authors to identify potential studies whereas the third review author (GJ) mediated any disagreement until a consensus was reached. Abstracts were screened using following search string: children AND intervention AND school AND (physical activity OR physical education OR extracurricular activity) AND (cognition OR academic performance OR academic achievement). All articles generated from the initial search were stored on Mendeley reference management software & researcher network (Elsevier, Amsterdam, Netherlands) which removed duplicate references.

Inclusion Criteria

Since the primary objective of the current study was to determine any impact and/or consequences of increased PA on children's behavior and AP, the reviewed interventions had to be published as articles in peer-reviewed scientific journals, as proceedings, or as doctoral dissertations with a focus on healthy school-aged children between 5 and 16 years of age, without disadvantages regarding socio economic standard and with evenly distributed sample in both genders.

The articles also needed to report an obvious measure of increased PA (expressed in minutes per week), including one or more of extracurricular or morning PA, PE, school sports, excluding professional sport activity, including standardized measures of AP (e.g., grade point average, standardized national tests, cognition and intelligence tests, validated tests from algebra, reading and writing).

TABLE 1 | All interventions included in study.

Author (year)	*N*	Age of children (years or school grade)	Intervention duration	Experimental design	Type of activity and *AP assessment*	Staff implementing intervention and measurements (HQ or LQ)	Intervention min/week	Effects on AP (ES)
Ahamed et al. (18)	288	9–11 years old** (4th and 5th grade)	16 months, 5 days/week; 15 min/day	CG and IG	Increased PA time; *Canadian achievement test*	Classroom teachers (LQ)	47	No effect (0.00)
Alesi et al. (33)	44	8–10 years old	6 months; 2 days/week; 75 min/day	CG and IG	Increased PA time; *Corsi block test, Forward digit span test, The backward digit span test*	PE teacher (HQ)	150	Significantly better executive functions in IG (1.62)
Ardoy et al. (34)	67	12–14 years old (II–V Tanner Grade)	17 weeks, 2 days/week; 55 min/day	CG and 2 IG. (1st IG had only increased PE time, 2nd IG had increased PE time, and intensity of PE lessons)	Enhanced PE and increased PA time; *IGF-M Intelligence Test, and school grades (mathematics, language, natural sciences, English)*	PE teachers (HQ)	110	Significantly better results in mathematics (0.47) and in GPA (2.60)
Beck et al. (35)	165	7.5 (±0.02) years old	6 weeks; 3 days/week; 60 min/day	CG and 2 IG (CG: non-motor enriched mathematical teaching; IG1: fine motor math group; IG2: gross motor math group)	Increased PA time (during academic narrated lessons); *standardized mathematical test, modified Eriksen Flanker test, CANTAB*	Classroom teachers (LQ)	180	No effect (0) after the last testing. Right after the intervention only normal math subgroup in gross motor math IG benefited compared to CG and fine motor IG
Bunketorp Käll et al. (36)	545	12 years old (5th grade)	3 years; 2 days/week; 30–45 min/day	CG and IG	Increased PA time; *Academic performance grades of mathematics, English, and Swedish language*	Not reported (LQ)	75***	No effect (0.00)
Chaddock-Heyman et al. (37)	32	8–9 years old	9 months; 5 days/week; 2 school periods/day	CG and IG	Increased PA time; *fMRI*	At university by research staff (HQ)	425***	No effect (0.00)
Coe et al. (38)	214	10–11 years old** (6th grade)	1 semester, 5 days/week, On average 19 min of MVPA/day	CG and IG. 1st group was assigned in PE in 1st semester; 2nd group was assigned to PE during 2nd semester	One semester without PE, other semester increased PE time; *Terra Nova Test and individual grades*	Not reported (LQ)	95	No effect (0.00)
Costigan et al. (39)	65	15.8 (±0.6) years old	8 weeks; 1(3)****days/week; 30(120)****min/day	CG and 2 IG (CG had normal PE-2 school hours/week; IG had high-interval PE)	Increased PA and enhanced PE; *The trail making test (TMT)*	PE teachers (HQ)	30	No effect (0.00)
Davis et al. (40)	94	7–11 ($M = 9.2$) years old	15 weeks, 5 days/week, 40 min/day	CG (no-exercise) and 2 IG (low-dose exercise group, high-dose exercise group)	Aerobic PA; average heart rate > 150 bpm; *CAS*	PE teachers, researchers (HQ)	200	Significantly better AP in high-dose exercise group (2.24)
Greeff et al. (41)	499	8.1 years old (2nd and 3rd grade)	2 years; 22 weeks/year; 3 days/week; 20–30 min/day	CG and IG	Increased PA time (during academic narrated lessons); *Golden stroop test, Digit Span backward, and Visual span backward test, M-WCST*	Primary and classroom teachers (LQ)	75***	No effect (0.00)

(Continued)

TABLE 1 | Continued

Author (year)	*N*	Age of children (years or school grade)	Intervention duration	Experimental design	Type of activity and *AP assessment*	Staff implementing intervention and measurements (HQ or LQ)	Intervention min/week	Effects on AP (ES)
Dwyer et al. (14)	~500 in 1st phase (1978); 216 in 2nd phase (1980)	10 years old	14 weeks, 5 days/week, 60 min/day	CG and 2 IG (fitness group and skill programme group)	Enhanced PE time and increased intensity of PA in skill programme group; *arithmetic and reading test*	Researchers (HQ)	225	No effect (0.00)
Ericsson (42)	251	6–9 years old; (1st, 2nd, and 3rd grades)	3 years, 3 days/week; 45 min/day	CG and 2 IG	Increased PE time (in CG normal curriculum-–2 h per week, in IG 5 h per week); *LUS, national tests in Swedish and mathematics, word, and reading test*	PE teachers (HQ)	135	Significantly better AP in both intervention groups (in national test in mathematics) (0.21)
Ericsson and Karlsson (43)	220	6–9 years old; (1st, 2nd, and 3rd grades) at baseline—follow-up till the 16 years of age	7–9 years, 3 days/week; 45 min/day	CG and IG	Increased PE time (in CG normal curriculum-–2 h per week, in IG 5 h per week); *LUS, national tests in Swedish and mathematics, word, and reading test*	PE teachers (HQ)	135	Significantly better AP in boys IG (1.5) and no effect in IG in girls (0.0)
Erwin et al. (44)	29	8–9 years old (*M* = 8.87) (3rd grade)	20 weeks; 5 days/week; 20 min/day	CG and IG	Increased PA time; *reading and mathematics fluency, school grades, standardized test scores*	Classroom teachers (LQ)	100	Significantly better AP on CBM scores (1, 24) and no effect on standardized tests (0.00) and teachers' grades (0.00)
Fedewa and Davis (45)	460	8–11 years old** (3rd-–5th grade)	8 months; 5 days/week; 20 min/day	CG and IG	Increased PA time (breaks); *Fluid intelligence (SPM), academic performance grades (mathematics and reading)*	Classroom teachers (LQ)	100	No effect (0.00)
Fisher et al. (46)	64	5–7 years old	10 weeks, 120 min/week	CG and IG	Aerobic PA; *CAS, CANTAB, ANT, Conner's Behavior Rating Scale*	Researchers, PE teachers and classroom teachers (HQ)	90	Significantly better AP in intervention group (in ANT and CANTAB and Conner's Behavioral Rating Scale) (0.14)
Gao et al. (47)	208	10–12 years old (*M* = 10, 3 years) (3rd–6th grade)	2 years; 3 days/week; 30 min/day	CG and IG	Increased PA time; *reading and math scores for Utah Criterion Referenced Test*	Classroom teachers (LQ)	90	No effect (0.00); nevertheless greater improvement on math scores of intervention children in Year 1 and 2, the difference was not statistically significant (0.00)
Hedges and Hardin (48)	152	6–7 years old (1st grade)	5 months, 5 days/week, 20 min/week	CG and IG	Increased PA time; *S.A.A.T*	Classroom teachers (LQ)	100	No effect (0.00)
Hillman et al. (49)	221	7–9 years old	9 months; 5 days/week; 2 school periods/day	CG and IG	Increased PA time; *Flanker task, RT, Switch task*	At university by research staff (HQ)	425***	Significantly better results in IG in inhibition (0.27), cognitive flexibility (0.35)

(Continued)

TABLE 1 | Continued

Author (year)	*N*	Age of children (years or school grade)	Intervention duration	Experimental design	Type of activity and *AP assessment*	Staff implementing intervention and measurements (HQ or LQ)	Intervention min/week	Effects on AP (ES)
Hollar et al. (50)	2,494	6–13 years old	2 years, 5 days/week, 10 min/day	CG and IG	Increased PA and lessons about healthy lifestyle, integrated and replicable nutrition; *FCAT (mathematics and reading)*	Researchers (HQ)	50	Significantly better AP in FCAT math scores (0.21)
Ismail (51)	142	10–12 years old	Academic year, 5 days/week, 60 min/day	CG and IG	Enhanced PE and increased PA with an emphasis on coordination and balance; *S.A.A.T and Otis test*	PE teachers (HQ)	225	Intervention group performed significantly better in AP (0.35)
Kamijo et al. (52)	36	7–9 years old	9 months; 5 days/week; 90 min/day	CG and IG	Increased PA time; *Sternberg cognitive task, EEG activity*	At university by research staff (HQ)	425***	Response accuracy was better in IG (0.73), three letter condition was significantly better in IG (0.65)
Katz et al. (53)	352	7–9 years old** (2nd–4th grade)	8 months; 5 days/week; 30 min/day	CG and IG	Increased PA time*; MAP, academic performance grades from communication, mathematics, and arts*	Classroom teachers (LQ)	150	No overall significant change was seen in math AP scores (0.00).
Koutsandreou et al. (54)	71	9–10 years old (3rd and 4th grade)	10 weeks; 3 days/week; 45 min/day	CG and 2IG (the motor-demanding exercise program and cardiovascular exercise program)	Increased PA time; *Letter Digit Span test*	Experienced exercise instructor (HQ)	135	No effect (0.00)
Kvalø et al. (55)	449	10–11 years old (5th grade)	10 months; 5/2 days/week; 20/45 min/day	CG and IG	Increased PA time (during academic narrated lessons, breaks and active homework); *Stroop test, verbal fluency test, digit span, and Trail Making test*	Classroom teachers (LQ)	188	Significantly increased executive function in intervention group (0.21)
Ludyga et al. (56)	36	12–15 years old	8 weeks; 5 days/week; 20 min/day	CG and IG	Increased PA time; *Sternberg cognitive task, EEG activity*	Experienced instructors (HQ)	100	No effect (0.00) in accuracy rates and significant impact on reaction time (0.79)
Mahar et al. (57)	342	5–11 years old	15 weeks, 5 days/week, 10 min/day	CG and IG	Increased PA (during academic narrated lessons); *knowledge test*	Classroom teachers (LQ)	50	No effect (0.00)
Mcclelland et al. (58)	348	7–13 years old	12 weeks; 5 days/week; 20 min/day	CG and IG	Increased PA time; *National examinations in mathematics, reading, and writing.*	Classroom teachers (LQ)	100	IG performed significantly better than CG (0.86) for national exams and (1.24) for progress through National Curriculum levels in reading, maths and writing.

(Continued)

TABLE 1 | Continued

Author (year)	*N*	Age of children (years or school grade)	Intervention duration	Experimental design	Type of activity and *AP assessment*	Staff implementing intervention and measurements (HQ or LQ)	Intervention min/week	Effects on AP (ES)
Mullender-Wijnsma et al. (59)	81	8.1 years old (2nd and 3rd grade)	22 weeks; 3 days/week; 20–30 min/day	CG and IG	Increased PA; *Tempo test Rekenen (speed test, arithmetic), Een-Minut Test, Reading*	Classroom teachers (LQ)	75	Mathematics (4.97) and reading (3.38) grades of 3nd grade children were significantly higher and mathematics grade of 2nd grade children were significantly lower (−5.17)
Mullender-Wijnsma et al. (60)	499	8.1 years old (2nd and 3rd grade)	44 weeks, 3 days/week, 45 min/day	CG and IG	Increased PA (during academic narrated lessons); *mathematic speed test and general mathematics skills test, reading, and spelling*	Qualified primary teachers at the beginning of the study, later classroom teachers (LQ)	135	Intervention group perform significantly better in AP: mathematic speed, general mathematics, and spelling (0.43)
Murray et al. (61)	893 (193)	8–11 years old	1.5 years; 5–20 min/day	CG and IG	Increased PA (during academic narrated lessons); *Stanford 10 reading comprehension and math problem-solving achievement tests*	Classroom teachers (LQ)	50***	Intervention group perform significantly better in math score and reading (0.31)
Peternelj et al. (62)	134	7–15 years old (1st–8th grade)	8 years; 2 (1st–6th grade) or 1 time/week (7th and 8th grade); 45 min/day	CG and IG	Increased PE time; Academic performance grades (mathematics and language), GPA	PE teachers (HQ)	78, 75***	Significant effect only in boys on the language (0.83) and GPA (0.54), whereas no effect in girls (0.00)
Reed et al. (63)	155	7–10 years old	4 months, 3 days/week, 30 min/day	CG and IG	Aerobic PA; *PACT, SPM, Fluid Intelligence Tests*	Researchers and classroom teachers (HQ)	90	Intervention group performed better in Fluid intelligence testing and in PACT tests (0.31)
Resaland et al. (64)	1,129	($M = 10.2$ years)	8 months;30 min/day (3 times/week); 15 min/day (every day)	CG and IG	Increased PA time (during academic narrated lessons, homework and breaks); *Standard Norwegian national tests (mathematics, reading, English)*	Classroom teachers (LQ)	165	No effect (0.00), some significant effects in subgroups (poorest in the baseline).
Riley et al. (65)	240	10–12 years old ($M = 11.13$) (5th and 6th grade)	6 weeks; 3 days/week; 60 min/day	CG and IG	Increased PA time (during academic narrated lessons); *math performance*	Classroom teachers (LQ)	180	No effect (0.00)
Sallis et al. (19)	655	10–11 years old** (5th and 6th grades)	2 years, 27–42 min/day	CG and 2 IG (group taught by professional PE teachers and group taught by untrained classroom teachers)	Enhanced PE; *Metropolitan achievement tests*	PE teachers and classroom teachers (HQ)	35.5	No effect (0.00)

(Continued)

TABLE 1 | Continued

Author (year)	*N*	Age of children (years or school grade)	Intervention duration	Experimental design	Type of activity and *AP assessment*	Staff implementing intervention and measurements (HQ or LQ)	Intervention min/week	Effects on AP (ES)
Shephard et al. (17)	546	6–12 years old** (1st grade-–6th grade)	6 years, 5 days/week, 60 min/day	CG and IG	Increased PA; *Standard provincial tests, teacher grades, WISC test*	PE teachers (HQ)	225	No effect (0.00); intervention group showed some insignificant improvements in AP grades and performed significantly better in Math Provincial Test Scores but significantly worse in overall score and English score.
Sjöwall et al. (66)	470	6–13 years old (1st–6th grade)	2 years; 3 days/week; 60 min/day	CG and IG	Increased PA time; *working memory, arithmetic test*	Activity leader (LQ)	120	No effect (0.00)
Spitzer and Hollmann (67)	44	12–13 years old [M = 12,5(IG) and 13 years (CG)] (6th grade)	4 months; 3 days/week; 45 min/day	CG and IG	Increased PA time; *academic performance grades from mathematics, German, and English language*	Classroom teacher (LQ)	135	No effect (0.00)
Tarp et al. (68)	855	12–14 years old (6th and 7th grade)	20 weeks; 5 days/week; 60 min/day	CG and IG	Increased PA time; *Eriksen flanker test for cognitive control, mathematics skills test (algebra, arithmetic, problem-solving, geometry)*	Researchers—external collaborator (also responsible for inviting schools) (HQ)	300	No effect (0.00)
Tuckman and Hinkle (69)	154	9–12 years old	12 weeks, 3 days/week, 30 min/day	CG and IG	Aerobic PA (running); *TDT*	Two experimenters and two undergraduate students (LQ)	90	No effect (0.00)
Niet et al. (70)	112	8–12 years old	22 weeks; 2 days/week; 30 min/day	CG and IG	Increased PA time (break time); *Stroop test, VMS, TMT, ToL*	PE teachers (HQ)	60	No effect (0.00); when taking baseline scores into account, intervention children showed small improvement in Stroop test but no significant differences were found on other executive functioning measures.

(Continued)

TABLE 1 | Continued

Author (year)	N	Age of children (years or school grade)	Intervention duration	Experimental design	Type of activity and AP assessment	Staff implementing intervention and measurements (HQ or LQ)	Intervention min/week	Effects on AP (ES)
Vazou et al. (71)	284	(4th and 5th grade)	8 weeks; 5 days/week; 25–50 min/day	CG and IG	Increased PA time (during academic narrated lessons); *Academic performance grades (mathematics)*	Classroom teachers (LQ)	185	Intervention group performed significantly better in math (0.68)
Zervas et al. (72)	26	11–14 years old	25 weeks, 3 days/week, 75 min/day	CG and IG	Aerobic PA; *Cognitrone test*	PE teachers (HQ)	225	Intervention group performed significantly better in Cognitrone test (2.01)

*Bpa, beats per minute; MVPA, moderate to vigorous PA; CG, control group; IG, intervention group; HQ, staff with higher professional qualifications; LQ, staff with lower professional qualifications; IGF-M, Medium version of the Spanish Overall Factorial Intelligence Test; CAS, Cognitive Assessment Treatment; M-WCST, modified Wisconsin card sorting test; WIAT-II, Wechsler Individual Achievement Test-2nd Edition; LUS, Reading development test; CANTAB, Cambridge Neuropsychological Test Battery; ANT, Attention Network Test; FCAT, Florida Comprehensive Achievement Test; S.A.A.T., Stanford Academic Achievement Test; MAP, Missouri Academic Performance; PACT, Palmetto Achievement Challenge Tests; SPM, Standard Progressive Matrices; WISC, Wechsler Intelligence Scale for Children; TDT, Test of divergent thinking; VMS, Visual Memory Span test; TMT, Trailmakig test; ToT, The tower of London test. **age was calculated using national primary and lower secondary school enrolment information; ***time was calculated using average minutes; ****overall intervention time.*

Only interventions longer than 6 weeks, with control and experimental groups, and with more than 25 participants were included in this review. Results with $p < 0.05$ were considered statistically significant. All AP outcomes have been recalculated according to the same scale—ES, considering one of the two criteria: (1) ES = 0, no effect; or (2) ES > 0.01, intervention group academically performing better than the control group. Interventions meeting all eligibility criteria are presented in **Table 1**.

Data Extraction and Statistical Analysis

One review author extracted data (VS), while the second (GS) and third (GJ) reviewer checked the entered data. Two review authors (VS and GS) extracted outcome data in duplicate, discussing and resolving discrepancies between them and consulted third (GJ) reviewer if necessary. Data supplied for included meta-analysis were checked for missing data and internal data consistency. Summary tables of entered data were checked with the trial protocol and latest trial report or publication. Any discrepancies or unusual patterns were checked with the study investigator. Hunter-Schmidt estimate was used for reducing the amount of bias and Fisher's z transformation was applied to samples' ES to display publication bias (31, 32). We also assessed publication bias with Egger bias test (73).

Chi-square statistical analysis were performed to establish the difference in the effects of interventions on AP in regards to the staff qualifications in PE teaching and exercise science. In the review, we differentiated between staff groups with higher professional qualifications, including exercise science researchers and PE teachers, and staff groups with lower professional qualifications, such as classroom teachers and students, who performed interventions and measurements.

The review includes only studies with enough data to calculate the standardized mean difference (ES) between the intervention and the control group's AP score. For this calculation, the Cohen's (74) and Rosenthal and Rosnow's (75) formulas were used: $ES = M_1 - M_2/SD_{pooled}$ (where $SD_{pooled} = \sqrt{[(SD_1^2 + SD_2^2)/2]}$) and $ES = 2t/\sqrt{df}$), where M_1 represents the intervention group, M_2 represents the control group, SD_{pooled} is the pooled standard deviation of both groups, SD_1 represents the standard deviation of the intervention group, and SD_2 represents standard deviation of the control group.

In studies that enabled the calculation of more ES, the average ES was used for further analysis. The ES of each intervention was converted to correlation (r_w) determined by Hunter-Schmidt approach (76), which suggests using pooled within-group SD, because it has less sampling error than the control group. In other words, the aforementioned method corrects ES for measurement error under the condition of equal ES. R_w was multiplied by the sample size of each study ($r_w \times N$), which represents the numerator and sum of sample sizes represents the denominator of the equation to calculate population effect (r_p). The generalizability of r_p was corrected using an artifact correction and variance sample ES, where the sampling error variance (V_{obs}) was based on the population correlation estimate (r_i) and the average sample size N. The variance due to sampling error was conducted using the equation: $V_s = (1\text{-}r_w^2)^2/(N\text{-}1)$,

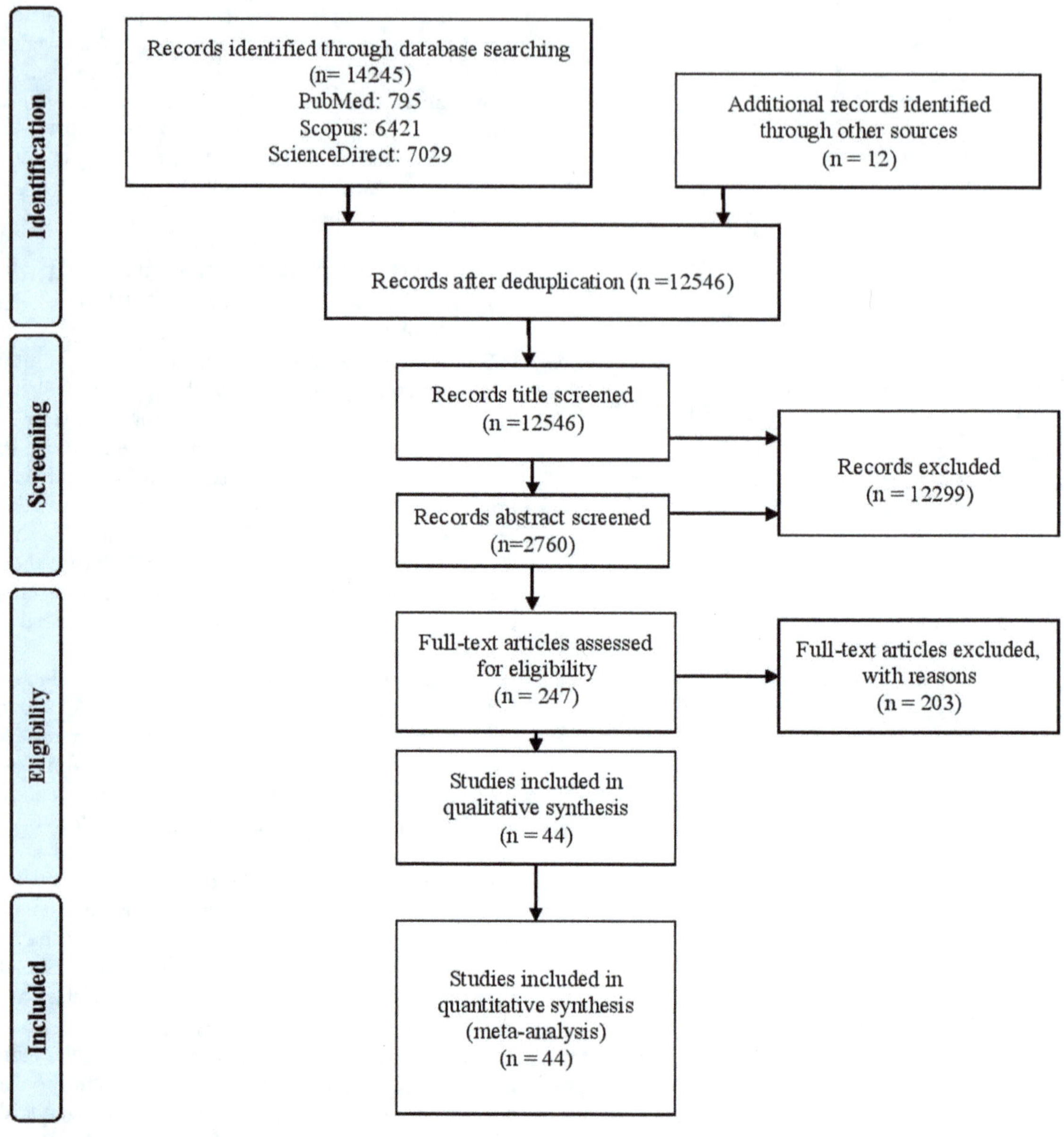

FIGURE 1 | The flow of articles through review.

where N is the sample size across studies. Estimates of the variance in ES have been calculated using the equation: $V_p = V_{obs}\text{-}V_s$. For weighted mean (r_w), 95% credibility interval: $CI_w = r_w + 1.96\sqrt{V_p}$ and I^{2and} Q statistics to measure heterogeneity of ES were calculated. Descriptors for the used magnitudes of ES were suggested by Cohen (74) and expanded by Sawilowsky (77).

Assessment of Bias Risk

The assessment of bias risk in the final sample ($n = 44$ studies) was conducted using the criteria previously used by Sneck et al. (78), including the criterion of power calculations. Each study received "0" (does not meet the criterion) or "1" (meets the criterion) based on an analysis of the reporting described in the original article. The Grades Research, Assessment, Development and Evaluation (GRADE) approach was applied to the meta-analysis to determine the quality of evidence; this involved grading the evidence based on a criteria for risk of bias, imprecision, inconsistency, indirectness and publication bias, in conformation with studies reported elsewhere (79, 80).

RESULTS

The flow of the review process is shown in **Figure 1**. Altogether 14,245 records were identified. After removing duplicates from

TABLE 2 | Descriptive statistics of the main characteristics of interventions included in the review.

	Number of participants			Duration of all interventions (week)			Intervention time (min/week)		
PA effect on AP	all	+	–	all	+	–	all	+	–
Min	26	26	29	6	8	6	30	50	30
Max	2,494	2,494	1,129	411	411	411	425	425	300
Median	211	142	215	25	28.5	22	115	135	100
Mean	240.5	281.8	294.2	60.6	73.2	69.8	144.5	170.9	118.3

All, presents all studies included in the meta-analysis; +, studies with positive effect on AP; –, studies with null or negative effect on AP.

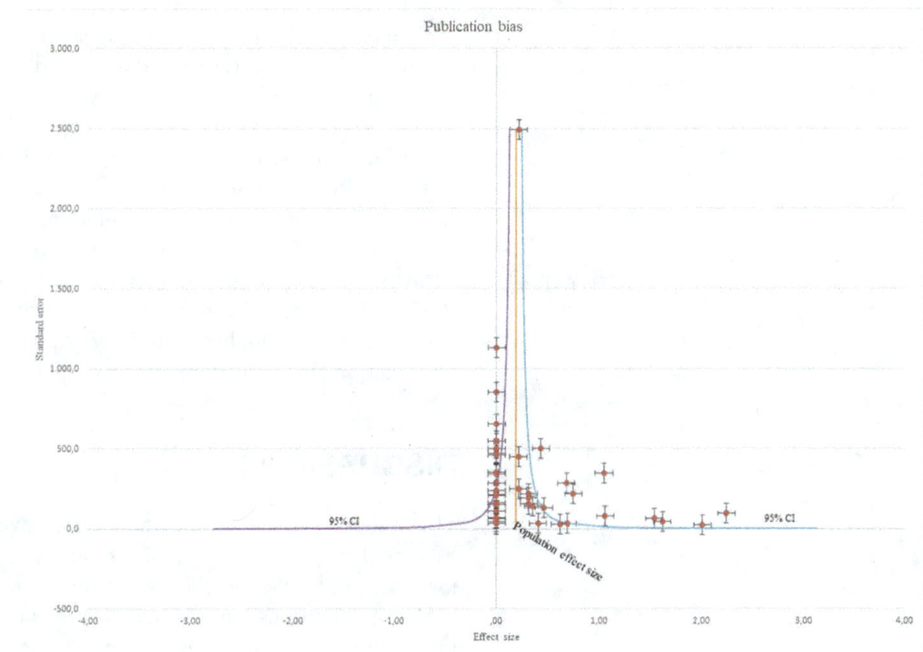

FIGURE 2 | Distribution of ES.

three different search engines, 591 abstracts with matching key words were identified, and 247 full-text papers were further reviewed. Among them, 68 were intervention studies with the control group. These were thoroughly reviewed, which left 44 intervention studies that met the final criteria for inclusion in the final review.

Altogether, 13,681 children participated in the interventions ($n = 44$) meeting the eligibility criteria. Present review covers over five decades of research studies, ranging from 1967 (51) to 2018 (56). All interventions, meeting all predefined criteria are presented in **Table 1**.

The mean of intervention time was 60.6 weeks and 144.5 min/week per intervention (**Table 2**). Duration of intervened time/week in studies with positive effect on AP was 170.9 min/week and 118.3 min/week in studies with no significant effect on AP. Duration of the average intervention time/week was 44.6% longer in studies with positive effect, also, the average study duration (weeks) was 4.9% longer in studies reporting a positive effect compared to studies with none or negative effect of increased PA on AP. Positive results of PA were evidenced in 20 interventions; of this, in 13 studies (65%) the interventions were performed by staff with higher professional qualifications. Negative or null effects on AP were reported in 24 interventions; of these in 9 studies (38%) the intervention(s) were performed by staff with higher professional qualifications (**Table 1**).

The Hunter-Schmidt method (76) for isolation and correction of sources of error, such as sampling error and reliability of measurement variables, was used. Unweighted mean effect of population is $r_u = 0.351$, whereas weighted mean effect or population effect size is $r_w = 0.181$. This means that groups with increased PA experienced a positive weak effect on AP compared to control groups. Since the variance across sample ES consists of the variance of ES and the sampling error, sampling error variance (V_{obs}) for every intervention and variance due to sampling error, using population effect (r_p), were calculated.

Variance due to sampling error ($Vs = 0.003$) and variance of population correlations ($V_p = 0.107$) were estimated. An average sample size of $N = 240$ yields a population effect size of $r_p = 0.181$with 95% confidence interval ranging from 0.083 and 0.279 and 80% credibility interval ranging from −0.237 and 0.600. Such

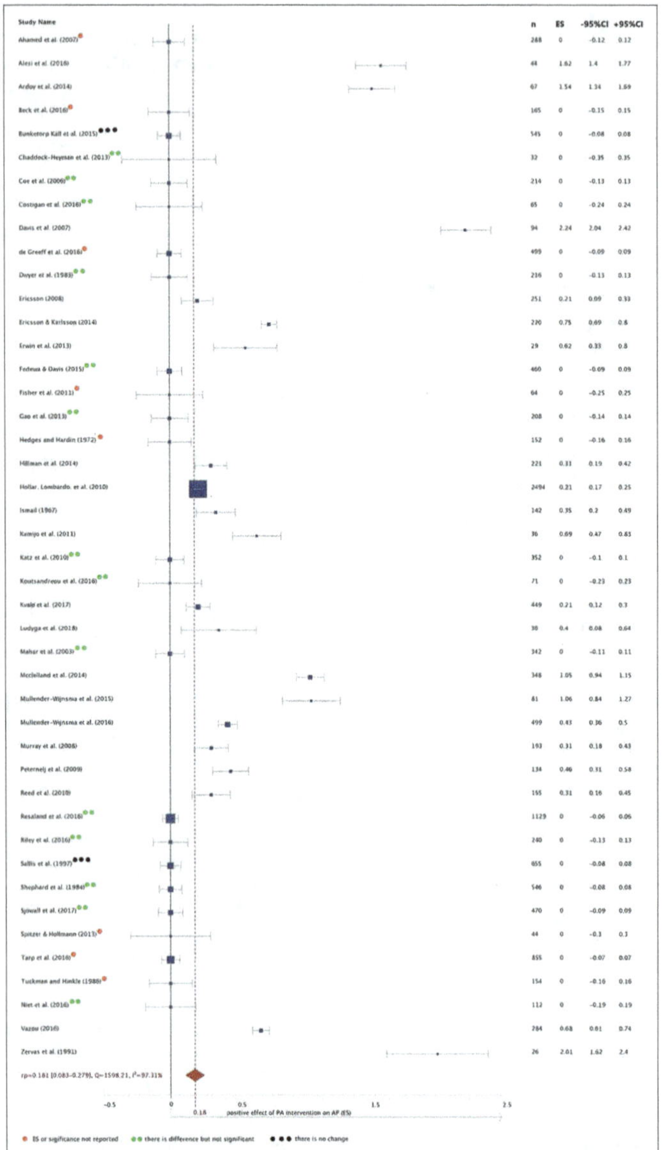

FIGURE 3 | Forest plot of all included studies.

reliable differences between studies that give rise to varying effects could be due to publication bias of included studies (31). The Egger bias test (73) provides significant evidence for publication bias (bias = 4.137, 95% CI: 0.805–7.469, $p = 0.019$). There were considerable differences between the ES's from all individual studies ($I^2 = 97\%$; Q = 1598.2; $p = 0.000$), in studies where staff with higher professional qualifications performed intervention ($I^2 = 97\%$; Q = 970.5; $p = 0.000$) and in studies where staff with lower professional qualifications performed intervention ($I^2 = 96\%$; Q = 622.8; $p = 0.000$). Distribution of ES in all eligible interventions and publication bias (**Figure 2**), and a forest plot of all included studies (**Figure 3**) are presented.

The positive effect of a PA intervention on AP was estimated in 13 out of 20 significant interventions in which staff with higher professional qualifications performed the intervention and measurements. The weighted mean effect of the population effect size in interventions, performed by staff with higher professional qualifications, is 0.22 and in interventions performed by staff with lower professional qualifications is 0.14. Chi-square statistics were calculated and showed a significant difference ($\chi^2 = 4.464$; $p = 0.035$) on AP between studies in which the intervention and measurement were performed by practitioners with higher professional qualifications compared to those conducted by staff with lower professional qualifications, or in studies that lacked this information. Cramer's V value (0.319) showed there is a strong association between staff qualification and its effect on AP ($p = 0.035$).

The results of the risk-of bias assessment analysis are shown in **Table 3**. Of the 44 studies, 29 were rated as having a low risk of bias (> 67% of total score) with average of 0.79 of total score and 15 were rated as having moderate risk of bias (between 33 and 67% of the total score) with average of 0.50 of total score. None of the studies was rated as having a high risk of bias. Only 11 studies (25 %) reported power calculations to determine sufficient sample size, of those reporting positive effects of PA on academic performance/cognition, power calculations were provided in five studies (34, 46, 49, 55, 60). The quality of evidence (GRADE) where staff with higher and lower qualifications performed intervention and measurements was moderate (**Table 4**).

DISCUSSION

This systematic review and meta-analysis investigated the impact of school-based PA interventions on the AP of primary and lower- secondary schoolchildren; it considered the amount of PA in the interventions and the qualifications of staff administering interventions in its analysis. The main findings of the study are that changes in AP itself is not caused solely by an increase in frequency and/or duration of PA, but studies must also take into consideration the intensity of PA administered. Secondly, and of equal import, is the significant positive effect observed when PA interventions are delivered by practitioners with higher professional qualifications, who were able to mediate higher PA intensity and focus of interventions.

Despite some promising results in the reviewed interventions (31, 33, 34, 37, 40, 42, 46, 49, 50, 52–55, 57, 58, 60, 61, 63, 71, 72), it is essential to emphasize that future research on the relationships between AP and PA should consider more qualitative aspects of PA, including intensity and types of activities. Namely, positive effects of AP may only accrue when of moderate-to-vigorous PA is increased (41, 42). Although the effects of PA on AP are seemingly well-documented in the literature most research and review studies have focused on the behavioral aspects of PA, such as frequency and duration, whereas PA intensity was hardly addressed, even though it is essential for properly elucidating the effects of exercise on cognition (43).

To avoid reporting sometimes misleading results of short interventions that are often affected by an initial increase in motivation of study participants (i.e., researchers, teachers, parents and children), only interventions longer than 6 weeks' duration were included for this analysis. The analysis showed that

TABLE 3 | Results of the risk-of bias assessment.

Author (year)	1. Randomization	2. Baseline comparable	3. Baseline values accounted for in analyses	4. Timing	5. Blinding of measuring	6. Validated outcome measures	7. Dropout analysis	8. Reporting of results	9. Power calculation	Total score of the risk of bias (decimal format)
Ahamed et al. (18)	1	1	1	1	0	1	1	1	0	7/9 (0.78)
Alesi et al. (33)	0	1	1	1	0	0	0	1	0	4/9 (0.44)
Ardoy et al. (34)	1	1	1	1	1	1	1	1	1	9/9 (1.00)
Beck et al. (35)	1	1	1	1	0	1	1	0	0	6/9 (0.67)
Bunketorp Käll et al. (36)	0	0	0	1	0	1	0	1	0	3/9 (0.33)
Chaddock-Heyman et al. (37)	1	1	1	1	1	1	1	1	0	8/9 (0.89)
Coe et al. (38)	1	0	0	1	0	1	1	1	0	5/9 (0.56)
Costigan et al. (39)	1	1	1	1	1	1	0	1	1	8/9 (0.89)
Davis et al. (40)	1	1	1	1	1	1	1	0	0	7/9 (0.78)
Greeff et al. (41)	1	1	1	1	1	1	0	1	1	8/9 (0.89)
Dwyer et al. (14)	1	1	1	1	1	1	0	1	0	7/9 (0.78)
Ericsson (42)	0	1	1	1	0	1	0	1	0	5/9 (0.56)
Ericsson and Karlsson (43)	0	1	1	1	1	1	0	1	0	6/9 (0.67)
Erwin et al. (44)	1	1	1	1	0	1	0	1	0	5/9 (0.56)
Fedewa and Davis (45)	1	0	1	1	0	1	0	1	0	5/9 (0.56)
Fisher et al. (46)	1	1	1	1	1	1	0	1	1	8/9 (0.89)
Gao et al. (47)	0	1	1	1	0	1	0	1	0	5/9 (0.56)
Hedges and Hardin (48)	0	1	1	1	0	0	0	1	0	4/9 (0.44)
Hillman et al. (49)	1	1	1	1	1	1	0	1	1	8/9 (0.89)
Hollar et al. (50)	0	1	1	1	0	1	1	1	0	6/9 (0.67)
Ismail (51)	0	1	1	1	0	0	0	1	0	4/9 (0.44)
Kamijo et al. (52)	1	1	1	1	0	1	0	1	0	6/9 (0.67)
Katz et al. (53)	1	1	1	1	0	1	1	1	0	7/9 (0.78)
Koutsandreou et al. (54)	1	1	1	1	1	1	1	1	0	8/9 (0.89)
Kvalø et al. (55)	1	1	1	1	1	1	1	1	1	9/9 (1.00)
Ludyga et al. (56)	1	1	1	1	0	1	0	1	1	7/9 (0.78)
Mahar et al. (57)	1	1	1	1	1	1	0	1	0	7/9 (0.78)
Mcclelland et al. (58)	0	1	1	1	0	0	0	1	0	4/9 (0.44)
Mullender-Wijnsma et al. (59)	1	0	1	1	0	1	1	1	0	6/9 (0.67)
Mullender-Wijnsma et al. (60)	1	0	1	1	0	1	1	1	1	7/9 (0.78)
Murray et al. (61)	1	1	1	1	0	1	0	1	0	6/9 (0.67)
Peternelj et al. (62)	1	1	1	1	0	1	0	1	0	6/9 (0.67)
Reed et al. (63)	1	0	0	1	1	1	1	1	0	7/9 (0.78)
Resaland et al. (64)	1	1	1	1	0	1	1	1	1	8/9 (0.89)
Riley et al. (65)	1	1	1	1	1	1	1	1	1	9/9 (1.00)

(Continued)

TABLE 3 | Continued

Author (year)	1. Randomization	2. Baseline comparable	3. Baseline values accounted for in analyses	4. Timing	5. Blinding of measuring	6. Validated outcome measures	7. Dropout analysis	8. Reporting of results	9. Power calculation	Total score of the risk of bias (decimal format)
Sallis et al. (19)	1	0	1	0	0	1	1	1	0	5/9 (0.56)
Shephard et al. (17)	0	1	1	1	0	0	0	1	0	4/9 (0.44)
Sjöwall et al. (66)	0	1	1	1	0	0	1	1	0	5/9 (0.56)
Spitzer and Hollmann (67)	0	1	1	1	0	0	0	1	0	4/9 (0.44)
Tarp et al. (68)	1	1	1	1	0	0	1	1	1	7/9 (0.78)
Tuckman and Hinkle (69)	1	1	1	1	0	0	1	1	0	6/9 (0.67)
Niet et al. (70)	0	1	1	1	0	1	0	1	0	5/9 (0.56)
Vazou et al. (71)	0	1	1	1	1	1	1	1	0	7/9 (0.78)
Zervas et al. (72)	1	1	1	1	0	1	0	1	0	6/9 (0.67)
Average of all studies	0.68	0.84	0.93	0.98	0.34	0.82	0.45	0.95	0.25	0.69

TABLE 4 | Summary of quality of evidence using the GRADE approach.

			Quality assessment					Effect	Quality of evidence—GRADE
Outcome	**Study design**	**No. of studies (no. of participants)**	**Risk of bias**	**Inconsistency**	**Indirectness**	**Imprecision**	**Other considerations**	**Rw (95 % CI)**	
Positive effect on AP where staff with higher professional qualifications performed intervention	15 randomized, 7 non-randomized	22 (6,536)	No serious risk of bias (15 low risk of bias, 4 moderate risk of bias).	*No serious inconsistency* I^2 = 97.8%	No serious indirectness.	No serious limitations.	None	0.22 (0.07–0.37)	⊕⊕⊕□ **MODERATE** (6 high, 13 moderate, 3 low)
Positive effect on AP where staff with lower professional qualifications performed intervention	15 randomized, 7 non-randomized	22 (7,145)	No serious risk of bias (2 moderate risk of bias, 5 high risk of bias).	*No serious inconsistency* I^2 = 96.6%	No serious indirectness.	No serious limitations.	None	0.14 (0.02–0.27)	⊕⊕⊕□ **MODERATE** (4 high, 14 moderate, 4 low)

GRADE, Grades of Research, Assessment, Development and Evaluation (GRADE Working Group).
⊕⊕⊕⊕ *(high): We have a lot of confidence that the true effect is similar to the estimated effect.*
⊕⊕⊕□ *(moderate): We believe that the true effect is probably close to the estimated effect.*
⊕⊕□□ *(low): We believe that the true effect might be markedly different from the estimated effect*
⊕□□□ *(very low): We believe that the true effect is probably markedly different from the estimated effect.*

in the longer-lasting interventions there was a greater decline in moderate-to vigorous PA across the intervention time.

Samples in interventions which reported positive PA impacts were larger than the ones in the interventions with negative or no impact; this should be taken into consideration when interpreting the results. The population effect (r_P) was shown to be small, which means that increased PA in experimental groups had only a small effect on AP compared to control groups. Since the connection between both variables was small, PA alone may not be the best predictor of children's AP. When researching the relationships between cognition and activity, researchers should start thinking about utilizing and reporting more stable measures, like the level of physical fitness, which is a marker outcome of habitual physical activity. For example, it has been shown that after-school PA improves cardiovascular endurance in children, which then mediates improvements in AP (81). A meta-analysis of published evidence on the relationship between physical fitness and AP between 2005 and 2015 asserts that cardiorespiratory fitness, speed-agility, motor coordination, and perceptual-motor skills are highly associated with AP (45), but the findings on the relationship between AP to strength and flexibility remain unclear in this regard. Indeed, it can be argued that physical fitness may be a better predictor of AP than PA. Several studies have identified a positive relationship between cardiorespiratory fitness, weight and AP (46–49) or with overall physical fitness (82). For example, researchers from Portugal have shown that cardiorespiratory fitness is independently related to AP; moreover, students with normal weight tended to have the best academic performance (52). The influence of moderators and mediators to PA, such as socioeconomic status, parental education (83), concentration (84) gender (85), personality (86), motivation, body-image, self-esteem (87), have also been shown to have an impact on AP.

In almost all analyzed interventions, the higher qualifications of the involved staff were shown to positively influence changes observed in AP. We know that PE lessons led by trained PE teachers provides more activity to students than ones led by generalized classroom teachers (25, 88–90). In general, the pedagogical qualifications of classroom teachers for delivering PE classes are far lower than those for of specialist PE teachers. The classroom teachers are of course qualified teachers, but with a rather limited training in PE teaching and exercise science, which requires specialist training to perform well. They often experience insufficient expertise and ability to organize PE with its distinctive content in an effective way (91). Breslin et al. (92) showed that the PE specialists show higher levels of self-determination toward exercise, are more autonomous in their decisions to be active, are more physically active and have a higher level of perceived qualification in delivering a PE lesson than the generalist teachers do. In addition, McKenzie et al. (89) reported that children taught by PE specialists spend 57% more time in moderate-to vigorous PA, with a concurrently increased emphasis on the promotion of physical fitness. This also has the important advantage of maintaining positive health-related behaviors that may last beyond childhood (93, 94).

Study Strengths and Limitations

The present review covers more than five decades worth of research studies, but analyses only PA interventions that have met the predefined criteria. Therefore, only interventions published in peer-reviewed scientific journals with a focus on primary and lower secondary school-children, evenly represented genders, exceeding 6 weeks and with reported ES or with data that enables the calculation of ES were included in the meta-analysis. The analysis did not: (i) distinguish between the published results that used moderate-to vigorous PA as a significant predictor that might affect AP and the ones that used low or vigorous physical activity; (ii) it did not take into consideration the differences between the results deriving from subjective or objective measures of PA; (iii) it did not take into consideration different instruments for assessing AP that were used in various studies, thus results cannot be generalized to different measures of AP; (iv) it did not take into consideration the differences between studies with large sample size that were able to detect even small differences and the ones with smaller sample sizes that could not, which can lead to potential bias; and it should always be noted that (v) statistically non-significant results are less-likely to be published, resulting in upwardly biased meta-analytically derived effect sizes for any analysis of this kind.

CONCLUSION

Parents are often concerned that time allocated to PA and sport may negatively affect children's AP. The present analysis shows that PA itself does not negatively affect AP; moreover, there are positive, (although relatively small) relationships between the two, and that changes in AP itself is not caused solely by an increase in frequency and/or duration of PA, but studies must also take into consideration the intensity of PA administered. Secondly, the significant positive effect of PA interventions are most observed when delivered by practitioners with higher professional qualifications who are able to mediate higher PA intensity in the interventions. Finally, in interventions with long durations, there are greater declines in moderate-to vigorous PA, suggesting a challenge to maintaining interventions across the intervention time-span. Finally, when reporting the monitoring, surveillance and evaluation of PA interventions, using physical fitness as criteria measure of PA is much more effective in terms of both the economic and organizational sense.

AUTHOR CONTRIBUTIONS

All authors listed have made a substantial, direct and intellectual contribution to the work, and approved it for publication.

ACKNOWLEDGMENTS

Prof. Jose Carlos Ribeiro is kindly acknowledged for reading the manuscript and giving helpful suggestions.

REFERENCES

Gunter KB, Almstedt HC, Janz KF. Physical activity in childhood may be the key to optimizing lifespan skeletal health. *Exerc Sport Sci Rev.* (2012) 40:13–21. doi: 10.1097/JES.0b013e318236e5ee

Janssen I, LeBlanc AG. Systematic review of the health benefits of physical activity and fitness in school-aged children and youth. *Int J Behav Nutr Phys Act.* (2010) 7:40. doi: 10.1186/1479-5868-7-40

Fernhall B, Agiovlasitis S. Arterial function in youth: window into cardiovascular risk. *J Appl Physiol.* (2008) 105:325– 33. doi: 10.1152/japplphysiol.00001.2008

Biddle SJH, Asare M. Physical activity and mental health in children and adolescents: a review of reviews. *Br J Sports Med.* (2011) 45:886– 95. doi: 10.1136/bjsports-2011-090185

Chaddock L, Pontifex MB, Hillman CH, Kramer AF. A review of the relation of aerobic fitness and physical activity to brain structure and function in children. *J Int Neuropsychol Soc.* (2011) 17: 975– 85. doi: 10.1017/S1355617711000567

Sibley BA, Etnier JL. The relationship between physical activity and cognition in children: a meta-analysis. *Pediatr Exerc Sci.* (2003) 15:243– 56. doi: 10.1123/pes.15.3.243

Castelli DM, Hillman CH, Buck SM, Erwin HE. Physical fitness and academic achievement in third-and fifth-grade students. *J Sport Exerc Psychol.* (2007) 29:239–52. doi: 10.1123/jsep.29.2.239

Chaddock L, Erickson KI, Prakash RS, VanPatter M, Voss MW, Pontifex MB, et al. Basal ganglia volume is associated with aerobic fitness in preadolescent children. *Dev Neurosci.* (2010) 32:249–56. doi: 10.1159/000316648

Kramer AF, Hahn S, Cohen NJ, Banich MT, McAuley E, Harrison CR, et al. Ageing, fitness and neurocognitive function. *Nature.* (1999) 400:418– 9. doi: 10.1038/22682

Kleim JA, Cooper NR, VandenBerg PM. Exercise induces angiogenesis but does not alter movement representations within rat motor cortex. *Brain Res.* (2002) 934:1–6. doi: 10.1016/S0006-8993(02)02239-4

Kramer AF, Erickson KI. Capitalizing on cortical plasticity: influence of physical activity on cognition and brain function. *Trends Cogn Sci.* (2007) 11:342–8. doi: 10.1016/j.tics.2007.06.009

Hillman CH, Erickson KI, Kramer AF. Be smart, exercise your heart: exercise effects on brain and cognition. *Nat Rev Neurosci.* (2008) 9:58– 65. doi: 10.1038/nrn2298

Bherer L, Erickson KI, Liu-Ambrose T. A review of the effects of physical activity and exercise on cognitive and brain functions in older adults. *J Aging Res.* (2013) 9:657508. doi: 10.1155/2013/657508

Dwyer T, Coonan WE, Leitch DR, Hetzel BS, Baghurst RA. An investigation of the effects of daily physical activity on the health of primary school students in South Australia. *Int J Epidemiol.* (1983) 12:308–13. doi: 10.1093/ije/12.3.308

Hollar D, Messiah SE, Lopez-Mitnik G, Hollar TL, Almon M, Agatston AS. Healthier options for public schoolchildren program improves weight and blood pressure in 6-to 13-year-olds. *J Am Diet Assoc.* (2010) 110:261– 7. doi: 10.1016/j.jada.2009.10.029

Donnelly JE, Greene JL, Gibson CA, Smith BK, Washburn RA, Sullivan DK, et al. Physical activity across the curriculum (PAAC): a randomized controlled trial to promote physical activity and diminish overweight and obesity in elementary school children. *Prev Med.* (2009) 49:336– 41. doi: 10.1016/j.ypmed.2009.07.022

Shephard RJ, Volle M, Lavallee H, LaBarre R, Jequier JC, Rajic M. Required physical activity and academic grades: a controlled study. In: Ilmarinen J, Välimäki I, editors. *Children and Sport.* Berlin: Springer (1984). p. 58– 63. doi: 10.1007/978-3-642-69465-3_8

Ahamed Y, MacDonald H, Reed K, Naylor PJ, Liu-Ambrose T, Mckay H. School-based physical activity does not compromise children's academic performance. *Med Sci Sports Exerc.* (2007) 39:371–6 doi: 10.1249/01.mss.0000241654.45500.8e

Sallis JF, McKenzie TL, Alcaraz JE, Kolody B, Faucette N, Hovell MF. The effects of a 2-year physical education program (SPARK) on physical activity and fitness in elementary school students. Sports, Play and Active Recreation for Kids. *Am J Public Health.* (1997) 87:1328–34. doi: 10.2105/AJPH.87.8.1328

Etnier JL, Salazar W, Landers DM, Petruzzello SJ, Han M, Nowell P. The influence of physical fitness and exercise upon cognitive functioning: a meta-analysis. *J Sport Exerc Psychol.* (1997) 19:249–77. doi: 10.1123/jsep.19.3.249

Trudeau F, Shephard RJ. Physical education, school physical activity, school sports and academic performance. *Int J Behav Nutr Phys Act.* (2008) 5:10. doi: 10.1186/1479-5868-5-10

Verstraete SJM, Cardon GM, De Clercq DLR, De Bourdeaudhuij IMM. Increasing children's physical activity levels during recess periods in elementary schools: the effects of providing game equipment. *Eur J Public Health.* (2006) 16:415–9. doi: 10.1093/eurpub/ckl008

Darling-Hammond L, Berry B. Highly qualified teachers for all. *Educ Leadersh.* (2006) 64:14–20.

Pantics N. *The meaning of teacher competence in contexts of change: in search of missing elements of a knowledge base for teacher education–moral purposes and change agentry* (doctoral dissertation), Utrecht, Netherlands, University of Utrecht (2011).

Daly-smith AJ, Zwolinsky S, Mckenna J, Tomporowski PD, Defeyter MA, Manley A. Systematic review of acute physically active learning and classroom movement breaks on children's physical activity, cognition, academic performance and classroom behaviour: understanding critical design features. *BMJ Open Sport Exerc Med.* (2018) 4:e000341. doi: 10.1136/bmjsem-2018-000341

Donnelly JE, Hillman CH, Castelli D, Etnier JL, Lee S, Tomporowski P, et al. Physical activity, fitness, cognitive function, and academic achievement in children: a systematic review. *Med Sci Sports Exerc.* (2016) 48:1197– 222. doi: 10.1249/MSS.0000000000000901

Singh AS, Saliasi E, Van Den Berg V, Uijtdewilligen L, De Groot RHM, Jolles J, et al. Effects of physical activity interventions on cognitive and academic performance in children and adolescents: a novel combination of a systematic review and recommendations from an expert panel. *Br J Sports Med.* (2018) 53:640–7. doi: 10.1136/bjsports-2017-098136

Xue Y, Yang Y, Huang T. Effects of chronic exercise interventions on executive function among children and adolescents: a systematic review with meta-analysis. *Br J Sport Med.* (2019) 53:1397–404. doi: 10.1136/bjsports-2018-099825

Watson A, Timperio A, Brown H, Best K, Hesketh KD. Effect of classroom- based physical activity interventions on academic and physical activity outcomes: a systematic review and meta-analysis. *Int J Behav Nutr Phys Act.* (2017) 14:114. doi: 10.1186/s12966-017-0569-9

Braaksma P, Stuive I, Garst RME, Wesselink CF, van der Sluis CK, Dekker R, et al. Characteristics of physical activity interventions and effects on cardiorespiratory fitness in children aged 6–12 years—A systematic review. *J Sci Med Sport.* (2018) 21:296–306. doi: 10.1016/j.jsams.2017. 07.015

Moher D, Liberati A, Tetzlaff J, Altman DG, PRISMA Group. Preferred reporting items for systematic reviews and meta-analyses: the PRISMA statement. *PLoS Med.* (2010) 6:e1000097. doi: 10.1371/journal.pmed.1000097

Moher D, Shamseer L, Clarke M, Ghersi D, Liberati A, Petticrew M, et al. Preferred reporting items for systematic review and meta-analysis protocols (PRISMA-P) 2015 statement. *Ann Intern Med.* (2009) 151:264– 9. doi: 10.7326/0003-4819-151-4-200908180-00135

Alesi M, Bianco A, Luppina G, Palma A. Improving children's coordinative skills and executive functions: the effects of a football exercise program. perceptual and motor skills. *Percept Mot Skills.* (2016) 122:27–46. doi: 10.1177/0031512515627527

Ardoy DN, Fernández-Rodríguez JM, Jiménez-Pavón D, Castillo R, Ruiz JR, Ortega FB. A physical education trial improves adolescents' cognitive performance and academic achievement: the EDUFIT study. *Scand J Med Sci Sports.* (2014) 24:e52–61. doi: 10.1111/sms.12093

Beck MM, Lind RR, Geertsen SS, Ritz C, Lundbye-Jensen J, Wienecke J. Motor-enriched learning activities can improve mathematical performance in preadolescent children. *Front Hum Neurosci*. (2016) 10:645. doi: 10.3389/fnhum.2016.00645

Bunketorp Käll L, Malmgren H, Olsson E, Lindén T, Nilsson M. Effects of a curricular physical activity intervention on children's school performance, wellness, and brain development. *J Sch Health*. (2015) 85:704– 13. doi: 10.1111/josh.12303

Chaddock-Heyman L, Erickson KI, Voss M, Knecht A, Pontifex MB, Castelli D, et al. The effects of physical activity on functional MRI activation associated with cognitive control in children: a randomized controlled intervention. *Front Hum Neurosci*. (2013) 12:72. doi: 10.3389/fnhum.2013.00072

Coe DP, Pivarnik JM, Womack CJ, Reeves MJ, Malina RM. Effect of physical education and activity levels on academic achievement in children. *Med Sci Sport Exerc*. (2006) 38:1515–9. doi: 10.1249/01.mss.0000227537.13175.1b

Costigan SA, Eather N, Plotnikoff RC, Hillman CH, Lubans DR. High- intensity interval training on cognitive and mental health in adolescents. *Med Sci Sports Exerc*. (2016) 48:1985–93. doi: 10.1249/MSS.0000000000000993

Davis CL, Tomporowski PD, Boyle CA, Waller JL, Miller PH, Naglieri JA, et al. Effects of aerobic exercise on overweight children's cognitive functioning: a randomized controlled trial. *Res Q Exerc Sport*. (2007) 78:510– 9. doi: 10.1080/02701367.2007.10599450

De Greeff JW, Hartman E, Bosker RJ, Doolaard S, Visscher C. Long-term effects of physically active academic lessons on physical fitness and executive functions in primary school children. *Health Educ Res*. (2016) 31:185– 94. doi: 10.1093/her/cyv102

Ericsson I. Motor skills, attention and academic achievements. An intervention study in school years 1–3. *Br Educ Res J*. (2008) 34:301– 13. doi: 10.1080/01411920701609299

Ericsson I, Karlsson MK. Motor skills and school performance in children with daily physical education in school–a 9-year intervention study. *Scand J Med Sci Sports*. (2014) 24:273–8. doi: 10.1111/j.1600-0838.2012. 01458.x

Erwin H, Fedewa A, Ahn S. Student academic performance outcomes of a classroom physical activity intervention : a pilot study. *Int Electron J Elem Educ*. (2013) 5:473–87.

Fedewa AL, Davis MC. A randomized controlled design investigating the effects of classroom-based physical activity on children's fluid intelligence and achievement. *School Psychol Int*. (2015) 36:135–53. doi: 10.1177/0143034314565424

Fisher A, Boyle JME, Paton JY, Tomporowski P, Watson C, McColl JH, et al. Effects of a physical education intervention on cognitive function in young children: randomized controlled pilot study. *BMC Pediatr*. (2011) 11:97. doi: 10.1186/1471-2431-11-97

Gao Z, Hannan P, Xiang P, Stodden DF, Valdez VE. Video game-based exercise, Latino children's physical health, and academic achievement. *Am J Prev Med*. (2013) 44:S240–6. doi: 10.1016/j.amepre.2012.11.023

Hedges WD, Hardin VB. Effects of a perceptual motor program on achievement of first graders. *Educ Leadersh Res Suppl*. (1972) 6:5231–2.

Hillman C, Pontifex MB, Castelli D, Khan NA. Effects of the FITKids randomized controlled trial on executive control and brain function. *Pediatrics*. (2014) 134:e1063–71. doi: 10.1542/peds.2013-3219

Hollar D, Lombardo M, Lopez-Mitnik G, Hollar TL, Almon M, Agatston AS, et al. Effective multi-level, multi-sector, school-based obesity prevention programming improves weight, blood pressure, and academic performance, especially among low-income, minority children. *J Health Care Poor Underserved*. (2010) 21:93–108. doi: 10.1353/hpu.0.0304

Ismail AH. The effects of a well-organized physical education programme on intellectual performance. *Research in Phys Educ*. (1967) 1:31–8.

Kamijo K, Pontifex MB, Leary KCO, Scudder MR, Wu C, Castelli DM, et al. The effects of an afterschool physical activity program on working memory in preadolescent children. *Dev Sci*. (2011) 14:1046– 58. doi: 10.1111/j.1467-7687.2011.01054.x

Katz DL, Cushman D, Reynolds J, Njike V, Treu JA, Walker J, et al. Putting physical activity where it fits in the school day: preliminary results of the abc (activity bursts in the classroom) for fitness program. *Prev Chronic Dis*. (2010) 7:A82.

KoutsandrÉou F, Wegner M, Niemann C, Budde H. Effects of motor versus cardiovascular exercise training on children's working memory. *Med Sci Sport Exerc*. (2016) 48:1144–52. doi: 10.1249/MSS.0000000000000869

Kvalø SE, Bru E, Brønnick K, Dyrstad SM. Does increased physical activity in school affect children's executive function and aerobic fitness? *Scand J Med Sci Sports*. (2017) 27:1833–41. doi: 10.1111/sms.12856

Ludyga S, Gerber M, Kamijo K, Brand S, Pühse U. The effects of a school-based exercise program on neurophysiological indices of working memory operations in adolescents. *J Sci Med Sport*. (2018) 21:833–8. doi: 10.1111/josh.12303

Mahar MT, Rowe DA, Kenny RK, Fesperman DN. Evaluation of the TAKE 10 classroom-based physical activity program. *Med Sci Sport Exerc*. (2003) 35:S135. doi: 10.1097/00005768-200305001-00742

Mcclelland E, Pitt A, Stein J. Enhanced academic performance using a novel classroom physical activity intervention to increase awareness, attention and self- control: putting embodied cognition into practice. *Improv Schools*. (2015) 18:83–100. doi: 10.1177/1365480214562125

Mullender-Wijnsma MJ, Hartman E, de Greeff JW, Bosker RJ, Doolaard S, Visscher C. Improving academic performance of school-age children by physical activity in the classroom: 1-year program evaluation. *J Sch Health*. (2015) 85:365–71. doi: 10.1111/josh.12259

Mullender-Wijnsma MJ, Hartman E, de Greeff JW, Doolaard S, Bosker RJ, Visscher C. Physically active math and language lessons improve academic achievement: a cluster randomized controlled trial. *Pediatrics*. (2016) 1:e20152743. doi: 10.1542/peds.2015-2743

Murray NG, Garza JC, Diamond PM, Hoelscher DM, Kelder S, Ward JL. Fitness and academic achievement among 3rd and 4th grade students in texas: 932. *Med Sci Sport Exerc*. (2008) 40:S96. doi: 10.1249/01.mss.0000321867.49584.bb

Peternelj B, Škof B, Strel J. Academic achievement of pupils in sport classes: pupils attending sport classes have higher final grades, but… *Kinesiologia Slovenica*. (2009) 15:5–16.

Reed JA, Einstein G, Hahn E, Hooker SP, Gross VP, Kravitz J. Examining the impact of integrating physical activity on fluid intelligence and academic performance in an elementary school setting: a preliminary investigation. *J Phys Act Heal*. (2010) 7:343–51. doi: 10.1123/jpah.7.3.343

Resaland GK, Aadland E, Moe VF, Aadland KN, Skrede T, Stavnsbo M, et al. Effects of physical activity on schoolchildren's academic performance: the Active Smarter Kids (ASK) cluster-randomized controlled trial. *Prev Med*. (2016) 91:322–8. doi: 10.1016/j.ypmed.2016.09.005

Riley N, Lubans DR, Holmes K, Morgan PJ. Findings from the EASY minds cluster randomized controlled trial : evaluation of a physical activity integration program for mathematics in primary schools. *J Phys Act Heal*. (2016) 13:198–206. doi: 10.1123/jpah.2015-0046

Sjöwall D, Hertz M, Klingberg T. No long-term effect of physical activity intervention on working memory or arithmetic in preadolescents. *Front Psychol*. (2017) 8:1–10. doi: 10.3389/fpsyg.2017. 01342

Spitzer US, Hollmann W. Trends in neuroscience and education experimental observations of the effects of physical exercise on attention, academic and prosocial performance in school settings. *Trends Neurosci Educ*. (2013) 2:1– 6. doi: 10.1016/j.tine.2013.03.002

Tarp J, Domazet SL, Froberg K, Hillman CH, Andersen LB, Bugge A. Effectiveness of a school-based physical activity intervention on cognitive performance in danish adolescents: lcomotion — learning, cognition and motion – a cluster randomized controlled trial. *PLoS ONE*. (2016) 11:e0158087. doi: 10.1371/journal.pone.0158087

Tuckman BW, Hinkle JS. An experimental study of the physical and psychological effects of aerobic exercise on schoolchildren. *Heal Psychol*. (1986) 5:197–207. doi: 10.1037/0278-6133.5.3.197

Niet AG Van Der, Smith J, Scherder EJA, Hartman E, Visscher C. Effects of a cognitively demanding aerobic intervention during recess on children's physical fitness and executive functioning. *Pediatr Exerc Sci*. (2016) 28:64–70. doi: 10.1123/pes.2015-0084

Vazou S. Intervention integrating physical activity with math : math performance, perceived competence, and need satisfaction. *J Sport Exercise Psy*. (2017) 15:508–22. doi: 10.1080/1612197X.2016.1164226

Zervas Y, Danis A, Klissouras V. Influence of physical exertion on mental performance with reference to training. *Percept Mot Skills*. (1991) 72:1215– 21. doi: 10.2466/pms.1991.72.3c.1215

Egger M, Smith GD, Schneider M, Minder C. Bias in meta- analysis detected by a simple, graphical test. *BMJ*. (1997) 15:629–34. doi: 10.1136/bmj.315.7109.629

Cohen J. *Statistical Power Analysis for the Behavioral Sciences*. Hillsdale, NJ: Lawrence Erlbaum Associates (1988).

Rosenthal R, Rosnow RL. *Essentials of Behavioral Research: Methods and Data Analysis*. New York, NY: McGraw-Hill (1991). p. 45.

Morris SB. Book Review: Hunter, JE, & Schmidt, FL (2004). Methods of Meta-Analysis: Correcting Error and Bias in Research Findings. Thousand Oaks, CA: Sage. *Organ Res Methods*. (2008) 11:184–7. doi: 10.1177/1094428106295494

Sawilowsky SS. New effect size rules of thumb. *J Mod Appl Stat Methods.* (2009) 8:597–9. doi: 10.22237/jmasm/1257035100

Sneck S, Viholainen H, Syväoja H, Kankaapää A, Hakonen H, Poikkeus AM, et al. Effects of school-based physical activity on mathematics performance in children: a systematic review. *Int J Behav Nutr Phys Act.* (2019) 16:109. doi: 10.1186/s12966-019-0866-6

Cumpston M, Li T, Page MJ, Chandler J, Welch VA, Higgins JP, et al. Updated guidance for trusted systematic reviews: a new edition of the Cochrane Handbook for Systematic Reviews of Interventions. *Cochrane Database Syst Rev.* (2019) 3:ED000142. doi: 10.1002/14651858.ED000142

Guyatt GH, Oxman AD, Kunz R, Atkins D, Brozek J, Vist G, et al. GRADE guidelines: 2. Framing the question and deciding on important outcomes. *J Clin Epidemiol.* (2011) 64:395–400. doi: 10.1016/j.jclinepi.2010.09.012

Fredericks CR, Kokot SJ, Krog S. Using a developmental movement programme to enhance academic skills in grade 1 learners. *South African J Res Sport Phys Educ Recreat.* (2006) 28:29–42. doi: 10.4314/sajrs.v28i1.25929

Rauner RR, Walters RW, Avery M, Wanser TJ. Evidence that aerobic fitness is more salient than weight status in predicting standardized math and reading outcomes in fourth-through eighth-grade students. *J Pediatr.* (2013) 163:344–8. doi: 10.1016/j.jpeds.2013.01.006

Yang XL, Telama R, Laakso L. Parents' physical activity, socioeconomic status and education as predictors of physical activity and sport among children and youths-A 12-year follow-up study. *Int Rev Sociol Sport.* (1996) 31:273– 91. doi: 10.1177/101269029603100304

Caterino MC, Polak ED. Effects of two types of activity on the performance of second-, third-, and fourth-grade students on a test of concentration. *Percept Mot Skills.* (1999) 89:245–8. doi: 10.2466/pms.1999.89.1.245

Fedewa AL, Ahn S. The effects of physical activity and physical fitness on children's achievement and cognitive outcomes: a meta-analysis. *Res Q Exerc Sport.* (2011) 82:521–35. doi: 10.1080/02701367.2011.10599785

Chamorro-Premuzic T, Furnham A. Neuroticism and "special treatment" in university examinations. *Soc Behav Personal an Int J.* (2002) 30:807– 11. doi: 10.2224/sbp.2002.30.8.807

Nelson MC, Gordon-Larsen P. Physical activity and sedentary behavior patterns are associated with selected adolescent health risk behaviors. *Pediatrics.* (2006) 117:1281–90. doi: 10.1542/peds.200 5-1692

Jurak G, Cooper A, Leskosek B, Kovac M. Long-term effects of 4-year longitudinal school-based physical activity intervention on the physical fitness of children and youth during 7-year follow-up assessment. *Cent Eur J Public Health.* (2013) 21:190–4. doi: 10.21101/cejph. a3823

McKenzie TL, Sallis JF, Faucette N, Roby JJ, Kolody B. Effects of a curriculum and inservice program on the quantity and quality of elementary physical education classes. *Res Q Exerc Sport.* (1993) 64:178– 87. doi: 10.1080/02701367.1993.10608795

Starc G, Strel J, Kovač M. *Telesni in Gibalni Razvoj Slovenskih Otrok in Mladine v Številkah: Šolsko Leto 2007/2008.* Ljubljana: Fakulteta za šport (2010).

Talbot M. Ways forward for primary physical education. *Phys Educ Matters.* (2008) 3:6–8.

Breslin G, Hanna D, Lowry RG, McKee D, Haughey T, Moore N. An exploratory study of specialist and generalist teachers: predicting self efficacy in delivering primary physical education. *Work Pap Heal Sci.* (2012) 1:1–9.

Manios Y, Kafatos I, Kafatos A, Team NCR. Ten-year follow-up of the Cretan Health and Nutrition Education Program on children's physical activity levels. *Prev Med.* (2006) 43:442–6. doi: 10.1016/j.ypmed.2006. 06.001

Whitehead M. *Physical Literacy: Throughout the Lifecourse.* New York, NY: Routledge (2010). doi: 10.4324/9780203881903

Designing and Validating a Basketball Learning and Performance Assessment Instrument (BALPAI)

Sergio J. Ibáñez[1], Sergio Martinez-Fernández[1,2], Sergio Gonzalez-Espinosa[1], Javier García-Rubio[1] and Sebastián Feu[3]*

[1] Faculty of Sport Science, University of Extremadura, Cáceres, Spain, [2] Cáceres Club Baloncesto, Cáceres, Spain, [3] Faculty of Education, University of Extremadura, Badajoz, Spain

***Correspondence:**
Javier García-Rubio
jagaru@unex.es

Introduction: The assessment of learning in basketball in the PE class, and in training sessions of young players, requires valid, reliable, and trustworthy tools. The purpose of this research was to design and validate the Basketball Learning and Performance Assessment Instrument (BALPAI) that assesses simultaneously decision making, technical execution and efficacy. The play actions are codified using a categorical system, awarding a score for each category (1 = inadequate action; 2 = neutral action 3 = adequate action). An example of a summative procedure for assessing decision making in dribbling is: (1) Dribbling to a place where there is defensive pressure and there is a free teammate able to receive the pass; (2) Dribbling to a place where there is defensive pressure or a free teammate able to receive the pass; (3) Dribbling through a space where there is no defensive pressure and no free teammate able to receive the pass.

Methods: A pilot study was performed following this procedure. A group of 13 experts participated in the assessment of the 33 elements (66 items) included in the BALPAI. Aiken's V formula was used to analyze content validity, and internal consistency was calculated using Cronbach's α. Inter-observer reliability was determined among three observers who used the BALPAI to record the play actions in a 3×3 basketball match ($N = 45$ possessions) and was calculated with the Multirater κfree, obtaining an almost perfect agreement with values between 0.84 and 1.

Results: The BALPAI has very high internal consistency (0.969), Interobserver reliability was almost perfect (>0.84 in all items) and Aiken's V coefficient (>0.71 in all items) attained a high value.

Conclusion: The BALPAI proved to be a valid tool, with high internal consistency and reliability that makes it possible to perform a complete assessment of basketball in PE classes.

Keywords: team sport, evaluation, validity, reliability, basketball, assessment

INTRODUCTION

A mandatory prerequisite for making a valid and reliable qualitative analysis is the organization of the information by competent analysts. A systematic observational strategy (SOS) has to be planned (Knudson and Morrison, 2002) that contains all the relevant information about human movements. Therefore, the designing of instruments for the assessment of team sports using observation has become increasingly important as a research topic in the last few years. Between the 60s and the 80s, objective tests were the predominant method for assessing motor skills (Lopez-Pastor et al., 2013).

These tests presented certain limitations for being applied to the different playing skills in invasion sports as they did not include decision making (Oslin et al., 1998), and actual play during games (Bar-Eli and Raab, 2006). Later, test focused on the speed decision-makings occurs in real game (Thiffault, 1980), and evolve to measure the accuracy of these decisions (French and Thomas, 1987). Advances in the assessment of game performance behaviors help PE teachers to draw solid conclusions about their interventions during team sports teaching. The development of valid and reliable instruments will help not only teachers, but also other students for peer assessment in classroom settings (Memmert and Harvey, 2008). Moreover, linking what is being taught to what will be assessed, helps students to focus on what is important, making the teaching-learning cycle more congruent (Grehaigne et al., 2005). Accordingly, specific research should be undertaken in the evolution and development of observation tools that overcomes these limitations.

Thus, several instruments have been developed to assess play performance using systematic observation (Morgan et al., 2014), like the *Game Performance Assessment Instrument* (GPAI) (Oslin et al., 1998), or the *Team Sport Assessment Procedure* (TSAP) (Gréhaigne et al., 1997). These instruments represent a starting point for the observation of different team sports, and were designed to offer tools for PE teachers to assess their students. Based on these tools, new specific ones have been developed for different sports like soccer (García-López et al., 2013), handball (Tallir et al., 2003), futsal (Gonzalez-Villora and da Costa, 2015), or basketball (Tallir et al., 2007; Chen et al., 2013; Folle et al., 2014). These tools including the observation and assessment of a greater number of offensive actions with the ball (for example: shooting technique, dribbling technique, passing and catching, in and out 1 × 1, etc.) and without the ball (for example: jump stop and pivoting, 2 × 2 and 3 × 3 game play, etc.). In fact, off-the-ball actions are essential to be successful (Oslin et al., 1998), due the quantity of game play that occurs away from the ball.

In basketball, the tactical instrument proposed by Tallir et al. (2007) is more complete that the one proposed by Chen et al. (2013), as it analyses three different components for each play action (decision making, execution of the motor skill and efficacy). In each one of these components, appropriate and inappropriate actions are defined using a system of categories. Thus, it specifies what decisions are *correct* and *incorrect*, what technical actions are executed *correctly* and *incorrectly* and finally if the results of the actions are *successful* or *unsuccessful*. However, the limitation of these aforementioned instruments is that they only observe and assess offensive actions, not taking into account defensive ones.

The tools for observation and evaluation of the game must not only be reliable and valid, but must also be designed so they do not generate doubts in the observers, possessing high inter and intra-observer reliability. For this reason, it is necessary to complement the designs and validation of tools with real-time testing by observers or coders (Painczyk et al., 2018). These instruments present limitations as they do not take into account all the phases of the game (offense and defense), all the playing skills (with and without the ball) or the three components of play actions (decision making, technical execution and efficacy). In addition, as Knudson and Morrison (2002) stated, although their book is primarily based on technique, it is necessary to establish the level of the analysis. These instruments should assess the long- or short-term improvement of a motor skill, called *Learning* and *Performance*. Short-term changes in motor skills refer to performance, whereas long-term changes are called learning. Therefore, the objectives of the present study were (i) to design and validate an instrument for the specific and overall assessment of basketball, and (ii) to assess its inter-observer reliability. This instrument should make it possible to evaluate the learning of the basic concepts of the game that can be used in a 3 × 3, because it can be used to evaluate students in school (basic learning) and young basketball players who are beginning their training (basic performance).

MATERIALS AND METHODS

Instrument

The measures tool, the Basketball Learning and Performance Assessment Instrument (BALPAI), e.g., the protocol to obtain the variables to be analyzed (see **Supplementary Annex 1**), includes a total of 11 play actions, 7 offensive play actions with and without the ball (Dribbling; Shooting; Passing; Receiving; Passing game; Occupying free spaces without the ball; Offensive rebound), and 4 on ball and off ball in defense (On ball defense; Off ball defense; Defensive help/defensive change; Defensive rebound). All these actions belong to the taxonomy of contents drawn up by Ibáñez (2002) for basketball training categories. Complex actions of the 3 × 3 game (pick and roll or pop, pin downs, hand-off, etc.) are not included, since the instrument has been designed to evaluate basic learning and performance. The inclusion of complex tactical actions, with multiple solutions, requires specific instruments, such as those designed to analyze the pick and roll (Gómez et al., 2015) or the inside pass (Courel-Ibáñez et al., 2016). The instrument assesses three differentiated components of play actions: decision making, technical execution and final efficacy. Each of these three components of the play action is codified according to its adequacy. Thus, each action is codified as: (i) Inadequate; (ii) Neutral; or (iii) Adequate. This codification proposal is different from the majority of existing instruments, as it is a development from two levels of assessment (appropriate/inappropriate; adequate/inadequate; successful/unsuccessful) to three, being similar to the one suggested by Folle et al. (2014), including an intermediate level of adequacy. The play actions are codified using a categorical system (**Supplementary Annex 1**), awarding a score for each category (1 = inadequate action; 2 = neutral action 3 = adequate action). Once all the play actions have been codified, the match participation and performance indicators are calculated for each player.

Two procedures were followed to establish the adequacy of the game action in each of the components of the instrument, [based on Chen et al. (2013) and Tallir et al. (2007)]: (i) the summative procedure, (ii) the levels procedure.

Summative Procedure

Two criteria were established to assess a game action. If the game action fulfills both established criteria, it is considered adequate; if it only fulfills one criterion it is considered neutral; and if it does not fulfill any criterion it is considered inadequate. An example of a summative procedure for assessing decision making in dribbling is: (1) Dribbling to a place where there is defensive pressure and there is a free teammate able to receive the pass; (2) Dribbling to a place where there is defensive pressure or a free teammate able to receive the pass; (3) Dribbling through a space where there is no defensive pressure and no free teammate able to receive the pass.

Levels Procedure

Three levels of adequacy were established for the action. Depending on how the action is observed, its level of adequacy is determined (inadequate, neutral or adequate). In addition, an example of the levels procedure for assessing final efficacy in shooting is: (1) The shot is blocked by a defender and/or does not touch the hoop or backboard; (2) The shot does not go through the hoop but touches the hoop or backboard; (3) The shot goes through the hoop.

After all the play actions have been codified, the indicators are calculated for participation in the game (PG), decision making (DM), technical execution (TE) and final efficacy (FE). The Performance Index (PI) in the game is calculated from these together with the decision-making performance index (DM-PI), the technical execution performance index (TE-PI), the final efficacy performance index (FE-PI); and the total performance index (Total-PI) (**Table 1**). These indices offer information on each of the analyzed dimensions and the game performance of the student or player.

Research Design

This research represents an instrumental investigation as it involves the design and validation of an instrument for its subsequent application (Ato et al., 2013). For this reason, this section is organized in two studies.

Study 1: Design and Validation of an Instrument for the Specific and Overall Assessment of Basketball

Participants

In this study, the selection of the sample was intentional, as all the subjects chosen had to fulfill determined inclusion criteria to be able to be identified as experts. These criteria were based on their experience in making judgments, their reputation in the community, their availability and motivation for participating in the study, and their impartiality and inherent qualities, like self-confidence and adaptability (Skjong and Wentworth, 2001). Thus all the experts had to fulfill at least four of the following six criteria: (i) have a Ph.D. in Sports Sciences; (ii) be or have been a university lecturer; (iii) have the highest federative qualification in a team sport; (iv) have 10 years' experience as a university lecturer; (v) have 10 years' experience as a team sport coach in any category, and (vi) have published articles on the topic of team sports (Blomqvist et al., 2005; Villarejo et al., 2014; García-Martín et al., 2016; Ortega-Toro et al., 2019). All the experts were from the same country (Spain), and did not have a direct relationship with the research team. None of the experts received any gratification for participating in the project, their intervention being voluntary. Participation was requested from 25 experts who met the aforementioned requirements, and a response was received from 13 (52% participation). All experts signed written informed consents prior to the development of the study.

Measures

Content validity, which is the degree to which each item represents the content (Thomas et al., 2015). This variable was measured by expert judgment. The group of experts evaluated both the degree of pertinence of each item to the object of study (Adequacy), and the degree of accuracy and correctness in its explanation (Wording). Both concepts were evaluated with a Likert-type scale from 1 to 10. They were also asked for a general qualitative evaluation of each item to express possible alternatives when they deemed it necessary (Villarejo et al., 2014; García-Martín et al., 2016). The validity of the instrument was measured with Aiken's V coefficient (Aiken, 1985).

Internal consistency or the reproducibility of the measure shows the internal reliability of the instrument A test cannot be valid if lacks of reliability. The have to be consistent to be trustworthy, results cannot depend on successive trials to achieve the same results (Thomas et al., 2015).

Procedures

For the first study, a literature review was previously conducted on designed instruments to assess performance in team sports in general and basketball in particular. The authors then defined all the items included in the first version of the tool. In the second stage of the study, the necessary criteria were established for being considered an expert. All the necessary documentation for the qualitative and quantitative assessment of the instrument was sent by email to 25 experts: a formal presentation of the study, the BALPAI and a template where they could make their assessments. Positive answers were received by email from the experts participating in the study. The experts were asked about: (i) the level of pertinence of the components of play actions (decision making, technical execution and final efficacy) and coding levels (inadequate action; neutral action; adequate action) to be evaluated; (ii) the level of comprehension of the components of play actions from the observational instrument; (iii) the need to include other play actions, or qualitative comments about play actions.

TABLE 1 | Calculation of indicators of participation and performance in the game.

	Decision making (DM)	Technical execution (TE)	Final Efficacy (FE)
PLAYER A	**Sum of points for decision making (Pts DM)**	**Sum of points for technical execution (Pts TE)**	**Sum of points for final efficacy (Pts FE)**
Participation in the game (PG)		PG = N° of total actions performed by player A	
Performance Index (PI)	PI-DM = Pts DM/PG	PI-TE = Pts TE/PG	PI-FE = Pts FE/PG
		Total PI = (PI-DM+PI-TE+PI-FE) /3	

After the assessment of the experts, the criteria were defined for the modification, elimination or approval of the items according to the value obtained for Aiken's (1985) V coefficient. The analysis of the internal consistency of the items was calculated with Cronbach's α based on the values provided by the experts for the two content validity variables of adequacy and wording of each item.

Study 2: Assessment the Instrument Inter-Observer Reliability

Participants

For reliability purposes, youth players were recorded and assessed. The youth participants were attending the same state school class. A total of 25 fifth graders students (14 boys aged 10.78 years and 11 girls aged 10.85 years), from two different class groups (13 students from group A and 12 students from group B) from a school in the southwest of Spain took part in the study. Teachers, students and experts were informed of the study protocol, the participation of both groups and the research purposes. The students were informed that they would be filmed for later analysis. The basketball half court matches were part of the Physical Education classes, included in a basketball program of 15 sessions (55 min each) (González-Espinosa et al., 2017). The games were filmed in the last two sessions. The teams were created for the study and they did not have prior experience as a team. The teams were balanced by considering technical-tactical skills of all the students involved (Gracia et al., 2014). Teams were formed together by the teacher and the research staff.

Measures

Inter-observer reliability, or internal reliability, understood as the degree of agreement among the observers. In this case, the agreement among different observers concerning the description of several events is assessed (Thomas et al., 2015). In order to achieve high levels of reliability, all observers have received training in the use of instrument.

Procedures

Finally, the level of inter-observer reliability of the instrument was determined among three observers who used the BALPAI to record the play actions in a 3 × 3 basketball match. Only one hoop is used in the game and when a defense rebound occurs, the ball have to be returned outside the traditional three point-line before start attacking (Montgomery and Maloney, 2018). The three observers who intervened in this phase fulfilled all the previously defined inclusion criteria for being considered expert and, in addition, have time availability. For the observers to attain a minimum of reliability and objectivity in the codification, it was necessary to reach an agreement among them to permit an increase in the accuracy of the recordings of this human behavior (Medina and Delgado, 1999). The three observers received five training sessions (Muñoz et al., 2018).

The last two corresponded to the test of reliability among the observers for which each one recorded all the play actions in a filmed 3 × 3 basketball match. This game modality offers the players a greater opportunity to participate more successfully than in more numerous game modalities (Martínez-Fernández et al., 2015). Games were recorded with a SONY Full HD 1080 video camera at 60 fps; allowing experts to use slow motion and watch the videos as many times as they needed. The experts collected the data using an excel sheet designed for this purpose. This test assessed six subjects at the same time. Thus, the reliability analysis was made on the first 15 possessions in a match of 5 min duration on the part of each observer. The teams were established randomly, to avoid the polluting variable of the game level. The sample that participated in this study was composed of six students, three students per team. For this study, a game was selected in which only boys played, to avoid the contaminating variable of gender. The same clips were evaluated by the experts, who had no relation with the players nor were known to them. The experts were able to watch the video clips using Gamebreaker software (Sylvan Advantage, Hartford, Vermont) as many times as they thought fit, until they could make an adequate judgment. This option was determined, as they were continuous game actions, occurring simultaneously.

The parents of the players were informed about the study and gave their written consent in accordance with the Declaration of Helsinki. The study, with a full description of the protocols regarding recruitment and participation of the experts, was approved by the Ethics Committee of the University of Extremadura (no. 67/2017).

DATA ANALYSIS

Firstly, content validity was calculated with Aiken's V coefficient (Aiken, 1985). Its value goes from 0 to 1, with the latter marking perfect concordance among the experts with regard to the contents assessed. Aiken's V coefficient score establishes which items should be eliminated, modified or retained. Aiken's V was calculated following the algebraic equation modified by Penfield and Giacobbi (2004).

$$V = \frac{\bar{X} - l}{k}$$

Calculations were made using the free software program Visual Basic 6.0 (Merino and Livia, 2009), which makes it possible to obtain three factors: the range of valuations (maximum valuation − minimum valuation), Aiken's V coefficient and the confidence intervals of 90, 95, and 99% using the score method (Penfield and Giacobbi, 2004).

The exact critical reference value for the acceptance of Aiken's V was calculated using the initial formula proposed by Aiken (1985), applying the central limit theorem for large samples (m > 25). The number of experts was 13 (n), the number of items 66 (m), with an answer range of 10 (c); applying the value of the constant of content validity of 95 and 99% (z).

$$\frac{z}{0.2\sqrt{\frac{3mn(c-1)}{(c+1)}}} + 0.5$$

The confidence level of 95% was considered to obtain the exact critical value for an item to be included and a value of 0.68 was attained. Similarly, the confidence level of 99% was considered to obtain the cut-off point for the modification of the tasks attaining a value of 0.75. **Table 2** shows the criteria used for the acceptance, modification or elimination of the items from the instrument.

Cronbach's α was then used for the analysis of internal consistency. This coefficient presents values between 0 and 1 and shows the reliability of the studied instrument. A value of 1 is perfect reliability but >0.70 is considered valid (Field, 2009). SPSS 21.0 software was used to analyze the internal consistency of the instrument (IBM SPSS Statistics for Windows. Armonk, NY: IBM Corp.).

Finally, the inter-rater agreement of the instrument was studied. As three raters intervened in the reliability analysis and the number of cases which had to be distributed in each of the categories of the instrument was unknown, it was necessary to use the *Free-Marginal Multirater Kappa* (*Multirater* κ_{free}) (Randolph, 2005). The computer application Online Kappa Calculator[1] was used for the interobserver reliability analysis. The variables analyzed were categorical. The following values were used to interpret the strength value of the Multirater κ_{free}: (i) a value of 0.00 or less was considered poor agreement; (ii) a value of 0.00 to 0.20 slight agreement; (iii) a value of 0.21 to 0.40 fair agreement; (iv) a value of 0.41 to 0.60 moderate agreement; (v) a value of 0.61 to 0.80 substantial agreement; and (vi) a value of 0.81 to 1 was considered almost perfect agreement (Landis and Koch, 1977; Altman, 1991).

RESULTS

Table 3 shows the mean values obtained for each of the items in the BALPAI instrument as well as the value of Aiken's V coefficient. These high values suggest a high content validity in our results.

The values obtained indicate that it was not necessary to eliminate any of the items according to the criteria established in the literature. A very demanding criterion was established for the elimination or modification of the items. However, there was no need to make any changes in Adequacy (A). Changes only had to be made in the Wording (W) of the following items: DM in dribbling; TE in shooting; DM in passing. The contributions that the group of experts made in their subjective valuations were used as a reference to carry out the necessary modifications. These modifications were made in all the items suggested with the aim of improving the instrument, despite not being necessary in some items. The instrument was sent back to the experts, who accepted the final version.

All the variables in the instrument attained a value for Cronbach's α of greater than 0.90 except Decision Making (0.87) (**Table 4**). The results of the internal consistency and IO reliability tests indicated high levels of reliability for this instrument. The analysis confirmed the high level of internal consistency.

Finally, **Table 5** shows the results regarding inter-observer reliability where all the items attained a value of above 0.81 and some equal to 1.

DISCUSSION

The purpose of the present study was to design an instrument for the specific and general assessment of basketball play. It had to assess offensive and defensive play actions, with and without the ball, and their three components. The results show that the BALPAI is the most complete of the existing instruments and has a high level of content validity, internal reliability and inter-observer reliability.

To validate the instrument, it was necessary to have expert opinion on its application (García-Martín et al., 2016). In the case of studies involving the judgment of experts a series of recommendations have to be taken into account, like those mentioned by Bulger and Housner (2007), Dunn et al. (1999), Escobar-Pérez and Cuervo-Martínez (2008) and Skjong and Wentworth (2001): the quality of the inclusion criteria, the number of experts necessary for this type of study, the preparation of the instructions and assessment templates, the procedure for collecting the quantitative and qualitative statistics as well as the adequate statistical analysis to give the instrument validity and reliability.

With regard to the sample of experts used in the investigation, several studies have established the range between two and twenty (Rubio et al., 2003), other researchers consider that ten is a reliable number (Hyrkäs et al., 2003), or three minimum, five acceptable, and ten, the ideal number (Lynn, 1986). In this study the number of experts who participated by offering their assessment of all the items in the instrument was 13, corresponding to 53% of the initially detected population according to demanding inclusion criteria, and fulfilling the requisites established in the literature.

The qualitative assessments of the experts are equally important when developing and perfecting the items of the instrument (Bulger and Housner, 2007; Carretero-Dios and Pérez, 2007; Padilla et al., 2007), and in this case, a deficiency was revealed in the quantification of the values of the questionnaire in some items. The experts' contributions were directed at

[1] http://justusrandolph.net/kappa/

TABLE 2 | Criteria for the acceptance, modification or elimination of the items.

		Wording		
		>0.75	[0.68–0.75]	<0.68
Adequacy	>0.75	Correct	Wording is modified	Wording is modified
	[0.68–0.75]	Adequacy is modified	Adequacy and Wording are modified	Adequacy and Wording are modified
	<0.68	Eliminated	Eliminated	Eliminated

TABLE 3 | Results of Aiken's V coefficient for the 11 variables of the BALPAI in each of the play action components.

	Dribbling						**Shooting**						**Passing**					
	DM*		**TE**		**FE**		**DM**		**TE***		**FE**		**DM***		**TE**		**FE**	
	A	**W**	**A**	**W**	**A**	**W**	**A**	**W**	**A**	**W**	**A**	**W**	**A**	**W**	**A**	**W**	**A**	**W**
M	7.57	7.50	8.50	8.14	8.57	8.71	9.00	8.29	8.50	7.36	8.07	9.07	8.14	7.57	8.29	8.07	9.15	9.50
V	0.79	0.72	0.83	0.79	0.84	0.86	0.89	0.81	0.83	0.71	0.79	0.90	0.79	0.73	0.81	0.79	0.91	0.94
	Receiving						**Passing and playing**						**Occupying free spaces**					
	DM*		**TE**		**FE**		**DM**		**TE***		**FE**		**DM***		**TE**		**FE**	
	A	**W**	**A**	**W**	**A**	**W**	**A**	**W**	**A**	**W**	**A**	**W**	**A**	**W**	**A**	**W**	**A**	**W**
M	8.86	8.14	8.86	8.29	8.57	9.50	8.08	8.08	9.07	8.50	9.29	8.50	9.07	8.21	8.93	8.64	8.79	8.71
V	0.87	0.79	0.87	0.81	0.84	0.94	0.79	0.79	0.90	0.83	0.90	0.83	0.90	0.80	0.88	0.85	0.87	0.86
	Offensive rebound						**Defensive rebound**						**On ball defense**					
	DM*		**TE**		**FE**		**DM**		**TE***		**FE**		DM*		**TE**		**FE**	
	A	**W**	**A**	**W**	**A**	**W**	**A**	**W**	**A**	**W**	**A**	**W**	**A**	**W**	**A**	**W**	**A**	**W**
M	9.21	8.86	8.93	9.14	8.86	8.71	9.36	9.21	9.21	8.79	9.36	9.07	9.29	8.93	9.36	8.50	9.00	9.00
V	0.91	0.87	0.88	0.90	0.87	0.86	0.93	0.91	0.91	0.87	0.93	0.90	0.92	0.88	0.93	0.83	0.89	0.89

	Off ball defense						**Assisting and recovery/defensive change**					
	DM*		**TE**		**FE**		**DM**		**TE***		**FE**	
M	9.21	8.21	8.93	8.64	9.21	8.79	8.57	8.21	8.50	8.14	9.14	8.65
V	0.91	0.80	0.88	0.85	0.91	0.87	0.84	0.80	0.83	0.79	0.90	0.85

*M, Arithmetic mean; V, Aiken's V; A, Adequacy; W, Wording; DM, Decision making; TE, Technical execution; FE, Final efficacy. * = Item where W was modified.*

TABLE 4 | Results of the analysis of the internal consistency of the instrument.

	Adequacy	**Wording**	**Offense**	**Defense**	**DM**	**TE**	**FE**	**Instrument**
α	0.959	0.950	0.953	0.933	0.876	0.917	0.921	0.969
N	33	33	42	24	22	22	22	66

DM, Decision making; TE, Technical execution; FE, Final efficacy; N, Number of items.

improving the wording, clarifying the expressions so that they did not generate doubts in the future codifiers. The value 2 did not correctly discriminate between the values one and three of the instrument. Thus, according to the suggestions of several experts, the value 2 was re-worded so that the difference with the other values was even clearer. Furthermore, although not as clearly as in the previous assessments, the experts indicated that the item on the technical execution of the shot led to misunderstandings in the way it was expressed. It was suggested that the description be modified, especially with regard to the part referring to "the starting point for the shot." Many of the assessments of the experts were reflections on the instrument which, in some cases, made it possible to define its items more clearly and accurately (Wiersma, 2001).

The content validity showed values in all the items of over 0.70 for Aiken's V, so that it was only necessary to modify the wording

TABLE 5 | Results of Interobserver reliability for each of the 11 variables in the BALPAI in each of the components of the play actions.

	Dribbling			Shooting			Passing			Receiving			Passing and playing			Occupying free spaces		
	DM	TE	FE	DM	TE	FE	DM	TE	FE	DM	TE	FE	DM	TE	FE	DM	TE	FE
Po	0.94	0.94	0.89	0.93	0.99	0.99	0.94	0.99	0.99	1	0.94	1	1	1	1	0.94	1	0.92
κ_{free}	0.92	0.92	0.84	0.90	0.99	0.99	0.92	0.99	0.99	1	0.91	1	1	1	1	0.91	1	0.88

	Offensive rebound			Defensive rebound			On Ball defense			Off ball defense			Assisting and recovery/defensive change		
	DM	TE	FE	DM	TE	FE	DM	TE	FE	DM	TE	FE	DM	TE	FE
Po	0.97	1	1	0.97	0.93	1	0.93	0.96	0.96	1	1	0.98	0.99	0.99	0.99
κ_{free}	0.96	1	1	0.96	0.90	1	0.90	0.95	0.95	1	1	0.97	0.99	0.99	0.99

Po, Percentage of global agreement; κ_{free}, Free-marginal kappa; DM, Decision making; TE, Technical execution; FE, Final efficacy; N, Number of items.

of three of the 66 items. The demands of inclusion, modification and exclusion criteria were increased, 95% confidence criterion was established for acceptance or elimination of an item, and 99% for its modification (Penfield and Giacobbi, 2004). Previous studies have had lower levels of demand (Ortega et al., 2008; García-Martín et al., 2016; García-Santos and Ibáñez, 2016). These items were reworded as in previous studies (Bulger and Housner, 2007; Ortega et al., 2008; Villarejo et al., 2014). When the internal consistency of the instrument was analyzed, it was seen that other tools (questionnaires, interviews, instruments...) that had already been published and validated, present lower values than those attained by the BALPAI, overall Cronbach's $\alpha = 0.97$ vs. Cronbach's $\alpha = 0.72$ of IOVAB for basketball referees (García-Santos and Ibáñez, 2016); vs. Cronbach's $\alpha = 0.94$ of Socio-emotional questionnaire (Gómez-Carmona et al., 2014); and vs. Cronbach's $\alpha = 0.96$ of programs for sports education in the school context (Gonzalez-Espinosa et al., 2017). The values for inter-observer reliability were over 0.84 in Kappa coefficient thus being perfect or nearly perfect (Altman, 1991; Landis and Koch, 1977). The BALPAI tool has demonstrated very good inter-observer reliability in its practical application, with values of the Kappa coefficient between 0.84 and 1 in the 11 variables and the three components of the play actions (decision making, technical execution and efficacy), considered as an almost perfect agreement (Landis and Koch, 1977; Altman, 1991). Painczyk et al. (2018) used Cohen's Kappa coefficient to determine the interobserver reliability of a match evaluation notational system in Rugby Union, with values lower than those found in this study. These results confirm the quality of the design of the tool, since the observers who have used it have shown great concordance evaluating game actions. All the analyses carried out confirmed the validity and reliability of the designed instrument.

Differences between instruments have been pointed out, but possible explanation for these differences have to be exposed. Painczyk et al. (2018) analyzed seven complete rugby union games, observing several performance indicators with different operational definitions. BALPAI variables and operational definitions used for reliability purposes in our study were smaller. In addition, BALPAI was design for make easier observations, in the number of variables analyzed as in player's skill level. Moreover, main concerns of reliability studies are the clear operational definitions of each variable (Painczyk et al., 2018; O'Donoghue, 2007) and the observers training processes (Liu et al., 2017). Researchers that carried out the BALPAI reliability analysis have participated in the development and validation of the instrument, showing a great understanding of variables and definitions. Moreover, these researchers have been defined as experts, that achieve better reliability values that inexperienced ones (Painczyk et al., 2018).

The importance of observational tools has been previously reported in other sports and contexts (Llobet-Martí et al., 2016). Other testing procedures have reported different approaches such as creativity or divergent thinking (Memmert, 2010). These approaches will have to be taken into consideration in future research. In addition, further research should also suggest the analysis of coaches in order to improve the learning process with the validation of observational tools (Nicholls and Worsfold, 2016).

LIMITATIONS

Basketball Learning and Performance Assessment Instrument contains many items and components, thus the assessment process can be quite hard. This process can be focused on a single item at a time, or two or several. As well as helping students to pay attention to important information that they should learn, it simplifies the assessment process for teachers and coaches. Moreover, before using the BALPAI, teachers and coaches must undergo a training period in how to implement it, leading to a better use and recognition of play behaviors that can be quite subjective.

CONCLUSION

The BALPAI, has shown, during this first phase of validation, to be a valid and reliable instrument for assessing learning in basketball in PE classes, and has proved to be more complete than previously published tools, on which its design was based. It also possesses a high level of reliability in the codification of the play actions.

Teachers can use BALPAI in their teaching programs in Physical Education as part of the evaluation. The use of this tool will make it possible to assess the progress of players in the educational context, assessing students' learning during the school year. In addition, teacher can assess different teaching programs, comparing studentsŕesults in both programs. The repetition of the assessment of students will make it possible to confirm if the intervention programs used in their training are effective.

ETHICS STATEMENT

This study have been approved by the Ethics Committee of the University of Extremadura.

AUTHOR CONTRIBUTIONS

SI: conceptualization, data collection, formal analysis, investigation, methodology, writing review, and editing. SM-F: data collection, formal analysis, investigation, writing original draft. SG-E: data collection, formal analysis and investigation. SF: supervision, writing review, and editing. JG-R: supervision, writing original draft, writing review, and editing.

REFERENCES

Aiken, L. R. (1985). Three coefficients for analyzing the reliability and validity of ratings. *Educ. Psychol. Meas.* 45, 131–142. doi: 10.1177/0013164485451012

Altman, D. G. (1991). *Practical Statistics for Medical Research*. London: Chapman & Hall.

Ato, M., López, J. J., and Benavente, A. (2013). Un sistema de clasificación de los diseños de investigación en psicología. *Anal. Psicol.* 29, 1038–1059.

Bar-Eli, M., and Raab, M. (2006). Judgment and decision making in sport and exercise: rediscovery and new visions. *Psychol. Sport Exerc.* 7, 519–524. doi: 10.1016/j.psychsport.2006.07.003

Blomqvist, M., Vänttinen, T., and Luhtanen, P. (2005). Assessment of secondary school students' decision-making and game-play ability in soccer. *Phys. Educ. Sport Pedagogy* 10, 107–119. doi: 10.1080/17408980500104992

Bulger, S. M., and Housner, L. D. (2007). Modified delphi investigation of exercise science in physical education teacher education. *J. Teach. Phys. Educ.* 26, 57–80. doi: 10.1123/jtpe.26.1.57

Carretero-Dios, H., and Pérez, C. (2007). Normas para el desarrollo y revisión de estudios instrumentales: consideraciones sobre la selección de tests en la investigación psicológica. *Int. J. Clin. Health Psychol.* 7, 863–882.

Chen, W., Hendricks, K., and Zhu, W. (2013). Development and validation of the basketball offensive game performance instrument. *J. Teach. Phys. Educ.* 32, 100–109. doi: 10.1123/jtpe.32.1.100

Courel-Ibáñez, J., McRnobert, A. P., Ortega, E., and Cárdenas, D. (2016). Inside pass predicts ball possession effectiveness in NBA basketball. *Int. J. Perform. Anal. Sport* 16, 711–725. doi: 10.1080/24748668.2016.11868918

Dunn, J. G., Bouffard, M., and Rogers, W. T. (1999). Assessing item content-relevance in sport psychology scale-construction research: issues and recommendations. *Meas. Phys. Educ. Exerc. Sci.* 3, 15–36. doi: 10.1207/s15327841mpee0301_2

Escobar-Pérez, J., and Cuervo-Martínez, A. (2008). Validez de contenido y juicio de expertos: una aproximación a su utilización. *Av. Medición* 6, 27–36.

Field, A. (2009). *Discovering Statistics Using SPSS*, 3rd Edn. Londres: Sage publications.

Folle, A., Quinaud, R. T., Barroso, M. L. C., Rocha, J. C. S., Ramos, V., and Nascimento, J. V. D. (2014). Construção e validação preliminar de instrumento de avaliação do desempenho técnico-tático individual no basquetebol. [Preliminary development and validation of an assessment instrument of basketball individual technical-tactical performance]. *Revista da Educação Física UEM* 25, 405–418. doi: 10.4025/reveducfis.v25i3.23085

French, K. E., and Thomas, J. R. (1987). The relation of knowledge development to children's basketball performance. *J. Sport Psychol.* 9, 15–32. doi: 10.1123/jsp.9.1.15

García-López, L. M., González-Víllora, S., Gutiérrez, D., and Serra, J. (2013). Development and validation of the game performance evaluation tool (GPET) in soccer. *Sport Rev. Eur. Cienc. Dep.* 2, 89–99.

García-Martín, A., Antúnez, A., and Ibáñez, S. J. (2016). Análisis del proceso formativo en jugadores expertos: validación de instrumento/analysis of expert players' training process: validation of tools. *Rev. Int. Med. Cienc. Ac.* 16, 157–182. doi: 10.15366/rimcafd2016.61.012

García-Santos, D., and Ibáñez, S. J. (2016). Diseño y validación de un instrumento de observación para la valoración de un árbitro de baloncesto (IOVAB). *Sport Rev. Eur. Cienc. Dep.* 5, 15–26.

Gómez, M. A., Battaglia, O., Lorenzo, A., Lorenzo, J., Jiménez, S., and Sampaio, J. (2015). Effectiveness during ball screens in elite basketball games. *J. Sports Sci.* 33, 1844–1852. doi: 10.1080/02640414.2015.1014829

Gómez-Carmona, P. M., Cervera, V., and Benito, P. J. (2014). Diseño y validación de un cuestionario socio-emocional para jóvenes futbolistas de élite. *Rev. Int. Med. Cienc. Ac.* 14, 545–559.

González-Espinosa, S., Ibáñez, S. J., and Feu, S. (2017). Design of two basketball teaching programs in two different teaching methods. *E-Balonmano. com* 13, 131–152.

Gonzalez-Espinosa, S., Ibáñez, S. J., Feu, S., and Galatti, L. (2017). Intervention programs for sports education in the school context, PETB and PEAB: preliminary study. *Retos* 31, 107–113.

Gonzalez-Villora, S., and da Costa, I. T. (2015). How to evaluate the soccer tactics? System of tactical assessment in soccer (fut-sat). *Educ. Fís. Dep.* 34, 467–505. doi: 10.17533/udea.efyd.v34n2a08

Gracia, F., García, J., Cañadas, M., and Ibáñez, S. J. (2014). Heart rate differences in small-sided games in formative basketball. *E-Balonmano.com* 10, 23–30.

Gréhaigne, J.-F., Godbout, P., and Bouthier, D. (1997). Performance assessment in team sports. *J. Teach. Phys. Educ.* 16, 500–516.

Grehaigne, J. F., Richard, J. F., and Griffin, L. (2005). *Teaching and Learning Team Sports and Games*. New York, NY: Routledge Falmer.

Hyrkäs, K., Appelqvist-Schmidlechner, K., and Oksa, L. (2003). Validating an instrument for clinical supervision using an expert panel. *Int. J. Nurs. Stud.* 40, 619–625. doi: 10.1016/s0020-7489(03)00036-1

Ibáñez, S. J. (2002). "Los contenidos de enseñanza del baloncesto en las categorías de formación," in *Novos Horizontes para o Treino do Basquetebol*, eds S. J. Ibáñez and M. Macías (Lisbon: FMH Edições), 111–135.

Knudson, V., and Morrison, S. (2002). *Qualitative Analysis of Human Momento*. Champaign, IL: Human Kinetics.

Landis, J. R., and Koch, G. G. (1977). The measurement of observer agreement for categorical data. *Biometrics* 33, 159–174.

Liu, H., Hopkins, W., Gomez, M. A., and Molinuevo, J. (2017). Inter-operator reliability of live football match statistics from OPTA sportsdata. *Int. J. Perf. Anal. Sport* 13, 803–821. doi: 10.1080/24748668.2013.11868690

Llobet-Martí, B., López-Ros, V., Barrera-Gómez, J., and Comino, J. (2016). Assessing novices' game performance in rugby union: the Rugby attack assessment instrument (RAAI). *J. Teach. Phys. Educ.* 35, 181–186. doi: 10.1123/jtpe.2014-0134

Lopez-Pastor, V. M., Kirk, D., Lorente-Catalan, E., MacPhail, A., and Macdonald, D. (2013). Alternative assessment in physical education: a review of international literature. *Sport Educ. Soc.* 18, 57–76. doi: 10.1080/13573322.2012.713860

Lynn, M. R. (1986). Determination and quantification of content validity. *Nurs. Res.* 35, 382–386.

Martínez-Fernández, S., García, J., and Ibáñez, S. J. (2015). Incidence of type of game mode in player participation in minibasket. *Rev. Psi Dep.* 24, 65–68.

Medina, J., and Delgado, M. Á (1999). Metodología de entrenamiento de observadores para investigaciones sobre EF y deporte en las que se utilice como método la observación. *Rev. Mot.* 5, 69–86.

Memmert, D. (2010). Game test situations: assessment of game creativity in ecological valid situations. *Int. J. Sport Psychol.* 41:94.

Memmert, D., and Harvey, S. (2008). The game performance assessment instrument (GPAI): some concerns and solutions for further development. *J. Teach. Phys. Educ.* 27, 220–240. doi: 10.1123/jtpe.27.2.220

Merino, C., and Livia, J. (2009). Intervalos de confianza asimeìtricos para el índice la validez de contenido: un programa visual basic para la V de Aiken. *Anal. Psicol.* 25, 169–171.

Montgomery, P. G., and Maloney, B. D. (2018). Three-by-three basketball: inertial movement and physiological demands during elite games. *Int. J. Sports Physiol. Perf.* 13, 1169–1174. doi: 10.1123/ijspp.2018-0031

Morgan, G., Muir, B., and Abraham, A. (2014). "Systematic observation," in *Res MethSport Coach*, eds L. Nelson, R. Groom, and P. Potrac (London: Routledge), 123–131.

Muñoz, J., Gamonales, J. M., León, K., and Ibáñez, S. J. (2018). Formación de codificadores y fiabilidad de los registros. Una aplicación al goalball / training of coders and reliability. an application to the goalball. *Rev. Int. Med. Cienc. Ac.* 18, 669–691.

Nicholls, S. B., and Worsfold, P. R. (2016). The observational analysis of elite coaches within youth soccer: the importance of performance analysis. *Int. J. Sports Sci. Coach.* 11, 825–831. doi: 10.1177/1747954116676109

O'Donoghue, P. (2007). Reliability issues in performance analysis. *Int. J. Perf. Anal. Sport* 7, 35–48. doi: 10.1080/24748668.2007.11868386

Ortega, E., Jimenez, J. M., Palao, J. M., and Sainz de Barranda, P. (2008). Diseño y validación de un cuestionario para valorar las preferencias y satisfacciones en jóvenes jugadores de baloncesto. *Cuad. Psicol. Dep.* 8, 39–58.

Ortega-Toro, E., García-Angulo, A., Giménez-Egido, J. M., García-Angulo, F. J., and Palao, J. M. (2019). Design, validation, and reliability of an observation instrument for technical and tactical actions of the offense phase in soccer. *Front. Psychol.* 10:22. doi: 10.3389/fpsyg.2019.00022

Oslin, J. L., Mitchell, S. A., and Griffin, L. L. (1998). The game performance assessment instrument (GPAI): development and preliminary validation. *J. Teach. Phys. Educ.* 17, 231–243. doi: 10.1123/jtpe.17.2.231

Padilla, J. L., Gómez, J., Hidalgo, M. D., and Muñiz, J. (2007). Esquema conceptual y procedimientos para analizar la validez de las consecuencias del uso de los test. *Psicothema* 19, 173–178.

Painczyk, H., Hendricks, S., and Kraak, W. (2018). Intra and inter-reliability testing of a south african developed computerised notational system among western province club rugby coaches. *Int. J. Sports Sci. Coach.* 13, 1163–1170. doi: 10.1177/1747954118796368

Penfield, R. D., and Giacobbi, P. R. (2004). Applying a score confidence interval to Aiken's item content-relevance index. *Meas. Phys. Educ. Exerc. Sci.* 8, 213–225. doi: 10.1207/s15327841mpee0804_3

Randolph, J. J. (2005). Free-marginal multirater kappa: an alternative to fleissñ fixed-marginal multirater kappa. *Paper Presented at the Joensuu University Learning and Instruction Symposium 2005*, Joensuu.

Rubio, D. M., Berg-Weger, M., Tebb, S. S., Lee, E. S., and Rauch, S. (2003). Objectifying content validity: conducting a content validity study in social work research. *Soc. Work Res.* 27, 94–104. doi: 10.1093/swr/27.2.94

Skjong, R., and Wentworth, B. H. (2001). Expert judgment and risk perception. *Paper Presented at the The Eleventh International Offshore and Polar Engineering Conference*, Stavanger.

Tallir, I. B., Lenoir, M., Valcke, M., and Musch, E. (2007). Do alternative instructional approaches result in different game performance learning outcomes? Authentic assessment in varying game conditions. *Int. J. Sport Psychol.* 38, 263–282.

Tallir, I. B., Musch, E., Lanoo, K., and Van de Voorde, J. (2003). Validation of video-based instruments for the assessment of game performance in handball and soccer. *Paper Presented at the 2nd International Conference Teaching Sport and Physical Education for Understanding*, Melbourne.

Thiffault, C. (1980). "Construction et validation d'une mesure de la rapidité de la pensée tactique des jouers de jockey sur glace (The construction and validation of a measure of tactical thought of ice jockey players)," in *Psychology of Motor Behavior and Sport*, eds C. H. Nadeau, W. R. Halliwell, K. M. Newell, and G. C. Roberts (Champaign, IL: Human Kinetics), 643–649.

Thomas, J. R., Silverman, S., and Nelson, J. (2015). *Research Methods in Physical Activity, 7E*. Champaing, IL: Human Kinetics.

Villarejo, D., Ortega, E., Gómez, M. Á., and Palao, J. M. (2014). Design, validation, and reliability of an observational instrument for ball possessions in rugby union. *Int. J. Perf. Anal. Sport* 14, 955–967. doi: 10.1080/24748668.2014.11868771

Wiersma, L. D. (2001). Conceptualization and development of the sources of enjoyment in youth sport questionnaire. *Meas. Phys. Educ. Exerc. Sci.* 5, 153–177. doi: 10.1207/s15327841mpee0503_3

Association between Physical Fitness and Anxiety in Children: A Moderated Mediation Model of Agility and Resilience

*Yansong Li [1], Xue Xia [2], Fanying Meng [3] and Chunhua Zhang [1]**

[1] School of Kinesiology, Shanghai University of Sport, Shanghai, China, [2] School of Psychology, Shanghai University of Sport, Shanghai, China, [3] Institute of Physical Education, Huzhou University, Huzhou, China

Correspondence:
Chunhua Zhang
zch20080808@126.com

Background: Anxiety is one of the most prevalent mental health problems in children. Although physical fitness as a predictor of mental health, the mechanisms underlying any association between physical fitness and anxiety in children have been understudied. Thus, the aim of the present study was to determine whether an association exists between physical fitness and anxiety and to explore the roles of agility and resilience in such an association.

Methods: This cross-sectional study investigated 269 children aged 7 to 12 years from three public primary schools in Shanghai (China). Physical fitness and agility were objectively measured, and resilience and anxiety were assessed using self-reported questionnaires. The moderated mediation model was examined using the SPSS PROCESS macro, in which the moderator variable was agility, and the mediator variable was resilience.

Results: Physical fitness was inversely associated with anxiety. Resilience partially and indirectly mediated this association, and agility moderated the association between physical fitness and resilience. Physical fitness had a greater impact on resilience in children with higher agility levels.

Conclusions: Agility moderated the mediation of resilience on the indirect, inverse association between physical fitness and anxiety; thus, incorporating methods to develop agility and resilience may lead to better outcomes for physical fitness programs designed to prevent or alleviate anxiety in children.

Keywords: children, physical fitness, agility, resilience, anxiety, moderated mediation

INTRODUCTION

Anxiety is one of the most prevalent mental health problems among children (1, 2), with an estimated prevalence up to 20% (3, 4). Anxiety in children has a negative impact on their school performance (5), social functioning (6), and quality of life (7). In addition, anxiety symptoms during childhood tend to be chronic and may lead to anxiety disorders and other serious psychopathological consequences that persist into later childhood and adulthood (1, 8, 9). Indeed, approximately half the anxiety disorders diagnosed in adults have an onset before 11 years of age (10). In addition to the potential long-term effects on individuals' growth and development, children's anxiety disorders place a burden on society via direct and indirect costs (11); public expenses are more than 20 times as high for a child with vs. without clinically relevant anxiety (12). Hence, to mitigate these negative consequences of childhood anxiety, identifying the factors that affect anxiety and their underpinning mechanisms may contribute to the development of effective prevention and treatment interventions to benefit individuals as well as society.

Previous research has shown various protective factors for anxiety, such as self-efficacy (13), coping style (14), and social support (15). A positive role for physical activity in the prevention of anxiety has also been shown in several types of recent studies (16–18). Physical fitness can be defined as the capacity to perform physical activity (19), and physical fitness is more predictive of health outcomes than is physical activity in children (20). Thus, given the established health benefits of physical activity broadly, increasing evidence indicates a need to explore physical fitness. Physical fitness is considered one of the most important health markers and predictors of future risk of mental health issues (21, 22). In addition, physical fitness also serves as a buffer against stress and stress-related disorders (23). Anxiety is a stress-related mental health problem, but the association between physical fitness and anxiety is still unclear (24, 25). Therefore, investigating the mechanisms underlying the role physical fitness plays in childhood anxiety is critically needed.

To date, it is not well-understood which factors are crucial for the maintenance of physical and mental health. Resilience is a relatively new construct that may be an important factor (26). Resilience is the ability to successfully adapt to stress, trauma, or adversity, enabling individuals to avoid stress-induced mental disorders, such as depression, posttraumatic stress disorder, and anxiety (27, 28). In this regard, exploring how to build resilience may be useful in assisting children affected by anxiety. On the other hand, physical fitness may confer resilience owing to its stress-buffering effects (23). Thus, from a stress perspective, physical fitness, and anxiety may be linked through resilience.

In addition, agility, as the main component of physical fitness, is a combination of physical qualities and cognitive components (22, 29). However, unlike studies examining other main components (e.g., cardiorespiratory fitness, muscular fitness), few studies have focused on the contribution of agility to mental health (19). Within the limited literature, agility was summarized as a major input that enables resilience (30). Research has also reported that regular exposure to diverse agility-type movement challenges may facilitate the movement efficiency of athletes and their resilience to numerous dimensions of movement stress (31). Thus, whether the benefits of physical fitness on childhood anxiety may be enhanced by resilience and the role that agility plays in these relationships warrant further attention.

Therefore, the present study examined the associations among physical fitness, agility, resilience, and anxiety in children. On the basis of previous research results, we proposed the following three hypotheses: (1) physical fitness is inversely associated with anxiety in children; (2) resilience mediates the association between physical fitness and anxiety; and (3) agility moderates the indirect effect of physical fitness on anxiety through resilience, with the association becoming stronger when agility is high and weaker when agility is low. Based on these hypotheses, we proposed a theoretical model to be tested (**Figure 1**). In the proposed model, physical fitness plays a role in enhancing resilience and ameliorating anxiety, and the influence of physical fitness on anxiety is mediated by resilience, with the strength of this mediation conditional depending on the level of agility.

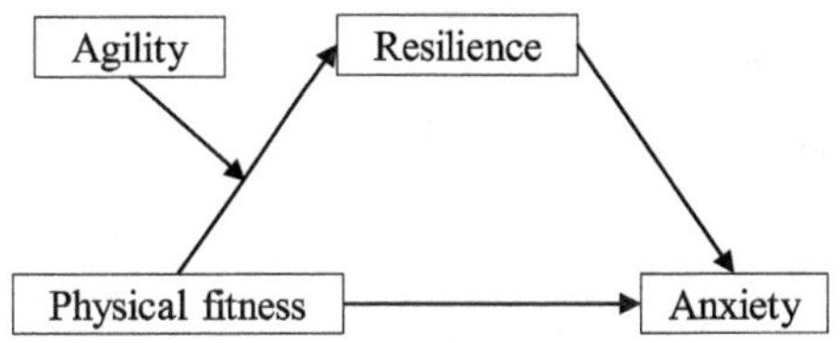

FIGURE 1 | The proposed moderated mediation model to be tested.

MATERIALS AND METHODS

Participants

The participants were selected from three primary schools in Shanghai (China). A sampling of schools was stratified according to physical fitness with three levels, with the first quartile being the lowest, followed by second and third quartiles, and the highest being the fourth quartile, as described and used in previous studies (32, 33). The current three schools were chosen for their representativeness of each level, considering the accessibility to our research team and the availability of the teachers to assist with logistics. Potential participants who had not received a diagnosis of any disease that made it impossible to complete the test and who understood each item in the questionnaires were included. Participants whose physical fitness test results exceeded the logical limits or whose questionnaires were considered invalid were excluded. After the aim of the study was explained, participants completed the objective measurements and self-reported questionnaires under the supervision of trained volunteers. Participants' names were substituted with codes in the data collection to protect privacy, and they were given an inexpensive gift as a token of appreciation. The results obtained from the tests were offered to the school administrators to provide suggestions for participants' physical activity and mental health.

Valid variables were obtained from 269 participants. The participants were in school grades 2 through 5 and comprised 126 boys and 143 girls, with ages ranging from 7–12 years (mean age = 9.75 years; SD = 1.17 years). The number (percentage) of participants by school grade was 72 (26.8%) in second grade, 67 (24.9%) in third grade, 66 (24.5%) in fourth grade, and 64 (23.8%) in fifth grade.

The study was conducted in accordance with the recommendations of the World Medical Association's

TABLE 1 | Fitness components and weights of CNSPFS scores in school-age children.

Second grade		Third and fourth grades		Fifth grade	
Fitness component	**Weight (%)**	**Fitness component**	**Weight (%)**	**Fitness component**	**Weight (%)**
BMI	15	BMI	15	BMI	15
Vital capacity of lung	15	Vital capacity of lung	15	Vital capacity of lung	15
50 m sprint	20	50 m sprint	20	50 m sprint	20
Sit and reach	30	Sit and reach	20	Sit and reach	10
Timed rope-skipping	20	Timed rope-skipping	20	Timed rope-skipping	10
		Timed sit-ups	10	Timed sit-ups	20
				50 m × 8 shuttle run	10

BMI, Body Mass Index; CNSPFS, Chinese National Student Physical Fitness Standard.

Declaration of Helsinki as revised in 1989 and was approved by the Shanghai University of Sport Ethics Committee (Shanghai, China). Written informed consent was obtained from the guardians of all participants.

Measures

Physical Fitness

To minimize variability, all physical fitness tests were conducted by trained volunteers from the Shanghai Research Center for Physical Fitness and Health of Children and Adolescents. The volunteers all majored in kinesiology and were already familiar with the testing methods.

Physical fitness was measured using the Chinese National Student Physical Fitness Standard (CNSPFS), a standardized test commonly used in Chinese schools (34). As indicated in the CNSPFS guidelines, the results of different fitness components were scored according to sex and school grade level. The total physical fitness score was composed of the product sum of the scores and weights of each component. The weights of the CNSPFS scores for each fitness component stratified by school grade are given in **Table 1**.

Agility

Agility was assessed using the side-step test, which is an effective and commonly used measure (35). For this test, the participant stood over a central line. At the start of the test, the participant moved laterally, side-stepping toward a far-right line (1 m from the central line) until the right foot crossed the far-right line. Once the right foot crossed that line, the participant changed directions and moved laterally, side-stepping to the left until the left foot crossed the far-left line (1 m from the central line). After reaching the far-left line, the participant moved laterally to return to the central line. This motion was repeated for 20 s, and one point was given for each line passed. The test was conducted twice, and the highest side-step score was recorded.

Resilience

Resilience was obtained using the Resilience Scale for Chinese Adolescents (RSCA), which has shown excellent psychometric properties and has been widely used in evaluating the resilience of Chinese children (36). It includes 27 items that have been classified into five factors: target concentration, emotional control, positive thinking, family support, and interpersonal assistance. Participants were asked to rate themselves on questions using a 5-point Likert scale ranging from a score of 1, indicating "not true at all," to 5, indicating "true nearly all the time." The total score for the RSCA ranged from 27 to 135, with a higher score indicating a higher level of resilience. Cronbach's alpha for this test in the present study was 0.74.

Anxiety

Anxiety was defined using the Chinese version of the Multidimensional Anxiety Scale for Children (MASC), a 39-item self-report scale for assessing children's anxiety (37). The items clustered into the following four scales: physical symptoms, harm avoidance, social anxiety, and separation anxiety. Response options ranged from 0, indicating "never true," to 3, indicating "often true." The total score (range, 0–117) was generated by adding the scores of all items; thus, a higher score reflected a greater degree of anxiety. Cronbach's alpha for this scale in this study was 0.89.

Statistical Analysis

The data were analyzed using SPSS, version 22.0, and the PROCESS macro program for SPSS (38). Both graphical (normal probability plots) and statistical (Kolmogorov–Smirnov test) methods were used to examine the nature of the variables, and all were found to fit a normal distribution. Thus, parametric statistics were used. Harman's single–factor test was conducted, and the results indicated that no serious method bias existed in the present study.

We conducted descriptive statistics for the main study variables (reported as means ± standard deviations) and Pearson correlation for bivariate associations (reported as values of r). We then used the PROCESS macro to perform a regression-based path analysis, which is similar to structural equation modeling but takes into consideration irregular sampling distributions (39). As noted by Edwards and Lambert (40), the distribution of the indirect effect can be non-normal even if the constituent variables are normal. Given this possibility, all regression coefficients were tested using the bias-corrected percentile Bootstrap method (41, 42). We tested the theoretical hypothesis model, controlled for age and sex, by estimating the 95% confidence intervals (CIs) for the mediation and

TABLE 2 | Descriptive statistics and correlations between variables.

Variable	Mean ± SD	1	2	3	4
(1). Physical fitness	81.50 ± 9.80	–			
(2). Agility	37.18 ± 9.03	0.408***	–		
(3). Resilience	93.10 ± 13.77	0.248***	0.267***	–	
(4). Anxiety	43.33 ± 19.18	−0.244***	−0.154*	−0.247***	–

*SD, standard deviation; *p < 0.05, ***p < 0.001.*

TABLE 3 | Mediation modeling results assessing the effect of physical fitness on anxiety.

Effect	Path	β	SE	t	LLCI	ULCI
Total effect	Physical fitness–anxiety	−0.256	0.060	−4.261***	−0.374	−0.137
Direct effect	Physical fitness–resilience	0.249	0.060	4.139***	0.131	0.367
	Resilience–anxiety	−0.190	0.060	−3.145**	−0.308	−0.071
	Physical fitness–anxiety	−0.208	0.061	−3.423**	−0.328	−0.089
Indirect effect	Physical fitness–resilience–anxiety	−0.047	0.019	-	−0.088	−0.013

*β, standardized coefficients; SE, standard error; LLCI and ULCI, lower level and upper level of the bias-corrected 95% bootstrap confidence interval; **p < 0.01, ***p < 0.001.*

moderation effects, with 5,000 resampled samples. When a 95% CI did not include 0, the result was considered statistically significant. We selected the Model 4 in PROCESS to examine the simple mediation effect of resilience on the association between physical fitness and anxiety. We then incorporated the proposed moderator variable (agility) into the model by conducting moderated mediation (also known as a conditional indirect effect) analysis using the Model 7 in PROCESS to determine whether the indirect path was conditionally moderated by the "strength" or value of agility. This model uses ordinary least squares regression to assess the conditional indirect effect and tests the effect with bootstrap CIs for different values of the moderating variable (agility) to determine whether the indirect effect varies. Before formal data analysis, all variables were standardized. Values of $p < 0.05$ were considered statistically significant.

RESULTS

Descriptive statistics and correlations of the study variables are shown in **Table 2**. We found that physical fitness, agility, and resilience were inversely correlated with anxiety; physical fitness was directly correlated with agility and resilience; and agility was directly correlated with resilience.

As shown in **Table 3**, the results of simple mediation model testing using Model 4 indicated that physical fitness was directly associated with resilience ($\beta = 0.249$, $t = 4.139$, $p < 0.001$). Resilience was inversely associated with anxiety ($\beta = -0.190$, $t = -3.145$, $p < 0.01$). The association between physical fitness and anxiety was also significant ($\beta = -0.208$, $t = -3.423$, $p < 0.01$). We also found a significant indirect effect of physical fitness on anxiety via resilience: the bootstrapping results indicated an indirect effect [$\beta = -0.047$; 95% CI: (-0.088, -0.013)]. The indirect effect accounted for 18.4% of the total effect, suggesting that resilience played a partial mediating role in the association between physical fitness and anxiety. These findings supported our first and second study hypotheses.

Moderated mediation analysis using Model 7 was conducted to assess whether anxiety was indirectly affected by physical fitness via mediation through resilience and whether this effect was conditionally moderated by agility. We hypothesized that children with higher agility scores would show a stronger association between physical fitness and resilience compared with those with lower agility scores. **Table 4** shows the results of the moderated mediation model test. The effect of the interaction between physical fitness and agility on resilience was statistically significant ($\beta = 0.167$, $t = 2.597$, $p < 0.05$). **Figure 2** illustrates the interaction at high (plus 1 SD) and low (minus 1 SD) levels of physical fitness and agility. The plots indicate the interaction between physical fitness and agility on resilience and suggested that for children with higher agility levels, there was a stronger positive association between physical fitness and resilience compared with children having lower agility levels.

The conditional indirect effect of physical fitness on anxiety through resilience at various values of agility was analyzed when the agility score was the sample mean and also at plus or minus 1 SD. The results revealed that the conditional indirect effect was significant at the mean and at a high level (plus 1 SD) of the moderator (agility), but not at a low level (minus 1 SD), and the bootstrap 95% CIs supported these results (see **Table 5**). In addition, the moderated mediation index was also statistically significant. These results supported our third study hypothesis because the association between physical fitness and the outcome variables became more evident as the moderator value increased.

DISCUSSION

In the present study, we used a moderated mediation model analysis to assist in understanding the mechanisms underlying any association between physical fitness and anxiety in children. Our results supported our three study hypotheses, namely, that

TABLE 4 | Moderated mediation modeling results assessing the effect of physical fitness on anxiety.

Outcome variable	Factor	β	SE	t	LLCI	ULCI	R^2	F
Resilience	Physical fitness	0.222	0.067	3.312**	0.090	0.353	0.119	7.129***
	Agility	0.144	0.068	2.119*	0.010	0.278		
	Physical fitness × agility	0.167	0.064	2.597*	0.040	0.293		
	Age	0.045	0.052	0.859	−0.058	0.147		
	Sex	−0.052	0.118	−0.444	−0.283	0.179		
Anxiety	Physical fitness	−0.208	0.061	−3.423**	−0.328	−0.089	0.109	8.061***
	Resilience	−0.190	0.060	−3.145**	−0.308	−0.071		
	Age	−0.052	0.050	−1.031	−0.150	0.047		
	Sex	0.187	0.118	1.586	−0.045	0.419		

*β, standardized coefficients; SE, standard error; LLCI and ULCI, lower level and upper level of the bias-corrected 95% bootstrap confidence interval; *p < 0.05, **p < 0.01, ***p < 0.001.*

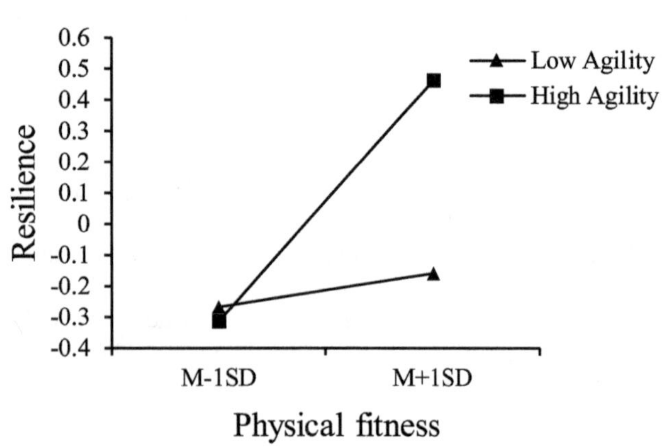

FIGURE 2 | Agility moderated the effect of physical fitness on resilience.

TABLE 5 | Moderated mediation effect of physical fitness on anxiety at specific conditional values of agility.

	Specific conditional values of agility			
	β	SE	LLCI	ULCI
−1 SD	−0.010	0.015	−0.046	0.017
Mean	−0.042	0.017	−0.077	−0.010
+1 SD	−0.074	0.030	−0.134	−0.017
	Index of moderated mediation			
	Index	**SE**	**LLCI**	**ULCI**
Agility	−0.032	0.016	−0.066	−0.003

β, standardized coefficients; SD, standard deviation; SE, standard error; LLCI and ULCI, lower level and upper level of the bias-corrected 95% bootstrap confidence interval.

(1) higher physical fitness levels were associated with lower anxiety levels in children, (2) resilience mediated physical fitness and anxiety, and (3) agility moderated the mediation of resilience on the association, which was stronger in children with higher levels of agility.

Our results suggested that higher levels of physical fitness were associated with lower anxiety levels in children. A plausible explanation for this finding is that individuals who display higher levels of physical fitness tend to have more positive perceptions of anxiety symptoms and thus feel less anxious (25). This supposition is supported by several studies that have shown that improvements in physical fitness are associated with reductions in levels of anxiety (43–45). However, Rodriguez-Ayllon et al. (19) found no relationship between physical fitness components and anxiety indicators. In addition to the demographic characteristics of the participants, these discrepant results may be because those previous studies focused on specific components of physical fitness (46), but physical fitness components relate in different ways to the various aspects of mental health (19). Our study results were based on the total physical fitness scores of children obtained by CNSPFS. This comprehensive outcome reflects the basic physical fitness of children and is an important basis for judging the overall level of physical fitness in children. Further analysis of physical fitness as a protective factor may provide a new approach for the prevention or intervention of childhood anxiety. Moreover, the fitness components, standards for evaluation, and score weights vary in the CNSPFS to adjust for the growth and development of children. Thus, incorporating interventions to reduce the level of anxiety through physical fitness programs that are appropriate at each age in children may lead to better outcomes.

Our mediation model revealed that resilience mediated the association between physical fitness and anxiety, indicating that establishing good physical fitness was conducive to resilience in children, which in turn ameliorates their anxiety. Physical fitness appears to confer resilience by blunting or optimizing neuroendocrine and physiological responses (e.g., the hypothalamic-pituitary-adrenal axis, the sympathetic nervous system) to physical and psychosocial stressors (23). In line with previous studies (47–49), our result is meaningful in that it supports physical fitness being an effective manner of building resilience in children. On the other hand, resilience can also indirectly reduce the negative effects of stress on anxiety through its mediation effect (50, 51). As a dynamic process, resilience is construed as an active adaptation mechanism that may help alleviate anxiety (27), which was observed in our study. In other words, resilience accounting for an important part of the variations in anxiety symptoms suggests that interventions should target ways to enhance resilience (50).

We speculate that a biological mechanism that might provide an explanation for our findings is that physical fitness may promote resilience by minimizing inflammation. The benefits of physical fitness may, in part, be attributed to anti-inflammatory effects via changes in body composition and skeletal muscle (23). On the other hand, Interleukin-8 as an inflammatory marker, has been suggested to be involved in the biological mechanisms mediating resilience to anxiety (52). Overall, resilience may serve as a "bridge" linking physical fitness and anxiety; thus, it would be insufficient to attempt to reduce anxiety in children by promoting physical fitness alone because resilience also plays an important role.

Our moderated mediation model offered a more detailed picture of the mechanisms that associated physical fitness with anxiety, providing a basis for improving anxiety in children using physical fitness via full consideration of the characteristics of agility. However, in research investigating the relationship between physical fitness and mental health, to the best of our knowledge, there is no in-depth analysis examining the importance of agility. Therefore, in our study, we used agility as an independent moderator to assess its influence. Interestingly, we found that physical fitness did not have a significant effect on resilience when the level of agility was low, but the positive effect of physical fitness occurred with the improvement of agility. More importantly, these results were confirmed in our physical fitness–anxiety model. These findings support our hypothesis that in relation to mental health, agility plays a critical role in the effects of physical fitness.

The self-efficacy based model of resilience suggests that executive function provides much of the capacity for resilience in individuals, with executive function enhancing self-efficacy to enable successful adjustment (53, 54). Additionally, executive function yields a greater propensity for resilience in children (55 56). On the other hand, recent evidence suggests that agility is a key component for executive function, and children with higher levels of agility have shown better performance in executive function (46, 57). Taken together, these findings indicate that executive function combines agility with resilience—which to some extent reflects the adaptation and coping ability of children (56)—to help explain the pathway between agility and resilience and provide a new perspective for further understanding how physical fitness affects resilience. More interestingly, the side-step test used in the present study is also considered useful for improving cardiorespiratory and muscular fitness (35). These main fitness components may all contribute to the promotion of resilience (19, 23). Therefore, the potential connections appear to demonstrate the value of agility, which should be taken into account for physical fitness to benefit resilience. To gain greater insight into the moderation effect of agility on the association between physical fitness and anxiety, both theoretical and empirical research studies are needed in the future.

Our study has some limitations that should be considered when interpreting our results. First, this study used a cross-sectional design, which prevented us from making any cause-and-effect conclusions. Therefore, longitudinal studies should be designed to validate the findings. Second, our study relied in part on self-reported data, which may affect the outcomes. Future studies should measure mental health objectively, such as through neuropsychological tests. Third, our findings were obtained from children in public primary schools, and whether the results are applicable to other populations will require further testing.

CONCLUSIONS

The current study offers some insight into the mechanisms underlying the association between physical fitness and anxiety. Physical fitness is a valuable factor, providing some protection against anxiety for children. This protective effect is partially mediated through the resilience, which is moderated by agility. The moderation effect may enable children with higher agility levels to show better outcomes in the association between physical fitness and anxiety. The analysis conducted in the present study using a moderated mediation model analysis expands on the current knowledge by providing evidence to support potential mechanisms. The results of this analysis suggest that incorporating methods to develop agility and to improve resilience may lead to better outcomes when designing physical fitness programs to prevent or alleviate anxiety in children.

ETHICS STATEMENT

The studies involving human participants were reviewed and approved by Shanghai University of Sport Ethics Committee. Written informed consent to participate in this study was provided by the participants' legal guardian/next of kin.

AUTHOR CONTRIBUTIONS

YL, FM, and CZ contributed to the conception and design of the study. XX and FM organized the database. YL and XX performed the statistical analysis and wrote the first draft of the manuscript. CZ revised the manuscript. All authors contributed to manuscript revision, read, and approved the submitted version.

ACKNOWLEDGMENTS

The authors thank all the participants, volunteers, teachers, and schools for their enthusiastic participation in this study.

REFERENCES

Cartwright-Hatton S, McNicol K, Doubleday E. Anxiety in a neglected population: prevalence of anxiety disorders in pre-adolescent children. *Clin Psychol Rev* (2006) 26:817–33. doi: 10.1016/j.cpr.2005.12.002

Lichtwarck-Aschoff A, van Rooij M. Are changes in children's communication patterns predictive of treatment outcomes for children with anxiety? *Clin Psychol Psychother*. (2019) 26:572–85. doi: 10.1002/cpp.2383

Chavira DA, Stein MB, Bailey K, Stein MT. Child anxiety in primary care: prevalent but untreated. *Depress Anxiety*. (2004) 20:155–64. doi: 10.1002/da.20039

Kendall PC, Safford S, Flannery-Schroeder E, Webb A. Child anxiety treatment: outcomes in adolescence and impact on substance use and depression at 7.4-year follow-up. *J Consult Clin Psychol*. (2004) 72:276–87. doi: 10.1037/0022-006X.72.2.276

Mazzone L, Ducci F, Scoto MC, Passaniti E, D'Arrigo VG, Vitiello B. The role of anxiety symptoms in school performance in a community sample of children and adolescents. *BMC Public Health*. (2007) 7:347. doi: 10.1186/1471-2458-7-347

Kertz SJ, Sylvester C, Tillman R, Luby JL. Latent class profiles of anxiety symptom trajectories from preschool through school age. *J Clin Child Adolesc Psychol*. (2019) 48:316–31. doi: 10.1080/15374416.2017.1295380

Kucian K, McCaskey U, O'Gorman Tuura R, von Aster M. Neurostructural correlate of math anxiety in the brain of children. *Transl Psychiatry*. (2018) 8:273. doi: 10.1038/s41398-018-0320-6

Bittner A, Egger HL, Erkanli A, Jane Costello E, Foley DL, Angold A. What do childhood anxiety disorders predict? *J Child Psychol Psychiatry*. (2007) 48:1174–83. doi: 10.1111/j.1469-7610.2007.01812.x

Green SA, Berkovits LD, Baker BL. Symptoms and development of anxiety in children with or without intellectual disability. *J Clin Child Adolesc Psychol*. (2015) 44:137–44. doi: 10.1080/15374416.2013.873979

Kessler RC, Berglund D, Demler O, Jin R, Merikangas KR. Lifetime prevalence and age-of-onset distributions of DSM-IV disorders in the national comorbidity survey replication. *Arch Gen Psychiatry*. (2005) 62:593–602. doi: 10.1001/archpsyc.62.6.593

Hoffman DL, Dukes EM, Wittchen HU. Human and economic burden of generalized anxiety disorder. *Depress Anxiety*. (2008) 25:72–90. doi: 10.1002/da.20257

Bodden DH, Dirksen CD, Bogels SM. Societal burden of clinically anxious youth referred for treatment: a cost-of-illness study. *J Abnorm Child Psychol*. (2008) 36:487–97. doi: 10.1007/s10802-007-9194-4

Sullivan TP, McPartland T, Price C, Cruza-Guet MC, Swan SC. Relationship self-efficacy protects against mental health problems among women in bidirectionally aggressive intimate relationships with men. *J Couns Psychol*. (2013) 60:641–7. doi: 10.1037/a0033406

Xiong W, Liu H, Gong P, Wang Q, Ren Z, He M, et al. Relationships of coping styles and sleep quality with anxiety symptoms among Chinese adolescents: a cross-sectional study. *J Affect Disord*. (2019) 257:108–15. doi: 10.1016/j.jad.2019.07.032

Hopkins PD, Shook NJ. A review of sociocultural factors that may underlie differences in African American and European American anxiety. *J Anxiety Disord*. (2017) 49:104–13. doi: 10.1016/j.janxdis.2017.04.003

Knappe F, Colledge F, Gerber M. Impact of an 8-week exercise and sport intervention on post-traumatic stress disorder symptoms, mental health, and physical fitness among male refugees living in a greek refugee camp. *Int J Environ Res Public Health*. (2019) 16:3904. doi: 10.3390/ijerph16203904

Schuch FB, Stubbs B, Meyer J, Heissel A, Zech P, Vancampfort D, et al. Physical activity protects from incident anxiety: a meta-analysis of prospective cohort studies. *Depress Anxiety*. (2019) 36:846–58. doi: 10.1002/da.22915

Yan W, Wang X, Kuang H, Chen Y, Baktash MB, Eskenazi B, et al. Physical activity and blood pressure during pregnancy: mediation by anxiety symptoms. *J Affect Disord*. (2020) 264:376–82. doi: 10.1016/j.jad.2019.11.056

Rodriguez-Ayllon M, Cadenas-Sanchez C, Esteban-Cornejo I, Migueles JH, Mora-Gonzalez J, Henriksson P, et al. Physical fitness and psychological health in overweight/obese children: a cross-sectional study from the activebrains project. *J Sci Med Sport*. (2018) 21:179–84. doi: 10.1016/j.jsams.2017.09.019

Bovet P, Auguste R, Burdette H. Strong inverse association between physical fitness and overweight in adolescents: a large school-based survey. *Int J Behav Nutr Phys Act*. (2007) 4:24. doi: 10.1186/1479-58 68-4-24

Ramos-Sepulveda JA, Ramirez-Velez R, Correa-Bautista JE, Izquierdo M, Garcia-Hermoso A. Physical fitness and anthropometric normative values among Colombian-Indian schoolchildren. *BMC Public Health*. (2016) 16:962. doi: 10.1186/s12889-016-3652-2

Ortega FB, Ruiz JR, Castillo MJ, Sjostrom M. Physical fitness in childhood and adolescence: a powerful marker of health. *Int J Obes*. (2008) 32:1–11. doi: 10.1038/sj.ijo.0803774

Silverman MN, Deuster PA. Biological mechanisms underlying the role of physical fitness in health and resilience. *Interface Focus*. (2014) 4:20140040. doi: 10.1098/rsfs.2014.0040

Kandola A, Vancampfort D, Herring M, Rebar A, Hallgren M, Firth J, et al. Moving to beat anxiety: epidemiology and therapeutic issues with physical activity for anxiety. *Curr Psychiatry Rep*. (2018) 20:63. doi: 10.1007/s11920-018-0923-x

Williams SE, Carroll D, Veldhuijzen van Zanten JJ, Ginty AT. Anxiety symptom interpretation: a potential mechanism explaining the cardiorespiratory fitness-anxiety relationship. *J Affect Disord*. (2016) 193:151–6. doi: 10.1016/j.jad.2015.12.051

Obbarius N, Fischer F, Obbarius A, Nolte S, Liegl G, Rose M. A 67-item stress resilience item bank showing high content validity was developed in a psychosomatic sample. *J Clin Epidemiol*. (2018) 100:1–12. doi: 10.1016/j.jclinepi.2018.04.004

Kalisch R, Muller MB, Tuscher O. A conceptual framework for the neurobiological study of resilience. *Behav Brain Sci*. (2015) 38:e92. doi: 10.1017/S0140525X15000023

Liu H, Zhang C, Ji Y, Yang L. Biological and psychological perspectives of resilience: is it possible to improve stress resistance? *Front Hum Neurosci*. (2018) 12:326. doi: 10.3389/fnhum.2018.00326

Sheppard JM, Young WB. Agility literature review: classifications, training and testing. *J Sports Sci*. (2006) 24:919–32. doi: 10.1080/02640410500 457109

Bowers C, Kreutzer C, Cannon-Bowers J, Lamb J. Team resilience as a second- order emergent state: a theoretical model and research directions. *Front Psychol*. (2017) 8:1360. doi: 10.3389/fpsyg.2017.01360

Liefeith A, Kiely J, Collins D, Richards J. Back to the future - in support of a renewed emphasis on generic agility training within sports-specific developmental pathways. *J Sports Sci*. (2018) 36:2250–5. doi: 10.1080/02640414.2018.1449088

Diez-Fernandez A, Martinez-Vizcaino V, Torres-Costoso A, Canete Garcia-Prieto J, Franquelo-Morales P, Sanchez-Lopez M. Strength and cardiometabolic risk in young adults: the mediator role of aerobic fitness and waist circumference. *Scand J Med Sci Sports*. (2018) 28:1801–7. doi: 10.1111/sms.13077

Garcia-Hermoso A, Esteban-Cornejo I, Olloquequi J, Ramirez-Velez R. Cardiorespiratory fitness and muscular strength as mediators of the influence of fatness on academic achievement. *J Pediatr*. (2017) 187:127–33 e3. doi: 10.1016/j.jpeds.2017.04.037

Zhu Z, Yang Y, Kong Z, Zhang Y, Zhuang J. Prevalence of physical fitness in Chinese school-aged children: findings from the 2016 physical activity and fitness in china-the youth study. *J Sport Health Sci*. (2017) 6:395–403. doi: 10.1016/j.jshs.2017.09.003

Thiebaud RS, Abe T, Bravo JC, Giovannitti N, Sullivan AP. Muscle activation and heart rate responses to a side-step interval exercise. *Clin Physiol Funct Imaging*. (2018) 38:285–90. doi: 10.1111/cpf.12413

Hu YQ, Gan YQ. Development and psychometric validity of the resilience scale for Chinese adolescents. *Acta Psychologica Sinica*. (2008) 40:902–12. doi: 10.3724/SP.J.1041.2008.00902

March JS, Parker JD, Sullivan K, Stallings P, Conners CK. The multidimensional anxiety scale for children (MASC): factor structure, reliability, and validity. *J Am Acad Child Adolesc Psychiatry*. (1997) 36:554–65. doi: 10.1097/00004583-199704000-00019

Hayes AF. *Introduction to Mediation, Moderation, and Conditional Process Analysis: A Regression-based Approach*. New York: The Guilford Press (2013).

Hayes AF, Montoya AK, Rockwood NJ. The analysis of mechanisms and their contingencies: PROCESS versus structural equation modeling. *Australas Mark J*. (2017) 25:76–81. doi: 10.1016/j.ausmj.2017.02.001

Edwards JR, Lambert LS. Material for methods for integrating moderation and mediation: a general analytical framework using moderated path analysis. *Psychol Methods*. (2007) 12:1–22. doi: 10.1037/1082-989X.12.1.1

MacKinnon DP, Lockwood CM, Hoffman JM, West SG, Sheets V. A comparison of methods to test mediation and other intervening variable effects. *Psychol Methods*. (2002) 7:83–104. doi: 10.1037/1082-989X.7.1.83

Zhou J, Yang Y, Qiu X, Yang X, Pan H, Ban B, et al. Serial multiple mediation of organizational commitment and job burnout in the relationship between psychological capital and anxiety in Chinese female nurses: a cross-sectional questionnaire survey. *Int J Nurs Stud*. (2018) 83:75–82. doi: 10.1016/j.ijnurstu.2018.03.016

Cordoba-Torrecilla S, Aparicio VA, Soriano-Maldonado A, Estevez-Lopez F, Segura-Jimenez V, Alvarez-Gallardo I, et al. Physical fitness is associated with anxiety levels in women with fibromyalgia: the al-Andalus project. *Qual Life Res.* (2016) 25:1053–8. doi: 10.1007/s11136-015-1128-y

Gordon BR, McDowell CP, Lyons M, Herring MP. Associations between grip strength and generalized anxiety disorder in older adults: results from the irish longitudinal study on ageing. *J Affect Disord.* (2019) 255:136–41. doi: 10.1016/j.jad.2019.05.043

Anyan F, Hjemdal O. Adolescent stress and symptoms of anxiety and depression: resilience explains and differentiates the relationships. *J Affect Disord.* (2016) 203:213–20. doi: 10.1016/j.jad.2016.05.031

Ma X, Wang Y, Hu H, Tao XG, Zhang Y, Shi H. The impact of resilience on prenatal anxiety and depression among pregnant women in Shanghai. *J Affect Disord.* (2019) 250:57–64. doi: 10.1016/j.jad.2019.02.058

Janelidze S, Suchankova P, Ekman A, Erhardt S, Sellgren C, Samuelsson M, et al. Low IL-8 is associated with anxiety in suicidal patients: genetic variation and decreased protein levels. *Acta Psychiatr Scand.* (2015) 131:269– 78. doi: 10.1111/acps.12339

Masten AS, Tellegen A. Resilience in developmental psychopathology: contributions of the project competence longitudinal study. *Dev Psychopathol.* (2012) 24:345–61. doi: 10.1017/S095457941200003X

Zhang Y, Zhang X, Zhang L, Guo C. Executive function and resilience as mediators of adolescents' perceived stressful life events and school adjustment. *Front Psychol.* (2019) 10:446. doi: 10.3389/fpsyg.2019.00446

Greenberg MT. Promoting resilience in children and youth: preventive interventions and their interface with neuroscience. *Ann N Y Acad Sci.* (2006) 1094:139–50. doi: 10.1196/annals.1376.013

Zotcheva E, Pintzka CWS, Salvesen O, Selbaek G, Haberg AK, Ernstsen L. Associations of changes in cardiorespiratory fitness and symptoms of anxiety and depression with brain volumes: the HUNT study. *Front Behav Neurosci.* (2019) 13:53. doi: 10.3389/fnbeh.2019.00053

Mora-Gonzalez J, Esteban-Cornejo I, Cadenas-Sanchez C, Migueles JH, Molina-Garcia P, Rodriguez-Ayllon M, et al. Physical fitness, physical activity, and the executive function in children with overweight and obesity. *J Pediatr.* (2019) 208:50–6. doi: 10.1016/j.jpeds.2018.12.028

Chen R, Fall K, Czene K, Kennedy B, Valdimarsdottir U, Fang F. Impact of parental cancer on IQ, stress resilience, and physical fitness in young men. *Clin Epidemiol.* (2018) 10:593–604. doi: 10.2147/CLEP.S152210

Hansen AM, Gullander M, Hogh A, Persson R, Kolstad HA, Willert MV, et al. Workplace bullying, sleep problems and leisure-time physical activity: a prospective cohort study. *Scand J Work Environ Health.* (2016) 42:26–33. doi: 10.5271/sjweh.3537

Jefferies P, Ungar M, Aubertin P, Kriellaars D. Physical literacy and resilience in children and youth. *Front Public Health.* (2019) 7:346. doi: 10.3389/fpubh.2019.00346

Obradović J. Physiological responsivity and executive functioning: implications for adaptation and resilience in early childhood. *Child Dev Perspect.* (2016) 10:65–70. doi: 10.1111/cdep.12164

Mora-Gonzalez J, Esteban-Cornejo I, Cadenas-Sanchez C, Migueles JH, Rodriguez-Ayllon M, Molina-Garcia P, et al. Fitness, physical activity, working memory, and neuroelectric activity in children with overweight/obesity. *Scand J Med Sci Sports.* (2019) 29:1352–63. doi: 10.1111/sms.13456

16

Self-Control in Aiming Supports Coping with Psychological Pressure in Soccer Penalty Kicks

José A. Navia[1], John van der Kamp[2,3], Carlos Avilés[4] and Jesús Aceituno[1]*

[1]Facultad de Ciencias de la Actividad Física y del Deporte, Departamento de Ciencias Sociales, de la Actividad Física y del Ocio, Universidad Politécnica de Madrid, Madrid, Spain, [2]Faculty of Behavioral and Movement Sciences, Department of Human Movement Sciences, Vrije Universiteit Amsterdam, Amsterdam, Netherlands, [3]Research Centre for Exercise, School and Sport, Windesheim University of Applied Sciences, Zwolle, Netherlands, [4]Facultad de Educación, Departamento de Didáctica de las Lenguas, Artes y Educación Física , Universidad Complutense de Madrid, Madrid, Spain

***Correspondence:**
José A. Navia
joseantonio.navia@upm.es

This study addressed the question whether coaches better allow athletes to self-control their decisions when under pressure or whether to impose a decision upon them. To this end, an experiment was conducted that manipulated the soccer kickers' degree of control in decision-making. Two groups of elite under-19 soccer players (n = 18) took penalty kicks in a self-controlled (i.e., kickers themselves decided to which side to direct the ball) and an externally controlled condition (i.e., the decision to which side to direct the ball was imposed upon the kickers). One group performed the penalty kick under psychological pressure (i.e., the present coaching staff assessed their performance), while the second group performed without pressure. Just before and after performing the kicks, CSAI-2 was used to measure cognitive and somatic anxiety and self-confidence. Further, the number of goals scored, ball placement and speed, and the duration of preparatory and performatory behaviors were determined. The results verified increased levels of cognitive and somatic anxiety after performing the kicks in the pressured group compared to the no-pressure group. In addition, degree of self-control affected the participants' performance, particularly in the pressured group. They scored more goals and placed the kicks higher in the self-controlled than in the externally-controlled condition. Participants also took more time preparing and performing the run-up in the self-controlled condition. Findings indicate that increased self-control helps coping with the debilitating effects of pressure and can counter performance deteriorations. The findings are discussed within the framework of self-control theories, and recommendations for practitioners and athletes are made.

Keywords: football (soccer), autonomy, anxiety, performance, penalties

INTRODUCTION

In the last decade or so, and particularly with the introduction of mobile gaze-trackers, soccer penalty kicking has attracted a growing interest among researchers. The soccer penalty kick provides a well-defined situation, granting researchers to study the (isolated) effects of constraints manipulation on interpersonal interactions in well-controlled (competitive) situations. At the same time, soccer penalty kicks, for example by winning or losing penalty shoot-outs in international soccer tournaments, have a tremendous socio-economic impact.

The probability of scoring a penalty kick is approximately 80% (Palacios-Huerta, 2003). This high success rate basically reflects the spatio-temporal demands of the situation; typically, a goalkeeper has less time available than they require to dive and intercept the ball (Van der Kamp et al., 2018). In other words, the advantage is clearly for the kicker (and should be, given that it was introduced as a punishment). The advantage for the penalty kicker comes with high expectancies of success. Such high expectancies can provoke adverse psychological effects, such as increased pressure and enhanced anxiety levels, which in turn may hamper performance. Psychological pressure is further increased when players are being evaluated or socially judged (reviews on Hill et al., 2010; Mesagno and Beckmann, 2017). Accordingly, when there is much at stake, and pressure is high, penalty takers' performance is negatively affected (Dohmen, 2008; Arrondel et al., 2019).

In addition, previous work has shown that soccer penalty kickers under pressure may behave in ways that can hinder performance maximization. Under pressure, players are more inclined to rush the preparation and the execution of the run-up toward the ball. Players who do show these avoidance coping behaviors converted 20% fewer penalties than those who take their time (Jordet et al., 2009). Research also shows that psychological pressure directly affects players' aiming. For example, in competition, penalty kicks are shot over four times more frequently toward lower zones of the goal than to the upper zones, despite the probability of scoring being significantly higher when the ball is directed toward upper areas of the goal (Bar-Eli and Azar, 2009; Almeida et al., 2016). Players seem to prefer the risk of a (low) ball being stopped by the goalkeeper over the risk of directing the (high) ball over the goal. Possibly, with respect to the latter failure, players may be apprehensive to be perceived as unskilled (Bar-Eli et al., 2009; Bar-Eli and Azar, 2009). In addition, experimental laboratory studies have indicated that increased anxiety negatively impacts attentional control and the aiming of the kick. Specifically, penalty takers looked longer toward the goalkeeper (and less toward the aiming location and/or the ball) and placed the penalties closer to the goalkeeper under high anxiety conditions (Wilson et al., 2009; c.f., Noël and Van der Kamp, 2012).

One influential account for explaining how athletes successfully cope to achieve their goals under pressure focusses on *perceived control* of the task, which refers to the athlete's beliefs about the degree of control they have over the task (Hanton et al., 2003; Jordet et al., 2006). Perceived control is conceptualized to consist of contingency expectations and self-competence. Contingency relates to the expectations of relationship between the athlete's action and the outcome, whereas self-competence perceptions relate the beliefs about the own ability (Skinner, 1996). Evidence suggests that increased anxiety can actually have a facilitative effect on performance provided the athletes maintain a good level of confidence of competence (Hanton and Connaughton, 2002; Hanton et al., 2003). Accordingly, with respect to soccer penalty kicks, Jordet et al. (2006) carried out retrospective interviews among elite players, who participated in a shoot-out during the European Championship for nation teams. They reported that penalty takers with relatively low perceived competence and contingency (i.e., players who attribute performance success to luck rather than skill) experienced enhanced cognitive anxiety and/or interpreted their somatic anxiety as more debilitative to their performance compared to players with high perceived competence and contingency. More recently, Wood and Wilson (2012) found that penalty kickers who followed a perceptual training (i.e., directing visual attention toward the aiming location prior to the kick) not only improved gaze but also reported enhanced perceived control of the task both with regard to contingency and self-competence. The enhanced perceived control was accompanied by an increment in the players' ability to cope with the pressure and to score. Yet, while these works show that perceived control is associated with the ability to cope with psychological pressure during penalty kicks (Jordet et al., 2006; Wood and Wilson, 2012; Wood et al., 2015), it has remained unclear to what extent the purported advantages of those (often retrospective) perceptions are underpinned by *actual control* of the task (rather than perceived control). Actual control is defined as the extent to which an individual can intentionally produce a desired outcome. Although actual control and perceived control are typically related, changes in actual control does entail modifications in objective control of context conditions and/or persons interactions or actions, unlike perceived control which might just be illusionary (Skinner, 1996).

One modality within actual control is an individual's autonomy in the control of and/or making decisions about intended actions, that is, the degree to which the individual can modulate the means that define task control. For example, self-controlled and externally controlled actions differ in the degree to which an athlete can choose (or not) pertinent aspects of task execution when trying to achieve the task goal. Typically, increasing self-control (e.g., having players decide upon amount of practice, the order of different practice trials, the use of models for observation, the use of assistive devices, or provision of feedback) enhances motor performance and/or learning (for overview, Wulf, 2007). For instance, in an early study by Janelle et al. (1997), which originated this line of research, participants showed better retention in the far-aiming task of ball throwing when they allowed to choose when to use evaluative video-feedback during practice in comparison to yoked counterparts who were not free to choose when to use feedback. Yet, these effects of self-control have not been thorougly investigated in elite players under condition of psychological pressure.

In soccer penalty kicks, Scurr and Hall (2009) manipulated the autonomy of players regarding the choice of the angle of approach during the run-up of kicks in no-pressure situations. In this case, the non-professional, intermediately skilled players showed similar kicking accuracy irrespective of whether they self-controlled the approach angle or whether it was pre-scribed or externally controlled. Other experimental studies in penalty kicking have used both self-controlled and externally controlled instructions for choosing the side and/or height for the placement of the ball (Morris and Burwitz, 1989; Furley et al., 2012), often in interaction with other penalty kick strategies (Castillo et al., 2010). Yet, these studies did not systematically manipulate and compare the efficacy of self- and externally controlled kicks.

In sum, the evidence indicates that with increased psychological pressure penalty kick performance deteriorates, among others because of poor decision-making about ball placement. It may therefore be anticipated that players would improve performance when they would follow instructions that would result in a more rational distribution of ball placement. However, the associated reduction of self-control over the task may adversely affect coping in pressure situations, which in turn would deteriorate performance. This has not been directly investigated. Hence, the present study manipulated the degree of autonomy of soccer penalty takers in choosing the aiming location (i.e., side and height). The players took penalty kicks in a self-controlled condition (i.e., they decided about the aiming location themselves) and in an externally controlled condition (i.e., the aiming location was imposed upon them). One group performed the kicks in a pressured condition and the second group in a no-pressure condition. It was predicted that self-control would lead to superior performance (i.e., goal scoring, ball placement and speed) and execution (i.e., preparatory and execution durations), in particular in the pressured group.

MATERIALS AND METHODS

Participants

Eighteen elite under-19 soccer players (*M* = 17.72 years old, SD = 0.83) volunteered to participate. Participants were all playing for a club that competes in the highest league in Spain for under-19 players (i.e., playing experience: *M* = 12.28 years, SD = 1.45). In addition, four goalkeepers, who were matched to the penalty takers in age (*M* = 17.40 years old, SD = 1.14), level (same league), and experience (*M* = 10.80 years, SD = 1.6) were recruited to act as actual goaltenders. Ethical approval was obtained from the local University's ethics committee, and all players provided written consent prior to the start of the experiment.

Equipment

The experiment was conducted on an outdoor artificial turf pitch. Dimensions of the goal (7.32 m × 2.44 m), ball type (size 5), and distance to the penalty mark (11 m) were in accordance with FIFA laws (IFAB, 2016). The goalmouth was fully covered with a canvas, which was divided in six equal areas of 2.44 m × 1.22 m (**Figure 1**, left). Each area was subdivided in 15 zones of 0.48 m × 0.40 m. Two cameras were employed to record the penalties. The first camera (Casio Exilim FH 100, Japan, 120 fps mode) was placed 2 m to the side and 1 m behind the penalty spot (**Figure 1**, left), in such way that recording perspective captured both the penalty taker's football contact and the outcome of the kick (i.e., the moment and location of the ball landing in the goal). A second camera (Casio Exilim FH 100, Japan, 30 fps mode) placed 3 m to the side and 2 m in front of the penalty spot recorded the preparatory actions of penalty takers (**Figure 1**, right). All recordings were analyzed with Kinovea V.0.8.25.

Finally, the anxiety of the players was assessed by means of the Competitive State Anxiety Inventory-2 (CSAI-2; Martens et al., 1990) in its revised Spanish version (CSAI-2R; Andrade et al., 2007). The questionnaire consists of 16 items (Likert-type scale from 1 to 4) distributed in three dimensions: (1) cognitive anxiety (five items), typified by negative self-images and self-doubts; (2) somatic anxiety (six items), which refers to physiological responses (e.g., increased heart rate, tense muscles, and clammy hands); and (3) self-confidence (five items) regarding the positive expectations of success (Andrade et al., 2007).

Procedure and Design

Data collection was carried out at the players' habitual training venue. Each participant received the same general instructions about the experimental session beforehand in the dressing room. They were, however, not told about the experimental conditions and/or the exact aims of the experiment. After having received the general instructions, they completed the CSAI-2R. After a self-selected warm up (i.e., lasting approximately 10 min), the participants performed four familiarization trials. Then, each participant took 10 experimental penalty kicks, and then, immediately afterward, completed the CSAI-2R once again.

The 10 experimental kicks were divided in five self-controlled and five externally controlled kicks. The players were encouraged to score as many of the 10 kicks as possible, whereas goalkeepers were told to do their very best to save them. In the self-controlled condition, the penalty takers were instructed to freely choose the area of the goal to which to aim the ball. In the externally

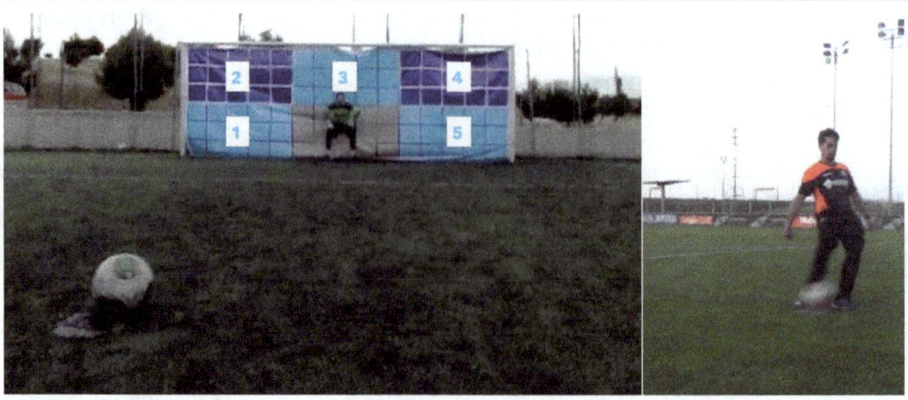

FIGURE 1 | Set up of the experiment depicting the perspective of the goal (left) and the penalty takers (right).

controlled condition, the experimenter instructed the players before the start of the run-up about the area of the goal where they had to place the ball, one shot toward each of the five outer areas (i.e., areas 1 to 5, **Figure 1**, left). The order of self-controlled and externally directed kicks was randomized using the Excel's "random" algorithm. In order to prevent that the goalkeeper became of aware of the two conditions, penalty takers followed the same routine regardless the condition. Players approached to researcher to take the ball from outside the penalty box and were shown that the goal area could be freely chosen or to which area to aim. By instructing them to pick a goal area before the start of the run-up, the procedure in the self-controlled condition promoted players to use the keeper-independent strategy (Van der Kamp, 2006; Noël et al., 2014). However, players were not explicitly instructed about it to prevent ironic effects (Bakker et al., 2006). In both conditions, there were no additional instructions regarding deception (Dicks et al., 2010) or run-up length (Van der Kamp, 2006), or angle of approach (Scurr and Hall, 2009). Finally, the players placed the ball on the penalty spot, prepared for the run-up, and executed the run-up to the ball and the kick.

Participants were ranked on the basis of the individual ability on penalty kicks and assigned to the pressure and no-pressure groups such that the two groups matched in ranking. To this end, information of the individual ability of the players was provided by the technical staff (i.e., coach and/or trainers) based on players' performance records, skill level, and previous involvement experience on competitive penalty kicks (Plessner et al., 2009). The pressure group performed the penalty kicks in the presence of the head coach and two members of the technical staff (i.e., assistant coach and physical trainer who took written notes of their performance) and were told that further decision regarding upcoming penalty shout outs of the team would be based on their performance (Note: players were fully debriefed after the experiment). By contrast, the no-pressure group took the penalty kicks only in the presence of the goalkeeper and researcher, and no further information on the importance of their performance was given.

Data Analysis

To verify anxiety, the cognitive, somatic, and self-confidence scores on the CSAI-2R were used. Performance was assessed offline from the video recordings. First, the number of penalties scored was counted. Second, the location of the kicks was determined by the area of the goal (i.e., at the center of the 15 smaller rectangles of the six areas) the ball contacted the canvas (or was intercepted) and calculated in vertical distance from the ground (i.e., height of the kick in cm) and horizontal distance from the goal center (i.e., extent of the kick in cm). Finally, the speed of the kick was calculated based on ball-flight time (i.e., differences between the moment of foot-ball contact and the moment the ball contacted the canvas or was intercepted) and the distance the ball travelled.

Two measures were used to calculate the duration of the preparatory and execution phase of the penalty kick (Jordet et al., 2009; Furley et al., 2012). The duration of the preparation phase was defined as the time between the placement of the ball on the penalty spot and the start of the run-up. The duration of the execution phase was defined as the time from the start of the run-up toward the ball until the football contact.

Statistics

To verify the effectiveness of the pressure manipulation, the ratings for anxiety were submitted to Mann-Whitney test to compare groups, whereas Wilcoxon tests were performed to compare differences between the two assessments before the experiment and immediately after. Effect sizes were expressed in r, with 0.1, 0.3, and 0.5 for small, medium, and large effects, respectively (Cohen, 1988). The remaining dependent variables were submitted to separate 2 (group: pressure vs. no-pressure) by 2 (autonomy: self-controlled vs. externally-controlled) Mixed Design Analysis of Variance (ANOVA). *Post hoc* comparisons were performed with t-test and Bonferroni corrections. Partial effect sizes of ANOVA's were expressed using (η_p^2), with values of 0.01, 0.06, and 0.14 representing small, medium, and large effects, respectively (Cohen, 1988). In case that the homogeneity and sphericity assumptions of the measures were not met, Mann-Whitney and Wilcoxon tests were conducted instead. IBM SPSS V. 24 was used to carry out statistical analysis.

RESULTS

Anxiety Measures

Figure 2 suggests that anxiety levels were similar between groups before taking the penalty kicks but lower for the

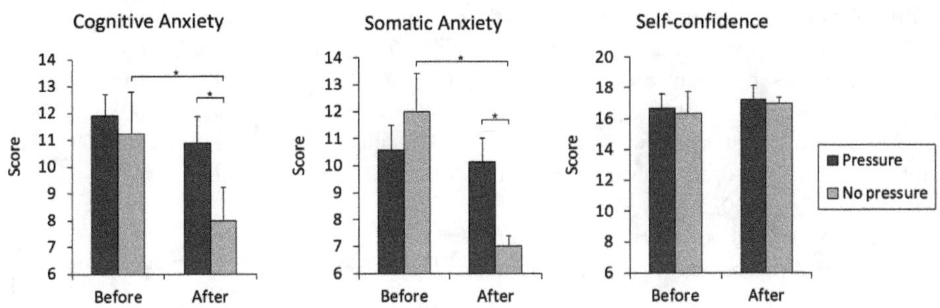

FIGURE 2 | Scores of CSAI-2R of the players before and after performing the penalty kicks. *$p < 0.05$.

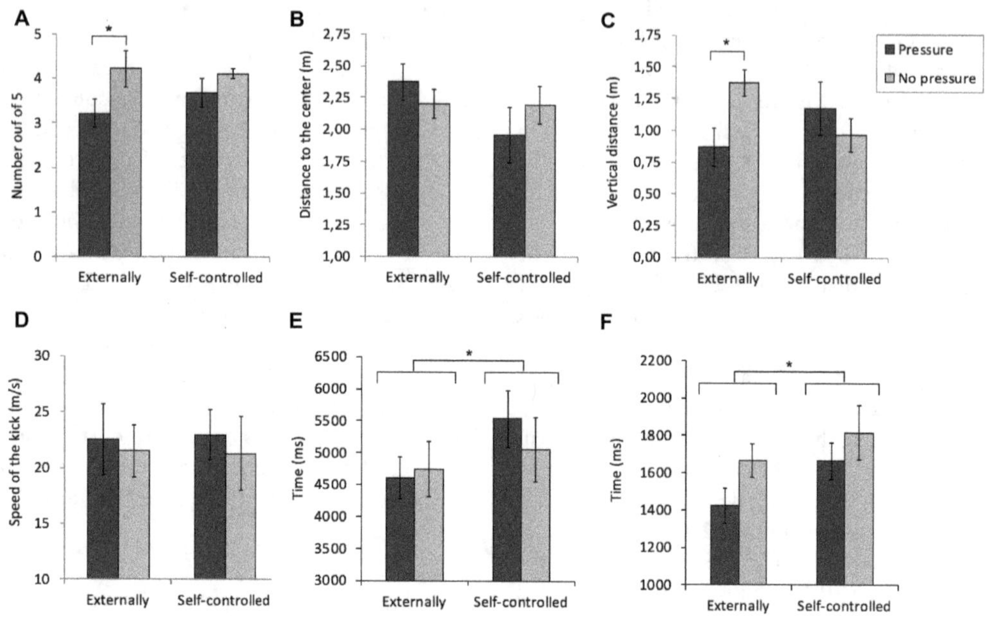

FIGURE 3 | Performance measures of the kicks **(A–D)** and penalty takers behavior **(E,F)**. Error bars represent standard error of the mean. *$p < 0.05$.

no-pressure group directly after the experiment. In other words, whereas participants of the pressure group reported moderately to high levels of anxiety throughout the experiment, these levels showed a steep drop for the no-pressure group. Accordingly, just before the experiment, no differences were found between groups for cognitive anxiety ($U = 39.50$, $p = 0.465$, $r = -0.02$), somatic anxiety ($U = 27.50$, $p = 0.129$, $r = -0.27$), or self-confidence ($U = 35.00$, $p = 0.333$, $r = -0.12$). However, immediately after the experiment, the no-pressure group showed significant lower levels of cognitive anxiety ($U = 20.00$, $p = 0.038$, $r = -0.43$), and somatic anxiety ($U = 17.50$, $p = 0.020$, $r = -0.49$) compared to pressure group (exact, unilateral). The self-confidence scores did not differ significantly between groups.

Furthermore, the no-pressure group significantly decreased both the cognitive anxiety ($z = -1.97$, $p = 0.047$, $r = -0.66$) and somatic anxiety ($z = -2.67$, $p = 0.004$, $r = -0.89$) during the experiment, whereas the pressure group maintained the scores over time (p's > 0.40). Differences in self-confidence across time were not found (**Figure 2**).

Performance Measures

Figure 3A shows that number of goals scored by the pressure group was lower than by the no-pressure group. Interestingly, it also suggests smaller differences between groups for the self-controlled compared to externally controlled condition. This was confirmed by Mann-Whitney test showing an effect of group on the number of goals scored only within the externally controlled condition ($U = 19.00$, $z = -1.97$, $p = 0.042$, $r = -0.46$) and not for the self-controlled condition ($U = 33.00$, $z = -0.79$, $p = 0.543$, $r = -0.19$). The remaining comparisons were not significant.

Autonomy had no effect on the horizontal extent (i.e., how far the ball was aimed from the goal center) as the mixed ANOVA did not reveal a significant main effect for autonomy, $F(1,16) = 2.30$, $p = 0.149$, $\eta_p^2 = 0.13$, and also not for group, $F(1,16) = 0.031$, $p = 0.862$, $\eta_p^2 < 0.01$, or their interaction, $F(1,16) = 1.98$, $p = 0.178$, $\eta_p^2 = 0.11$ (**Figure 3B**). With respect to vertical distance, the effects of autonomy and group seem to interact (**Figure 3C**). Accordingly, mixed ANOVA did not found an effect for autonomy, $F(1,16) = 0.12$, $p = 0.74$, $\eta_p^2 = 01$, and group, $F(1,16) = 1.04$, $p = 0.323$, $\eta_p^2 = 0.06$, but did reveal a significant interaction between autonomy and group ($F(1,16) = 4.81$, $p = 0.043$, $\eta_p^2 = 0.23$). *Post hoc* comparisons indicated that the pressure group placed the kicks lower than the no-pressure group but only in externally controlled condition (**Figure 3C**). In addition, we considered for the externally controlled condition to what degree the participants adhered to the instructions regarding the to-be-kicked height[1]. One-sample t-tests revealed that the pressure group aimed the kicks lower than instructed, $t(8) = -3.18$, $p = 0.013$, $df = -0.47$, $d = -1.05$, while no such difference with the instructed height was found for the no-pressure group, $t(8) = 0.30$, $p = 0.773$, $df = 0.03$, $d = 0.11$ (**Figure 3C**).

The speed of the kicks ranged between 17.9 and 28.2 m/s. Mixed ANOVA did not reveal significant effects of autonomy, $F(1,16) = 0.026$, $p = 0.875$, $\eta_p^2 < 0.01$, group, $F(1,16) = 1.39$, $p = 0.256$, $\eta_p^2 = 0.08$, or the interaction between the two factors, $F(1,16) = 0.28$, $p = 603$, $\eta_p^2 = 0.02$ (see **Figure 3D**).

Penalty takers took less time to prepare the kick in the externally controlled than during self-controlled condition, but

[1]During externally-directed condition, three kicks were intended towards the upper areas of the goal (areas 2, 3 and 4, **Figure 1**, left) and two kicks towards the lower areas (1 and 5). Taking the midpoints of the upper (1.83 m) and lower areas (0.61 m), the weighted average of the instructed height is 1.34 m.

this was not affected by pressure (**Figure 3E**). Accordingly, mixed ANOVA showed a main effect with a large effect size for autonomy on preparation time, $F(1,16) = 7.76$, $p = 0.013$, $\eta_p^2 = 0.33$, but no effects for group, $F(1,16) = 0.08$, $p = 0.776$, $\eta_p^2 < 0.1$, or between autonomy and group, $F(1,16) = 1.87$, $p = 0.191$, $\eta_p^2 = 0.10$) were found. Finally, **Figure 3F** illustrates the duration of the execution phase. Again, the duration for the externally controlled condition was shorter than in the self-controlled condition, $F(1,16) = 11.64$, $p = 0.004$, $\eta_p^2 = 0.42$. The mixed ANOVA did not reveal further effects of group, $F(1,16) = 1.84$, $p = 0.194$, $\eta_p^2 = 0.10$, or the interaction between the two factors, $F(1,16) = 0.60$, $p = 0.451$, $\eta_p^2 = 0.04$, on the run-up time.

DISCUSSION

This study examined the effect of actual self-control on coping with psychological pressure in a soccer penalty kick situation. To this end, we compared *in situ* performance of two groups of young, elite soccer players in conditions with different degrees of autonomy with respect to choosing the aiming location. Psychological pressure was effectively modulated by requiring them to take the penalty kicks in the presence of members of training staff, who–purportedly–would selectively evaluate their performances.

Research has shown that increased psychological pressure negatively affects the rate of scoring in penalty kicking (Dohmen, 2008; Wilson et al., 2009; Arrondel et al., 2019). In particular, increased pressure is associated with a hasted preparation and execution (Jordet et al., 2009) and sub-optimal ball placement (Bar-Eli and Azar, 2009; Almeida et al., 2016). The present study confirmed this: performances of the pressured group was worse compared to the no-pressure group. Importantly, however, this difference in performance was not found for the self-controlled condition. By contrast, in externally controlled condition, players under pressure actually showed signs of unsuccessful coping. They scored less goals and placed the kicks lower. Thus, the reduction in autonomy seems to be related to a reduction in the players' ability to cope with anxiety, possibly resulting in the observed drop in performance.

This finding is in line with studies that examined individual self-control or autonomy in the performance and learning of motor skills. Typically, self-control in deciding when to obtain feedback or assistance has been shown to enhance learning and performance (e.g., Janelle et al., 1997). In our study, although participants were enticed to follow a goalkeeper-independent strategy (i.e., aim the ball toward an early chosen location, irrespective of the goalkeeper's actions; Van der Kamp, 2006) in all instances, the reduction of autonomy in the externally controlled condition made the task constraints even more strict (i.e., the kicker was not allowed to change ball direction even if the goalkeeper would very clearly move in one direction long before the kick was completed). Consequently, penalty takers may have experienced a reduction of the control over the task during externally controlled kicks. The benefits of self-control have been explained by referring to motivational effects of increased autonomy, as indicated by concomitant increase in task interest, engagement, satisfaction, and self-efficacy (Sanli et al., 2013; Wulf and Lewthwaite, 2016). We did not gauge the motivational beliefs of the players in detail. Yet, we did find that the current participants' ratings of self-confidence remained high across the entire experiment and equally so in both groups. It stands to reason, therefore, that the observed benefits of self-control or autonomy in coping with pressure should also be attributed to an increase in *actual* control on task performance –and not exclusively– to a change in perceived control or other motivational beliefs. Although we meant to elicit a goalkeeper-independent strategy (see above), it cannot be ruled out that sometimes (and more often under pressure) they switched to a goalkeeper-dependent strategy. This might (partly) explain the observed advantage in self-controlled condition in the pressured group. If so, that would be contrary to previous experimental work that showed a clear advantage of GK-independent strategy (Van der Kamp, 2006; Noël and Van der Kamp, 2012; c.f., Noël et al., 2014), or at least it raises further questions on how autonomy affects the degree of adherence to either a goalkeeper independent or dependent strategy. For instance, a kicker may intend to aim to a beforehand chosen area (i.e., independent strategy) unless she/he recognizes that the goalkeeper clearly moves in advance (e.g. longer than 600 ms before ball contact, Van der Kamp, 2011) toward that intended location.

The results also showed that durations of the different phases in the penalty kick sequence was affected to a greater extent by the degree of autonomy than by psychological pressure. The pressure group did not show a significant hastening behavior (c.f., Jordet et al., 2009), but they did significantly reduce the preparation and run-up times in the externally controlled compared to the self-controlled condition. For the preparatory phase, this may be due to absent and/or reduced decision-making and planning behaviors in the externally controlled condition. During run-up phase, the slightly extra time might suggest adaptive behaviors to the actual situation, such as, responding to the goalkeeper (see above).

For future work, we recommend to include more qualitative measures (e.g., extra measures as perceived control or contingency, but also including confrontation interviews; Jordet et al., 2006) to find out in more detail what players experience in in the different conditions. For instance, whether the anxiety levels are linked to the degree of autonomy control, or how the players experience cope with pressure during the performance of the penalty kicks. In this sense, note that anxiety levels of the penalty takers were already high in the period that preceded the kicks. The group exposed to pressure maintained those levels moderately high, whereas perceived anxiety of the no-pressure group dropped. This particular fluctuation of anxiety is consistent with previous observations among expert penalty takers (Jordet and Elferink-Gemser, 2012). In this respect, it is obviously also important to verify whether adopting self-control in soccer training programs indeed can effectively increase penalty kicking performance in competitive environments.

Future research may also want to more forcefully instruct penalty takers on the strategy to be adopted (i.e., goalkeeper-independent), as well as consider the interaction between goal achievement (intended vs. reached location) and degree of autonomy control of actions. Finally, as is often the case in studies that involve elite players, the present study is low in the number of participants. Although we had the opportunity to include more, but lower skilled participants, we decided against this in order to ensure the high technical ability of participants. Hence, it is important not to overgeneralize the current findings to other groups.

CONCLUSION

This is the first experimental evidence that *actual* task control can influence coping with psychological pressure in soccer penalty kicking. Reduced degree of task control in the soccer penalty kicks can enhance the debilitating effects of high pressure as performance was shown to deteriorate when strictly following instruction of others about the aiming location. In addition, a reduced degree of autonomy also was found to result in more rushed behaviors in penalty kickers, irrespective of pressure. Finally, a coach may be inclined to forcefully instruct the players about the distribution of the penalty kicks, especially in a penalty shoot-out. However, such instructions may reduce the degree of task control and, consequently, hinder rather than improve performance, especially in stressful situations. Therefore, and based on the current observations, it seems more advisable to leave to the penalty takers themselves to choose the aiming location.

ETHICS STATEMENT

This study was carried out in accordance with the recommendations of Comité de Ética de la UPM with written informed consent from all subjects. All subjects gave written informed consent in accordance with the Declaration of Helsinki. The protocol was approved by the Comité de Ética de la UPM.

AUTHOR CONTRIBUTIONS

JN and JA contributed to the design of the study and data collection. JN performed data analysis. JK led the writing of the paper, and CA and JN significantly contributed to writing process.

REFERENCES

Almeida, C. H., Volossovitch, A., and Duarte, R. (2016). Penalty kick outcomes in UEFA club competitions (2010-2015): the roles of situational, individual and performance factors. *Int. J. Perform. Anal. Sport* 16, 508–522. doi: 10.1080/24748668.2016.11868905

Andrade, E., Lois, G., and Arce, C. (2007). Propiedades psicométricas de la versión española del inventario de ansiedad competitiva CSAI-2R en deportistas. *Psicothema* 19, 150–155.

Arrondel, L., Duhautois, R., and Laslier, J.-F. (2019). Decision under psychological pressure: the shooter's anxiety at the penalty kick. *J. Econ. Psychol.* 70, 22–35. doi: 10.1016/j.joep.2018.10.008

Bakker, F., Oudejans, R., Binsch, O., and Van der Kamp, J. (2006). Penalty shooting and gaze behavior: unwanted effects of the wish not to miss. *Int. J. Sport Psychol.* 37, 265–280.

Bar-Eli, M., and Azar, O. H. (2009). Penalty kicks in soccer: an empirical analysis of shooting strategies and goalkeepers' preferences. *Soccer Soc.* 10, 183–191. doi: 10.1080/14660970802601654

Bar-Eli, M., Azar, O. H., and Lurie, Y. (2009). (Ir)rationality in action: do soccer players and goalkeepers fail to learn how to best perform during a penalty kick? *Prog. Brain Res.* 174, 97–108. doi: 10.1016/S0079-6123(09)01309-0

Castillo, J. M., Oña, A., Raya, A., Bilbao, A., and Serra, E. (2010). Tactical skills and ball speed during a field simulation of penalty kick strategies in soccer. *Percept. Mot. Skills* 111, 947–962. doi: 10.2466/05.23.24.27.PMS.111.6.947-962

Cohen, J. (1988). *Statistical power analysis for the behavioural science.* 2nd edn. (New York: Academic Press).

Dicks, M., Button, C., and Davids, K. (2010). Availability of advance visual information constrains association-football goalkeeping performance during penalty kicks. *Perception* 39, 1111–1124. doi: 10.1068/p6442

Dohmen, T. J. (2008). Do professionals choke under pressure? *J. Econ. Behav. Organ.* 65, 636–653. doi: 10.1016/j.jebo.2005.12.004

Furley, P., Dicks, M., Stendtke, F., and Memmert, D. (2012). "Get it out the way. The wait's killing me." hastening and hiding during soccer penalty kicks. *Psychol. Sport Exerc.* 13, 454–465. doi: 10.1016/j.psychsport.2012.01.009

Hanton, S., and Connaughton, D. (2002). Perceived control of anxiety and its relationship to self-confidence and performance. *Res. Q. Exerc. Sport* 73, 87–97. doi: 10.1080/02701367.2002.10608995

Hanton, S., O'Brien, M., and Mellalieu, S. D. (2003). Individual differences, perceived control and competitive trait anxiety. *J. Sport Behav.* 26, 39–55.

Hill, D. M., Hanton, S., Matthews, N., and Fleming, S. (2010). Choking in sport: a review. *Int. Rev. Sport Exerc. Psychol.* 3, 24–39. doi: 10.1080/17509840903301199

IFAB (2016). *Laws of the game.* (Zurich: FIFA).

Janelle, C. M., Barba, D. A., Frehlich, S. G., Tennant, L. K., and Cauraugh, J. H. (1997). Maximizing performance feedback effectiveness through videotape replay and a self-controlled learning environment. *Res. Q. Exerc. Sport* 68, 269–279. doi: 10.1080/02701367.1997.10608008

Jordet, G., and Elferink-Gemser, M. T. (2012). Stress, coping, and emotions on the world stage: the experience of participating in a major soccer tournament penalty shootout. *J. Appl. Sport Psychol.* 24, 73–91. doi: 10.1080/10413200.2011.619000

Jordet, G., Elferink-Gemser, M. T., Lemmink, K. A., and Visscher, C. (2006). The "Russian roulette" of soccer?: perceived control and anxiety in a major tournament penalty shootout. *Int. J. Sport Psychol.* 37, 281–298.

Jordet, G., Hartman, E., and Sigmundstad, E. (2009). Temporal links to performing under pressure in international soccer penalty shootouts. *Psychol. Sport Exerc.* 10, 621–627. doi: 10.1016/j.psychsport.2009.03.004

Martens, R., Burton, D., Vealey, R. S., Bump, L. A., and Smith, D. E. (1990). "Development and validation of the competitive state anxiety inventory-2" in *Competitive anaxiety in sport.* eds. R. Martens, R. S. Vealey, and D. Burton (Champaign: Human Kinetics), 117–190.

Mesagno, C., and Beckmann, J. (2017). Choking under pressure: theoretical models and interventions. *Curr. Opin. Psychol.* 16(Suppl. C), 170–175. doi: 10.1016/j.copsyc.2017.05.015

Morris, A., and Burwitz, L. (1989). Anticipation and movement strategies in elite soccer goalkeepers at penalty kicks. *J. Sports Sci.* 7, 79–80.

Noël, B., Furley, P., Van der Kamp, J., Dicks, M., and Memmert, D. (2014). The development of a method for identifying penalty kick strategies in association football. *J. Sports Sci.* 33, 1–10. doi: 10.1080/02640414.2014.926383

Noël, B., and Van der Kamp, J. (2012). Gaze behaviour during the soccer penalty kick: an investigation of the effects of strategy and anxiety. *Int. J. Sport Psychol.* 41, 1–20.

Palacios-Huerta, I. (2003). Professionals play minimax. *Rev. Econ. Stud.* 70, 395–415. doi: 10.1111/1467-937X.00249

Plessner, H., Unkelbach, C., Memmert, D., Baltes, A., and Kolb, A. (2009). Regulatory fit as a determinant of sport performance: how to succeed in a soccer penalty-shooting. *Psychol. Sport Exerc.* 10, 108–115. doi: 10.1016/j.psychsport.2008.02.001

Sanli, E., Patterson, J., Bray, S., and Lee, T. (2013). Understanding self-controlled motor learning protocols through the self-determination theory. *Front. Psychol.* 3. doi: 10.3389/fpsyg.2012.00611

Scurr, J., and Hall, B. (2009). The effects of approach angle on penalty licking accuracy and kick kinematics with recreational soccer players. *J. Sports Sci. Med.* 8, 230–234.

Skinner, E. A. (1996). A guide to constructs of control. *J. Pers. Soc. Psychol.* 71, 549–570. doi: 10.1037/0022-3514.71.3.549

Van der Kamp, J. (2006). A field simulation study of the effectiveness of penalty kick strategies in soccer: late alterations of kick direction increase errors and reduce accuracy. *J. Sports Sci.* 24, 467–477. doi: 10.1080/02640410500190841

Van der Kamp, J. (2011). Exploring the Merits of Perceptual Anticipation in the Soccer Penalty Kick. *Motor Control* 15, 342–358.

Van der Kamp, J., Dicks, M., Navia, J. A., and Noël, B. (2018). Goalkeeping in the soccer penalty kick. *Ger. J. Exerc. Sport Res.* 48, 169–175. doi: 10.1007/s12662-018-0506-3

Wilson, M., Wood, G., and Vine, S. J. (2009). Anxiety, attentional control, and performance impairment in penalty kicks. *J. Sport Exerc. Psychol.* 31, 761–775. doi: 10.1123/jsep.31.6.761

Wood, G., Jordet, G., and Wilson, M. R. (2015). On winning the "lottery": psychological preparation for football penalty shoot-outs. *J. Sports Sci.* 33, 1758–1765. doi: 10.1080/02640414.2015.1012103

Wood, G., and Wilson, M. R. (2012). Quiet-eye training, perceived control and performing under pressure. *Psychol. Sport Exerc.* 13, 721–728. doi: 10.1016/j.psychsport.2012.05.003

Wulf, G. (2007). Self-controlled practice enhances motor learning: implications for physiotherapy. *Physiotherapy* 93, 96–101. doi: 10.1016/j.physio.2006.08.005

Wulf, G., and Lewthwaite, R. (2016). Optimizing performance through intrinsic motivation and attention for learning: the OPTIMAL theory of motor learning. *Psychon. Bull. Rev.* 23, 1382–1414. doi: 10.3758/s13423-015-0999-9

17

Physical Activity and Sedentary Behavior of Children in Afterschool Programs: An Accelerometer-Based Analysis in Full-Day and Half-Day Elementary Schools in Germany

Arvid Kuritz[1*], *Christoph Mall*[2], *Melina Schnitzius*[2] *and Filip Mess*[2]

[1] *Department of Sport Science, University of Konstanz, Konstanz, Germany,* [2] *Department of Sport and Health Sciences, Technical University of Munich, Munich, Germany*

Correspondence:
Arvid Kuritz
arvid.kuritz@uni-konstanz.de

Background: Regular physical activity (PA) and reduced sedentary behavior (SB) are positively related to children's health and considered as pillars of a healthy lifestyle. Full-day schools with their afterschool programs (ASPs) have an impact on children's daily PA and SB. Studies investigating PA and SB in ASPs, which compare PA and SB between the organizational forms full-day and half-day schools, are rare. The aim of this study is to describe elementary school children's PA and SB during ASPs and to compare the results to other time periods of the day, e.g., teaching hours and leisure time. Additionally, PA and SB of children in full-day and half-day schools are compared. Further, relevant factors influencing the achievement of the World Health Organization's (WHO's) PA guidelines for children, e.g., time spent in ASPs, are investigated.

Methods: PA and SB of 332 German students (n = 198 full-day school children; n = 134 half-day school children) from 11 different elementary schools were measured via accelerometry for 5 consecutive days within one school week in 2017. PA and SB during ASPs and other times of the day were analyzed via one-way and factorial ANOVA, correlation, and logistic regression.

Results: Children attending full-day schools show the highest percentage of moderate-to-vigorous PA (MVPA) (13.7%) and the lowest percentage of SB (49.5%) during ASPs, in comparison with teaching hours and leisure time. In the afternoon hours, full-day school children show 20 min less SB than half-day school children. Children spending more time in ASPs obtain significantly more SB (r = 0.23) and less MVPA (r = −0.15). Further, they less likely reach WHO's PA guidelines odds ratio (OR = 0.98).

Conclusion: Peers and the choice as well as offer of extracurricular activities promote PA in ASPs. Media availability leads to higher SB in leisure time. ASPs help to be more active and less sedentary. Time spent in ASPs should be limited, so that full-day school children still have the possibility to join other PA offers in leisure time. ASP time should contain a certain minimum amount of MVPA in line with ASP guidelines.

Keywords: physical activity, sedentary behavior, full-day school, after-school program, children, accelerometry

INTRODUCTION

Physical inactivity and sedentary behavior (SB) are determinants of poor health (1). On the contrary, a basic level of physical activity (PA) is one pillar of a healthy lifestyle. There is manifold evidence for health benefits resulting from regular PA (2, 3) and reduced SB (1). Especially for children, regular PA and reduced SB are important health factors. Based on Dahlgren and Whitehead's (4, 5) model of *Social Determinants of Health*, behavior patterns such as PA and SB are significantly influenced by the social network and living as well as working conditions. For children, these living and working conditions are primarily the family, the commune they grow up in, and the school they attend. Considering the amount of time children spend at school on weekdays, the factor *school* contributes substantially to children's daily PA as well as SB and therefore their health.

In industrialized countries, almost every child is enrolled in school, and school has the most intensive and continuous impact on children aged 6–15 (6). Overall, in Germany, two organizational forms of school exist: full-day schools and half-day schools. The main difference is the amount of time spent at school. Children at half-day schools on average stay 5 h in school. Children at full-day schools on average spend 7–8 h in school. Time beyond teaching hours is usually spent in extracurricular activities of afterschool programs (ASPs). This extra time in full-day schools also provides a large amount of free time for PA, and this can reduce SB. In Europe, most countries offer full-day school programs (7). In the USA, extracurricular activities are usually part of the school system. The organizational form of Germany's school system, especially considering elementary schools, currently changes from half-day to full-day schools. Full-day schools feature diverse characteristics: mandatory vs. voluntary attendance, partly rhythmization of lessons and ASPs as well as a varying overall duration. Parents can typically choose if their children attend a full-day or half-day class within one school. All full-day schools offer a variety of ASPs. Sports activities are the most frequent offers in German full-day school ASPs (8, 9). Federal regulations ensure that either teachers or trained staff organize and guide ASPs or observe free play. Children typically have to sign up for an activity for one term. Age groups are usually mixed. A standard school day in German full-day schools starts with teaching in the morning until lunch break, followed by rarely more teaching or time for homework and extracurricular activities in the afternoon. Prolonged attendance at full-day schools compared with half-day schools impacts children's lifestyle and leisure behavior as well as health behavior depending on the organizational form or ASPs' duration. Full-day schools providing PA offers within ASPs in a low-threshold way can help to reach guidelines for PA and SB, independent of social network (4, 5) or participation in organized sports (10). Full-day schools can therefore influence health-related behavior patterns.

The World Health Organization (WHO) recommends at least 60 min of moderate-to-vigorous PA (MVPA) daily for children aged 5–17 (11). These *Global Recommendations on Physical Activity for Health* (WHO PA GL) are a marker for a healthy lifestyle in the meaning of daily PA. Besides the WHO PA GL, there are several recommendations, policies, or guidelines regarding the amount of PA in ASPs (12). These requirements postulate that up to 60 min of MVPA should take place in ASPs (13–15). It is also recommended that 20–50% of PA in ASPs should be MVPA (14). Most organizations, e.g., the United States National Afterschool Association, call for 30 min MVPA in ASPs (14). This means that ASPs should provide half of the recommended MVPA (12). The WHO PA GL states physical inactivity or SB as evidence of poor health. Specific recommendations regarding SB for children aged 5–17 are missing. In Germany, *National Recommendations for Physical Activity and Physical Activity Promotion* (16) recommends as little as possible and a maximum of 60 min daily sitting, using a screen media or SB. Guidelines for ASPs also recommend a screen time of <60 min (13–15). Screen time should be limited to homework, research, or digital learning (14). The California Department of Education also recommends a maximum 60 min of SB in ASPs (13).

Several studies investigated PA and SB in the school context, especially considering full-day school's ASPs: Beets et al. (17) showed in their study with more than 1,000 elementary school children attending 97 ASPs in South Carolina, USA, operated by the Young Men's Christian Association (YMCA), that only one quarter reached the 30-min guideline of PA in ASPs. On average, children spent 21.4 min in MVPA and 64.3 min in SB at baseline. In the study, ASP staff qualification was also investigated with the assumption that trained staff can increase students' MVPA during ASPs. Regarding children's overall PA in combination with ASP's, PA helps to identify active periods within 1 day. De Meester et al. (10) investigated daily PA of 1,526 Belgian students and compared participants of extracurricular school-based sports offerings with non-participants via questionnaire. Participants were significantly more physically active than non-participants, even after controlling for outer school sports participation. They concluded that ASP participation is linked to higher PA levels. Therefore, full-day school may contribute to an active and healthy lifestyle. Pau et al. (18) measured PA and SB via accelerometry in 169 Italian elementary school children. They compared full-day and half-day school children's PA and SB in different time periods. In the afternoon time period, where ASPs take place for full-day attendants, children spent significantly less time in SB and more time in MVPA than did half-day school children spending the afternoon hours outside school. Van Stralen et al. (19) investigated in a cross-European cross-sectional survey (The ENERGY project) PA and SB during the school day. Ten- to 12-year-old European school children spent on average 65% of their time at school in SB and 5% in MVPA. Van Stralen et al. found significant differences in SB and MVPA for boys and girls. Boys showed less SB and higher amounts of MVPA than did girls. In Messing et al. (20) systematic review of reviews considering PA promotion among children and adolescents, few studies analyzed time in ASPs and identified these programs as effective health promoter. Regarding associations between PA and ASPs, especially programs focusing on PA and/or sports were categorized as effective. Other studies investigated PA and SB in students or in school, respectively, but without specific reference to full-day school or ASPs. Systematic reviews from Parrish et al.

(21) or Atkin et al. (22) provided an overview of studies and results in this field. The analyzed studies either took place during recess or lunch break (21) or examined additionally implemented short-term interventions to promote PA and reduce SB in school (22). For this reason, comparisons with these findings are limited to the field of PA and SB in ASPs in full-day schools.

Overall, most studies in this field analyzed children's daily PA and SB, without differentiating between times of the day. Research analyzing PA and SB in ASPs and its potential influence on daily PA as well as studies comparing full-day school and half-day school are rudimentary. Studies investigating PA and SB in German full-day schools accurately and with device-based measurements, such as accelerometry, are missing. Only one international study (18) compared full-day and half-day school children's PA and SB via accelerometry. Considering this state of studies, questions about full-day schools' or particularly ASP's contribution to children's PA and SB cannot be answered clearly. Further, a comparison between PA and SB in half-day and full-day school children is still pending. Against this background, this study has three major aims:

1. the description of PA and SB of children attending full-day schools during time spent in ASPs, and additionally, the comparison of PA and SB in ASPs with PA and SB during teaching hours and leisure time;
2. the comparison of full-day school and half-day school children's PA and SB during the afternoon hours; and
3. the investigation of the impact of full-day school specific factors on the achievement of WHO PA GL.

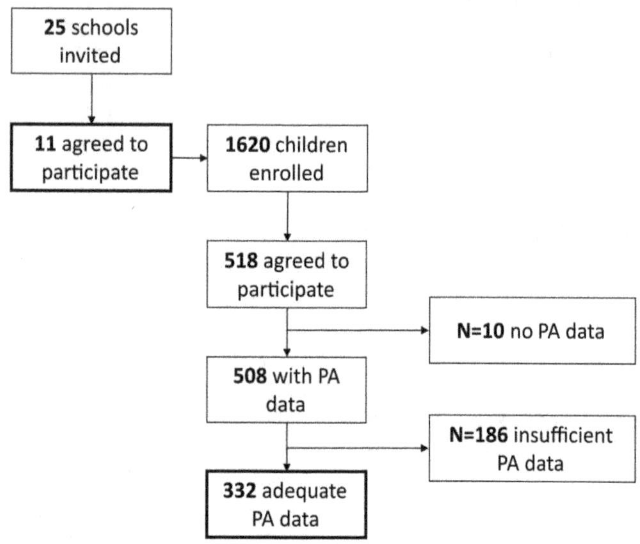

FIGURE 1 | Flow chart of the sample selection process.

MATERIALS AND METHODS

Study Design

This study was part of the project *Physical Activity in Full-Day School Children* funded by the German Federal Ministry of Education, Youth and Sports Baden Württemberg from 2014 to 2018. The study was performed from May to July 2017 in elementary schools with either a mandatory or voluntary full-day school branch located in the federal state of Baden-Württemberg, Germany. To minimize weather condition-related differences in PA and SB, data were collected in spring and summer. Regional weather conditions (hours of sunshine, temperature, and daily rainfall) were documented and checked using data from the German Weather Service.

In the first step, 25 schools—officially registered, accredited, and therefore supported by the Federal Ministry of Education, Youth and Sports Baden-Württemberg in their first year as full-day school—were asked to join the study. Eleven schools (44%) agreed to participate. Overall, 1,620 children from grade 1 to 4 were enrolled in the 11 participating schools. In the second step, principals and class teachers handed out an information letter about the study. Parents were asked to fill out the included reply form to accept or decline their children's participation in the study. Regardless of their affiliation to half-day or full-day school, all children of grade 1 to grade 4 were invited to participate. Data were collected by accelerometry for device-based measurement of PA and SB and by paper–pencil questionnaire (23).

Abbreviations: PA, physical activity; SB, sedentary behavior; WHO, World Health Organization; ASP, after-school program; WHO PA GL, Global Recommendations on Physical Activity for Health; MVPA, moderate-to-vigorous physical activity; LPA, light physical activity; OR, odds ratio.

Participants and Data Collection

In total, 508 children were equipped with accelerometers and paper–pencil questionnaires. The test period was a regular week without special events (e.g., federal youth games, excursions, and sports meetings). Because of broken devices (n = 10) and lack of wear time (n = 186), the final sample included 332 children with adequate data for 5 consecutive school days (**Figure 1**). The reason to exclude students with insufficient data is based on the study of Rich et al. (24) determining minimum wear time for accelerometer data. A measurement reliability coefficient of 0.92 can be achieved by a wear time of at least 6 h/day on 5 days. Children's age ranged from 6.69 to 12.3 years with an average of 8.97 (SD = 1.2) years. Sex, organizational form of school, and grade level were well-distributed. **Table 1** shows detailed sample characteristics.

Measures

Participating children wore a tri-axial accelerometer (ActiGraph® GT3X, GT3X+ or, GT3XBT, Acticorp Co., Pensacola, USA) at the left hip with an elastic belt. Robusto and Trost's (25) study highlighted a strong agreement between the different models of applied ActiGraph accelerometer monitors. Children were asked to wear the accelerometer as soon as they got up in the morning and only remove it during water-based activities, at night and in exceptional cases because of the

TABLE 1 | Sample and characteristics.

N	332
Age (mean, SD)	8.97 (±1.2)
Age (range)	6.69–12.3
Sex	
Female	172 (51.8%)
Male	160 (48.2%)
Organizational form	
Half-day school	134 (40.4%)
Full-day school	198 (59.6%)
Grade level	
1st	77 (23.2%)
2nd	88 (26.5%)
3rd	90 (27.1%)
4th	62 (18.7%)
Mixed-age classes	15 (4,5%)
Students per school	30.18 (±14.0)

risk of injury, e.g., while performing contact sports such as martial arts.

Data collection by accelerometer was set to 10-s epoch length and started 1–2 h after distribution to avoid increased PA results because of curiosity for device and study. ActiLife Software v6.11.9 was used for data processing. Wear time validation was calculated using Troiano (26) defaults. Time intervals of at least 60 consecutive minutes of zero counts were defined as non-wear time. For PA level calculation and identification of SB, Pulsford's cut points for children (27) were used. Therefore, counts per minute of the vertical axis were classified as SB (SB $<$ 100), light PA (LPA $\leq$ 2,240), moderate PA (MPA $\leq$ 3,840), and vigorous PA (VPA $\geq$ 3,841).

Socio-demographic data (date of birth and sex) were collected via paper–pencil questionnaire, which was an adapted version of the *Motorik-Modul activity questionnaire MoMo-AFB* (23). Children filled out the questionnaire together with their parents or guardians. In the questionnaire, parents and children were asked if the child attended full-day or half-day school. If attending full-day school, ASP end time or time leaving school should be specified for each day separately. Additional information about class and ASP schedules or other school-based information was given by the schools' principals or teaching staff.

Data Preparation and Data Analyses

PA and SB data were divided into different time periods throughout the day and summarized for 5 consecutive school days from Monday to Friday. Individual timetables were created, based on class schedule and ASP attendance information. A typical school day was divided into teaching hours and leisure time for half-day school children and teaching hours, ASPs, and leisure time for full-day school children. To compare PA and SB in the afternoon hours between full-day and half-day school children, an additional time period named *non-teaching* time was created. Children attending full-day schools stay in school for extracurricular activities in ASPs. Leisure time with activities free of choice started after ASPs. *Non-teaching* time for full-day school children included ASPs and leisure time. Children in half-day schools left school after teaching hours. The remaining time awake was leisure time and therefore equal to *non-teaching* time. Valid wear time was checked for full day recording (as mentioned above) and double-checked for each period of the day to ensure at least 50% wear time in each time period. On average, daily wear time amounted to 11.92 (SD = 2.3) hours and 49.7% (SD = 9.5) for a whole day; 4.06 (SD = 0.7) hours in teaching hours, which equates to 89.3% (SD = 12.8) for daily teaching hours, 2.46 (SD = 1.0) hours and 91.6% (SD = 14.4) in ASPs, 6.72 (SD = 2.1) hours and 50.6% (SD = 13.5) in leisure time, and 7.75 (SD = 1.9) hours and 54.1% (SD = 12.5) in *non-teaching* time.

After raw data to PA and SB data with ActiLife® software were converted, Microsoft® Excel® for Office 365 MSO was used to prepare data.

Comparisons of children's PA and SB in different time periods (e.g., ASPs and leisure time) within the day were conducted by repeated measure factorial ANOVA with sex and grade as independent variables. Analyses comparing full-day and half-day school children or subgroups differentiated by school affiliation were fulfilled by one-way ANOVA, to identify the interaction effect between sex and grade, a factorial ANOVA was conducted. For multiple comparisons, Tukey's *post-hoc* test was used. Effect size eta squared was categorized based on Cohen (28): small, $\eta^2 < 0.06$; medium, $\eta^2 = 0.06$ to 0.14; and large, $\eta^2 > 0.14$. If sphericity was missing, Greenhouse–Geisser correction was applied. Correlations between variables were calculated via Pearson correlation coefficient. Prediction for school's organizational form attendance and WHO PA GL achievement was checked with chi-squared test for the whole sample. The subsample of full-day school children was analyzed by logistic regression to identify general (sex and age) and specific full-day school predictors (number of days per week in ASPs, duration of ASPs in minutes per day, minutes of MVPA in ASPs per day, and reaching the guideline of 20% MVPA in ASPs) as independent variables, which were given as odds ratio (OR) to achieve the WHO PA GL (dependent variable). Significance was assessed at $\alpha = 0.05$ for all analyses. All statistical tests were conducted using IBM® SPSS® Statistics (version 26).

RESULTS

Children's Physical Activity and Sedentary Behavior in After-School Programs

The following results refer to the subgroup of participants attending full-day school ($n = 198$) and taking part in ASPs on at least 1 and up to 5 days of the week. Over two thirds of students attending full-day school participate on three (31.8%) or four (37.4%) afternoons in ASPs. The number of days varies in the full range from one (6.6%) or two (7.1%), up to five (17.2%) days attending full-day school programs within a school week with an average of 3.52 (SD = 1.1) days weekly. On average, children spend 162.88 (SD = 57.0) minutes per day in ASPs.

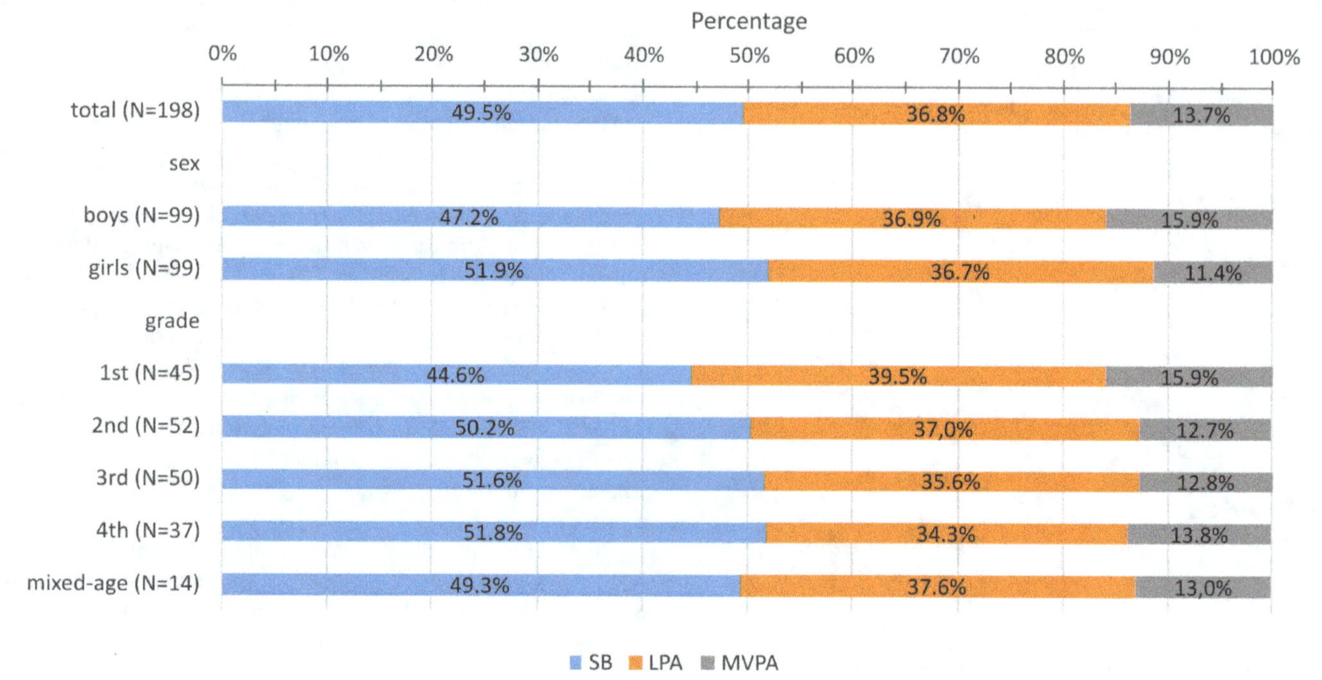

FIGURE 2 | Percentages of physical activity and sedentary behavior in after-school program time of full-day school children.

The maximum duration of ASPs time is 5 h/day. Summarizing all school days within 1 week, we found that children attend extracurricular activities in ASPs for 9 h 42 min (M = 582.45 min, SD = 285.7) on average.

Figure 2 shows the constitution of SB, LPA, and MVPA in ASPs for the full-day school subgroup—differentiated by sex and grade (and therefore indirectly by age). In ASPs, factorial ANOVA reveals no significant interaction for grade and sex [$F_{(4,188)} = 1.32$, $p = 0.263$, $\eta^2 = 0.03$] in percentage of SB. Both factors individually show significant differences: boys' SB is lower than girls' [$F_{(1,198)} = 8.34$, $p < 0.001$, $\eta^2 = 0.04$]. Differentiated by grade, there is a significant difference of SB in ASPs [$F_{(4,198)} = 4.24$, $p = 0.003$, $\eta^2 = 0.08$]. Tukey's *post-hoc* multiple comparisons show that only first graders show significantly less SB than do second, third, and fourth graders. Considering the percentage of time spent in MVPA during ASPs, only sex shows a significant difference [$F_{(1,198)} = 28.19$, $p < 0.001$, $\eta^2 = 0.13$]. There are neither significant differences between grades [$F_{(4,198)} = 1.99$, $p = 0.107$, $\eta^2 = 0.04$] nor an interaction effect [$F_{(4,188)} = 0.65$, $p = 0.625$, $\eta^2 = 0.01$]. Significant differences with large effects are found for school affiliation in both percentage in SB [$F_{(10,198)} = 5.42, p < 0.001, \eta^2 = 0.23$] and MVPA [$F_{(10,198)} = 3.53, p < 0.001, \eta^2 = 0.16$]. *Post-hoc* results reveal that only one school stands out with a highly active ASP. This school is the only one in the sample where full-day school is mandatory for all children. PA and SB data of this school ($n = 27$) show that children spend on average 18.4% (SD = 8.2) of ASPs time in MVPA (overall: M = 13.7%, SD = 6.2), which differs significantly in comparison with four schools in a multiple comparison. In 39.0% (SD = 10.0) of ASP time, children of this school are sedentary (overall: M = 49.5%, SD = 9.9), which is significantly different to eight schools.

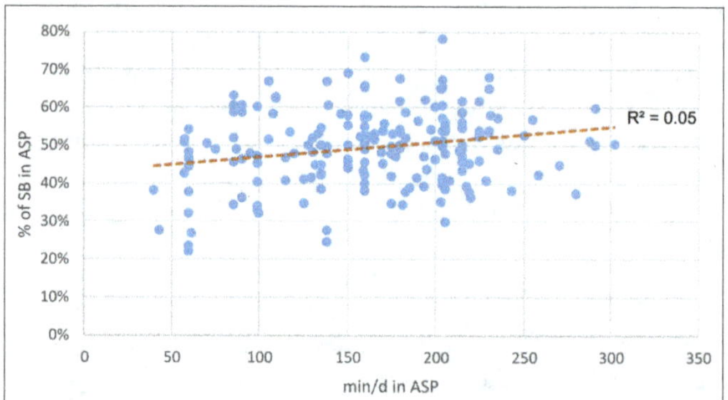

FIGURE 3 | Duration of after school program (ASP) correlated to percentage of time in sedentary behavior in ASP.

Children attending full-day school stay on average 2 h 43 min (M = 162.88 min, SD = 57.0) per school day at school for extracurricular activities in ASPs. Regarding the duration, there is a small positive correlation for SB ($r = 0.23$, $p = 0.001$) and a slightly negative correlation for MVPA percentages ($r = -0.15$, $p = 0.037$) as seen in **Figures 3, 4**. This shows that children who spend more minutes per day in ASPs show a higher percentage of SB and a lower percentage of MVPA than do children who spend less time in ASPs.

For children attending full-day school, ASP (SB: M = 49.5%, SD = 9.9; MVPA: M = 13.7%, SD = 6.2) time is significantly

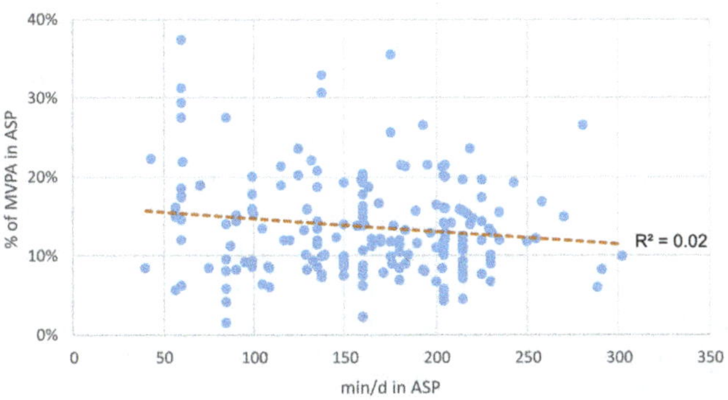

FIGURE 4 | Duration of after school program (ASP) correlated to percentage of time in moderate-to-vigorous physical activity (MVPA) in ASP.

the most active and least sedentary time of the day than are teaching hours (SB: M = 61.6%, SD = 7.0; MVPA: M = 8.4%, SD = 2.9) and leisure time (SB: M = 57.9%, SD = 7.6; MVPA: M = 10.1%, SD = 3.5) with the highest percentage of MVPA and lowest percentage of SB. Considering SB, interaction effects of the repeated measure factorial ANOVA are significant for the time periods differentiated by sex, but not by grade or by sex and grade. For percentages of MVPA, significant interaction effects can be found for sex as well as grade, but not for grade and sex (see **Tables 2**, **3**). Descriptive data can be found in **Supplementary Tables A, B.**

Comparison of Full-Day and Half-Day School Children's Physical Activity and Sedentary Behavior in the Afternoon Hours

During *non-teaching* time children attending full-day schools (M = 256.84 min, SD = 76.45) spend significantly less minutes in SB than children in half-day schools (M = 276.60 min, SD = 89.0): $F_{(1,332)} = 4.67$, $p = 0.031$, $\eta^2 = 0.01$. The difference in minutes of MVPA in the *non-teaching* time is not significant; half-day school children (M = 47.57 min, SD = 19.59) spend 1.7 min less in MVPA than children attending full-day schools (M = 49.26 min, SD = 18.60): $F_{(1,332)} = 0.63$, $p = 0.427$, $\eta^2 < 0.01$. Considering girls and boys separately, the affiliation to school's organizational forms do not differ in boys' SB [$F_{(1,160)} = 0.33$, $p = 0.570$, $\eta^2 < 0.01$) or MVPA [$F_{(1,160)} = 0.33$, $p = 0.565$, $\eta^2 < 0.01$). The difference in minutes of SB in the *non-teaching* time for girls aggregates to almost 30 min. Girls in half-day schools show SB for 290.47 (SD = 87.19) minutes and girls in full-day schools for 260.73 (SD = 85.29) min [$F_{(1,172)} = 5.02$, $p = 0.026$, $\eta^2 = 0.03$). As reported for boys' PA, there are no significant differences in girls' MVPA [$F_{(1,172)} = 0.06$, $p = 0.801$, $\eta^2 < 0.01$). Regarding subgroups divided by grade, there is a difference in second graders: half-day school children in second grade spend significantly more time in SB during *non-teaching* time than full-day school children [$F_{(1,88)} = 5.75$, $p = 0.019$, $\eta^2 = 0.06$). For all other grades, differences in SB and PA between full-day and half-day school children are not significant.

TABLE 2 | Differences of percentages in time spent in sedentary behavior (SB) in different periods of the day in full-day school children ($n = 198$).

	Test for difference	p	η^2
Setting[a]	$F_{(1.87,351.47)} = 138.86$	< 0.001	0.43
Setting × grade[a]	$F_{(7.48,351.47)} = 1.89$	0.066	0.04
Setting × sex[a]	$F_{(1.87,351.47)} = 4.03$	0.021	0.02
Setting × grade × sex[a]	$F_{(7.48,351.47)} = 1.43$	0.189	0.03

[a]*Sphericity not given, Greenhouse–Geisser correction.*

TABLE 3 | Differences of percentages in time spent in moderate to vigorous physical activity (MVPA) in different periods of the day in full-day school children ($n = 198$).

	F	p	η^2
Setting[a]	$F_{(1.66,312.60)} = 83.94$	< 0.001	0.31
Setting × grade[a]	$F_{(6.65,312.60)} = 2.38$	0.024	0.05
Setting × sex[a]	$F_{(1.66,312.60)} = 8.41$	0.001	0.04
Setting × grade × sex[a]	$F_{(6.65,312.60)} = 0.70$	0.667	0.02

[a]*Sphericity not given, Greenhouse–Geisser correction.*

The Global Recommendations on Physical Activity for Health: The Influence of Specific Full-Day School and General Variables

In this study, 59.9% of participants reach the recommended 60 min of MVPA daily according to the WHO PA GL (11). A chi-squared test shows that significantly more boys (73.8%) than girls (47.1%) can be categorized as active in the meaning of the WHO ($\chi^2(1) = 24.53$, $p < 0.001$, $\varphi = 0.27$). Attendance to full-day or half-day school does not show any significant difference in the percentage of children reaching the WHO PA GL: full-day school 62.1%, half-day school 56.7% ($\chi^2(1) = 0.97$, $p = 0.324$, $\varphi = 0.05$).

The logistic regression model with six predictors reaches a likelihood of 79.1%. The OR is displayed in **Table 4**. Sex as a significant predictor in this model shows that boys are more than twice as much likely (OR = 2.16) than girls to reach the WHO PA GL. Age and number of days per week attending ASPs do not show any significant predictions. The likelihood to reach the WHO PA GL decreases (OR = 0.98) when duration of ASPs increases. Vice versa, an increased number of minutes of MVPA in ASPs helps to increase the likelihood of reaching the guideline (OR = 1.26). Reaching the ASP guideline of 20% MVPA of total time in ASPs does not show a significant influence on the dependent variable.

DISCUSSION

After-School Program as Highly Active Time of the Day

Germany's change from the traditional half-day to a full-day school system may bring along changes in children's lifestyle, leisure time, and PA as well as SB habits. Hence, the first aim

TABLE 4 | Logistic regression and odds ratio (OR) for reaching the Global Recommendations on Physical Activity for Health (WHO PA GL).

Variable	OR	95% CI		*p*-value
		Low	High	
Sex (ref. girl)	ref.			0.048
Boy	2.16	1.01	4.63	
Age	0.94	0.67	1.31	0.696
Number of days per week in ASP (ref. 1 day)	ref.			0.605
2 days	4.18	0.50	35.19	0.188
3 days	2.05	0.39	10.73	0.394
4 days	2.51	0.47	13.44	0.281
5 days	1.46	0.24	8.83	0.684
Duration of ASP (min/day)	0.98	0.97	0.99	< 0.001
Minutes of MVPA in ASP (min/day)	1.26	1.16	1.36	< 0.001
Reaching the guideline of 20% MVPA in ASP	0.39	0.08	2.01	0.259

Total assumption: $\chi^2(9) = 84.91$, $p < 0.001$. Effect size: Nagelkerke's $R^2 = 0.48$.

of this study was to describe and analyze PA and SB in ASPs of children attending full-day schools and compare the results considering ASPs with other times of the day. Girls as well as children in higher grades show more SB and less MVPA in ASPs than boys or children in lower grades, respectively. These well-known differences (29) may lead to a policy of organizing ASPs in full-day schools: it is essential to offer various activities in ASPs to address all children independent of sex or age. In elementary schools, age-appropriate activities, specifically for older children in grades 3 and 4, may motivate this age group to be physically active and by this decrease their SB time. Additionally, results showed that ASP time is characterized by high percentages of MVPA as well as low percentages of SB. ASPs therefore depict the most active time of the day in comparison with teaching hours or leisure time. Three points may explain this highly active time: first, at German full-day schools, most ASP activities involve sports, games, or play. Almost every school provides at least one PA-based offer within its full-day school program (8, 9). Second, children attending ASPs have access to facilities that allow or promote PA, e.g., schoolyards. Access to facilities promotes PA and therefore reduces SB (30, 31). In the case of full-day schools, availability and access to the schoolyard or in some cases the school's own gym may help to encourage children for PA (32). Third, leisure time at home is often characterized by SB in the form of screen usage (33). At school, screen usage is restricted to educational purposes, which the *National Afterschool Association* (14) also recommends for ASPs. Time for highly active offers in ASPs seem to be limited. Prolonged attendance in ASP correlates with a higher percentage of time spent in SB. One reason might be full-day schools' organization. In this sample, federal requirements ask for 7–8 h in school on 3–4 days. Further, many full-day schools offer privately organized and fee-based voluntary childcare exceeding after-school hours. In this time beyond the federal required ASPs, less children are present. Consequently, there is less variety of organized activities, and the possibility to play freely with other children that brings along PA decreases. The lack of peers or offers therefore may be reason for the higher percentage of SB in prolonged ASPs. Furthermore, there may be an infrastructural reason for less PA and more SB in prolonged ASPs: schools and sports clubs typically share facilities. As sports clubs' activities take place in the later afternoon hours, the availability of gyms and playing fields (e.g., soccer pitches or athletics fields) for activities in ASPs is limited. This double usage of sports facilities is a limiting factor for extracurricular activities in ASPs (34) in general and in prolonged ASPs in particular. Because of these reasons, it can be assumed that staying in full-day schools for an extended time may involve an unorganized and SB-based waiting for pickup by parents or guardians.

Comparison of Full-Day and Half-Day School Children's Physical Activity and Sedentary Behavior

The second major aim of this study was to compare PA as well as SB of children in full-day and half-day schools during the afternoon hours in the *non-teaching* time period. Children attending full-day schools showed less SB than children in half-day schools in the afternoon hours. For the same time period, this study did not find significant differences in MVPA. The results can confirm Pau et al. (18) results regarding lower SB, but not regarding higher MVPA among full-day school children in comparison with half-day school children. According to Dahlgren and Whitehead's (4, 5) model, living conditions and the social network are different in full-day and half-day school children's *non-teaching* time. On the one hand, in ASPs, peers and space for free play or organized extracurricular activities are available. This enables full-day school children to spend their time less sedentary and more active in ASPs as compared with half-day school children who potentially spend the early afternoon at home. On the other hand, referring data of this study, Spengler et al. (35) showed that full-day school children are less engaged in organized sports outside school than are half-day school children. Furthermore, weekly duration of training in sports clubs is significantly higher in half-day school children compared with full-day school children. This may explain that there is no significant difference in MVPA between children attending full-day and half-day schools in the afternoon hours. Against this background, it seems that Züchner and Arnoldt's (36) hypothesis considering the changes in children's sports club activities in connection with full-day school attendance can be accepted: a shift of PA in leisure time from sports club activities to ASPs for full-day school children seems possible. ASPs may be a chance to increase MVPA and decrease SB of children who do not participate in organized sports activities in their leisure time (10). With the aim to reduce SB and increase PA, three policies seem promising: first, half-day school children could join ASPs to reduce their SB in the early afternoon, independent of participation in organized sports. Second, children attending ASPs in full-day schools should be motivated to participate in club sports or to join free play in the late afternoon. And third, schools should provide an obligatory PA time during ASPs but in accordance to a designated duration of ASPs. Therefore, a guideline for PA and SB in ASPs should include both absolute and relative values as recommendations for PA and SB. This finding can also decline critics' assumption that full-day school will only increase SB.

After-School Program in Full-Day Schools and the Global Recommendations on Physical Activity for Health

The third aim of this study was to identify potential and specific full-day school factors that influence the achievement of WHO PA GL. The schools' organizational form did not influence reaching the boundary value of 60 min MVPA daily. Analyzing predictors identified gender in favor of boys, shorter duration of ASPs, and higher number of minutes of MVPA in ASPs as beneficial to reach WHO PA GL. The gender effect in favor of boys is comparable with that of the study of Beets et al. (29). Combining these findings, quantity and quality of ASPs are relevant for children's PA and should be adjusted. This means that beyond the obligatory lunch (federal requirements) and time for homework, ASPs should provide time to be active in extracurricular activities. Prolonged attendance without activities may lead to sedentariness and by this decreases the possibility to reach WHO PA GL.

Future Research and Practical Implications

Future research should investigate children's PA and SB longitudinally. PA and SB development or changes over time comparing different organizational forms could be displayed. Transitions from half-day to full-day school or vice versa may bring along changes in lifestyle habits, sports club participation, and other factors influencing daily PA and SB. This study's results considering PA and SB only show children's behavior in spring and summer season with mostly good weather conditions. Comparisons between other seasons of the year or the influence of weather conditions for full-day and half-day school children's PA and SB would be interesting, too. This study analyzed device-based measured PA and SB via accelerometry. ASP content was not observed. To identify offers in ASPs that lead to higher or lower PA, ASP content should be analyzed in combination with PA and SB data. As research in physical education classes explains quality of teaching content and staff qualification, these aspects should be investigated in ASPs likewise. Examining the optimal duration and content of ASPs benefitting children's daily PA and SB requires multiple findings regarding the abovementioned topics. Including children's and parents' or guardians' socioeconomic status may (a) help to identify specific subgroups or (b) highlight the school's organizational form influence on children's PA and SB. Compared with sports clubs, full-day schools with optional sports activities reach more children. A potential influence of socioeconomic issues on children's sports activities may be much smaller in full-day schools' ASPs than in organized activities in sports clubs. Additionally, activities in ASPs could have a recruitment effect on club sports (36).

Findings of this study may lead to the following practical implications: time in ASPs should be limited in duration and not exceed the late afternoon. Full-day schools should offer a variety of extracurricular activities in ASPs for the time children stay in school. Children attending full-day school should still have the possibility to participate in organized sports, e.g., organized by sports clubs. Therefore, full-day schools and sports clubs should cooperate. Because of a lack of teachers, providing extracurricular activities for the whole time in ASPs is a problem for many schools. Including sports club coaches in ASPs may help to offer more activities during ASPs and at the same time enable sports clubs' recruitment of interested children to participate in organized sports. The compliance of PA-based ASP guidelines may help to lead children not engaged in organized sports to more PA and less SB.

Strengths and Limitations

A strength of this study is the device-based measurement of PA and SB via accelerometry with a sample size of $N = 332$ distributed over 11 elementary schools. Accelerometer-based PA and SB data underlies the chosen algorithms to calculate wear time and cut points. Algorithms used in this study were chosen by best fitting arguments. Comparisons with studies using other algorithms should be done carefully (37). Although, Robusto and Trost (25) as well as the producer postulate that the ActiGraph® models used in this study are completely compatible, a doubtless comparison of data seems to be only possible using totally identical device models. This study was conducted in the federal state of Baden-Württemberg, Germany. Therefore, the sample is not representative and is subjected to regional conditions. Schools' participation was voluntary. It can be assumed that schools declined their participation because of bad circumstances, e.g., schoolyards under construction, shortage of teachers, or the apprehension to achieve bad results and to be marked as *low PA school*. Further, children's participation was voluntary. The relatively low participation rate (31.8%) may be attributed to the considerable effort for parents, managing questionnaire completion, and accelerometer recording for a whole week. Although parents were informed about privacy and the Federal Ministry's approval of the study, data collection via accelerometry might still be seen critically by some parents.

ETHICS STATEMENT

The studies involving human participants were reviewed and approved by Ethics Commitee of the University of Konstanz (approval number: 08/2019). Written informed consent to participate in this study was provided by the participants' legal guardian/next of kin.

AUTHOR CONTRIBUTIONS

AK and FM coordinated the whole project and developed the study design. AK collected data and wrote the paper with substantial contributions from CM and MS. AK and CM performed the data preparation and statistical analysis. MS performed the final proofreading. All authors provided feedback on drafts and approved the final manuscript.

ACKNOWLEDGMENTS

We would like to thank the Federal Ministry of Education, Youth and Sports Baden-Württemberg for their cooperation. Further, we would like to thank all school staff, children, and their parents or guardians who participated in the study; Pia Breffka for her work in the project in data collection and preparation; and Sarah Spengler and Matthias Rabel for their feedback and input concerning data management and publication planning within the project.

REFERENCES

Lee D-c, Ellingson L. Physical inactivity and ill health. In: Draper N, Stratton G, editors. *Physical Activity: A Multi-Disciplinary Introduction*. London; New York, NY: Routledge (2019). p. 46–65.

Lahart I, Metsios G, Kite C. Physical activity and health. In: Draper N, Stratton G, editors. *Physical Activity: A Multi-Disciplinary Introduction*. London; New York, NY: Routlege (2019). p. 66–94.

Warburton DE, Nicol CW, Bredin SS. Health benefits of physical activity: the evidence. *Can Med Assoc J.* (2006) 174:801–9. doi: 10.1503/cmaj.051351

Dahlgren G, Whitehead M. *Policies and Strategies to Promote Social Equity in Helath.* Stockholm: Institute for Future Studies (1991).

Vonneilich N, von dem Knesebeck O. Sozialepidemiologische grundlagen der gesundheitswissenschaften. In: Haring R, editor. *Gesundheitswissenschaften·* Berlin: Springer (2018). p. 1–11.

Story M, Nanney MS, Schwartz MB. Schools and obesity prevention: creating school environments and policies to promote healthy eating and physical activity. *Milbank Q.* (2009) 87:71–100. doi: 10.1111/j.1468-0009.2009.00548.x

Allemann-Ghionda C. Ganztagsschule im internationalen Vergleich - von der Opposition zur Arbeitsteilung zwischen Staat und Familie? In: Hansel T, editor. *Ganztagsschule Halbe Sache - großer Wurf? Schulpädagogische Betrachtung eines Bildungspolitischen Investitionsprogramms.* Herbolzheim: Centaurus (2005). p. 199–223.

Kuritz A, Dinkelacker M, Mess F. Bewegung und Sport in Ganztagsschulen: Eine systematische Literaturübersicht zum aktuellen Forschungsstand in Deutschland. *Sportwissenschaft.* (2016) 46:162–78. doi: 10.1007/s12662-016-0406-3

Neuber N, Kaufmann N, Salomon S. Ganztag und Sport. In: Schmidt W, Neuber N, Rauschenbach T, Brandl-Bredenbeck HP, Süßenbach J, Breuer C, editors. *Dritter Deutscher Kinder- und Jugendsportbericht Kinder- und Jugendsport im Umbruch.* Schorndorf: Hofmann (2015). p. 416–43.

De Meester A, Cardon G, De Bourdeaudhuij I, Haerens L. Extracurricular school-based sports as a stepping stone toward an active lifestyle? Differences in physical activity and sports-motivation between extracurricular school- based sports participants and non-participants. *J Teach Phys Educ.* (2017) 36:485–97. doi: 10.1123/jtpe.2016-0035

World Health Organization. *Global Recommendations on Physical Activity for Health.* Geneva: World Health Organization, (2010).

Weaver RG, Beets MW, Huberty J, Freedman D, Turner-Mcgrievy G, Ward D. Physical activity opportunities in afterschool programs. *Health Promot Pract.* (2015) 16:371–82. doi: 10.1177/1524839914567740

California Department of Education (CDE). *California After School Physical Activity Guidelines.* Sacramento, CA: California Department of Education (CDE) (2009). Available online at: https://www.cde.ca.gov/ls/ex/documents/paguidelines.pdf (May 3, 2020).

National Afterschool Association (NAA). *The NAA HEPA Standards 2.0.* Oakton, VA (2011). Available online at: https://indd.adobe.com/view/ 681ce31e-c7b2-4ab2-983d-d644ffb6b71d (May 3, 2020).

YMCA of the USA. *The YMCA's Healthy Eating and Physical Activity Standards for Early Learningand AfterschoolPrograms: YMCA of the USA.* (2014). Available online at: https://www.ymcamn.org/sites/default/ files/Healthy-Eating-and-Physical%20Activity-Standards.pdf?openyts= 1530403200172 (May 3, 2020).

Rütten A, Pfeifer K, Banzer W, Ferrari N, Füzéki E, Geidl W, et al. *National Recommendations for Physical Activity and Physical Activity Promotion* Erlangen: FAU University Press (2016).

Beets MW, Weaver RG, Turner-McGrievy G, Saunders RP, Webster CA, Moore JB, et al. Evaluation of a statewide dissemination and implementation of physical activity intervention in afterschool programs: a nonrandomized trial. *Transl Behav Med.* (2017) 7:690–701. doi: 10.1007/s13142-017-0484-2

Pau M, Corona F, Leban B, Piredda S, Vacca MM, Mura G. Influence of school schedules on physical activity patterns in primary school children: a case study in Italy. *J Phys Act Health.* (2017) 14:501–5. doi: 10.1123/jpah.2016-0492

van Stralen MM, Yildirim M, Wulp A, te Velde SJ, Verloigne M, Doessegger A, et al. Measured sedentary time and physical activity during the school day of European 10- to 12-year-old children: the ENERGY project. *J Sci Med Sport.* (2014) 17:201–6. doi: 10.1016/j.jsams.2013.04.019

Messing S, Rütten A, Abu-Omar K, Ungerer-Röhrich U, Goodwin L, Burlacu I, et al. How can physical activity be promoted among children and adolescents? A systematic review of reviews across settings. *Front Public Health.* (2019) 7:55. doi: 10.3389/fpubh.2019.00055

Parrish A-M, Okely AD, Stanley RM, Ridgers ND. The effect of school recess interventions on physical activity. *Sports Med.* (2013) 43:287– 99. doi: 10.1007/s40279-013-0024-2

Atkin AJ, Gorely T, Biddle SJ, Cavill N, Foster C. Interventions to promote physical activity in young people conducted in the hours immediately after school: a systematic review. *Int J Behav Med.* (2011) 18:176– 87. doi: 10.1007/s12529-010-9111-z

Schmidt S, Will N, Henn A, Reimers A, Woll A. Der Motorik- Modul Aktivitätsfragebogen MoMo-AFB: Leitfaden zur Anwendung und Auswertung. In: *KIT Scientific Working Papers*, Karlsruhe (2016) 53.

Rich C, Geraci M, Griffiths L, Sera F, Dezateux C, Cortina-Borja M. Quality control methods in accelerometer data processing: defining minimum wear time. *PLoS ONE.* (2013) 8:e67206. doi: 10.1371/journal.pone.00 67206

Robusto KM, Trost SG. Comparison of three generations of ActiGraph^{TM} activity monitors in children and adolescents. *J Sport Sci.* (2012) 30:1429– 35. doi: 10.1080/02640414.2012.710761

Troiano RP. Large-scale applications of accelerometers: new frontiers and new questions. *Med Sci Sports Exerc.* (2007) 39:1501. doi: 10.1097/mss.0b013e318150d42e

Pulsford RM, Cortina-Borja M, Rich C, Kinnafick FE, Dezateux C, Griffiths LJ. Actigraph accelerometer-defined boundaries for sedentary behaviour and physical activity intensities in 7 year old children. *PLoS ONE.* (2011) 6:e21822. doi: 10.1371/journal.pone.0021822

Cohen J. *Statistical Power Analysis for the Behavioral Sciences.* Hillsdale, NJ: Erlbaum (1988).

Beets MW, Shah R, Weaver RG, Huberty J, Beighle A, Moore JB. Physical activity in after-school programs: comparison with physical activity policies. *J Phys Act Health.* (2015) 12:1–7. doi: 10.1123/jpah.12.1.1

Sallis JF, Prochaska JJ, Taylor WC. A review of correlates of physical activity of children and adolescents. *Med Sci Sports Exerc.* (2000) 32:963– 75. doi: 10.1097/00005768-200005000-00014

Van Der Horst K, Paw MJ, Twisk JW, Van Mechelen W. A brief review on correlates of physical activity and sedentariness in youth. *Med Sci Sports Exerc.* (2007) 39:1241–50. doi: 10.1249/mss.0b013e318059bf35

Ajja R, Clennin MN, Weaver RG, Moore JB, Huberty JL, Ward DS, et al. Association of environment and policy characteristics on children's moderate- to-vigorous physical activity and time spent sedentary in afterschool programs. *Prev Med.* (2014) 69:S49–54. doi: 10.1016/j.ypmed.2014. 09.010

Marques A, Sallis JF, Martins J, Diniz J, Da Costa FC. Correlates of urban children's leisure- time physical activity and sedentary behaviors during school days. *Am J Hum Biol.* (2014) 26:407–12. doi: 10.1002/ajhb.22535

Laging R, Dirks F. Sport- und Bewegungsangebote an Ganztagsschulen: zur Bedeutung von Kooperationen. *Bewegung und Sport in der Ganztagsschule - StuBSS: Ergebnisse der qualitativen Studie: Studie zur Entwicklung von Bewegung, Spiel und Sport in der Ganztagsschule (StuBSS)*. Hohengehren: Schneider-Verl (2014). p. 206–49.

Spengler S, Kuritz A, Rabel M, Mess F. Are primary school children attending full-day school still engaged in sports clubs? *PLoS ONE*. (2019) 14:e0225220. doi: 10.1371/journal.pone.0225220

Züchner I, Arnoldt B. Sport von Kindern und Jugendlichen in Ganztagsschule und Sportverein. *Schulpädagogik heute*. (2012) 3:121–35. doi: 10.2307/j.ctvss3zr9.11

Anedda B, Niessner C, Burchartz A, Oriwol D, Schmidt S, Woll A. Processing accelerometer data of children and adolescents - influence of wear time algorithm, epoch length and cut-off points on age specific subgroups. In: Murphy M, Boreham C, de Vito G, Tsolakidis E, editors. *Book of Abstracts of the 23rd Annual Congress of the European College of Sport Science - 4th - 7th July 2018, Dublin - Ireland*. Cologne: European College of Sport Science (2018). p. 129.

18

Competitive Psychological Disposition and Perception of Performance in Young Female Soccer Players

Aurelio Olmedilla[1], Roberto Ruiz-Barquín[2], Francisco Javier Ponseti[3], Francisco Javier Robles-Palazón[4] and Alexandre García-Mas[5]*

[1] Department of Personality, Evaluation and Psychological Treatment, University of Murcia, Murcia, Spain, [2] Department of Developmental and Educational Psychology, Autonomous University of Madrid, Madrid, Spain, [3] Department of Pedagogy, University of the Balearic Islands, Mallorca, Spain, [4] Department of Physical Activity and Sport, University of Murcia, Murcia, Spain, [5] Department of Psychology, University of the Balearic Islands, Mallorca, Spain

***Correspondence:**
Aurelio Olmedilla
olmedilla@um.es

The athletes' psychological disposition is a factor that is increasingly considered by researchers as a key to sports performance, even as a mediator between the physical, technical and tactical abilities of the athlete and their competitive performance, thus acquiring great relevance in training and in sports performance. The purpose of this study is to analyze the psychological characteristics of young soccer players and their relation to their performance perception, made both by the player herself and by their coaches. The sample is composed of 108 women (*M* age = 15.53, *SD* age = 1.05), with ages between 13 and 17 years (13 years, $n = 1$, 14 years, $n = 18$, 15 years, $n = 36$, 16 years, $n = 29$, 17 years, $n = 24$), and with a sport practice experience of 7.27 years on average ($SD = 2.64$). For to address this aim, we used the Psychological Characteristics related to the Sport Performance Questionnaire (CPRD) and the Psychological Skills Inventory for Sports (PSIS). In addition, regarding the evaluation of performance perception, an *ad hoc* short questionnaire was created, composed by one question addressed to the player and one directed to the coach. The results indicate that the group of players of the under-16 category obtained higher scores in all the psychological dimensions than the U-18 players, showing significant differences in Team Cohesion ($p < 0.048$). Regarding the degree of congruence between the player's psychological features, and the player's and coach's performance perceptions, the results show statistically significant and negative correlations between the Team Cohesion factor and the athlete's own outcome perception for the match #1 ($r_{xy} = -0.479$; $p < 0.001$), and match #2 ($r_{xy} = -0.402$; $p < 0.01$). The results of this study may contribute to establish the differences between different constellations of psychological characteristics according to the categories of competition and their relationship with the perception of performance. This knowledge can be used by sports professionals: coaches, psychologists, physical educators, etc., in order to help athletes to reach their maximum performance.

Keywords: psychological profile, performance perception, mental skills, football, women

INTRODUCTION

Soccer is a high-intensity intermittent team sport that requires technical, tactical and physical skills (Stolen et al., 2005), as well as psychological (Gledhill et al., 2017; Olmedilla et al., 2018b) for optimal performance. Soccer is one of the most researched sports in the scientific literature (Reilly et al., 2000; Datson et al., 2014). However, most of studies have been conducted traditionally with male soccer player samples, and only recent studies have analyzed female soccer player cohorts (Vescovi and McGuigan, 2008). Nowadays, female soccer has a great participation in United States (Markovits and Hellerman, 2003) and begins to be considered an attractive sport by women athletes in Europe and other countries around the world (Wright, 2014). Therefore, a greater research about the main factors related to the female soccer players' performance is clearly required.

Starting from the theoretical model of Gagné (2004) (Differentiated Model of Gift and Talent, GMGT) to work simultaneously with personality traits, acquired skills and psychology requirements for the sports competition, it has been considered that the psychological disposition is one of the factors that have been strongly added to this analysis (Olmedilla and Dominguez-Igual, 2016; González, 2017). Considered as intermediary between players' physical, technical and tactical abilities (Morris, 2000; Castilla and Ramos, 2012; Abdullah et al., 2016; Swann et al., 2017), psychological disposition is one of the keys for the sport performance due to the influence that it would have in the player's competitive success (Anderson et al., 2014; Arthur et al., 2017). In this sense, some studies have found that physiological variables represent between 45 and 48% of the sport performance, and when the psychological variables were added, the proportion of variance explained increased around 79–85% in certain sports like wrestling (Nagle et al., 1975; Silva et al., 1981; Bali, 2015; Abdullah et al., 2016; Olmedilla et al., 2017a).

One of the approaches for studying the role of the psychological variables in sport performance is based on the personality traits (Mahoney and Avener, 1977; Gould et al., 1981; Burnik et al., 2005; Rasmus and Kocur, 2006; Cabrita et al., 2014), as the recent published study by Danielsen et al. (2017) where a relationship was found between the influence of mental toughness and the level of competition in female soccer players. Another approach studies differences between athletes and non-athlete population. For instance, Malinauskas et al. (2014) found higher scores in Consciousness in athletes than in non-athlete population, and greater Extraversion in team sportspeople in comparison with athletes from individual sports. Steca et al. (2018) found that athletes with better success in their careers revealed higher punctuations in all the Big-Five personality dimensions.

Given that these results do not show clearly a specific personality profile to distinguish between athletes and non-athlete population (Weinberg and Gould, 2014), neither result really useful for the sport performance, researchers have focused on the study of the relationship between athletes' mental strategies, abilities and behaviors, and their subsequent performance (Romero et al., 2010; Álvarez et al., 2014; García-Naveira et al., 2015). This approach has been able to provide a better knowledge of the most relevant psychological characteristics for athletes, as well as to explain the differences between diverse sport participants and/or tactical positions in the same sport (Olmedilla et al., 2015). Also as they indicate Baillie et al. (2014, p. 406) "personality may also play a central role in determining the goodness of the fit between an athlete or team and a (psychologist) practitioner," it could serve to distinguish male soccer players from female soccer players, and thus establish working hypotheses about the most appropriated psychological intervention to assist the sport performance; the knowledge of an athlete's psychological profile enables a better understanding, the improvement of the communication procedures with himself and the increase in training effectivity (Martínez-Ferreiro, 2016), and it will result in better mental preparation and better psychological skills acquisition related to the sport success (Bahrololoum et al., 2012; Olmedilla et al., 2018c).

In recent years the number of works that show an especial attention in the study of the relationship between psychological factors and sport performance in female soccer has increased considerably (Danielsen et al., 2017). Specifically, the main psychological factors studied have been self-esteem and anxiety control (Williams, 2017), the prediction of the goal orientations suggesting coach's specific actions (Granero-Gallegos et al., 2015; Domínguez-Escribano et al., 2017), some mental health indicators as depression and anxiety (Junge and Feddermann-Demont, 2016; Olmedilla et al., 2018a), and mood states (Arroyo del Bosque et al., 2016). Thus, it seems interesting the suggestion made by Rutkowska and Bergier (2015), who emphasized the importance of examining the women soccer players' psychological profile due to the relevant information derived from this evaluation for improving training programs, primarily in mental training and in soccer players close to the professional level of performance (Martín-García, 2003).

In summary, sport performance is determined by a physical, technical and tactical systematic practice, necessary to achieve an elite level in soccer (Haugaasen et al., 2014). The same practice should be applied to the psychological training, strengthening the psychological resources for the sport competition; in this sense, the review published by Gledhill et al. (2017) stated 48 social and psychological factors linked to the talent development in soccer (e.g., adaptive lifestyle choices, practice and play behaviors). Similarly, there is a clear need to use women soccer players given the lack of studies that analyze this population in comparison with their male counterparts. Therefore, the main purposes of the current study were: (1) to describe the psychological characteristics of a Spanish sample of female young soccer players, and (2) to determine the differences between under-16 and under-18 age-groups, as well as their relation and congruence with perception of performance by the soccer player herself and her coach.

MATERIALS AND METHODS

Participants

The sample was formed by 108 players that participated in the National Championship of Autonomic Selections of Spain of female soccer, in the categories under-16 and under-18. Mean age was 15.53 ± 1.05 years and mean of years practicing the sport was 7.27 ± 2.64 years, and 1.75 ± 0.92 years of experience in the highest category. The female players train an average of almost 3 sessions a week (2.98), lasting between 1 and 3 h each session, 102.64 ± 17.42 min on average and a total weekly training time of 304.44 ± 74.26 min on average.

Measures

Psychological variables were assessed using the Psychological Characteristics Related to Sport Performance Questionnaire (CPRD, Gimeno et al., 2001), based on the Psychological Skills Inventory for Sports (PSIS, Mahoney et al., 1987; Mahoney, 1989). The questionnaire consists of 55 items graded in a 5-option Likert scale (from totally disagree to totally agree). It also includes a response option "I do not understand" to avoid missing answers.

Characteristics related to the Sport Performance Questionnaire includes five subscales: Stress Control (SC), Influence of Performance Evaluation (IPE), Motivation (M), Team Cohesion (TCOH), and Mental Skills (MSK), showing acceptable values of internal consistency for the total scale ($\alpha = 0.85$) and for most of the subscales ($\alpha SC = 0.88$; $\alpha IPE = 0.72$; $\alpha M = 0.67$; $\alpha TCOH = 0.78$; $\alpha MSK = 0.34$). According to the authors, the low internal consistency of MSK is probably related to it tapping a wide range of different skills but authors still keep the subscale due to the factorials loads showed by the items of this factor.

Stress Control consists of 20 items and refers athlete's responses to potentially stressful situations and other training and competition demands. Higher scores denote athlete has management skills to cope with sport-related stress. IPE consists of 12 items and regards to athlete's responses to situations in which he/she or people close to him/her judges his/her performance. It also includes an assessment about antecedents of athlete's performance judgment. Higher scores mean the athlete can control the impact of performance judgment. M consists of eight items referring to basic motivation to sport performance and achievement, as well as to the regular training and competition activities. Higher scores indicate strong motivation and commitment to competitive sport practice. MSK consists of nine items and assess the use of different mental skills which are related to sport performance. Higher scores express better psychological resources to improve his/her performance. TCOH includes six items and assesses the extension the athlete feels attracted and identified with the sport group. This scale has not been used in this study due to the nature of the target sports.

To assess the perception of performance, an *ad hoc* instrument was created with a question addressed to the player, and a question addressed to the coach, and in both cases they had to answer on a liker scale of 0 (I played very badly) to 10 (I played very well).

Procedure

After the corresponding author's institution IRB approval (UM1551/2017), athletes were contacted by Football Federation of the Region of Murcia (FFRM) and football sport clubs. The researchers explained to both parents and athletes about the objectives and use of the information, and those who voluntarily participated signed an informed consent. In the cases in which the players were under 18 years of age, the signature of the parents was required. The data collection was made during the National Championship of Women's Autonomous Soccer Teams held in Murcia (Spain) in December 2017. In the Championship participated the selections of Balearic Islands, Castilla la Mancha and the Region of Murcia in both categories. Authorization was requested to the Football Federation of the Region of Murcia (organizer of the event) and the coordinators of the different selections were informed about the objectives of the study. The CPRD questionnaire was administered in the accommodation hotel of the selections and during the leisure time between competitions. The evaluation of the perception of the performance was carried out right at the end of each game (from a total of two matches), asking first the players about their performance in the match, and then the coach of each team about the performance of each of their players in the match.

Data Analysis

The analysis of data used have been: measures of tendency of central (means); dispersion measures (standard deviation); frequency analysis; normality tests using the Kolmogorov–Smirnov test; analysis of difference of means for two independent samples by the Mann–Whitney U; mean difference analysis for two correlational samples using the Wilcoxon W statistic; correlational analysis using Spearman's correlation coefficient. Statistical analyzes were carried out using the statistical package SPSS 22.0.

RESULTS

Table 1 shows the descriptive analysis of the total sample of soccer players, and the application of the normality test (Kolmogorov–Smirnov) for the five factors, of which Team Cohesion ($p < 0.001$) and Motivation ($p < 0.01$) are not distributed normally.

Figure 1 shows the scores obtained by the players in each of the factors of the CPRD, compared with and the average scores of a general sample of athletes in the study from Gimeno (1999) with the same tool. It is noteworthy that in all the factors, the scores coming from the group of female soccer players are higher than to those from the general sample, highlighting the Motivation factor ($c = 85$, M = 23.86, $SD = 4.04$), Stress Control ($c = 65$; $M = 51.26$, $SD = 11.15$), and Team Cohesion ($c = 65$, $M = 19.94$, $SD = 2.85$), while the Influence of the Performance Evaluation ($c = 55$, $M = 25.83$, $SD = 6.70$) and Mental Ability (c = 55, $M = 21.37$, $SD = 4.09$) values are on the average.

Table 2 shows the descriptive values from the players' self-evaluation of the performance in match 1. The answer rate was 81.5% ($n = 88$), while it was 82.4% for the second match ($n = 89$). When observing the coaches evaluations, it was initially of 83.3% ($n = 90$) in the first game, and of 84.3% ($n = 91$) in the second one. Of these last two evaluation, only 66.67% ($n = 72$) and 66.76% ($n = 73$) of valid cases have been finally considered, due to the

TABLE 1 | Descriptive values of the five factors of the CPRD questionnaire and application of the Kolmogorov–Smirnov normality test.

	M	*SD*	Minimum	Maximum.	Centil	K–S	Sig.
SC	51.26	11.16	24.00	80.00	65	0.076	0.155
IPE	25.83	6.70	11.00	44.00	55	0.080	0.085†
M	23.86	4.04	10.00	32.00	85	0.110	0.003**
MSK	21.37	4.09	11.00	33.00	55	0.073	0.200
TCOH	19.94	2.85	4.00	24.00	65	0.186	0.000***

SC, Stress Control; IPE, Influence of Performance Evaluation; M, Motivation; MSK, Mental Skills; TCOH, Team Cohesion. †$p < 0.10$; **$p < 0.01$; ***$p < 0.001$.

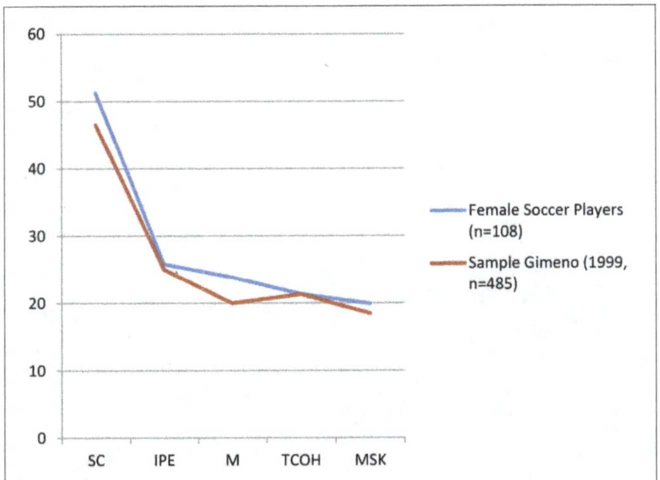

FIGURE 1 | Comparative graph between the average scores of a general sample of athletes (Gimeno, 1999), and the scores of female soccer players in the present study.

elimination of 18 evaluations of match 1 and 18 from the match 2 due to observed answers biases (extreme scores given without discrimination of variability in scores).

We may observe also that the players' self-evaluations are very similar between the two games, although this short difference is significant in favor of the first match ($z = -3.606$, $p < 0.001$). Regarding the evaluations made by the coaches, they are somewhat higher than those made by the athletes, finding significant differences between the performance evaluations made between the first and second match ($z = -2.295$, $p < 0.05$). Unlike athletes, coaches give a better rating to the performance obtained in the 2nd game than the one from the first game.

Table 3 shows the descriptive values and the differences of means between the under-16 and under-18 categories.

The under-16 category players obtain higher scores than the players of the under-18 category in all the factors, although only statistically significant differences appears in Team Cohesion ($p < 0.05$.), and a tendency toward significance in the Motivation factor ($p < 0.05$).

Table 4 shows the players' performance self-evaluations, the coaches' evaluations and the scores obtained in the five factors of the CPRD, considering independently the under-16 category and the under-18 category.

In the under-16 category, only correlations are found between the two coaches' evaluations (match 1 and match 2; rho = 0.500, $p < 0.01$), and a tendency to statistical significance ($p < 0.10$) between the perception of the players in match 1 and the Mental Ability factor. On the contrary, in the under-18 category multiple results with statistical significance appears. There are important correlations between the perception of the players' performance in match 1 and match 2 (rho = 0.702, $p < 0.001$). Also, significant correlations –with medium values- were found between the player's perception of their performance in game 1 and the coaches' perception in that same game (rho = 0.405; $p < 0.05$), obtaining values significantly higher when considering the second match (rho = 0.445; $p < 0.01$).

Regarding to the CPRD factors, the Team Cohesion obtains significant inverse correlations of medium values when correlated with the players' perception in matches 1 (rho = −0.479; $p < 0.001$) and 2 (rho = −0.402; $p < 0.01$). The same factor have a significant negative tendency (rho = −0.273; $p < 0.10$) correlated with coaches' evaluation in match 2. Added to this, there is a positive correlation with tendency to the significance between the Motivation factor and the coach's evaluation in the first game (rho = −0.264; $p < 0.10$).

DISCUSSION

Studying the psychological profile of female soccer players, as was indicated by Rutkowska and Bergier (2015), is extremely important, and also can provide many interesting ideas about the specific nature of women's youth soccer.

It can also show where improvements can be made in sports training programs, specifically in mental training, especially in those players who will soon become part of professional football (MacNamara and Collins, 2017). In this vein, the objectives of this

TABLE 2 | Descriptive values and means differences between players' and coaches' perceptions of performance in the two games (Wilcoxon W).

	N	*M*	*SD*	Minimum	Maximum	Average rank	Total ranks	*Z*	*p*
PP-1	88	7.182	1.2158	4.0	9.5	30.34	1153.00	−3.006	0.000***
PP-2	89	7.006	1.6140	2.0	9.5	20.75	332.00		
N valid	87								
CP-1	72	7.347	1.4551	0.0	9.0	29.08	523.50	−2.295	0.022*
CP-2	73	7.795	1.6726	4.0	10.0	28.22	1072.50		
N valid	71								

PP, Players' perceptions; CP, Coaches' perceptions. *$p < 0.05$; ***$p < 0.001$.

TABLE 3 | Descriptive values and analysis of means differences of the two subgroups ($n = 54$ each group).

		M	*SD*	Average rank	Total ranks	W Wilcoxon	*Z*	Sig.
SC	Under-16	52.22	12.04969	56.97	3076.50	2809.500	−0.821	0.412
	Under-18	50.30	10.20660	52.03	2809.50			
IPE	Under-16	26.65	6.92591	58.51	3159.50	2726.500	−1.332	0.183
	Under-18	25.02	6.42663	50.49	2726.50			
M	Under-16	24.52	4.00820	59.77	3227.50	2658.500	−1.756	0.079†
	Under-18	23.20	4.00179	49.23	2658.50			
MSK	Under-16	21.74	3.59866	57.53	3106.50	2779.500	−1.008	0.313
	Under-18	21.00	4.53914	51.47	2779.50			
TCOH	Under-16	20.37	2.43633	60.38	3260.50	2625.500	−1.975	0.048*
	Under-18	19.50	3.16675	48.62	2625.50			

SC, Stress Control; IPE, Influence of Performance Evaluation; M, Motivation; MSK, Mental Skills; TCOH, Team Cohesion. †$p < 0.10$; *$p < 0.05$.

TABLE 4 | Correlation values regarding the under-16 category ($n = 29$) and under-18 ($n = 44$) using the Spearman's Rho statistic.

	Under-16				Under-18			
	PP-1	PP-2	PE-1	PE-2	PP-1	PP-2	PE-1	PE-2
PP-1	1.000				1.000			
PP-2	0.286	1.000			0.702***	1.000		
	0.141				0.000			
PE-1	0.126	0.057	1.000		0.405*	0.215	1.000	
	0.516	0.774			0.014	0.207		
PE-2	−0.037	0.118	0.500**	1.000	0.351*	0.445**	0.360*	1.000
	0.850	0.535	0.007		0.036	0.007	0.018	
SC	−0.126	0.231	−0.278	−0.288	0.142	0.242	−0.003	−0.120
	0.514	0.220	0.144	0.123	0.359	0.113	0.987	0.445
IPE	−0.303	0.254	−0.244	−0.086	−0.108	−0.007	−0.081	−0.237
	0.110	0.176	0.202	0.650	0.487	0.966	0.605	0.127
M	0.253	0.125	−0.255	−0.203	−0.040	−0.006	0.264†	−0.162
	0.185	0.510	0.182	0.283	0.798	0.971	0.087	0.299
MSK	0.331†	0.026	0.008	−0.154	−0.173	−0.052	0.038	−0.104
	0.079	0.891	0.969	0.416	0.261	0.738	0.809	0.506
TCOH	0.003	−0.101	0.109	−0.097	−0.479***	−0.402**	−0.101	−0.273†
	0.989	0.595	0.574	0.611	0.001	0.007	0.518	0.076

PP, Players' perceptions; CP, Coaches' perceptions; SC, Stress Control; IPE, Influence of Performance Evaluation; M, Motivation; MSK, Mental Skills; TCOH, Team Cohesion. †$p < 0.10$; *$p < 0.05$; **$p < 0.01$; ***$p < 0.001$.

study have been to describe the psychological characteristics of young female soccer players, determine the differences between the under-16 and under-18 categories, showing their relationship and congruence with the perception of performance, from both the players and coaches.

The results show that the scores of the young soccer players in the CPRD are higher than those of the general sample of athletes, especially in the scales of M, SC, and TCOH. Specifically in M they have a score that can be considered as quite high, that is, the players in the sample studied seem to have an adequate motivational state to meet the demanding requirements of sports practice and the competition, which coincides with other studies on female soccer players (Muñoz et al., 2018), in which the basic motivation found was intrinsical, related to the game itself and by being part of a team, although these features have fluctuations depending on the competition level (Domínguez-Escribano et al., 2017).

Both in the SC and in TCOH subscales the scores obtained are moderately high, which in principle seems to indicate that the players tend to control well the potential stress inherent to the competition, and that they have a good disposition to work with the team. Regarding the scores obtained in IPE and MSK, the results indicate that they are on the average, which in the first case indicates that the players can be negatively affected by the evaluation that other people (or indeed themselves) make of their performance, and in the second case indicates that the players do not have full consolidated psychological skills, needed for to perform optimally. This last factor affects the need to propose psychological intervention programs tailored to the specific needs and characteristics of athletes, depending on the competition level, gender, etc. In the same vein, Slimani et al. (2016) performed a systematic review finding some very interesting data showing the differences in cognitive/psychological training interventions, and their effectiveness, depending on whether they are directed toward practices or competition, age, competition level and the players' position.

Considering that the players have a similar level of performance in their respective categories, it is clear they show some overestimation of their skills (mainly perceived in the under-16 category), perhaps due to a fewer competitive experience, a lower self-awareness of psychological limitations, and less exposure to experiences related to the performance in competition demands. Also, from an evolutionary perspective, players of 14 and 15 years old are in the middle of the adolescence, where variables such as self-concept and self-knowledge are under construction, and therefore, may have a minor adjustment of their psychological skills to deal with situations of stress and promote self-confidence (Sarkar and Fletcher, 2014; González-Campos et al., 2015; Gómez-Espejo et al., 2017).

On the other hand, with respect to the second objective, the results indicate that the under-16 players obtain higher scores than the under-18 players in all the factors, showing statistically significant differences in TCOH and a tendency to statistical significance in M. In any case, the most relevant differences are in the TCOH scale, where perhaps the younger players have a better disposition to work inside the team, while the U18 players have other aspects of personal competence could work against the teamwork; and on the M scale, which in this case may be better understandable due to other major competitive factors, such as being near the end of the youth stage in the case of the U-18, when some of the players could to be thinking about alternatives outside the practice of competitive football, or that the perceived pressure is inadequately managed, generating anxiety and worry. These data are in accord with what other found in other studies (Pan and Zhu, 2003), where at a higher level of psychological competitiveness, lower is the level of worry and anxiety and better the performance.

Finally, regarding the third objective, and taking into account the whole sample, the results indicate that the players' self-evaluations are very similar between match 1 and match 2, although this difference is significant in favor of match 1. In other words, they perceived that they have played the first match better than the second. Interestingly, the evaluations made by the coaches are somewhat higher than those made by the players themselves, finding significant differences between the assessments made between the match 1 and 2; unlike the players, the coaches give a better rating to the performance obtained in match 2. In this sense, some studies (Møllerløkken et al., 2017) have also found differences between the perception of players and coaches regarding the motivational climate, meaning that players of both sexes perceived that the motivational climate was more oriented toward the performance and less toward the domain compared to coaches. In both cases, these findings may improve our understanding of the coach-player relationship, and may be important in understanding the players' motivational style. Indeed, Reid and Crust (2012) examined the perceptions of elite soccer players and coaches about the psychological drive and how it relates to objective performance, finding that teammates and spectators can have a greater impact on the momentum in female football than with the male soccer.

When analyzing the data by categories, the results indicate that in the under-16 category, only correlations are found between the coaches' evaluation of first and second matches. On the other hand, in the under-18 category there are quite relevant correlations between the perception of the player's performance between the two matches; between the players' and coach performance perception match 1 and the perception, indeed reaching higher significant values when considering the second game. In this last case, the under-18 players' great experience could explain, in part, the correlation of their performance perception with that of their coach, since in the under-16 category that lack of experience could play against a more realistic self-evaluation, differing more with the most experienced coach evaluation.

Furthermore, this fact supports the fact that the TCOH factor obtains significant inverse correlations -of medium values- when is correlated with the player's self-perception both in the first and second matches, and when at the same time obtain a significant negative tendency with the coach's evaluation in the second game. In short, these results indicate that the under-18 players have performance perceptions more adjusted to the expert criterion (from the coaches) than the under-16; the higher experience in the under-18 players' sport practice could explain these differences between these both groups.

Finally, the CPRD questionnaire seems to be a very appropriate instrument to describe the relevant psychological characteristics related to sports performance, and to provide very valuable information, both from a group and individual point of view, serving as a basis for implementing training programs and specific psychological training for the team or individual level. As indicated by Olmedilla et al. (2017a) the knowledge of the psychological characteristics of young athletes can be very valuable so that, together with the physical and anthropometric indicators, they allow their coaches to individualize the training processes and thus optimize them.

The present study provides fundamentally some knowledge about the psychological variables of women's competitive soccer, showing psychological differences in two youth sports categories where the player's experience and age may have great relevance (Ruiz, 2005), as well as the relationships between the load of practice and/or competitions regarding players' mood, psychological well-being and physiological well-being (Lowe, 2017; McFadden et al., 2017; Tharawadeepimuk and Wongsawat, 2017), especially in view of the possibility of evaluating and intervening on a psychological level in women's football teams (Olmedilla et al., 2018b).

The results of this study can help to establish the differences between different constellations of psychological characteristics related with performance levels and their relationship with the subjective perception of performance. This knowledge can be used by sports professionals: coaches, psychologists, physical educators, etc., to help athletes achieve their maximum performance, and to implement effective intervention programs for sports performance (MacNamara et al., 2010; Bennett and Maynard, 2016; Gledhill et al., 2017); personal growth and athletes' dual-career (Llames and García-Dantas, 2017), or even athletes' injury prevention (Olmedilla et al., 2017b).

Limitations and Future Research Directions

In the present study, the participating regional teams have been analyzed in the final phase of the national 11 women's soccer championship in the under-16 and under-18 categories, with 3 teams in each category. The non-randomized selection of the participants, the specific context of the competition and the small sample size of the current research imply that the results obtained cannot be generalized, and that they cannot be compared with other performance levels.

On the other hand, it would be interesting to collect data from a greater number of matches, and perhaps to include practices, in order to determine the differences in the player's and coaches' perception of performance between the two situations. In addition, the coaches' evaluation carried out is individual and not peer-reviewed, and in subsequent studies it should be good to carry out inter-judge analyzes obtaining a more reliable expert criterion regarding the data analysis.

Likewise, there is a great dispersion in the number of hours and days of practice in the players assessed, what is a representation of the reality of female soccer in Spain; so it could be interesting to study more homogeneous groups in future approaches. Regarding future research developments, should be interesting made up studies where specific changes of psychological skills in different female sports teams may be analyzed. Likewise, it would be convenient to establish comparisons with male athletes, aiming to tailoring accurately eventual psychological interventions addressed to each epidemiological segment (such as gender, sport type, athletes' age, and level of performance).

CONCLUSION

The scores of the young soccer players in the CPRD are higher than those of the general sample of athletes, especially in the scales of M, SC, and TCOH.

The under-16 category players' obtained higher scores than the under-18 category players' in all factors, showing statistically significant differences in TCOH, and a tendency to statistical significance in M.

The players' self-perception of their performance is very similar between match 1 and match 2, although the small difference is significant in favor of match 1.

The players' performance made by their coaches is somewhat higher than those made by the players themselves.

ETHICS STATEMENT

This study was carried out in accordance with the recommendations of the Declaration of Helsinki. The protocol was approved by the Comité de Ética de la Universidad de Murcia (reference: UM 1551/2017). All subjects gave written informed consent in accordance with the Declaration of Helsinki.

AUTHOR CONTRIBUTIONS

AO and AG-M contributed with the conception and design of the study. AO and RR-B organized the database. RR-B and FP performed the statistical analysis. AO wrote the first draft of the manuscript. FP, AG-M, RR-B, and FR-P wrote the sections of the manuscript. FR-P was in charge of the formal aspects of the work. All authors contributed to the revision of the manuscript, and read and approved the presented version.

REFERENCES

Abdullah, M. R., Musa, R. M., Maliki, A. B. H. M., Kosni, N. A., and Suppiah, P. K. (2016). Role of psychological factors on the performance of elite soccer players. *J. Phys. Educ. Sport* 16:170. doi: 10.7752/jpes.2016.01027

Álvarez, O., Estevan, I., Falcó, C., Hernández-Mendo, A., and Castillo, I. (2014). Perfil de habilidades psicológicas en taekwondistas universitarios y su relación con el éxito en competición. *Cuad. Psicol. Dep.* 14, 13–20. doi: 10.4321/s1578-84232014000300002

Anderson, R., Hanrahan, S. J., and Mallett, C. J. (2014). Investigating the optimal psychological state for peak performance in Australian elite athletes. *J. Appl. Sport Psychol.* 26, 318–333. doi: 10.1080/10413200.2014.885915

Arroyo del Bosque, R., Irazusta, S., and González-Rodríguez, O. (2016). *Impacto del Resultado Post-Partido en el Estado de Ánimo en Jóvenes Jugadoras de Fútbol* Ph.D. thesis, Universidad del País Vasco País Vasco, SP.

Arthur, R. A., Fitzwater, J., Roberts, R., Hardy, J., and Arthur, C. A. (2017). Psychological skills and "the paras": the indirect effects of psychological skills on endurance. *J. Appl. Sport Psychol.* 29, 449–465. doi: 10.1080/10413200.2017.1306728

Bahrololoum, H., Hassani, A., Reza, M., and Akbari, A. (2012). The relationship between the emotional intelligence and mental skills in iranian elite Male Volleyball Players. I. *J. Acad. Res. Bus. Soc. Sci.* 2, 123–130.

Baillie, P. H. F., Davis, H., and Ogilvie, B. C. (2014). "Working with Elite Athletes," in *Exploring Sport and Exercise Psychology*, 3rd Edn, eds J. van Raalte and B. Brewer (Washington DC: APA), 401–425. doi: 10.1037/14251-018

Bali, A. (2015). Psychological factors affecting sports performance. *Int. J. Phys. Educ. Sports Health* 1, 92–95.

Bennett, J., and Maynard, I. (2016). Performance blocks in sport: recommendations for treatment and implications for sport psychology practitioners. *J. Sport Psychol. Action* 8, 60–68. doi: 10.1080/21520704.2016.1227414

Burnik, S., Jug, S., Kajtna, T., and Tusak, M. (2005). Differences in personality traits of mountain climbers and nonathletes in Slovenia. *Acta Univ. Palacki. Olomuc. Gymn.* 35, 13–17.

Cabrita, T., Rosado, A., de la Vega, R., and Serpa, S. (2014). Relaciones entre identidad atlética y personalidad en el deporte de competición. *Rev. Psicol. Dep.* 23, 247–253.

Castilla, J. F., and Ramos, L. C. (2012). Rendimiento deportivo, estilo de liderazgo y evitación experiencial en jóvenes futbolistas almerienses. *J. Sport Psychol.* 21, 137–142.

Danielsen, L. D., Rodahl, S. E., Giske, R., and Høigaard, R. (2017). Mental toughness in elite and sub-elite female soccer players. *Int. J. Appl. Sports Sci.* 29, 77–85. doi: 10.24985/ijass.2017.29.1.77

Datson, N., Hulton, A., Andersson, H., Lewis, T., Weston, M., Drust, B., et al. (2014). Applied physiology of female soccer: an update. *Sports Med.* 44, 1225–1240. doi: 10.1007/s40279-014-0199-1

Domínguez-Escribano, M., Ariza-Vargas, L., and Tabernero, C. (2017). Motivational variables involved in commitment of female soccer players at different competitive levels. *Soccer Soc.* 18, 801–816. doi: 10.1080/14660970.2015.1067789

Gagné, F. (2004). Transforming gifts into talents: the DMGT as a developmental theory. *High Abil. Stud.* 15, 119–147. doi: 10.1080/1359813042000314682

García-Naveira, A., Ruiz-Barquín, R., and Ortín, F. J. (2015). Optimismo y competitividad en jóvenes atletas de rendimiento. *Rev. Latinoam. Psicol.* 47, 124–135. doi: 10.1016/j.rlp.2014.08.001

Gimeno, F. (1999). *Variables Psicológicas Implicadas En El Rendimiento Deportivo: Elaboración Y Estudios Sobre La Aplicación Del Cuestionario "Características Psicológicas Relacionadas Con El Rendimiento Deportivo" (CPRD).* Doctoral thesis, National Distance Education University, Madrid, SP.

Gimeno, F., Buceta, J. M., and Pérez-Llantada, M. C. (2001). El cuestionario "características psicológicas relacionadas con el rendimiento deportivo" (CPRD): características psicométricas. *Análise Psicol.* 1, 93–133. doi: 10.14417/ap.346

Gledhill, A., Harwood, C., and Forsdyke, D. (2017). Psychosocial factors associated with talent development in football: a systematic review. *Psychol. Sport Exerc.* 31, 93–112. doi: 10.1007/s40279-017-0851-7

Gómez-Espejo, V., Aroca, B., Robles-Palazón, F. J., and Olmedilla, A. (2017). Formación integral en la cantera del real murcia CF: tutorías psicológicas. *Rev. Psicol. Apl. Dep. Ejerc. Físico* 2, 1–11.

González, J. (2017). Diseño del entrenamiento mental del tenista. De lo científico a la aplicado. *Rev. Psicol. Apl. Dep. Ejerc. Físico* 2, 1–14. doi: 10.5093/rpadef2017a5

González-Campos, G., Valdivia-Moral, P., Zagalaz, M. L., and Romero, S. (2015). La autoconfianza y el control del estrés en futbolistas: revisión de estudios. *Rev. Iberoam. Psicol. Ejerc. Dep.* 10, 95–101.

Gould, D., Weiss, M., and Weinberg, R. S. (1981). Psychological characteristics of successful and less successful big ten wrestlers. *J. Sport Psychol.* 3, 69–81. doi: 10.1123/jsp.3.1.69

Granero-Gallegos, A., Gómez-López, M., Abraldes, J. A., and Baena-Extremera, A. (2015). Predicción de las orientaciones de meta en el fútbol femenino. *J. Sport Health Res.* 7, 31–42. doi: 10.1163/9789401202084_005

Haugaasen, M., Toering, T., and Jordet, G. (2014). From childhood to senior professional football: a multi-level approach to elite youth football players' engagement in football-specific activities. *Psychol. Sport Exerc.* 15, 336–344. doi: 10.1016/j.psychsport.2014.02.007

Junge, A., and Feddermann-Demont, N. (2016). Prevalence of depression and anxiety in top-level male and female football players. *BMJ Open Sport Exerc. Med.* 2:e000087. doi: 10.1136/bmjsem-2015-000087

Llames, R., and García-Dantas, A. (2017). Entrenamiento psicológico deportivo aplicado a una estudiante de oposición. *Rev. Psicol. Dep.* 26, 98–103.

Lowe, A. C. (2017). *Physiological and Psychological Well-Being During the Spring Season in Female Soccer Players.* Master's Thesis, Louisiana State University, Lousiana.

MacNamara, A., Button, A., and Collins, D. (2010). The role of psychological characteristics in facilitating the pathway to elite performance part 1: identifying mental skills and behaviors. *Sport Psychol.* 24, 52–73. doi: 10.1123/tsp.24.1.52

MacNamara, Á, and Collins, D. (2017). "Psychological characteristics of developing excellence," in *Sport Psychology for Young Athletes*, eds C. J. Knight, C. G. Harwood, and D. Gould (London: Routledge).

Mahoney, M. J. (1989). Psychological predictors of elite and non-elite performance in Olympic weightlifters. I. *J. Sport Psychol.* 20, 1–12.

Mahoney, M. J., and Avener, M. (1977). Psychology of the elite athlete: an exploratory study. *Cogn. Ther. Res.* 1, 135–141. doi: 10.1007/BF01173634

Mahoney, M. J., Gabriel, T. J., and Perkins, T. S. (1987). Psychological skills and exceptional athletic performance. *Sport Psychol.* 1, 181–199. doi: 10.1123/tsp.1.3.181

Malinauskas, R., Dumciene, A., Mamkus, G., and Venckunas, T. (2014). Personality traits and exercise capacity in male athletes and non-athletes. *Percep. Motor Skills* 118, 145–161. doi: 10.2466/29.25.PMS.118k13w1

Markovits, A. S., and Hellerman, S. L. (2003). Women's soccer in the United States: yet another American "exceptionalism". *Soccer Soc.* 4, 14–29. doi: 10.1177/2325967119829212

Martínez-Ferreiro, J. (2016). *Inteligencia Emocional y Rendimiento Deportivo en el Futbol Femenino de Alta Competición.* Doctoral thesis, Universidad de Valladolid, Valladolid, SP.

Martín-García, G. (2003). La mujer futbolista desde la perspectiva psicológica. *Cuad. Psicol. Dep.* 3, 7–15.

McFadden, B. A., Walker, A. J., Sanders, D. J., Hofacker, M., Bello, M., Poyssick, A., et al. (2017). Workload-related psychological and physiological changes in female college soccer players during a competitive season. *Med. Sci. Sports Exerc.* 49:577. doi: 10.1249/01.mss.0000518503.47781.ba

Møllerløkken, N. E., Lorås, H., and Pedersen, A. V. (2017). A comparison of players' and coaches' perceptions of the coach-created motivational climate within youth soccer teams. *Front. Psychol.* 8:109. doi: 10.3389/fpsyg.2017.00109

Morris, T. (2000). Psychological characteristics and talent identification in soccer. *J. Sports Sci.* 18, 715–726. doi: 10.1080/02640410050120096

Muñoz, S. P., Calle, R. C., Muñoz, A. S., Cayetano, A. R., de Mena Ramos, J. M., Blanco, J. M. F., et al. (2018). ¿Por qué juego al fútbol si soy una mujer?: Motivaciones para jugar al fútbol. *Retos* 34, 183–188.

Nagle, F. J., Morgan, X. P., Hellickson, R. O., Serfass, R. C., and Alexander, J. F. (1975). Sporting success traits in Olympic contenders. *Phys. Sportsmed.* 3, 31–34. doi: 10.1080/00913847.1975.11948293

Olmedilla, A., and Dominguez-Igual, J. (2016). Entrenamiento psicológico para la mejora de la atención y la autoconfianza en un futbolista. *Rev. Psicol. Apl. Dep. Ejerc. Físico* 1, 1–11. doi: 10.5093/rpadef2016a4

Olmedilla, A., García-Mas, A., and Ortega, E. (2017a). Psychological characteristics for sport performance in young players of football, Rugby, and Basketball. *Acci. Psicol.* 14, 7–16. doi: 10.5944/ap.14.1.19249

Olmedilla, A., Rubio, V. J., Ortega, E., and García-Mas, A. (2017b). Effectiveness of a stress management pilot program aimed at reducing the incidence of sports injuries in young football (soccer) players. *Phys. Ther. Sport* 24, 53–59. doi: 10.1016/j.ptsp.2016.09.003

Olmedilla, A., Ortega, E., de los Fayos, E. G., Abenza, L., Blas, A., and Laguna, M. (2015). Perfil psicológico de los jugadores profesionales de balonmano y diferencias entre puestos específicos. *Rev. Latinoam. Psicol.* 47, 177–184. doi: 10.1016/j.rlp.2015.06.005

Olmedilla, A., Ortega, E., Robles-Palazón, F. J., Salom, M., and García-Mas, A. (2018a). Healthy practice of female soccer and futsal: identifying sources of stress, anxiety and depression. *Sustainability* 10:2268. doi: 10.3390/su10072268

Olmedilla, A., Sánchez-Aldeguer, M. F., Almansa, C. M., Gómez-Espejo, V., and Ortega, E. (2018b). Entrenamiento psicológico y mejora de aspectos psicológicos relevantes para el rendimiento deportivo en jugadoras de fútbol. *Rev. Psicol Apl. Deporte Ejerc. Físico* 3, 1–11. doi: 10.5093/rpadef2018a2

Olmedilla, A., Torres-Luque, G., García-Mas, A., Rubio, V. J., Ducoing, E., and Ortega, E. (2018c). Psychological profiling of triathlon and road cycling athletes. *Front. Psychol.* 9:825. doi: 10.3389/fpsyg.2018.00825

Pan, G. P., and Zhu, J. M. (2003). A research on the top female soccer players' psychological characteristics in competition. *Sports Sci. Res.* 24, 32–34.

Rasmus, P., and Kocur, J. (2006). Personality traits and competition skills in adolescent tennis players. *Physic. Educ. Sport* 50, 93–95.

Reid, J., and Crust, L. (2012). "Psychological momentum in elite female soccer: perceptions of players and coaches," in *Proceedings of the BASES Student Conference 2012, 16-17 April 2012*, (London: University of East London).

Reilly, T., Bangsbo, J., and Franks, A. (2000). Anthropometric and physiological predispositions for elite soccer. *J. Sports Sci.* 18, 669–683. doi: 10.1080/02640410050120050

Romero, A. E., Zapata, R., García-Mas, A., Brustad, R. J., Garrido, R., and Letelier, A. (2010). Estrategias de afrontamiento y bienestar psicológico en jóvenes tenistas de competición. *Rev. Psicol. Dep.* 19, 117–133.

Ruiz, R. (2005). Análisis de las diferencias de personalidad en el deporte del judo a nivel competitivo en función de la variable sexo y categoría de edad deportiva. *Cuad. Psicol. Dep.* 5, 29–48.

Rutkowska, K., and Bergier, J. (2015). Psychological gender and emotional intelligence in youth female soccer players. *J. Hum. Kinet.* 47, 285–291. doi: 10.1515/hukin-2015-0084

Sarkar, M., and Fletcher, D. (2014). Psychological resilience in sport performers: a review of stressors and protective factors. *J. Sports Sci.* 32, 1419–1434. doi: 10.1080/02640414.2014.901551

Silva, J. M., Shultz, B. B., Haslam, R. W., and Murray, D. F. (1981). A psychophysiological assessment of elite wrestlers. *Res. Q. Exerc. Sport* 52, 348–358. doi: 10.1080/02701367.1981.10607882

Slimani, M., Bragazzi, N. L., Tod, D., Dellal, A., Hue, O., Cheour, F., et al. (2016). Do cognitive training strategies improve motor and positive psychological skills development in soccer players? Insights from a systematic review. *J. Sports Sci.* 34, 2338–2349. doi: 10.1080/02640414.2016.1254809

Steca, P., Baretta, D., Greco, A., D'Addario, M., and Monzani, D. (2018). Associations between personality, sports participation and athletic success. a comparison of Big Five in sporting and non-sporting adults. *Pers. Individ. Dif.* 121, 176–183. doi: 10.1519/JSC.0b013e3182719123

Stolen, T., Chamari, K., Castagna, C., and Wisloff, U. (2005). Physiology of soccer: an update. *Sports Med.* 35, 501–536. doi: 10.2165/00007256-200535060-00004

Swann, C., Crust, L., Jackman, P., Vella, S. A., Allen, M. S., and Keegan, R. (2017). Psychological states underlying excellent performance in sport: toward an integrated model of flow and clutch states. *J. Appl. Sport Psychol.* 29, 375–401. doi: 10.1080/10413200.2016.1272650

Tharawadeepimuk, K., and Wongsawat, Y. (2017). Quantitative EEG evaluation for performance level analysis of professional female soccer players. *Cogn. Neurodyn.* 11, 233–244. doi: 10.1007/s11571-017-9427-3

Vescovi, J. D., and McGuigan, M. R. (2008). Relationships between sprinting, agility, and jump ability in female athletes. *J. Sports Sci.* 26, 97–107. doi: 10.1080/02640410701348644

Weinberg, R. S., and Gould, D. (2014). *Foundations of Sport and Exercise Psychology*. Champaign: Human Kinetics.

Williams, K. T. (2017). *Physiological and Psychological Characteristics of First Division Female Football Players*. Doctoral thesis, University of Johannesburg, Johannesburg SA.

Wright, M. D. (2014). Neuromuscular training in girl's football-the challenge of applying evidence based practice in an FA center of excellence. *J. Sports Sci.* 32, s93–s100.

19

The Mediating Role of the Self-Concept between the Relationship of the Body Satisfaction and the Intention to be Physically Active in Primary School Students

Pedro Antonio Sánchez-Miguel[1], Patxi León-Guereño[2], Miguel Angel Tapia-Serrano[1], David Hortigüela-Alcalá[3], Miguel A. López-Gajardo[4] and Mikel Vaquero-Solís[1]*

[1] Faculty of Teaching Training, University of Extremadura, Cáceres, Spain, [2] Faculty of Psychology and Education, University of Deusto, Donostia-San Sebastian, Spain, [3] Department of Specific Didactics, Faculty of Education, University of Burgos, Burgos, Spain, [4] Faculty of Sports Sciences, University of Extremadura, Cáceres, Spain

***Correspondence:**
Pedro Antonio Sánchez-Miguel
pesanchezm@unex.es

The aim was to analyze the extent to which anthropometric values, in line with body image and physical ability, predict physical self-concept, and the latter, in turn, predicts the practice and intention to pursue physical activity. A total of 302 participants, 150 males and 152 females were recruited from different primary schools in Extremadura (Spain). The age of the participants ranges from 10 to 13 years old (M = 11.74; SD = 0.86). The indirect effects of the model showed significant relationship between physical condition ($p = 0.001$) and PA levels, according to the perception of self-concept [$\beta = 0.231$, 95% BcCI = (0.055, 0.212)]. However, anthropometric variables proved not to be related to any significant extent ($p < 0.05$). The second level covered the indirect effects between the intention to be physically active and self-concept, which showed a significant relationship between the perception of self-concept ($p = 0.000$) and the intention to be physically active. Last, the third level showed significant relationships between physical condition ($p = 0.001$) and the intention to pursue physical activity. The present investigation concluded that physical condition, anthropometric variables, and body image predict the perception of physical self-concept in adolescents. Finally, this article highlights the importance of body image perception, anthropometric values, and physical condition in the intention of being physically active. In addition, it highlights the mediating role of physical self-concept to develop physical activity.

Keywords: body image, physical fitness, physical condition, youths, primary school

INTRODUCTION

Adolescence is characterized by being a stage in which major biological and psychological changes take place that define what a person will be like in adulthood (1). Studies show a decline in physical activity (PA) during this stage (2, 3), and this is a cause for concern given the physical and psychosocial benefits gained from doing PA (4), such as improvements in cardiovascular fitness, anthropometric values, bone structure, reduction in symptoms associated with depression and anxiety, and an improvement in psychological well-being. Along these lines, the adolescent stage is characterized by being a critical period in the development of the body image and one's perception of physical self-concept, whereby poor development of these constructs may give rise to problems linked to depression, anxiety, eating disorders, and imbalances in the perception of the body image and self-concept (5–7). In this respect, Casas et al. (8) stress the importance of detecting any factors that may contribute to an improvement in mental health in young people, drawing attention to the influence of body weight. With this in mind, Fernández-Bustos et al. (9) consider the body mass index (BMI) to be a major predictor of body image and self-esteem as well as body dissatisfaction in both men and women (10).

In keeping with the above, body image is a key element in the shaping of one's self-concept (11), and in this sense, body image reflects how individuals think, are viewed and act (12). Añez et al. (13) show its relationship with PA and draw attention to the fact that a poor body image may act as a barrier to pursuing physical activity. Moreover Neumark-Sztainer et al. (14), explain that adolescents with low body satisfaction are less likely to commit themselves to physical activity, instead of being more likely to spend their time indulging in sedentary activities such as watching TV, playing video games, or using the phone, etc. Likewise, attention is drawn to the moderating role of gender in associating body image with PA, by showing a positive association between the two in the case of the male gender (15). Conversely, there is no clear evidence of physical exercise in body image in the case of the female gender (16).

Additionally, body image is a factor that has a great impact on psychological well-being, which determines how self-concept is shaped, in particular, during adolescence (11). Numerous studies refer to a positive relationship between body satisfaction and self-concept (17, 18). Basing ourselves on the hierarchical and multidimensional model of general self-concept (19), physical self-concept (20) comprises the sum of specific domains: perceived competence, physical condition, physical appeal, and strength, while Sonstroem et al. (21) go on to add self-esteem. Previous studies have tended to relate physical self-concept to physical activity (9, 22, 23), the intention to pursue physical activity, social support (24), body image (25), physical condition (26), and anthropometric values such as BMI (27).

In terms of theoretical models that attempt to provide an explanation about the determining factors that the pursuit of physical activity entails, Fernández-Bustos et al. (9) explain that both physical activity and BMI predict body image, physical self-concept, and general self-concept. In this regard, Garn et al. (28) and Zamani Sani et al. (29) draw attention, respectively, to reciprocity and direct and indirect links to physical and psychological mechanisms. Similarly, Jekauc et al. (30) focus on the importance of motor skills in predicting self-concept and, ultimately, PA, while Moreno et al. (24), Fernandez-Rio et al. (31), and Grao Cruces et al. (32) point out that it is physical self-concept that predicts the intention to be physically active. Last, Li et al. (33) propose a model in which social support (parents and peers) predicts physical self-concept, and the latter, in turn, predicts physical activity.

For all the aforementioned reasons, the present research tests a model based on four levels, in which anthropometric values, in line with body image and physical ability (level 1), predict self-concept (level 2), which will, in turn, predict physical activity (level 3), and this last-mentioned will predict the intention to pursue it (level 4). Some authors differ in how they test their models, drawing attention to distinct variables when predicting self-concept and the relationship this has to the previously mentioned variables.

Hence, this work constitutes an attempt to provide a new approach that may offer an explanation about the physical and psychological mechanisms associated with the practice of, and intention to, pursue PA. For this reason, the aim of this research is to analyze the extent to which anthropometric values, in line with body image and physical ability, predict physical self-concept, and the latter, in turn, predicts the practice and intention to pursue PA. To this end, anthropometric values, physical condition, and body image are thought to provide a positive prediction of the perception of self-concept, physical activity, and the intention to pursue the latter, while the perception of self-concept is likewise thought to act as mediator between anthropometric values, physical condition, body image, and the intention to pursue physical activity.

MATERIALS AND METHODS

Participants

A total number of 302 Spanish students from eight different primary schools in Extremadura, Spain, agreed to participate on a voluntary basis: males ($n = 150$) and females ($n = 152$), ranging in age from 10 to 13 years old ($M = 11.74$; $SD = 0.86$). All data was collected during normal school hours. The sample was selected according to the relevant research, respecting accessibility and involvement on the part of the schools. Moreover, taking into account that the highest levels of physical inactivity were evidenced in adolescents (7), we would like to cover school ages in order to test the relationships between the different variables. Data was collected from February 2018 to May 2018 in Cáceres. The sample was selected through hierarchical cluster sampling, considering the distance of the schools, whether the teaching staff was available, and the time required for the researcher to travel.

Instruments

Anthropometric Variables

Body Mass Index

The body mass index was established by obtaining weight and height, and by applying the following formula: weight (kg)/height (m)^2. Height and weight were established using the SECA 884 stadiometer model.

Waist-to-Height Ratio (WHtR)

The waist height perimeter was used, in which previous research has related to cardiometabolic markers (34). *WHtR* was calculated by dividing waist circumference (in cm) by height (in cm) (35).

Physical Condition Variables

Aerobic capacity

This was assessed using the 6-min walk test (6MWT), which was standardized by the American Thorax Society (36). A single 6MWT was undertaken along a flat, straight corridor over a hard surface, and the stimulus was used during the test. The children were given instructions to stop if they felt upset or uncomfortable. The maximum recorded distance (6MWD) was determined at the end of the test in order to assess the children's cardiorespiratory level. With a view to establishing comparisons, raw data was used owing to a possible bias in obtaining an equation in order to estimate the mean peak VO2 from the mean 6MWD in the children who took part (37).

Psychosocial Variables

Body image

The Stunkard Figure Rating Scale (**Figure 1**) was used to assess self and ideal body sizes. The Stunkard Scale consists of nine silhouette figures that increase in size from very thin (a value of 1) to very obese (a value of 9) (38). Self-body size refers to the number of the figure selected by participants in response to the prompt "Choose the figure that reflects how you think you look." Ideal body size refers to the number of the figure chosen in response to the prompt "Choose your ideal figure." For self-body size and ideal body size, dummy variables were created for the underweight, normal weight, overweight, and obese body size categories. This scale evidenced good validity and reliability (39), and body size satisfaction was subsequently calculated. The ensuing value is defined as the difference between one's perceived self-body size and perceived ideal body size. A body size satisfaction value was created for each participant by subtracting the number of the figure indicated as being the ideal body size from the number of the figure selected as the self-body size.

Self-concept perception

The Spanish version (40) of the Physical Self-Perception Profile (41) was used to assess physical self-concept. The complete instrument comprises 28 items that assess five factors: fitness (five items, e.g., "I feel very confident about continuously practicing and maintaining my physical form." $\alpha = 0.78$; $\Omega = 0.78$); perceived competence (four items, e.g., "I am very good at nearly all sports." $\alpha = 0.78$; $\Omega = 0.79$); physical strength (six items, e.g., "I am the first to put myself forward in situations that require strength." $\alpha = 0.68$; $\Omega = 0.65$); appearance (nine items, e.g., "I feel very satisfied with how I am physically." $\alpha = 0.72$; $\Omega = 0.74$); and self-esteem (four items, e.g., "I don't feel very self-confident in terms of physical appearance" $\alpha = 0.65$; $\Omega = 0.65$). Responses were rated on a Likert-type scale from 1 (*strongly disagree*) to 4 (*strongly agree*). The instrument evidenced acceptable internal consistency.

Physical activity

Physical activity was assessed using the Physical Activity Questionnaire for Adolescents: (PAQ-A) (42). This questionnaire comprises nine items that assess the physical activity pursued by the adolescent over the past 7 days, using a five-point Likert scale: during their free time, during physical education classes and also at different times during class days (lunchtime, afternoons, and evenings), and during the weekend. The result is a score from 1 to 5 that enables the level of physical activity to be graded (43), and their final score is obtained using the arithmetic mean of eight of the nine items, as the last item assesses whether the participant had been ill over the last week (43). Last, the Cronbach's alpha coefficient obtained for this sample was ($\alpha = 0.79$; $\Omega = 0.78$).

Intention to be physically active

This was assessed using an item in which the participant was asked: *Do you intend to practice sport in the future?* The response options were represented by a five-point Likert scale ranging from 1 (*totally disagree*) to 5 (*totally agree*).

Procedure

Parents and school supervisors were informed by letter about the nature and purpose of the study, and written informed consent was provided. The study obtained permission from the University Ethics Committee, which adheres to the code of ethics established by the World Medical Association (Declaration of Helsinki), and the protocol was approved by the Ethics Committee of the University of Extremadura (89/2016). All participants were treated in accordance with guidelines set out by the American Psychological Association (APA), ensuring trust and anonymity in terms of student responses. Before commencing the data collection process, permission was requested via a letter of consent addressed to parents and teachers, in which the following were to be assessed: What the study consisted of, the anthropometric and psychometric variables that would be assessed and, last, an assurance that all responses would be anonymous and would not compromise the identity of the participants. The participants completed the questionnaires during physical education class in the presence of the teacher, who told them that it was not an assessment test, and that they should be sincere with their answers. While they were completing them, researchers called the students in order from the list to weigh and measure them, subsequently noting down the weight and height in the relevant space on the questionnaire. The results obtained from the tests were passed on to the teacher if they asked for them.

Statistical Analysis

The SPSS 23.0 statistical package was used to carry out data analysis (see **Supplementary Material**). Likewise, different tests were used to determine the nature of this data—the Kolmogorov–Smirnov test and Levene's test—which provided scores over 0.05, whereby a decision was made to produce parametric statistics. Descriptive statistics were then provided together with a correlation analysis.

The MPLUS 7.0 statistical package was also used to ascertain predictive capacity (structural equation model) regarding the intention to pursue physical activity, and last, the indirect effects of the structural equations were then calculated.

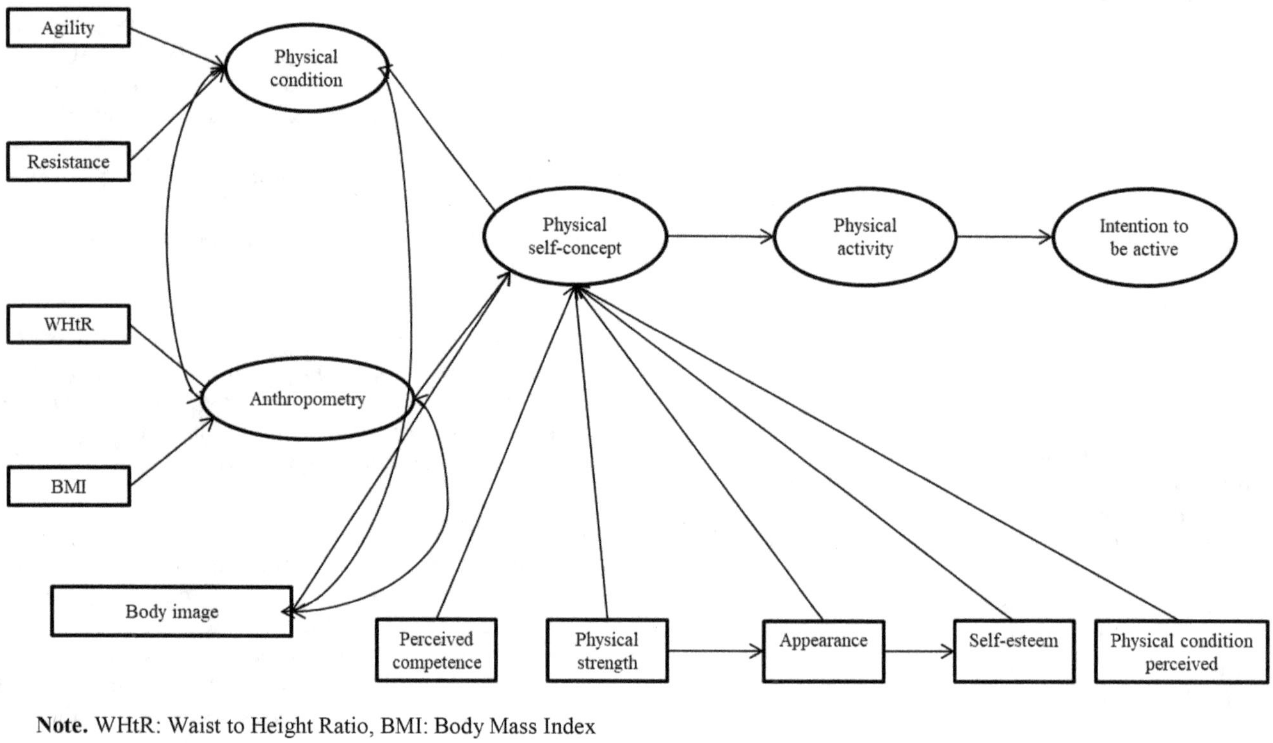

FIGURE 1 | Hypothesized model. WHtR, waist-to-height ratio; BMI, body mass index.

RESULTS

Table 1 shows the descriptive statistics and bivariate correlations of all the variables involved in the study, in which significant positive relationships between the intention to pursue physical activity, the time spent on extra-curricular activities, and the dimensions of perceived self-concept are provided. Likewise, it is shown how physical activity is positively related to the perception of self-concept and cardiovascular fitness, and negatively related to agility, anthropometric variables, and the perception of body image. The global score regarding the perception of self-concept also has a significant negative relationship with all those variables that refer to anthropometric values (BMI, waist–height perimeter), body image, and levels of physical condition (agility), except for resistance.

Structural Equation Model

A structural equation model was hypothesized with the following structure (**Figure 1**). This model was formed from three latent variables: physical condition (agility and resistance), anthropometric variables (waist–height perimeter and body mass index), and self-concept (self-esteem, strength, and perceived competence). Variables pertaining to physical activity, extra-curricular time, and intention to be physically active were also used, with the last mentioned acting as a dependent variable of the model.

The initial model showed the following adjustment indexes—$MRL\chi^2 = 372.295$, $p < 0.05$, $df = 66$, CFI $= 0.74$, TLI $= 0.68$, SRMR $= 0.12$, and RMSA $= 0.12$—whereby we decided to restructure the model in accordance with previous literature (9, 22, 24, 30, 33). Thus, the modification indexes suggest new forms of interaction to us: on the one hand, a correlation between body image and anthropometric variables, which provided us with the following adjustment indexes—$MRL\chi^2 = 248.954$, $p < 0.05$, $df = 66$, CFI $= 0.84$, TLI $= 0.80$, SRMR $= 0.084$, and RMSA $= 0.09$—and, on the other, a regression in which perceived appearance would predict self-esteem, namely, $MRL\chi^2 = 154.238$, $p < 0.05$, $df = 66$, CFI $= 0.92$, TLI $= 0.89$, SRMR $= 0.072$, and RMSA $= 0.073$. This last-mentioned modification provides us with nearly acceptable adjustment indexes, although a decision was made to make a final modification in which perceived appearance would predict strength. The final model (**Figure 2**) offered some good adjustment indexes: $MRL\chi^2 = 125.535$, $p < 0.05$, $df = 66$, CFI $= 0.94$, TLI $= 0.92$, SRMR $= 0.054$, and RMSA $= 0.059$.

Invariance of the model was then tested in terms of gender. To do so, a first step was taken in which it was noted how the model adapted according to participants' gender. The results showed how the model is better explained in the female gender $MRL\chi^2 = 64.433$, $p < 0.05$, CFI $= 0.98$, TLI $= 0.98$, SRMR $= 0.046$, and RMSA $= 0.027$, than in the male gender $MRL\chi^2 = 131.375$, $p < 0.05$, CFI $= 0.91$, TLI $= 0.88$, SRMR $= 0.072$, and RMSA $= 0.092$. In this respect, the model explains how anthropometric variables, physical condition, and self-concept can be considered greater predictors of the intention to pursue physical activity in the male gender than in the female gender.

TABLE 1 | Descriptive statistics and correlation analysis.

	1	2	3	4	5	6	7	8	9	10	11	12	13
1. INPFA	–	0.37**	0.17**	0.33**	0.19**	0.11	0.32**	0.32**	−0.05	0.10	−0.03	−0.061	−0.11*
2. PPC	–	–	0.41**	0.69**	0.43**	0.22**	0.53**	0.75**	0.30**	0.26**	−0.24**	0.38**	−0.26**
3. PAP	–	–	–	0.30**	0.44**	0.59**	0.18*	0.73**	−0.20**	0.11*	−0.05	−0.25**	−0.17**
4. PC	–	–	–	–	0.51**	0.21**	0.52**	0.75**	−0.25**	0.25**	−0.32**	−0.28**	−0.22**
5. PS	–	–	–	–	–	0.34**	0.31**	0.74**	0.04	0.16**	−0.13**	−0.07	−0.01
6. SEL	–	–	–	–	–	–	0.12*	0.66*	−0.10	0.06	−03	−0.13	−0.10
7. PA	–	–	–	–	–	–	–	0.46**	−0.11**	0.21**	−0.16**	−0.19**	−0.12*
8. GS_SC	–	–	–	–	–	–	–	–	−0.22**	0.23**	−0.21**	−0.30**	−21**
9. BMI	–	–	–	–	–	–	–	–	–	−0.17**	0.25**	0.58**	0.73**
10. TM6	–	–	–	–	–	–	–	–	–	–	−0.46**	−0.13*	−0.09
11. Agil	–	–	–	–	–	–	–	–	–	–	–	17**	23**
12. Body_I	–	–	–	–	–	–	–	–	–	–	–	–	54**
13. Wai_hei	–	–	–	–	–	–	–	–	–	–	–	–	–
M	4.6	3.8	3.7	3.5	3.3	3.9	3.2	3.7	18.6	15.8	13.1	3.3	42.4
SD	0.69	0.84	0.70	0.86	0.84	0.96	0.67	0.61	3.00	3.93	1.69	1.13	4.64
Ω	–	0.78	0.72	0.78	0.68	0.65	0.79	–	–	–	–	–	–
Ω	–	0.78	0.74	0.79	0.65	0.65	0.78	–	–	–	–	–	–

INPFA, intention to pursue physical activity; PPC, perceived physical condition; PAP, perceived appearance; PC, perceived competence; PS, perceived strength; SEL, self-esteem; PA, physical activity; GS_SC, self-concept global score; BMI, body mass index; TM6, 6-min test; Agil, agility; Body_I, body image; Wai_hei, waist–height perimeter. $*p < 0.01$, $**p < 0.001$.

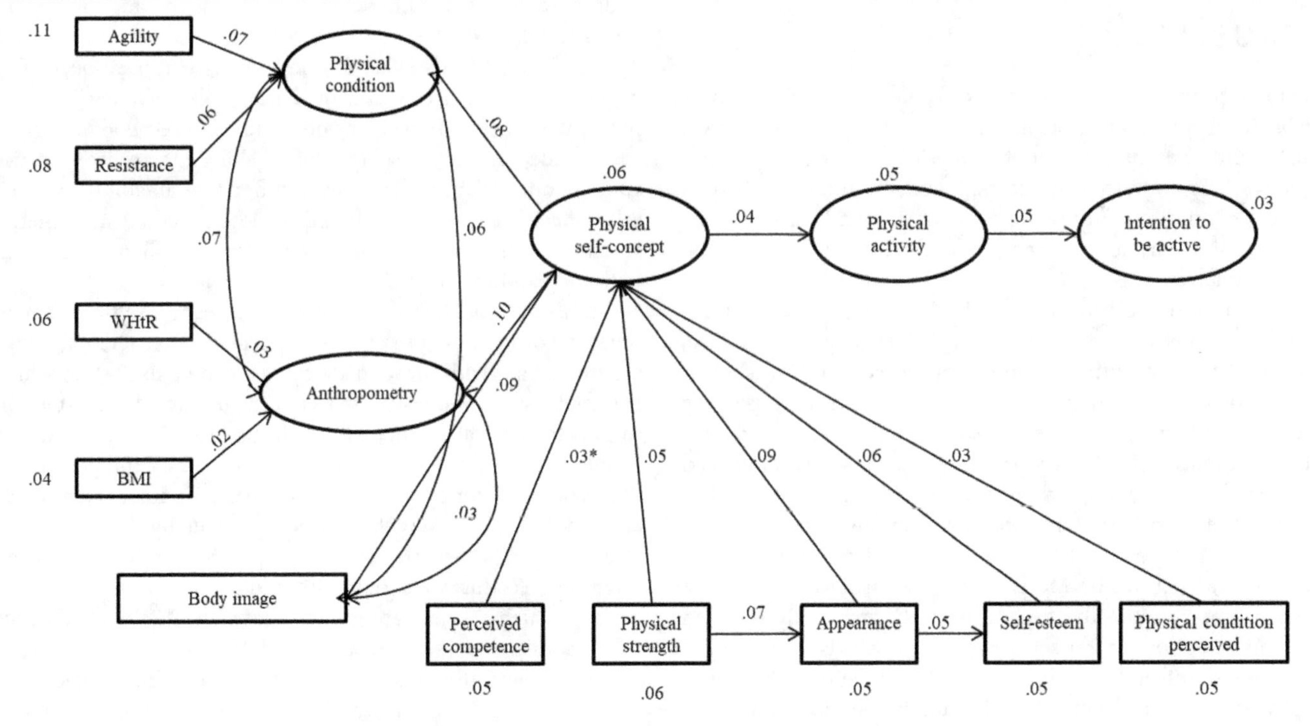

Note. WHtR: Waist to Height Ratio, BMI: Body Mass Index

FIGURE 2 | Final model. WHtR, waist-to-height ratio; BMI, body mass index.

Indirect effects among variables were calculated on several levels according to the hypothesized model. The first level showed the indirect effects among all the variables situated between the pursuit of physical activity and physical condition, anthropometric variables, and body image. In this sense, the analysis of indirect effects evidenced significant relationships between physical condition ($p = 0.001$) and PA levels, according to the perception of self-concept [β = 0.231, 95% BcCI = (0.055, 0.212)], in a similar way to how body image showed significant relationships between physical condition ($p = 0.003$) and levels of physical activity, according to the perception of self-concept [β = 0.172, 95% BcCI = (0.058, −0.295)]. However, anthropometric variables proved not to be related to any significant extent ($p < 0.05$) to physical activity, according to the perception of self-concept. The second level covered the indirect effects between the intention to be physically active and self-concept, which showed a significant relationship between the perception of self-concept ($p = 0.000$) and the intention to be physically active, according to physical activity [β = 0.196, 95% BcCI = (0.036, −0.543)]. Last, the third level showed significant relationships between physical condition ($p = 0.001$) and the intention to pursue physical activity, according to the level of that activity [β = 0.074, 95% BcCI = (0.022, −0.362)], in the same way that body image proved to be significantly related ($p = 0.007$) to the intention to be physically active, according to the level of physical activity [β = −0.055, 95% BcCI = (0.020, −0.708)]. For their part, anthropometric variables proved not to be significantly related to the intention to pursue physical activity ($p < 0.05$).

DISCUSSION

The main purpose of this study was to analyze the relationships established between anthropometric values, body image, physical ability, and the intention to be physically active. A further objective was to test a structural equation model in which physical conditions, anthropometric values, body image, self-concept, and physical activity explain the intention to be physically active.

In terms of the relationships established, a significant positive relationship between the intention to be physically active, physical activity, and the perception of self-concept was shown, and to this end, Zamani Sani et al. (29) showed positive associations between physical activity and self-concept, also drawing attention to the fact that this association is influenced by different key factors such as body image, body mass index, and physical form. In terms of the relationships established between self-concept and the intention to be physically active, the study carried out by Moreno et al. (24) showed significant relationships between the two. Conversely, our study revealed that the intention to pursue physical activity is negatively—albeit not significantly—related to anthropometric values, and to physical form in terms of agility, unlike physical resistance, with which a positive relationship was found. This is in line with previous studies in which attention was drawn to the perception of physical condition as being the most determining factor in being active (44, 45). As for the negative relationship with anthropometric values, our results are in line with those found by Centeio et al. (46), in which physical ability acted as a mediator with the intention to be physically active, although the intention to pursue physical activity may vary depending on the strategies we implement. In this respect, García-Hermoso et al. (47) point out that the intention to be physically active might be improved by activities such as walking or cycling to school. Likewise, the overall perception of self-concept was negatively and significantly related to anthropometric values, and agility to physical form, although this proved not to be the case with resistance. In this sense, Reigal-Garrido et al. (48) draw attention to the fact that the study of aerobic capacity is a determining factor in the perception of self-concept.

In terms of the structural equation model, our model showed that physical condition, anthropometric variables, and body image predict the perception of physical self-concept as backed up by previous literature on the subject. As for the predictive role of physical condition, Garn et al. (23) draw attention to the fact that overall physical self-concept is predicted by multiple improvements that take place in physical condition. Thus, the fact might be interpreted that improvements taking place via specific exercises involving speed, strength, and resistance would have a direct influence on self-concept, as shown by Lemoyne et al. (49) in university students. On the other hand, and in terms of the predictive role of anthropometric values (BMI and waist–height perimeter), our results are in keeping with those found in the study by Fernández-Bustos et al. (9), where a model was shown in which BMI predicted physical activity and self-concept. A difference should also be highlighted in the role taken on by body image in the model put forward by Fernández-Bustos et al. (9) and ours. In this respect, they provided body image with a mediating role between BMI and physical activity (50), whereas our study showed body image to be an independent construct which, alongside anthropometric values and variables associated with physical ability, predict self-concept. Therefore, it should be noted that anthropometric variables such as BMI are associated with body dissatisfaction in both men and women (10).

Last, our model showed the role played by self-concept in pursuing or intending to pursue physical activity. These findings are in keeping with those made by Moreno et al. (24), in which it was shown that physical self-concept predicted the intention to pursue physical activity, although the intention that a subject should remain physically active is influenced by the perception of physical self-concept, as this is positively modified via physical activity (51), and also with the findings made by Fernandez-Rio et al. (31), in which the pursuit of physical activity predicted intention. To this, we should also add the importance of other variables such as motivation and enjoyment that will influence the intention to pursue such activity (52).

Nonetheless, the results obtained should be treated with caution, as the present research is subject to certain limitations such as its transversal design, which does not enable cause–effect relationships to be established, and the small number of participants, whereby these conclusions are not able to be transferred to a different population. Thus, this research draws the conclusion that the intention to pursue and practice physical activity is predicted by body image, anthropometric values, physical condition, and the perception of physical self-concept. In this respect, those individuals who evidence having a healthy body image accompanied by suitable anthropometric values and physical condition will be more likely to have a perception of self-concept and, therefore, be more inclined to pursue physical activity. Future studies should replicate this same hypothesized model, increasing the sample size. On another hand, it should focus on stipulating profiles of physical self-concept and being more specific about these relationships, rather than referring to a high or low degree of self-concept, as this might give rise to incongruences when establishing such relationships. In this regard, there may, on the one hand, be individuals who have a great perception of strength and physical competence, who maintain more significant relationships with tests associated with physical ability, while on the other, other types of individual may have a better self-esteem and perception of themselves and be more closely related to variables such as body image.

ETHICS STATEMENT

This study was conducted in accordance with the Declaration of Helsinki, and the protocol was approved by the Ethics Committee of the University of Extremadura (89/2016). Written informed consent to participate in this study was provided by the participants' legal guardian/next of kin.

AUTHOR CONTRIBUTIONS

PS-M, PL-G, ML-G, and MT-S contributed conception and design of the study. DH-A and MV-S organized the database. PS-M and MV-S performed the statistical analysis and wrote the first draft of the manuscript. PS-M, MT-S, and MV-S wrote sections of the manuscript. All authors contributed to manuscript revision, read, and approved the submitted version.

ACKNOWLEDGMENTS

This study was funded by the European Community and Ministry of Economy of Extremadura (IB16193). The work has been done as part of the multidisciplinary training program for the promotion of physical activity and other healthy habits in sedentary adolescents. We gratefully acknowledge the financial support of the Ministry of Economy and Infrastructures and European Community. The authors wish to thank the schools, children and their parents who generously volunteered to participate in the study. We also acknowledge all the staff members involved in the fieldwork for their efforts and great enthusiasm.

REFERENCES

Richter LM. Studying adolescence. *Science.* (2006) 312:1902– 5. doi: 10.1126/science.1127489

Inchley J, Currie D, Young T, Samdal O, Torsheim T. Growing up unequal gender and socioeconomic differences in young people's health and well- being; health behaviour in school-aged children study, international report fro. *Health Policy Child Adolesc.* (2016) 7:13–212.

Wassenaar TM , Wheatley CM, Beale N, Salvan P, Meaney A, Possee JB, et al. Effects of a programme of vigorous physical activity during secondary school physical education on academic performance, fitness, cognition, mental health and the brain of adolescents (Fit to Study): study protocol for a cluster- randomised trial. *Trials.* (2019) 20:189. doi: 10.1186/s13063-019-3279-6

Brown HE, Pearson N, Braithwaite RE, Brown WJ, Biddle SJH. Physical activity interventions and depression in children and adolescents: a systematic review and meta-analysis. *Sports Med.* (2013) 43:195–206. doi: 10.1007/s40279-012-0015-8

McClure AC, Tanski SE, Kingsbury J, Gerrard M, Sargent JD. Characteristics associated with low self-esteem among uS adolescents. *Acad Pediatr.* (2010) 10:238–44.e2. doi: 10.1016/j.acap.2010.03.007

Hallal PC, Andersen LB, Bull FC, Guthold R, Haskell W, Ekelund U, et al. Global physical activity levels: surveillance progress, pitfalls, and prospects. *Lancet.* (2012) 380:247–57. doi: 10.1016/S0140-6736(12)60646-1

Sánchez-Miguel PA, González JJP, Sánchez-Oliva D, Alonso DA, Leo FM. The importance of body satisfaction to physical self-concept and body mass index in Spanish adolescents. *Int J Psychol.* (2018) 54:521–9. doi: 10.1002/ijop.12488

Casas AG, Garcia PLR, Guillamon AR, Garcia-Canto E, Soto JJP, Marcos MLT, et al. Nivel de condición física y su relación con el estatus de peso corporal en escolares. *Nutr Hosp.* (2015) 31:393–400. doi: 10.3305/nh.2015.31.1.8074

Fernández-Bustos JG, Infantes-Paniagua Á, Cuevas R, Contreras OR. Effect of physical activity on self-concept: theoretical model on the mediation of body image and physical self-concept in adolescents. *Front Psychol.* (2019) 10:1537. doi: 10.3389/fpsyg.2019.01537

Molina-García J, Castillo I, Queralt A, Álvarez O. Precursors of body dissatisfaction and its implication for psychological well-being in young adults. *Univers Psychol.* (2019) 18:1–11. doi: 10.11144/Javeriana.upsy18-2.pbdi

Fenton C, Brooks F, Spencer NH, Morgan A. Sustaining a positive body image in adolescence: an assets-based analysis. *Health Soc Care Commun.* (2010) 18:189–98. doi: 10.1111/j.1365-2524.2009.00888.x

Thompson JK, Heinberg LJ, Altabe M, Tantleff-Dunn S. *Exacting Beauty: Theory, Assessment, and Treatment of Body Image Disturbance.* Washington, DC: American Psychological Association (1999). doi: 10.1037/10312-000

Añez E, Fornieles-Deu A, Fauquet-Ars J, López-Guimerà G, Puntí-Vidal J, Sánchez-Carracedo D. Body image dissatisfaction, physical activity and screen-time in Spanish adolescents. *J Health Psychol.* (2018) 23:36– 47. doi: 10.1177/1359105316664134

Neumark-Sztainer D, Goeden C, Story M, Wall M. Associations between body satisfaction and physical activity in adolescents: implications for programs aimed at preventing a broad spectrum of weight-related disorders. *Eat Dis.* (2004) 12:125–37. doi: 10.1080/10640260490444989

Bassett-Gunter R, McEwan D, Kamarhie A. Physical activity and body image among men and boys: a meta-analysis. *Body Image.* (2017) 22:114– 28. doi: 10.1016/j.bodyim.2017.06.007

McIntosh-Dalmedo S, Devonport TJ, Nicholls W, Friesen AP. Examining the effects of sport and exercise interventions on body image among adolescent girls: a systematic review. *J Sport Behav.* (2018) 41:245–69.

Buchanan NCT, Bluestein BM, Nappa AC, Woods KC, Depatie MM. Exploring gender differences in body image, eating pathology, and sexual harassment. *Body Image.* (2013) 10:352– 60. doi: 10.1016/j.bodyim.2013.03.004

Fernández-Bustos JG, González-Martí I, Contreras O, Cuevas R. Relación entre imagen corporal y autoconcepto físico en mujeres adolescentes. *Revista Latinoamericana de Psicologia.* (2015) 47:25–33. doi: 10.1016/S0120-0534(15)30003-0

Shavelson RJ, Hubner JJ, Stanton GC. Self-concept: validation of construct interpretations. *Rev Educ Res.* (1976) 46:407– 41. doi:10.3102/00346543046003407

Fox KR, Corbin CB. The physical self-perception profile: devlopment and preliminary validation. *J Sport Exerc Psychol.* (1989) 11:408–30. doi: 10.1123/jsep.11.4.408

Sonstroem RJ, Harlow LL, Josephs L. Exercise and self-esteem: validity of model expansion and exercise associations. *J Sport Exerc Psychol.* (1994) 16:29–42. doi: 10.1123/jsep.16.1.29

Revuelta L, Esnaola I, Goñi A. Relaciones entre el autoconcepto físico y la actividad físico-deportiva adolescente. *Revista Internacional de Medicina y Ciencias de La Actividad Fisica y Del Deporte.* (2016) 16:561–81. doi: 10.15366/rimcafd2016.63.010

Garn AC, Moore EW, Centeio EE, Kulik N, Somers C, McCaughtry N. Reciprocal effects model of children's physical activity, physical self-concept, and enjoyment

Psychol Sport Exerc. (2019) 45:101568. doi: 10.1016/j.psychsport.2019.101568

Moreno JA, Moreno R, Cervelló E. El autoconcepto físico como predictor de la intención de ser físicamente activo. *Psicología y Salud.* (2007) 17:261–7. doi: 10.25009/pys.v17i2.710

Sánchez-Miguel PA, Leo FM, Amado D, Hortigüela-Alcalá D, Tapia-Serrano MA, De La Cruz-Sánchez E. Children's physical self-concept and body image according to weight status and physical fitness. *Sustainability.* (2020) 12:782. doi: 10.3390/su12030782

Balsalobre FJB, Sánchez GFL, Suárez AD. Relationships between physical fitness and physical self-concept in Spanish adolescents. *Proc Soc Behav Sci.* (2014) 132:343–50. doi: 10.1016/j.sbspro.2014.04.320

Linares-Manrique M, Linares-Girela D, Schmidt-Rio-valle J, Mato-Medina O, Fernández-García R, Cruz-Quintana F. Relación entre autoconcepto físico, ansiedad e imc en estudiantes universitarios Mexicanos. *Revista Internacional de Medicina y Ciencias de La Actividad Fisica y Del Deporte.* (2016) 16:497– 519. doi: 10.15366/rimcafd2016.63.007

Garn AC, Morin AJS, Martin J, Centeio E, Shen B, Kulik N, et al. A reciprocal effects model of children's body fat self-concept: relations with physical self-concept and physical activity. *J Sport Exerc Psychol.* (2016) 38:255–67. doi: 10.1123/jsep.2015-0255

Zamani Sani SH, Fathirezaie Z, Brand S, Pühse U, Holsboer-Trachsler E, Gerber M, et al. Physical activity and self-esteem: testing direct and indirect relationships associated with psychological and physical mechanisms. *Neuropsychiatr Dis Treat.* (2016) 12:2617–25. doi: 10.2147/NDT.S116811

Jekauc D, Wagner MO, Herrmann C, Hegazy K, Woll A. Does physical self-concept mediate the relationship between motor abilities and physical activity in adolescents and young adults? *PLoS ONE.* (2017) 12:e0168539.doi: 10.1371/journal.pone.0168539

Fernandez-Rio J, Cecchini JA, Méndez-Gimenez A, Mendez-Alonso D, Prieto JA. Self-regulation, cooperative learning, and academic self- efficacy: interactions to prevent school failure. *Front Psychol.* (2017) 8:22. doi: 10.3389/fpsyg.2017.00022

Grao Cruces A, Fernández Martínez A, Teva Villén M, Nuviala Nuviala Autoconcepto físico e intencionalidad para ser físicamente activo en los participantes del programa escuelas deportivas. *J Sport Health Res.* (2017) 9:15–26.

Li R, Bunke S, Psouni E. Attachment relationships and physical activity in adolescents: the mediation role of physical self-concept. *Psychol Sport Exerc.* (2016) 22:160–9. doi: 10.1016/j.psychsport.2015.07.003

Ashley-Martin J, Ensenauer R, Maguire B, Kuhle S. Predicting cardiometabolic markers in children using tri-ponderal mass index: a cross-sectional study. *Archiv Dis Childhood.* (2019) 104:577–82. doi: 10.1136/archdischild-2018-316028

McCarthy HD, Ashwell M. A study of central fatness using waist-to-height ratios in UK children and adolescents over two decades supports the simple message– 'keep your waist circumference to less than half your height'. *Int J Obes.* (2006) 30:988–92. doi: 10.1038/sj.ijo.0803226

Crapo RO, Casaburi R, Coates AL, Enright PL, MacIntyre NR, McKay RT, et al. ATS statement: guidelines for the six-minute walk test. *Am J Respir Crit Care Med.* (2002) 166:111–7. doi: 10.1164/ajrccm.166.1. at1102

Ross RM, Murthy JN, Wollak ID, Jackson AS. The six minute walk test accurately estimates mean peak oxygen uptake. *BMC Pulmonary Med.* (2010) 10:31. doi: 10.1186/1471-2466-10-31

Stunkard AJ, Sørensen T, Schulsinger F. Use of the Danish Adoption Register for the study of obesity and thinness. *Res Public Assoc Res Nervous Mental Dis.* (1983) 60:115–20.

CarraÇa EV, Markland D, Silva MN, Coutinho SR, Vieira PN, Minderico CS, et al. Physical activity predicts changes in body image during obesity treatment in women. *Med Sci Sports Exerc.* (2012) 44:1604– 12. doi: 10.1249/MSS.0b013e31824d922a

Murcia J, Gimeno E, Lacárcel J, Pérez L. Physical self-concept of Spanish schoolchildren: differences by gender, sport practice and levels of sport involvement. *J Educ Hum Dev.* (2007) 1:1–17.

Fox KR. *The Physical Self-perception: Profile Manual.* Northern Illinois University Press (1990).

Kowalski KC, Crocker PRE, Donen RM. *The Physical Activity Questionnaire for Older Children (PAQ-C) and Adolescents (PAQ-A) Manual, Vol. 87.* College of Kinesiology, University of Saskatchewan (2004) 1–38.

Martínez-Gómez D, Martínez-de-Haro V, Pozo T, Welk GJ, Villagra A, Calle ME, et al. Fiabilidad y validez del cuestionario de actividad física PAQ-A en adolescentes españoles. *Revista Española de Salud Pública.* (2009) 83:427–39. doi: 10.1590/S1135-57272009000300008

Lubans DR, Cliff DP. Muscular fitness, body composition and physical self-perception in adolescents. *J Sci Med in Sport.* (2011) 14:216– 21. doi: 10.1016/j.jsams.2010.10.003

Grao-Cruces A, Nuviala A, Fernandez-Martinez A, Perez-Turpin JA. Association of physical self-coc, life satisfaction and Mediterranean diet in adolescents. *Kinesiology.* (2014) 46:3–11.

Centeio EE, Cance JD, Barcelona JM, Castelli DM. Relationship between health risk and school attendance among adolescents. *Am J Health Educ.* (2018) 49:28–32. doi: 10.1080/19325037.2017. 1360810

García-Hermoso A, Saavedra JM, Escalante Y, Domínguez AM. The intention to be physically active in sedentary obese children: a longitudinal study. *Behav Sci.* (2018) 8:9. doi: 10.3390/bs8010009

Reigal-Garrido RE, Becerra-Fernández CA, Hernández-Mendo A, Martín-Tamayo I. Relación del autoconcepto con la condición física y la composición corporal en una muestra de adolescents. *Anales de Psicologia.* (2014) 30:1079–85. doi: 10.6018/analesps.30.3.157201

Lemoyne J, Valois P, Guay F. Physical self-concept and participation in physical activity in college students. *Med Sci Sports Exerc.* (2014) 47:142– 50. doi: 10.1249/MSS.0000000000000378

Mak KK, Cerin E, McManus AM, Lai CM, Day JR, Ho SY. Mediating effects of body composition between physical activity and body esteem in Hong Kong adolescents: a structural equation modeling approach. *Eur J Pediatr.* (2016) 175:31–7. doi: 10.1007/s00431-015-2586-5

Crocker PRE, Eklund RC, Kowalski KC. Children' s physical activity and physical self-perceptions. *J Sports Sci.* (2000) 18:383–94. doi: 10.1080/02640410050074313

Franco E, Coterón López J. The effects of a physical education intervention to support the satisfaction of basic psychological needs on the motivation and intentions to be physically active. *J Hum Kinetics.* (2017) 59:5– 15. doi: 10.1515/hukin-2017-0143

20

Comparing the Pathway to Success in European Countries Competing in the Swimming World Championships

Inmaculada Yustres[1], Jesús Santos del Cerro[2], Fernando González-Mohíno[1,3], Michael Peyrebrune[4] and José María González-Ravé[1]*

[1]Department of Physical Activity and Sport Sciences, University of Castilla-La Mancha, Toledo, Spain, [2]Department of Statistics, University of Castilla-La Mancha, Toledo, Spain, [3]Departamento de Educación, Facultad de Educación y Lenguas, Universidad Nebrija, Madrid, Spain, [4]Department of Exercise and Health Sciences, School of Sport, Exercise and Health Sciences, Loughborough University, Leicestershire, United Kingdom

***Correspondence:**
José María González-Ravé
josemaria.gonzalez@uclm.es

Purpose: This study aimed to compare the performance progression model of the European countries that participated in the World Championships (WCs) from 2006 to 2017. Data from all championships were compared between the top five (1–5) and the next five (6–10) countries on the medal table. The study also identifies the ages of peak performance in senior swimmers, the annual ratio of progression and the effect of junior performance on senior success by these groups of countries. We hypothesized that: (1) countries with swimmers achieving better performances at the Junior WCs would also be higher in the medal ranking at the Senior WCs and (2) a higher annual performance progression in their swimmers increases the chances of countries being ranked in the top 5 at the Senior World Championships.

Methods: Participant's data from all Junior and Senior WCs between 2006 and 2017 were obtained from FINA. The final, filtered database included 629 swimmers after removing those participating only in the Junior WCs and selecting swimmers from the top 10 countries. One-way ANOVA, F test, and decision tree methods were used to examine differences between the top (1–5) and the next best (6–10) countries on the medal table for first participation age, annual progress, and best-time in junior and senior championships.

Results: There was no difference ($p = 0.492$ and $p = 0.97$) between 1–5 and 6–10 ranked countries for best senior time and annual progression, respectively. Countries ranked in the top 5 at the Senior WCs had swimmers with faster times at the Junior WCs ($p > 0.001$). Decision tree analysis found that best-time at the Junior WC had the greatest explanatory capacity (94%).

Conclusion: European countries with swimmers who perform best at the Junior WCs are also likely to be in the top 5 countries that win medals at the Senior WCs.

Keywords: talent, swimming, progression model, youth, junior

INTRODUCTION

The short (25 m pool) and long course (50 m pool) swimming World Championships (Cs) are run by FINA. Since 2001, the long course Championships have been held every 2 years in the odd years, while the long course after the Summer Olympics every 4 years. Since 2006, European (as a whole), American, and Australian swimmers are regularly the top nations ranked by number of medals won. Although the USA and Australia have been studied in a number of investigations (Trewin et al., 2004; Allen et al., 2014), little is known about the performances of the European countries. As nationality seems to play a key role in achieving the top positions at the WCs, a more detailed analysis of the performance of European countries is warranted.

Due to the increasing competition between nations for medals at major international events such as the World Championships and Olympic Games (Bosscher et al., 2006), many national sporting organizations have invested their available resources more effectively by identifying talented athletes well in advance (Vaeyens et al., 2009; Allen et al., 2015). Talent identification programs aim to identify athletes with high potential for success in senior elite sport (Allen et al., 2014). As a result, the best young athletes are routinely selected into talent development programs (Boccia et al., 2017) based primarily on their age-related competition performance (Lloyd et al., 2015). The concept of developing talent in youth is the goal of many coaches and sports systems. Developing talent at youth level to improve senior performance is the goal of many coaches and sporting organizations. Consequently, an increasing number of national governing bodies have adopted long-term development models in an attempt to provide a structured approach to the training of youth athletes (Svendsen et al., 2018).

Well-designed training plans can enhance performance by improving physiological parameters and enhancing technique (Morais et al., 2014). Details of these plans and their effects on performance are scarce. Many different factors contribute to performance in swimming (Morais et al., 2014) and other sports (Morais et al., 2017), although very little is known about their relative contribution, their progression as athletes develop and the interaction of these factors.

Longitudinal performance assessment is important to help coaches to define realistic goals and monitor training methods (Pyne et al., 2004). One way to achieve this is by tracking the swimmers' performance for a given period of time and analyzing the progression between competitions and seasons. This information can be used to: (1) describe and estimate the progression and the variability of performance during and between seasons; (2) estimate chronological points that predict swimmer's performances throughout their career or a given time frame; and (3) determine a swimmer's probability to reach finals or win medals in important competitions (Costa et al., 2010).

If early sporting success is a pre-requisite for senior elite success (Neeru et al., 2013; Green, 2015), it is clear that maximizing sporting talent is an important goal of long-term development models. Some studies have described athlete development as an ascending scale and depicted improvements using a pyramid or linear model (Barreiros et al., 2014; Green, 2015). However, this assumption appears contentious given the low conversion rates of junior to senior athletes when focusing on specific groups (Durand-Bush and Salmela, 2002; Barreiros et al., 2014).

Consequently, the lack of studies that have focused on the general paths to success followed by international elite swimmers suggests there is a need to track the improvement and development of junior elite athletes. Performance models that provide useful information and minimize the drop out from junior to senior swimming would be extremely valuable (Costa et al., 2011; Allen et al., 2014). In addition, such predictive models can ensure that elite youth athletes are provided with a strategic plan to develop their maximal potential, thereby maximizing participation rates between junior and senior ages and improve long-term sports performance.

No studies have investigated trends in participation, age, and performance in European swimmers at the swimming WCs. In addition, the differences between the more successful and less successful teams have not been studied. The aim of the present study therefore was to compare the general performance progression model of the European countries that participate in the World Championships (WCs) from 2006 to 2017. Data compare the five best (1–5) and the next five best (6–10) European countries from a general medal ranking created with data from all the years analyzed. In addition, we identify the ages of peak performance in senior swimmers, the annual ratio of progression, and the effect of junior performance on senior success in these two groups of European countries.

MATERIALS AND METHODS

Subjects and Design

Authors have no conflicts of interest to disclose. The Castilla-La Mancha University Ethical Committee approved this research dated November 30th 2016. This retrospective study was conducted with public data, and hence no informed consent was obtained. Results and birth dates were obtained from http://www.fina.org/ and http://www.omegatiming.com/ and processed by the authors. All historical data were retrieved from official results websites for the 2007, 2009, 2011, 2013, 2015, and 2017 Senior WCs and 2006, 2008, 2011, 2013, 2015, and 2017 Junior WCs. The age of the swimmers participating in Junior WCs must be between 14–17 and 15–18 years for women and men, respectively.

The final, filtered database (628 swimmers) included swimmers who swam in the Senior WCs (C3) and both Junior and Senior WCs (C1). The analysis was accomplished from top to bottom, trying to analyze where the swimmers who participate in the Absolute World Championship come from.

Mean ± standard deviations were identified by swim strokes, distances, and gender for a more appropriate standardization of the times. Each entry contains the full name, race time, position, age, country, gender, distance, swimming stroke, and year of competition. The distances analyzed were 50, 100, 200, 400, 800, and 1,500 m freestyle; 50, 100, and 200 m backstroke/breaststroke/butterfly, and 200 and 400 m individual medleys.

Procedure

The times have been standardized by means of Ztime scores in order to compare swimmers' times without influencing the variables gender, swim stroke, and distance. The, Ztime score was created by using the annual best performance of each swimmer.

$$Z_{ij} = \frac{X_{ij} - \overline{X}_i}{\sigma_i}$$

where j = individual i = group by gender, swim stroke, and distance.

The following variables have been defined within the model: the top five countries (1) European countries that have had the best results in medal rankings at the WCs (1–5: France, Italy, United Kingdom, Russia, and Sweden); and the next five (0) in the medal rankings (6–10: Hungary, Netherlands, Germany, Denmark, and Poland).

The criteria followed to subdivide the countries between the five best and 6th to 10th has been to develop a general ranking medal with the whole amount of European countries participating in the World Championships. For this purpose, we searched on internet the information about the ranking medal for each World Championship, and a general ranking was created integrating all this information. A total of 10 European countries had participated in all the World Championships analyzed in this study. Therefore, noticing the differences between the positions obtained by the five best and 6th to 10th countries, authors decided to subdivide the countries in that way.

The following variables were analyzed for statistical significance: (1) best-time Senior or peak performance at Senior level (BS): best-standardized performance in its senior stage; (2) minimum age (MA): age in years in which swimmers made their first World Championship; (3) best-time Junior (BJ): the best-standardized performance at the Junior competition; and (4) progress (P): an annual average of the interannual variations of standardized performances. As swimmers can participate in many events in a championship, the z scores of each of their performances were calculated and their minimum scores identified at Junior and Senior level. Both scores were then subtracted and divided by the number of championships.

Statistical Analysis

Mean ± standard deviation was used to characterize swimmers from both groups (1–5 vs. 6–10 countries). Graphical and analytical descriptive statistical measures were used to identify differences between groups of countries in BS, BJ, and P. One-way ANOVA and F test were used to determine the differences and relationships between performances at the Junior and Senior WCs.

Non-parametric tests were also used to estimate the previous patterns with a classification methodology based on decision trees which enabled the identification of the significant aspects in order to achieve the best performances at the swimming WCs. The total sample was divided into a learning sample that was used to estimate both models and a test sample that allowed the estimated models to be validated. All analyses were performed with the software R.

RESULTS

Descriptive average values between the top five (1–5) and the next five (6–10) countries are shown in **Table 1**.

TABLE 1 | Descriptive average values between top and non-top countries.

N = 628	Top countries	Non-top countries
% Swimmers	40.13	59.87
% Males	46.28	53.72
% Females	45.24	54.76
Mean age of best performance in senior	22.70 ± 3.50	22.15 ± 3.70
MA	21.11 ± 3.72	20.83 ± 3.81

"MA" minimum age: age in years in which swimmers involved in this study competed their first world championship competition.

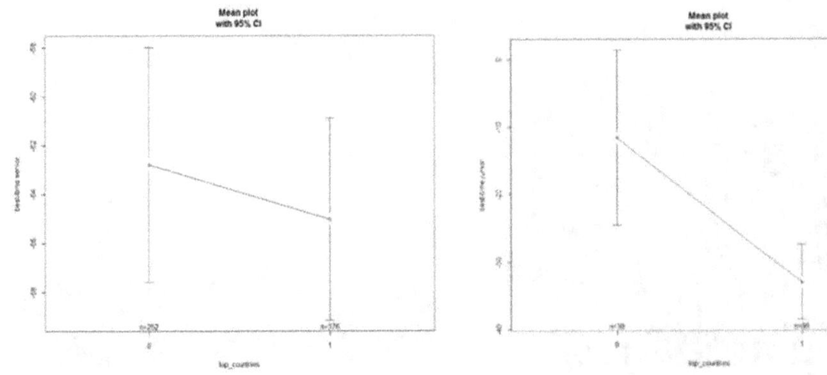

FIGURE 1 | Differences between top and non-top countries in best-time senior and best-time junior.

No significant differences were found ($p = 0.492$) between the 1–5 and 6–10 countries (**Figure 1**).

As best time at senior level (BS) was not a discriminant factor in achieving 1–5 country status, further analyses were carried out to answer the hypothesis of the study.

We accept hypothesis (1) countries with swimmers achieving better performances at the Junior WCs would also be higher in the medal ranking at the Senior WCs as BJ was significantly higher in 1–5 vs. 6–10 countries ($p < 0.001$; $F = 12.86$, **Figure 1**).

Despite this, we reject hypothesis (2) a higher annual performance progression in their swimmers increases the chances of countries being ranked in the top 5 at the Senior World Championships as no differences ($p = 0.97$; $F = 0.001$) were found (**Figure 2**).

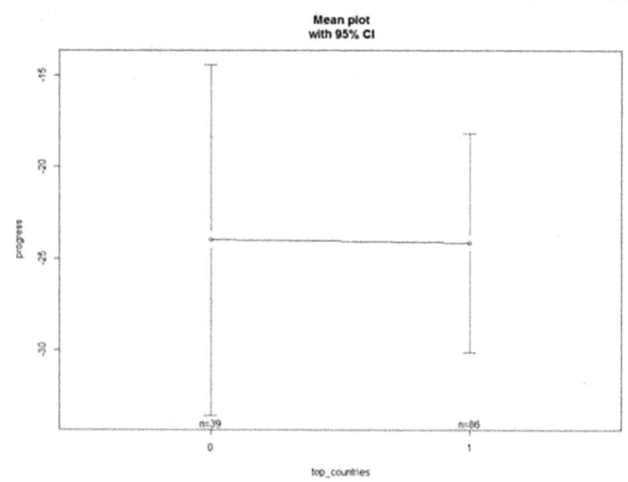

FIGURE 2 | Differences between top and non-top countries in annual progression performance.

The deviation analysis carried out by the decision tree model found that BJ had the greatest explanatory capacity (94%). In addition, both P and MA (3%) carry much less importance.

Therefore, the first relevant classification variable according to the estimated tree is BJ. If the score is below −0.025, there is a high probability (63%) of becoming one of the top (1–5) countries (**Figure 3**).

The confusion matrix, validation sample, and accuracy of the conditional inference tree are shown in **Table 2**.

DISCUSSION

The main objective of the study was to compare the performance progression model of the top 10 European countries that participate in all World Championships (WCs) from 2006 to 2017. The swimmers' performance in Junior WCs was significantly better in European countries ranked 1–5 than those ranked between 6 and 10 in the Senior WCs.

Previous studies have also suggested that Senior competitive level prediction increases markedly from the age of 16 (Costa et al., 2011; Neeru et al., 2013; Green, 2015). Svendsen et al. (2018) found that race performance at Junior level was found to be a strong predictor of subsequent success in senior elite cyclists. In swimming, Yustres et al. (2017) showed that 45.0%

TABLE 2 | Confusion matrix with the validation sample.

	Predicted	
Actual	**No**	**Yes**
No	1	10
Yes	4	23
Accuracy	0.63	

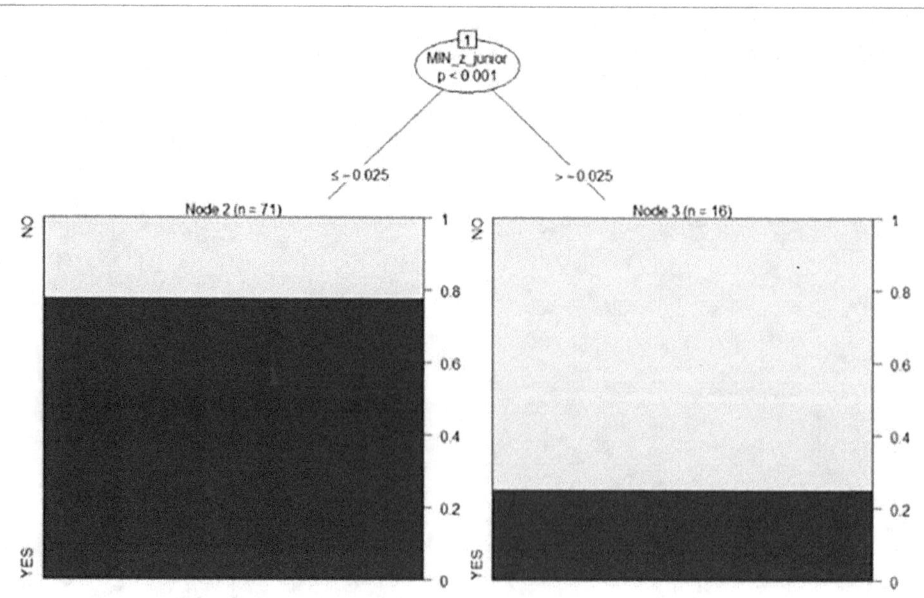

FIGURE 3 | Conditional inference tree.

of Russian and 53.9% of Australian swimmers who achieved medals at the Junior WCs qualified for the finals in Senior WCs. Consequently, it seems that recruiting and developing swimmers from an early age will be advantageous in maximizing performance in Senior swimmers.

While this strategy appears logical, contradictory evidence from the German elite sport system showed that athletes recruited to talent-development squads at young ages exited the system the earliest, and the use of athlete support services was not substantially related to greater attainment of senior success. These observations were corroborated by Sokolovas et al. (2006), who found that most of the top American swimmers at the age of 17–18 were not ranked in the country's top-100 at younger ages.

Allen et al. (2014) indicated that national swimming federations might improve the performance success by targeting resources towards larger groups of swimmers several years out from an international event. Concentrating on training processes and creating independence may help swimmers create an intrinsic motivation to succeed rather than an early specialized program that offers the benefit of early access to Sports Science and other resources.

Longitudinal performance prediction in National federations is increasingly popular to identify the characteristics necessary for winning medals at major events such as the World Championships or Olympic Games. Results from this study showed that an optimal annual progression in performance from Junior to Senior does not improve the chances of becoming a top-ranked country in the medal table at the Senior WCs. This indicates that on average, swimmers from all countries improve at a similar rate and the ones who start from a higher level at the Junior WCs are still in the top 5 at the Senior WCs. This supports the study by Trewin et al. (2004) who found no differences in mean progression rates between nations when analyzing the variability of competitive performance between FINA world-rankings and Olympic performances. This appears to be a conflicting area for research.

In contrast to our results, Pyne et al. (2001) found that lower ranked athletes with greater rates of performance improvement will increased their chances of winning a medal more than highly ranked athletes in future International competitions. Hopkins et al. (1999) also observed that an athlete in contention for a medal has to improve their performance by approximately one-half of the typical race to-race variation in performance (expressed as a standard deviation) to substantially increase their chances of success. In addition, improvements of this magnitude (~1% per year) should be considered when estimating performance times for future competitions (Pyne et al., 2004).

Longitudinal monitoring of performance progress must be able to differentiate between "normal" increases in performance caused by maturation and training, and "unnatural" improvement caused by doping (Hopker et al., 2018). Seasonal performance variability could become a useful indicator in targeting possible offenders. Previous studies suggested a coefficient of variation ranging from 1 to 1.5% in track and field athletics (Malcata and Hopkins, 2014) and 1% for elite rowing athletes (Smith and Hopkins, 2011). This confounding variable could be one reason why the annual rate of progression is not critical in becoming a top 5 country in the medal table at the Senior WCs.

In this study, there were no differences in minimum age (MA) between the top 5 countries and the next 5 on the WCs medal table. This suggests that national governing bodies would be advised to focus on maximizing swimmer's performance at the Junior level over early exposure to Senior International competition.

Yustres et al. (2017) found a close relationship ($p < 0.001$) between the position obtained at Senior level and the number of years remaining competing in World Championships. Swimmers tend to be older when they achieve their best performance. It would appear that a greater number of experiences at international level will increase the chances of achieving better performances at the Senior WCs. It is likely that a better Junior performance level and competing for longer at Senior international level will increase the chances of success for counties aiming to be ranked in the top 5 at the Senior WCs.

In this study, we support the hypothesis that European countries with swimmers achieving an optimal performance at the Junior WCs have a better chance of success at the Senior WCs. We rejected the hypothesis that the swimmer's annual performance progression is critical to Nations being a top-ranked European country in the medal table at the Senior WC. Future studies might analyze the evolution of the best junior swimmers competing the Junior World Championships to really determine how many will reach the World Championships of absolute category, identifying further contributory factors in helping countries to develop athletes and predict success at the Senior WCs. Besides, some other variables that could explain our main aim can be analyzed. However, it was not possible in our study due to the limited relevant information that we have about some other explicative variables.

CONCLUSION

Countries with swimmers achieving an optimal performance in the Junior WCs will have a better chance of reaching the top 5 position in the medal ranking at the Senior WCs.

Average best time at the Senior WCs and an optimal annual progression performance from Junior to Senior do not affect the chances of becoming a top-ranked (1–5) country in the medal table at the Senior WCs.

This comparison between the performance progression model of European countries shows that countries aiming to reach the top positions in the medal should not focus on annual progression rates, the age of first performance, or the age of peak performance at Senior level. However, there is a 63% chance of swimmers who succeed at the Junior WCs that will also help their countries to achieve a top 5 medal ranking at the Senior WCs.

AUTHOR CONTRIBUTIONS

IY, JG-R, and JS conceptualized, designed and performed the experiments. IY, JG-R, JS, and FG-M analyzed and interpreted the data. IY, JG-R, MP, and FG-M edited and critically reviewed the manuscript. IY, JG-R, MP, and JS wrote the manuscript.

ACKNOWLEDGMENTS

This is a short text to acknowledge the contributions of specific colleagues, institutions, or agencies that aided the efforts of the authors.

REFERENCES

Allen, S., Vandenbogaerde, T., and Hopkins, W. (2014). Career performance trajectories of Olympic swimmers: benchmarks for talent development. *Eur. J. Sport Sci.* 14, 643–651. doi: 10.1080/17461391.2014.893020

Allen, S., Vandenbogaerde, T., Pyne, D., and Hopkins, W. (2015). Predicting a nation's Olympic-qualifying swimmers. *Int. J. Sports Physiol. Perform.* 10, 431–435. doi: 10.1123/ijspp.2014-0314

Barreiros, A., Côté, J., and Fonseca, A. M. (2014). From early to adult sport success: analysing athletes' progression in national squads. *Eur. J. Sport Sci.* 14(Supp. 1), S178–S182. doi: 10.1080/17461391.2012.671368

Boccia, G., Moisè, P., Franceschi, A., Trova, F., Panero, D., La Torre, A., et al. (2017). Career performance trajectories in track and field jumping events from youth to senior success: the importance of learning and development. *PLoS One* 12:1. doi: 10.1371/journal.pone.0170744

Bosscher, V., de Knop, P., van Bottenburg, M., and Shibli, S. (2006). A conceptual framework for analysing sports policy factors leading to international sporting success. *Eur. Sport Manag. Q.* 6, 185–215. doi: 10.1080/16184740600955087

Costa, M., Marinho, D., Bragada, J., Silva, A., and Barbosa, T. (2011). Stability of elite freestyle performance from childhood to adulthood. *J. Sports Sci.* 29, 1183–1189. doi: 10.1080/02640414.2011.587196

Costa, M., Silva, A. J., Marqués, M., Bragada, J. A., and Barbosa, T. (2010). Tracking the Performance of World-Ranked Swimmers. *J. Sports Sci. Med.* 9, 411–417.

Durand-Bush, N., and Salmela, J. (2002). The development and maintenance of expert Athletic performance: perceptions of World and Olympic champions. *J. Appl. Sport Psychol.* 14, 154–171. doi: 10.1080/10413200290103473

Green, B. (2015). Building sport programs to optimize athlete recruitment, retention and transition: toward a normative theory of sport development. *J. Sport Manag.* 19, 233–253. doi: 10.1123/jsm.19.3.233

Hopker, J., Schumacher, Y. O., Fedoruk, M., Mørkeberg, J., Bermon, S., Iljukov, S., et al. (2018). Athlete performance monitoring in anti-doping. *Front. Physiol.* 9:232. doi: 10.3389/fphys.2018.00232

Hopkins, W. G., Hawley, J. A., and Burke, L. M. (1999). Design and analysis of research on sport performance enhancement. *Med. Sci. Sports Exerc.* 31, 472–485. doi: 10.1097/00005768-199903000-00018

Lloyd, R. S., Oliver, J. L., Faigenbaum, A. D., Howard, R., De Ste Croix, M. B. A., Williams, C. A., et al. (2015). Long-term athletic development: part 1: a pathway for all youth. *J. Strength Cond. Res.* 29, 1439–1450. doi: 10.1519/JSC.0000000000000756

Malcata, R. M., and Hopkins, W. G. (2014). Variability of competitive performance of elite athletes: a systematic review. *Sports Med.* 44, 1763–1774. doi: 10.1007/s40279-014-0239-x

Morais, J. E., Marques, M. C., Marinho, D. S., Silva, A. J., and Barbosa, T. M. (2014). Longitudinal modeling in sports: young swimmers' performance and biomechanics profile. *Hum. Mov. Sci.* 37, 111–122. doi: 10.1016/j.humov.2014.07.005

Morais, J. E., Silva, A. J., Marinho, D. A., Lopes, V. P., and Barbosa, T. M. (2017). Determinant factors of long-term performance development in young swimmers. *Int. J. Sports Physiol. Perform.* 12, 198–205. doi: 10.1123/ijspp.2015-0420

Neeru, J., Dugas, L., and LaBella, C. (2013). Sports specialization in young athletes: evidence-based recommendations. *Sports Health* 5, 251–257. doi: 10.1177/1941738112464626

Pyne, D. B., Lee, H., and Swanwick, K. (2001). Monitoring the lactate threshold in world-ranked swimmers. *Med. Sci. Sports Exerc.* 33, 291–297. doi: 10.1097/00005768-200102000-00019

Pyne, D., Trewin, C., and Hopkins, W. (2004). Progression and variability of competitive performance of Olympic swimmers. *J. Sports Sci.* 22, 613–620. doi: 10.1080/02640410310001655822

Smith, T. B., and Hopkins, W. G. (2011). Variability and predictability of finals times of elite rowers. *Med. Sci. Sports Exerc.* 43, 2155–2160. doi: 10.1249/MSS.0b013e31821d3f8e

Sokolovas, G., Vilas-Boas, J. P., Alves, F., and Marques, A. (2006). Analysis of USA swimming's all-time top 100 times. Biomechanics and Medicine in Swimming X. *Rev. Port. Cien. Desp.* 11, 315–317. https://bibliotecadigital.ipb.pt/bitstream/10198/3571/3/BMS2010_BMS_XI_final_lowres-co%CC%81pia.pdf

Svendsen, I. S., Tønnesen, E., Tjelta, L. I., and Orn, S. (2018). Training, performance and physiological predictors of a successful elite senior career in junior competitive road cyclists. *Int. J. Sports Physiol. Perform.* 20, 1–6. doi: 10.1123/ijspp.2017-0824

Trewin, C. B., Hopkins, W. G., and Pyne, D. B. (2004). Relationship between world-ranking and Olympic performance of swimmers. *J. Sports Sci.* 22, 339–345. doi: 10.1080/02640410310001641610

Vaeyens, R., Lenoir, M., Williams, A. M., and Philippaerts, R. M. (2009). Talent identification and promotion programmes of Olympic athletes. *J. Sports Sci.* 27, 1367–1380. doi: 10.1080/02640410903110974

Yustres, I., Martín, R., Fernández, L., and González-Ravé, J. M. (2017). Swimming championship finalist positions on success in international swimming competitions. *PLoS One* 12:11. doi: 10.1371/journal.pone.0187462

Effects of Installing Height-Adjustable Standing Desks on Daily and Domain-Specific Duration of Standing, Sitting and Stepping in 3rd Grade Primary School Children

Ole Sprengeler[1], *Antje Hebestreit*[1*], *Hannah Gohres*[2], *Jens Bucksch*[3] and *Christoph Buck*[4]

[1] Department of Epidemiological Methods and Etiologic Research, Leibniz Institute for Prevention Research and Epidemiology - BIPS, Bremen, Germany, [2] School of Public Health, Bielefeld University, Bielefeld, Germany, [3] Department of Sociological and Human Sciences, Heidelberg University of Education, Heidelberg, Germany, [4] Department of Biometry and Data Management, Leibniz Institute for Prevention Research and Epidemiology - BIPS, Bremen, Germany

***Correspondence:**
Antje Hebestreit
hebestr@leibniz-bips.de

Specialty section:

Background: Aim of this intervention study was to evaluate whether availability of standing desks in classrooms may reduce sitting time and enhance standing and stepping time during lessons and breaks. Further, we evaluated if differences in standing desk use differed by physical fitness (PF) levels of children.

Methods: To assess sitting, standing and stepping during a typical school week in 3rd grade primary school children ($N = 52$), activPAL monitors were used at baseline: T0, 1st follow-up: T1 and 2nd follow-up: T2. At baseline, PF was measured using the standing long jump and the 6-min jog-walk to assign children as having low PF (LPF) or high PF (HPF). Standing desks were assigned randomly to intervention and control groups at T1 (group 1) and T2 (group 2) with a cross-over design. Changes of sitting, standing and stepping were analyzed to investigate intervention effects at follow-up, using linear mixed models.

Results: At baseline, children spent about 60 and 30% of time sitting during lessons and breaks, respectively. After installing standing desks (T1), significantly lower proportions of sitting were observed in the intervention group 1 [−13.1%, 95%-CI: (−20.5; −5.72)] and the control group 2 [−9.78%, 95%-CI: (−17.3; −2.28)]. Compared to the baseline measurement (T0), lower proportions of sitting were particularly expressed during school breaks in group 1 and 2 after intervention in T1 [group 1: −10.3%, 95%-CI: (−16.4; −4.25)] or in T2 [group 2: −8.59%, 95%-CI: (−15.2; −1.94)]. In general, children with higher physical fitness were less sedentary and more active, but intervention effects did not differ by fitness levels.

Conclusion: Standing desks provide an opportunity to reduce sedentary time during lessons and breaks at school in primary school children, but do not directly increase PA of high intensity such as stepping. Future studies should consider potential bandwagon effects caused by structural interventions.

Keywords: objective measurement, lessons, breaks, leisure time activity, physical fitness

BACKGROUND

The World Health Organization (WHO) recommends that children and adolescents between 5 and 17 years should engage in moderate-to-vigorous physical activity (MVPA) for at least 60 min every day (1), but only one fifth of German school children (2) meet this recommendation. Regarding sedentary behavior, the WHO recommends that children and adolescents should limit the amount of time spent being sedentary, in particular the amount of recreational screen time. However, associations between sedentary behavior and child health are still discussed controversially (3–5), but there is evidence that sedentary behavior tracks from childhood to adulthood underpinning importance of health promotion activities targeting the reduction of sitting time already early in life (6). Possible health benefits resulting from the reduction of sedentary time in childhood may relate to a healthier weight status, blood pressure, metabolism, fitness, self-esteem and social behavior and may even improve academic performance (7). A large number of studies observed a gradient between time spent sedentary and worsening of health, but evidence is inconclusive with regard to a clear dose-response relationship. For screen time, adverse health effects are observed from up to 2 h. (8) This is alarming insofar as primary school children are sitting ~6.5 h at school (9–12), particularly German children and adolescents spent up to 9 h sedentary during a typical school day (13) and sitting duration increases as children get older (9–12, 14).

In recent years, multiple strategies aiming to decrease daily sedentary time and motivate children to move more during the day have been discussed (15). One strategy to reduce sitting time during school hours was addressed but still requires deeper investigation: the installation of height-adjustable standing desks (in the following named simply "standing desks"). Although some reviews have been published in this field (16, 17), research findings are contradicting and do not yet allow to draw final conclusions. Recent studies showed that implementing standing desks in schools could significantly decrease durations of sitting per day, without any disadvantages such as reduced concentration during lessons at school (16–19). On the contrary, positive effects of standing desks were observed in primary children rather than in secondary school children (20).

Only few high-quality studies have been conducted in this fieldwhere only about half of them included control groups as highlighted by Minges et al. (16). Additionally, short follow-up duration and unreliable sensors to distinguish between sitting and standing time (e.g., Actigraph accelerometers) were also highlighted as limitations by Sherry et al. (17). In general, three main obstacles are known in research to investigate sitting and standing in children with standing desks provided at school. First, recent studies can afford only a low number of standing desks due to the high costs of this structural intervention strategy. Second, mostly the duration of sitting/standing during the total day or during total school hours is analyzed rather than assessing how sitting/standing changes during lessons and breaks, respectively, if standing desks are (un-) available. Third, researchers focused on durations of sitting and standing until now, but did not investigate potential factors associated with the acceptability or use of standing desks.

Hence, the aim of this study was to investigate whether the availability of standing desks in primary school children leads to less sitting and more standing and stepping time during school hours—particularly during lessons and breaks—and whether shorter vs. longer standing time during school hours affected leisure time activities of children after school. Further, we explored possible differences in the effects of standing desk use with regard to the physical fitness (PF) levels of children prior to the intervention.

METHODS

Study Sample

The study was conducted in one primary school in Ludwigsburg, Germany. All 59 children of the entire third grade, distributed into three classes, were invited to participate in the study (**Figure 1**). Parents were informed during a parent evening and by provision of study information. Parents were asked for written informed consent; additionally, all children were asked for oral consent prior to the assessment. In total, written informed consent was provided by parents of 54 children. The study was carried out in accordance with the Declaration of Helsinki, and the study protocol was approved by the institutional review board of the University of Bremen (19.09.2017).

Study Design

This case-crossover study was carried out between January and March 2018. Since the case-crossover design is useful to evaluate brief and changing exposures, it was chosen to ensure an identical environment and reduce confounding (e.g., by schedule, or weather) for intervention and control group (21). At baseline (T0, January 2018), all measurements were applied in all children (**Figure 1**). Baseline measurements for all children included: objective measurement of sitting, standing and physical activity (PA), anthropometry and PF as well as a parental questionnaire assessing socioeconomic status. After completion of the baseline survey (T0), a total of 32 standing desks were equally distributed among the three classes. The standing desks were assigned randomly to half of all children in each class (intervention group at T1, referred to as group 1), whilst the other half of the children worked at their traditional working desks (control group at T1, referred as group 2). In the third week after installing the standing desks, the first follow-up examinations (T1, February 2018) included the identical measurements conducted at T0 (except anthropometry and PF) in all participating children. After the T1 measurements were completed, standing desks were assigned to those children, who belonged to the control group previously (group 2, now intervention group at T2). The remaining children (group 1: intervention group at T1, now control group at T2) were assigned to the traditional working desk at this time. Again, after a washout period of 2 weeks, the second follow-up was conducted (T2, March 2018), including the identical measurements from T1 and T0. In summary, to address the crossover design in the analyses, groups were distinguished as having the intervention, i.e., having

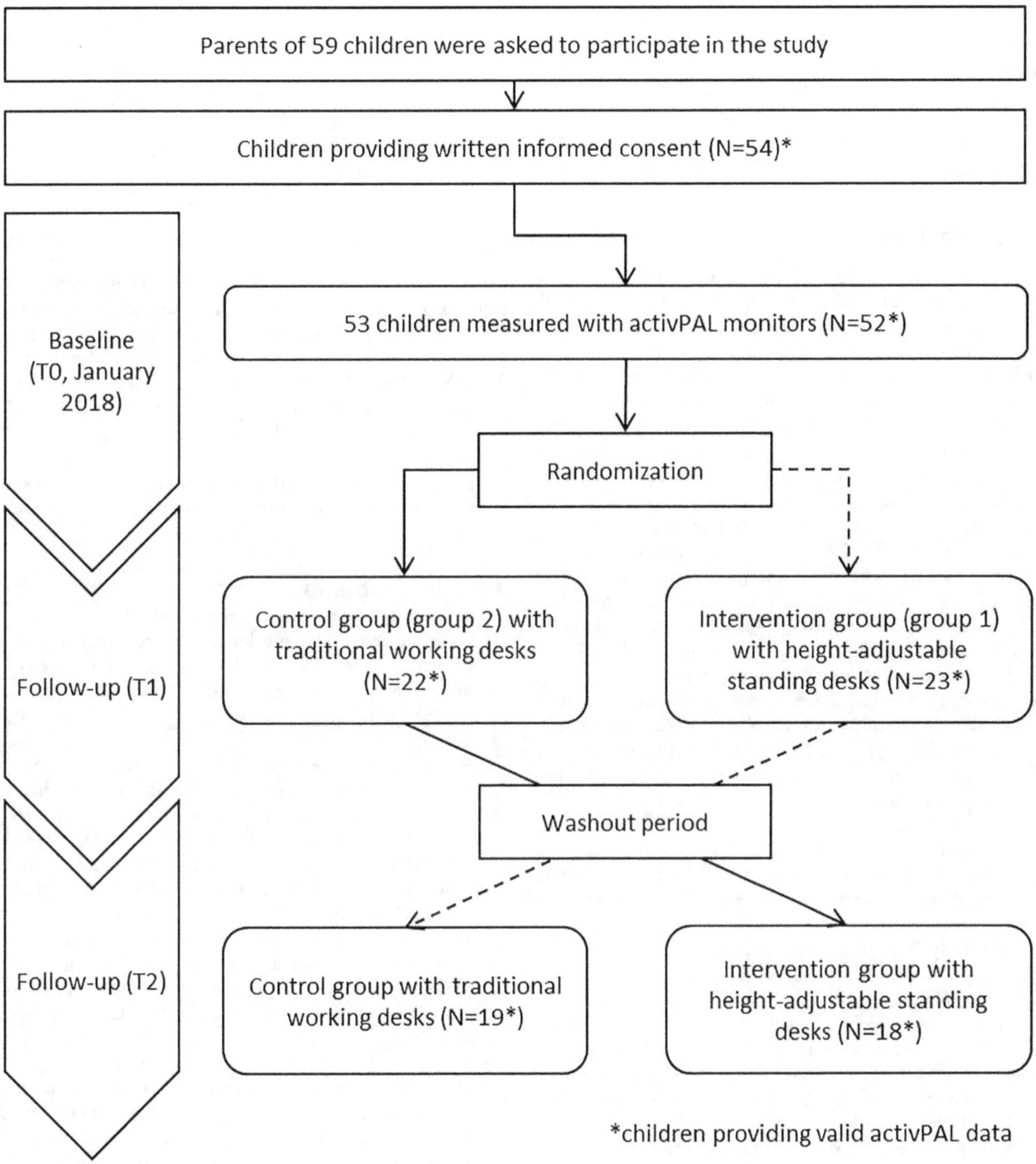

FIGURE 1 | Study design and number of participants.

standing desks designated to half of the children within each classroom, between baseline and first follow-up (group 1) and between first and second follow-up, for the other half of the classroom (group 2).

Height-Adjustable Standing Desks

The city of Ludwigsburg provided 32 standing desks (Rondo-Lift-KF ($N = 21$) and SitAndStand ($N = 11$) by VS Middle East, height-adjustable between 69–113 cm and 70–115 cm, respectively). Children were able to sit at the desks with their usual chairs at minimum height. Desk bases had lockable castors and were freely movable. Spatial arrangement was carried out by the teachers so that children who choose to stand did not bother the view of sitting children. In general, children with standing desk were allowed to lift and lower their standing desks at its own discretion; they were not reminded or encouraged to stand during lessons. The height of the standing position was not assessed.

Activity Behavior

Sitting, standing and PA were assessed by activPAL inclinometer (PAL Technologies Ltd., Glasgow, UK). At each survey period, the devices were distributed during physical education classes. Study personnel instructed verbally how to use the devices and directly helped attaching the devices at the mid-point on the front of the right thigh. Additionally, all children received an information sheet explaining the handling of the device, in order to inform their parents. All participating children were asked to wear the devices for 24 h on 10 consecutive days (except during swimming and bathing). To assess standing, sitting and stepping in primary children, activPAL monitors have been proven to be valid and reliable (22–25). We derived PA intensities from counts in 15 s epochs within the daily time frame of 6:30 am to 8:30 pm in order to reduce bias through inaccurate estimates of get up or sleep times. We restricted the analysis to children with PA data of at least 2 days with at least 10 h of measured time. The measured duration of PA was considered per domain i.e., lessons, school breaks and leisure time and generated using exact time stamps of the respective weekly schedule of each class for each child. Further, daily information on PA intensities was cleaned with regard to extreme values in steps and sedentary time, i.e., days with <1,000 steps and/or a sedentary time of more than 90% of the measured time were excluded. Eventually, we averaged habitual PA, i.e., stepping, standing, and sitting, over weekdays (not weekend days) for children providing at least 3 days of valid measurements at each survey. Time spent sitting, standing and stepping was measured by the devices and later processed in minutes per day. In order to describe the distribution of activity intensities per day and domain, i.e., lessons, school breaks or leisure time, minutes per day spent sitting, standing or stepping were summed up based on all weekdays and for any specific domain. This duration was then divided by the total measured minutes per weekday and domain, respectively. Accelerometry data derived from the activPAL3-software (activPAL Professional v7.2.29, PAL Technologies Ltd., Glasgow UK) was processed using R Version 3.5.1 and particularly R-packages dplyr, ggplot2, and scales.

Parental Questionnaire and School Information

Sex and age of all participating children were obtained by the written informed consent. The parent completing the questionnaire answered questions about the highest level of education and highest professional qualification of both parents. Both were classified according to the international standard classification of education (ISCED) (26), which were categorized as low (ISCED level 1 or 2), medium (ISCED levels 3 or 4), and high (ISCED level 5 or higher) and using the maximum of both parents (if data available) as an indicator of the family educational status. Parents were also asked if their child participated in organized youth sports. Teachers provided the class-specific schedules to facilitate the assignment of objectively measured activity and sedentary behaviors to the timing of school breaks and lessons throughout the school day.

Anthropometry

Anthropometric measurements were carried out by trained study personnel using standardized instruments. Height was measured using a telescopic stadiometer (Seca 225, seca, Birmingham, UK) to the nearest 0.1 cm (27). Body mass was measured using the TANITA BC 420 SMA, a digital weighing scale (TANITA, Tokyo, Japan) that was previously used in young children (28). We calculated BMI as weight in kilograms divided by squared height in meters and categorized weight status of children as overweight or obese according to the German reference system by Kromeyer-Hausschild using the 90th percentile for the age 8, 9 and 10 (29).

Physical Fitness

In order to briefly classify the participants into children with less or more ability to stand longer as a potential confounder, two motor tests (standing long jump and 6-min jog-walk) were conducted to assess components of physical fitness (explosive strength and endurance capacity).

Both PF tests were conducted after a typical warm-up at the beginning of physical education lessons. The standing long jump test was used to assess the lower-limb explosive strength. Children had to jump off a marked line with both feet and to land on both feet at the same time, if possible. The recorded value was the difference (in cm) between the marked line and the last heel mark (30). To assess endurance capacity, we applied the 6-min jog-walk, a quick and convertible test during physical education lessons to assess the maximal oxygen uptake. Children had to run a 54 m round as often as possible within 6 min. They were allowed to walk if they could not run anymore. The test has proven to moderately correlate with a spiroergometry in children aged 8–10 years (31). The PF at baseline was categorized into high PF (HPF) for children who at least performed more than of 17 rounds in the 6-min jog-walk or jumped more than 128 cm in the standing long jump test and low PF (LPF), if none of the above applied. Since only two motor tests were conducted and in order to enable a specific classification within our sample, the median values of our results was chosen as cutoffs (17 rounds, 128 cm) for low and high PF.

Statistical Analysis

We calculated descriptive statistics, such as mean and standard deviation (SD) as well as range for continuous variables in this study and proportions for categorical variables with regard to the overall study sample and stratified by PF levels.

We used linear mixed models to investigate the effect of the implementation of standing desks in classrooms on PA, i.e., sitting, standing, and stepping in children. Linear mixed models provide the flexibility to model the time and intervention effect, i.e., the interaction, while accounting for repeated measurements by means of a random residual effect and particularly based on unbalanced data, i.e., incorporating the complete sample despite loss to follow up.

Outcome variables, sitting, standing, and stepping were considered as continuous dependent variables in the linear mixed models. For each PA outcome we modeled the exposition to the intervention a) for each group over time using two main effects for the survey wave and group assignment and b) the interaction of survey wave with group assignment (group 1 at T1 and group 2 at T2) which are presented as the actual intervention effect. Outcome variables were modeled using total school time data as well as considering the domain-specific data during lessons, school breaks, and leisure time. Further, all models were adjusted for sex, age, weight status, PF, parental education and class. Mixed models were also conducted stratified by PF to assess whether effects of the intervention differed by children's PF levels at T0. From each of these linear mixed models, least-square means (LSM) and 95% confidence limits (95% CI) of dependent PA variables were estimated for each group ($k = 2$) per survey ($t = 3$) as well as all possible fifteen ((k*t−1)!) LSM-differences of mean PA variables and the 95% CI for each combination of survey wave and group assignment. This way, both direct intervention effects (group 1: T1 - T0, group 2: T2 - T0) and potential indirect effects, either between group assignment or over survey waves could be identified. Normality of outcome variables was assessed using residual and Q-Q plots. Confidence intervals were estimated considering the sidak adjustment for multiple testing within each regression model. Significance level was set to $\alpha = 0.05$, however we did not adjust for multiple testing with regard to number of regression models.

RESULTS

Among the total of 53 participating children at baseline, 52 participants provided valid activPAL data of at least 2 days with at least 10 h per day (**Figure 1**). Of those, 61.5% were girls ($N = 17$) (**Table 1**). The average age of all participating children was 8.4 years (SD: 0.7) and the proportion participating in organized youth sports was 76.9%. About one fourth of the study sample was categorized as having overweight or obesity (23%). About twice as many children were categorized as having low fitness levels than having high fitness levels. Further, children with higher fitness levels ran about four rounds more during the 6 min run and achieved ~30 cm more distance at the standing long jump than the less fit children. In general, children spent about 7 h per day and about half of their leisure time sitting. Almost two thirds of the time in school lessons were spent sedentary, whereas in school breaks only one third was spent sitting. In contrast, at least 70% of school breaks was spent active in children either with low and high fitness levels (**Table 1**). Total daily sitting time revealed only small differences between fitness level, whereas children with higher fitness level had 30 min longer stepping duration per day (168.4 min/day), compared to children with lower fitness level.

Table 2 presents results of linear mixed models showing estimated means (Est) with 95% confidence intervals (95% CI) of PA variables during lessons for group assignment and survey wave as well as differences of survey waves per group to identify intervention effects. Estimated proportions of sitting, standing and stepping during lessons varied substantially per survey wave and intervention group (**Table 2**).

Across survey waves, group 1 almost persistently showed less sedentary and more active pattern during lessons, compared to group 2. Between T0 and T1, sitting time significantly decreased between T0 and T1 in the intervention group [group 1: −13.1, 95%CI (−20.5; −5.72)], but also in the control group [group 2: −9.78, 95%CI (−17.3; −2.28)]. In addition, standing time significantly increased after the first intervention in T1 [group 1: 11.6, 95%CI (4.85, 18.3) as well as in the control group (group 2: 8.63, 95%CI (1.78; 15.5)].

Table 3 presents PA patterns during school breaks. At both follow-ups (T1 and T2), about ten percentage points less sitting during breaks were found in all children in both groups. Compared to T0, in group 1 significantly lower proportions of sitting [−10.3%, 95%-CI: (−16.4; −4.25)] and higher proportions of standing: [6.20%, 95%-CI: (1.37; 11.0)] were measured during school breaks at T1. Similarly, group 2 showed lower proportions of sitting [−8.59%, 95%-CI: (−15.2; −1.94)] and higher proportions of standing [8.08%, 95%-CI: (2.78; 13.4)] after the intervention in T2.

Table 4 summarizes PA patterns during leisure time. In group 1, slightly higher values (1–4 percentage points) have been observed regarding the time standing and stepping across all survey periods, compared to group 2. No intervention effect was observed regarding sitting, standing or stepping during leisure time.

Regarding overall PA per day, group 1 accumulated less sitting time and more standing and stepping time per day, across all survey periods, compared to group 2 (**Table 5**). Regarding the total time per day spent sitting, standing and stepping, no intervention effects were observed across survey periods and groups.

Results of linear mixed models stratified by fitness levels are presented in **Supplemental Tables 1–4**. Basically, children with higher fitness levels spent between 44 and 47% of their leisure time per day with sitting, whereas children with low fitness levels spent more than half of their leisure time sedentary (53–54%). At T0, children with high fitness levels spent four to seven percentage points less sitting during breaks [group 1: 26.1%, 95%-CI: (19.7; 32.6), group 2: 24.3%, 95%-CI: (12.0; 36.6)], compared to children showing low fitness levels [group 1: 30.3% 95%-CI: (25.0; 35.7), group 2: 31.4%, 95%-CI: (26.7; 36.0)]. Children with higher fitness levels of the intervention group at T1 (group 1) increased their standing time about twice as much [15.7%, 95%-CI: (4.04; 27.3)], compared to children of group 1 with low fitness levels [7.79%, 95%-CI: (−1.20; 16.8)].

TABLE 1 | Study characteristics and total as well as domain-specific time during spent sitting, standing and stepping on weekdays in school children at baseline ($N = 52$).

	All (N = 52)		Fitness level			
			Low (n = 32)		High (n = 16)	
	N	%	N	%	N	%
Sex						
Male	20	38.5	12	33.3	8	50
Female	32	61.5	24	66.6	8	50
Sports Club member	40	76.9	26	72.2	14	87.5
Weight status						
Normal weight	41	78.9	25	69.4	16	100
Overweight/obese	11	21.1	11	30.6		
ISCED categories						
Low (0–2)	8	15.4	6	16.7	2	12.5
Medium (3,4)	16	30.8	13	36.1	3	18.8
High (5+)	28	53.9	17	47.2	11	68.8
	Mean (SD)	**Range**	**Mean (SD)**	**Range**	**Mean (SD)**	**Range**
Age (years)	8.4 (0.7)	(8–10)	8.4 (0.7)	(8–10)	8.2 (0.4)	(8,9)
Body Mass Index	17.7 (3.4)	(12.3–27.5)	18.5 (3.8)	(12.3–27.5)	16.1 (1.5)	(14.1–19.2)
Fat Free Mass (kg)	24.7 (4.0)	(18.5–36)	25 (4.3)	(18.5–36)	24.0 (3.3)	(19.2–32.8)
Six min run (rounds)	16.0 (2.6)	(10–21)	14.7 (1.8)	(10–17)	18.6 (1.7)	(16–21)
Standing long jump (cm)	115.4 (21.1)	(62–153)	104 (14.8)	(62–127)	137.4 (12.1)	(119–153)
Overall						
Sitting time (min/day)	419.9 (62.1)	(294–556)	423.2 (62.2)	(301–556)	412.5 (63.4)	(294–531)
Standing time (min/day)	232.7 (49.9)	(114–354)	234.1 (54.2)	(114–354)	229.5 (40.40)	(154–299)
Stepping time (min/day)	147.6 (33.8)	(58–220)	138.4 (27.6)	(58–220)	168.4 (38.1)	(93–216)
Domain lessons						
Sitting (%)	58.2 (14.0)	(30.8–83.3)	58.2 (13.1)	(30.8–81.9)	58.3 (16.2)	(33.1–83.3)
Standing (%)	30.8 (12.4)	(11.7–57.6)	30.8 (12.0)	(11.8–57.6)	30.5 (13.6)	(11.7–54.0)
Stepping (%)	11.3 (3.2)	(4.0–20.0)	10.9 (3.1)	(4.0–20 0)	11.1 (3.4)	(5.0–16.2)
Domain school breaks						
Sitting (%)	28.0 (8.3)	(9.5–53.3)	29.2 (8.5)	(9.5–53.3)	25.4 (7.2)	(11.5–44.0)
Standing (%)	34.1 (5.8)	(23.3–46.1)	34.2 (5.6)	(24.4–46.1)	34.0 (6.3)	(23.5–43.3)
Stepping (%)	37.8 (9.1)	(13.9–56.4)	36.6 (9.1)	(13.9–54.0)	40.6 (8.7)	(26.6–56.4)
Domain leisure time						
Sitting (%)	50.4 (11.4)	(23.3–85.4)	51.7 (11.5)	(25.8–85.4)	47.3 (10.8)	(23.3–66.0)
Standing (%)	30.5 (8.2)	(8.1–50.2)	30.9 (9.1)	(8.1–50.2)	29.5 (5.8)	(22.2–40.8)
Stepping (%)	19.2 (6.8)	(3.9–36.3)	17.4 (5.8)	(3.9–32.2)	23.2 (7.5)	(11.4–36.3)

DISCUSSION

The present study aimed to investigate whether installing height-adjustable standing desks affects proportions of sitting, standing and stepping on typical school days and in particular domains (lessons, breaks and leisure time). By measuring PF levels at baseline, we were able to investigate whether potential intervention effects in primary school children differed by PF levels, since the latter indicates increased motivation and capability for PA. We observed significant shorter durations of sitting and longer durations of standing during lessons at T1 in both, the control group (group 2) and the intervention group (group 1). This observation that not only children with but also children without standing desks increased standing during lessons, might be explained by a bandwagon effect, which is a common phenomenon in intervention studies (32). In particular during breaks, positive intervention effects, i.e., significant lower sitting and higher standing durations were observed in both groups after each intervention at T1 and T2, respectively, compared to the baseline measurement (T0).

In general, children with higher fitness levels were found to accumulate more standing time during the day. Further, children having higher fitness levels were more active (up to 7 percentage points more stepping/day) and less likely to have an

TABLE 2 | Results of linear mixed models in terms of estimated means of sitting, standing, and stepping time in percentage (%) of total time during lessons per intervention group and survey as well as differences of least-square means (LSM) for direct intervention effects (group 1: T1 – T0, group 2: T2 – T0) and differences across all surveys for $N = 134$ observations of $n = 48$ children.

		Sitting time in % during lessons		Standing time in % during lessons		Stepping time in % during lessons	
Group	**Survey**	**Estimate**	**95% CI**	**Estimate**	**95% CI**	**Estimate**	**95% CI**
Group 1							
	T0	58.4	(51.7; 65.0)	30.5	(25.6; 36.3)	11.2	(9.67; 12.7)
	T1	45.3	(38.3; 52.3)	42.0	(35.8; 48.2)	12.8	(11.2; 14.3)
	T2	56.0	(48.8; 63.1)	31.5	(25.1; 37.8)	12.6	(11.0; 14.2)
	Mean differences						
	T1 - T0	**−13.1**	**(−20.5; −5.72)**	**11.6**	**(4.85; 18.3)**	**1.57**	**(0.10; 3.05)**
	T2 - T0	−2.40	(−10.2; 5.44)	0.99	(−6.16; 8.15)	1.45	(−0.12; 3.02)
	T2 - T1	**10.7**	**(2.47; 18.9)**	**−10.6**	**(−18.1; −3.09)**	−0.12	(−1.77; 1.53)
Group 2							
	T0	60.8	(53.4; 68.1)	28.7	(22.3; 35.2)	10.5	(8.85; 12.2)
	T1	51.0	(43.4; 58.6)	37.4	(30.7; 44.1)	11.7	(9.96; 13.4)
	T2	57.1	(49.2; 65.0)	31.8	(24.8; 38.8)	11.2	(9.44; 13.0)
	Mean differences						
	T1 - T0	**−9.78**	**(−17.3; −2.28)**	**8.63**	**(1.78; 15.5)**	1.16	(−0.34; 2.66)
	T2 - T0	−3.69	(−11.8; 4.40)	3.02	(−4.36; 10.4)	0.69	(−0.93; 2.31)
	T2 - T1	6.09	(−2.06; 14.3)	−5.61	(−13.1; 1.83)	−0.47	(−2.09; 1.16)

TABLE 3 | Results of linear mixed models in terms of Estimated means of sitting, standing, and stepping time in percentage (%) of total time during school breaks per intervention group and survey as well as differences of least-square means (LSM) for direct intervention effects (group 1: T1 – T0, group 2: T2 – T0) and differences across all surveys for $N = 134$ observations of $n = 48$ children.

		Sitting time in % during breaks		Standing time in % during breaks		Stepping time in % during breaks	
Group	**Survey**	**Estimate**	**95% CI**	**Estimate**	**95% CI**	**Estimate**	**95% CI**
Group 1							
	T0	28.7	(24.7; 32.8)	34.7	(37.1; 44.6)	36.7	(32.6; 40.8)
	T1	18.4	(14.0; 22.8)	40.9	(37.1; 44.6)	40.8	(36.4; 45.2)
	T2	17.0	(12.4; 21.6)	39.8	(35.9; 43.6)	43.2	(38.7; 47.7)
	Mean differences						
	T1 - T0	**−10.3**	**(−16.4; −4.25)**	**6.20**	**(1.37; 11.0)**	4.12	(−1.14; 9.37)
	T2 - T0	**−11.8**	**(−18.2; −5.31)**	5.11	(−0.03; 10.3)	**6.52**	**(0.92; 12.1)**
	T2 - T1	**−1.45**	**(−8.19; 5.29)**	−1.09	(−6.47; 4.29)	2.40	(−3.46; 8.26)
Group 2							
	T0	29.5	(25.1; 34.0)	30.9	(27.1; 34.6)	39.8	(35.3; 44.2)
	T1	17.7	(13.0; 22.4)	38.7	(34.7; 42.6)	43.8	(39.1; 48.4)
	T2	20.9	(15.9; 25.9)	38.9	(34.7; 43.2)	40.2	(35.3; 45.1)
	Mean differences						
	T1 - T0	**−11.8**	**(−18.0; −5.63)**	**7.82**	**(2.90; 12.7)**	4.01	(−1.34; 9.37)
	T2 - T0	**−8.59**	**(−15.2; −1.94)**	**8.08**	**(2.78; 13.4)**	0.44	(−5.33; 6.21)
	T2 - T1	3.23	(−3.52; 9.97)	0.26	(−5.11; 5.63)	−3.57	(−9.40; 2.26)

overall sedentary lifestyle (<50% sitting on average school days), compared to children with low fitness levels. To summarize, standing desks were able to reduce sitting, but did not enhance PA in terms of stepping. After installing standing desks, overall PA was not affected across survey periods and intervention effects did not differ by fitness levels. We also might preclude potential selection bias in terms of PA levels and body composition since basic characteristics of our study sample were comparable to other study populations (20). In particular, the proportion of overweight children was around 20% which is similar to other studies (33, 34) and most primary school children spent up to 10 h sedentary per day (17).

TABLE 4 | Results of linear mixed models in terms of Estimated means of sitting, standing, and stepping time in percentage (%) of total time during leisure time on weekdays per intervention group and survey as well as differences of least-square means (LSM) for direct intervention effects (group 1: T1 – T0, group 2: T2 – T0) and differences across all surveys for $N = 134$ observations of $n = 48$ children.

		Sitting time in % during leisure time		Standing time in % during leisure time		Stepping time in % during leisure time	
Group	**Survey**	**Estimate**	**95% CI**	**Estimate**	**95% CI**	**Estimate**	**95% CI**
Group 1							
	T0	51.4	(46.3; 56.6)	31.3	(27.7; 34.8)	17.3	(14.4; 20.2)
	T1	52.1	(46.6; 57.6)	30.2	(26.4; 34.0)	17.7	(14.6; 20.8)
	T2	50.9	(45.2; 56.6)	29.9	(26.0; 33.9)	19.2	(15.9; 22.4)
	Mean differences						
	T1 - T0	0.69	(−6.25; 7.62)	−1.04	(−5.71; 3.64)	0.36	(−3.73; 4.46)
	T2 - T0	−0.54	(−7.91; 6.84)	−1.33	(−6.31; 3.64)	1.83	(−2.53; 6.19)
	T2 - T1	−1.22	(−8.94; 6.50)	−0.30	(−5.51; 4.91)	1.47	(−3.09; 6.03)
Group 2							
	T0	55.2	(49.6; 60.9)	28.9	(24.9; 32.8)	15.9	(12.8; 19.1)
	T1	55.9	(50.1; 61.8)	28.5	(24.4; 32.6)	15.5	(12.2; 18.8)
	T2	58.7	(52.4; 64.9)	26.1	(21.8; 30.4)	15.2	(11.7; 18.7)
	Mean differences						
	T1 - T0	0.71	(−6.36; 7.77)	−0.32	(−5.09; 4.44)	−0.39	(−4.57; 3.78)
	T2 - T0	3.45	(−4.16; 11.1)	−2.75	(−7.88; 2.39)	−0.71	(−5.20; 3.79)
	T2 - T1	2.74	(−4.96; 10.4)	−2.42	(−7.61; 2.77)	−0.32	(−4.24; 4.87)

TABLE 5 | Results of linear mixed models in terms of Estimated means of sitting, standing, and stepping time in min./day of weekdays per intervention group and survey as well as differences of least-square means (LSM) for direct intervention effects (group 1: T1 – T0, group 2: T2 – T0) and differences across all surveys for $N = 134$ observations of $n = 48$ children.

		Average sitting time min./day		Average standing time min./day		Average stepping time min./day	
Group	**Survey**	**Estimate**	**95% CI**	**Estimate**	**95% CI**	**Estimate**	**95% CI**
Group 1							
	T0	422.9	(392.3; 453.5)	235.3	(212.1; 258.5)	140.3	(126.2; 154.4)
	T1	391.1	(358.7; 423.6)	260.4	(235.9; 285.0)	144.9	(129.9; 156.0)
	T2	416.7	(383.5; 450.0)	231.9	(206.7; 257.0)	149.9	(134.4; 165.3)
	Mean differences						
	T1 - T0	−31.7	(−67.7; 4.24)	25.1	(−1.60; 51.9)	4.62	(−12.9; 22.1)
	T2 - T0	−8.90	(−44.4; 32.1)	−9.76	(−55.1; 35.6)	9.56	(−9.07; 28.2)
	T2 - T1	25.5	(−14.5; 65.7)	−28.5	(−58.4; 1.30)	4.94	(−14.6; 24.5)
Group 2							
	T0	445.0	(411.2; 478.8)	217.7	(192.1; 243.3)	128.3	(112.7; 143.9)
	T1	425.6	(390.6; 460.6)	241.6	(215.1; 268.2)	131.1	(114.9; 147.3)
	T2	457.6	(421.0; 494.1)	212.9	(185.2; 240.6)	123.6	(106.6; 140.6)
	Mean differences						
	T1 - T0	−19.4	(−56.0; 17.3)	23.9	(−3.29; 51.2)	2.85	(−15.0; 20.7)
	T2 - T0	12.6	(−26.9; 52.0)	−4.80	(−34.2; 24.5)	−4.65	(−23.9; 14.6)
	T2 - T1	31.9	(−7.91; 71.7)	−28.7	(−58.3; 0.86)	−7.50	(−26.9; 11.9)

Similar to our findings, Verloigne et al. recently found a short-term intervention effect leading to decreased sitting time by installing standing desks in primary school children, but also highlighted that alternative study designs need to be explored and encouraging the continuous use of standing desks is necessary (20). In general, the observed high proportions spent sitting during lessons are typical for school children since they were obviously forced to sit about two thirds during lessons. However, children were likely to compensate their sedentary lesson time with activities such as standing and stepping during breaks (<30% sedentary). However, no compensatory effects such as lower or higher activity during leisure time was observed after installing standing desks, which is in line with the reviews of Kidokoro et al. (35) as well as Silva et al. (36). In contrast to our results, Kidokoro et al. found children to accumulate about 20 min more high-intensity PA per day, when having standing desks (35).

Since most standing desk interventions do not integrate strategies to increase high-intensity PA such as MVPA, such strong increases of MVPA are uncommon if the intervention was not focused on enhancing PA. Furthermore, the applied devices to assess PA (Actigraph accelerometers) are not the most robust monitor to reliably distinguish between sitting and standing (37).

Recent studies questioned the long-term effects of cost-effective structural interventions, that aim to change behavior without study personnel that regularly motivates to be physically active (38). Such an intervention was conducted by Silva et al. (36) who combined standings desks with teacher training and motivation sessions (36). By incorporating students and parents, they achieved significant decreases of sitting (−7%) and increase of standing (+30%) during school hours. This indicates beneficial effects for complementary behavioral strategies to maintain the use of standing desks as a change of daily lifestyle.

Strengths and Limitations

Main strength of this study was the objective PA measurement using activPAL monitors and the standardized study protocol. These devices have recently been shown to reliably quantify sitting and standing time in children (37). Since we wanted to particularly investigate within-day differences in specific domains rather than describing the "habitual" PA of a typical week by using accelerometry, we decided to use an uncommon inclusion criteria of 2 valid days of 10 h in order not to loose more participants. Further, we explored an alternative study design using the cross-over design that has rarely been evaluated (39). We may however not preclude that other intervention effects might be observed only by the cross-over design, since another study ($N = 27$) with a traditional control group (another classroom) showed significant decreases (∼10%) of sitting time (18). Due to the cross-over study design, whose advantages have recently been highlighted by Ee et al. (39), we were able to preclude effects by season and different teachers confounding the intervention effects. Until now, PF levels have not been highlighted as a potential confounder in recent reviews on this topic (16, 17). However, we need to acknowledge that PF was derived by assessing important, but only two components (explosive strength and endurance capacity) of PF. An important limitation is the follow-up duration of 3 months that only enables to summarize the observed effects that all children reduced sitting and increased standing time from baseline to T1 as a case of short-term reactivity. Finally, the small sample size was due to the limited number of standing desks affordable, which indeed is typical for most studies evaluating standing desks interventions (17, 35). Since our study was only conducted in the 3rd grade of one primary school, caution should be taken when generalizing our findings and more confounders appear to be relevant.

CONCLUSION

Providing height-adjustable standing desks in primary schools offers the opportunity to replace sedentary time during school hours by more active behavior such as standing during lessons and particularly during school breaks. When evaluating the compliance and effects of standing desk interventions, psychological (e.g., bandwagon effect) physiological (e.g., PF) should be taken into account in future studies. To increase and maintain the use of standing desks in primary children and working in a standing position during lessons needs to accompanied by motivational strategies.

ETHICS STATEMENT

The studies involving human participants were reviewed and approved by Institutional review board of the University of Bremen (19.09.2017). Written informed consent to participate in this study was provided by the participants' legal guardian/next of kin.

AUTHOR CONTRIBUTIONS

OS, AH, HG, and JB designed the study. OS and AH trained the study personnel. HG and JB conducted the field experiments. OS and CB drafted the manuscript and analyzed the data. All authors revised the paper and approved the final version.

ACKNOWLEDGMENTS

The authors thank all participating children, parents, the primary school Osterholzschule and their teachers for supporting the present study. In particular, we need to thank the City of Ludwigsburg for providing the height-adjustable standing desks. The authors would also like to thank everyone who helped with the data collection. The publication of this article was funded by the Open Access Fund of the Leibniz Association.

REFERENCES

WHO. *Global Recommendations on Physical Activity for Health.* Geneva: World Health Organization (2010).

Demetriou Y, Hebestreit A, Reimers AK, Schlund A, Niessner C, Schmidt S, et al. Results from Germany's 2018. Report card on physical activity for children and youth. *J Phys Act Health.* (2018) 15:S363–5. doi: 10.1123/jpah.2018-0538

Suchert V, Hanewinkel R, Isensee B. Sedentary behavior and indicators of mental health in school-aged children and adolescents: a systematic review. *Prev Med.* (2015) 76:48–57. doi: 10.1016/j.ypmed.2015. 03.026

Chinapaw MJ, Proper KI, Brug J, van Mechelen W, Singh AS. Relationship between young peoples' sedentary behaviour and biomedical health indicators: a systematic review of prospective studies. *Obesity Rev.* (2011) 12:e621–32. doi: 10.1111/j.1467–789X.2011. 00865.x

Chinapaw M, Altenburg T, Brug J. Sedentary behaviour and health in children - evaluating the evidence. *Prev Med.* (2015) 70:1–2. doi: 10.1016/j.ypmed.2014.10.029

Biddle SJ, Pearson N, Ross GM, Braithwaite R. Tracking of sedentary behaviours of young people: a systematic review. *Prev Med.* (2010) 51:345–51. doi:10.1016/j.ypmed.2010.07.018

World Health Organization. *WHO Guidelines on Physical Activity and Sedentary Behaviour for Children and Adolescents, Adults and Older Adults.* World Health Organization (2020).

Carson V, Hunter S, Kuzik N, Gray CE, Poitras VJ, Chaput JP, et al. Systematic review of sedentary behaviour and health indicators in school-aged children and youth: an update. *Appl Physiol Nutr Metab.* (2016) 41(6 Suppl. 3):S240–65. doi: 10.1139/apnm-2015–0630

Cooper AR, Goodman A, Page AS, Sherar LB, Esliger DW, van Sluijs EM, et al. Objectively measured physical activity and sedentary time in youth: the International children's accelerometry database (ICAD). *Int J Behav Nutr Phys Act.* (2015) 12:113. doi: 10.1186/s12966-015- 0274–5

Tremblay MS, LeBlanc AG, Kho ME, Saunders TJ, Larouche R, Colley RC, et al. Systematic review of sedentary behaviour and health indicators in school-aged children and youth. *Int J Behav Nutr Phys Act.* (2011) 8:98. doi: 10.1186/1479–5868-8–98

Harding SK, Page AS, Falconer C, Cooper AR. Longitudinal changes in sedentary time and physical activity during adolescence. *Int J Behav Nutr Phys Act.* (2015) 12:44. doi: 10.1186/s12966–015-0204–6

Janssen X, Mann KD, Basterfield L, Parkinson KN, Pearce MS, Reilly JK, et al. Development of sedentary behavior across childhood and adolescence: longitudinal analysis of the gateshead millennium study. *Int J Behav Nutr Phys Act.* (2016) 13:88. doi: 10.1186/s12966-016- 0413–7

Sprengeler O, Wirsik N, Hebestreit A, Herrmann D, Ahrens W. Domain- specific self-reported and objectively measured physical activity in children. *Int J Environ Res Public Health.* (2017) 14:242. doi: 10.3390/ijerph140 30242

Konstabel K, Veidebaum T, Verbestel V, Moreno LA, Bammann K, Tornaritis M, et al. Objectively measured physical activity in European children: the IDEFICS study. *Int J Obes.* (2014) 38(Suppl. 2):S135–43. doi: 10.1038/ijo.2014.144

Rütten A, Abu-Omar K, Messing S, Weege M, Pfeifer K, Geidl W, et al. How can the impact of national recommendations for physical activity be increased? Experiences from Germany. *Health Res Policy Syst.* (2018) 16:121. doi: 10.1186/s12961–018-0396–8

Minges KE, Chao AM, Irwin ML, Owen N, Park C, Whittemore, et al. Classroom standing desks and sedentary behavior a systematic review. *Pediatrics.* (2016) 137:1–18. doi: 10.1542/peds.2015- 3087

Sherry AP, Pearson N, Clemes SA. The effects of standing desks within the school classroom: a systematic review. *Prev Med Rep.* (2016) 3:338–47. doi:10.1016/j.pmedr.2016.03.016

Clemes SA, Barber SE, Bingham DD, Ridgers ND, Fletcher E, Pearson N, et al. Reducing children's classroom sitting time using sit-to-stand desks: findings from pilot studies in UK and Australian primary schools. *J Public Health.* (2016) 38:526–33. doi: 10.1093/pubmed/ fdv084

Hinckson EA, Aminian S, Ikeda E, Stewart T, Oliver M, Duncan S, et al. Acceptability of standing workstations in elementary schools: a pilot study. *Prev Med.* (2013) 56:82–5. doi: 10.1016/j.ypmed.2012. 10.014

Verloigne M, Ridgers ND, De Bourdeaudhuij I, Cardon G. Effect and process evaluation of implementing standing desks in primary and secondary schools in Belgium: a cluster-randomised controlled trial. *Int J Behav Nutr Phys Act.* (2018) 15:94. doi: 10.1186/s12966–018- 0726–9

Maclure M, Mittleman MA. Should we use a case-crossover design? *Ann Rev Public Health.* (2000) 21:193–221. doi: 10.1146/annurev.publhealth.2 1.1.193

Ridgers ND, Salmon J, Ridley K, O'Connell E, Arundell L, Timperio Agreement between activPAL and actiGraph for assessing children's sedentary time. *Int J Behav Nutr Phys Act.* (2012) 9:15. doi: 10.1186/1479- 5868-9–15

Aminian S, Hinckson EA. Examining the validity of the activPAL monitor in measuring posture and ambulatory movement in children. *Int J Behav Nutr Phys Act.* (2012) 9:119. doi: 10.1186/1479–5868-9–119

Alghaeed Z, Reilly JJ, Chastin SF, Martin A, Davies G, Paton JY. The influence of minimum sitting period of the activPAL on the measurement of breaks in sitting in young children. *PLoS ONE.* (2013) 8:e71854. doi: 10.1371/journal.pone.0071854

Bassett DR, Jr, John D, Conger SA, Rider BC, Passmore RM, et al. Detection of lying down, sitting, standing, and stepping using two activPAL monitors. *Med Sci Sports Exerc.* (2014) 46:2025–9. doi: 10.1249/MSS.0000000000 000326

UNESCO. *International Standard Classification of Education.* (2010). Available online at: www.uis.unesco.org (accessed March 15, 2020).

Nagy P, Kovacs E, Moreno LA, Veidebaum T, Tornaritis M, Kourides Y, et al. Percentile reference values for anthropometric body composition indices in European children from the IDEFICS study. *Int J Obes.* (2014) 38(Suppl. 2):S15–25. doi: 10.1038/ijo.2014.131

Bammann K, Sioen I, Huybrechts I, Casajus JA, Vicente-Rodriguez G, Cuthill R, et al. The IDEFICS validation study on field methods for assessing physical activity and body composition in children: design and data collection. *Int J Obes.* (2011) 35(Suppl. 1):S79–87. doi: 10.1038/ijo. 2011.38

Kromeyer-Hauschild K, Wabitsch M, Kunze D, Geller F, Geiß HC, Hesse V, et al. Perzentile für den body-mass-index für das kindes- und jugendalter unter heranziehung verschiedener deutscher stichproben. *Monatsschrift Kinderheilkunde.* (2001) 149:807–18. doi: 10.1007/s001120170107

De Miguel-Etayo P, Gracia-Marco L, Ortega FB, Intemann T, Foraita R, Lissner L, et al. Physical fitness reference standards in European children: the IDEFICS study. *Int J Obes.* (2014) 38(Suppl. 2):S57–66. doi: 10.1038/ijo.2014.136

Lawrenz W, Stemper T. Vergleich von 6-Minuten-Lauf-Test und maximaler sauerstoffaufnahme von 8–10- jährigen schulkindern. *Deutsche Zeitschrift für Sportmedizin.* (2012) 2012:102–5. doi: 10.5960/dzsm.2012.012

Howard J. *Cognitive Errors and Diagnostic Mistakes.* Cham: Springer International Publishing AG, part of Springer Nature (2019).

Ahrens W, Pigeot I, Pohlabeln H, De Henauw S, Lissner L, Molnar D, et al. Prevalence of overweight and obesity in European children below the age of 10. *Int J Obes.* (2014) 38(Suppl. 2):S99–107. doi: 10.1038/ijo.20 14.140

Garrido-Miguel M, Oliveira A, Cavero-Redondo I, Alvarez- Bueno C, Pozuelo-Carrascosa DP, Soriano-Cano A, et al. Prevalence of overweight and obesity among European preschool children: a systematic review and meta-regression by food group consumption. *Nutrients.* (2019) 11:1698. doi: 10.3390/nu110 71698

Kidokoro T, Shimizu Y, Edamoto K, Annear M. Classroom standing desks and time-series variation in sedentary behavior and physical activity among primary school children. *Int J Environ Res Public Health.* (2019) 16:1892. doi: 10.3390/ijerph16111892

Silva DR, Minderico CS, Pinto F, Collings PJ, Cyrino ES, Sardinha LB. Impact of a classroom standing desk intervention on daily objectively measured sedentary behavior and physical activity in youth. *J Sci Med Sport.* (2018) 21:919–24. doi: 10.1016/j.jsams.2018.01.007

Ridley K, Ridgers ND, Salmon J. Criterion validity of the activPAL and actiGraph for assessing children's sitting and standing time in a school classroom setting. *Int J Behav Nutr Phys Act.* (2016) 13:75. doi: 10.1186/s12966–016-0402-x

Abu-Omar K, Rütten A, Messing S, Pfeifer K, Ungerer-Röhrich U, Goodwin L, et al. The German recommendations for physical activity promotion. *J Public Health.* (2018) 27:613–27. doi: 10.1007/s10389-018-0 986–5

Ee J, Parry S, Oliveira BI, McVeigh JA, Howie E, Straker L. Does a classroom standing desk intervention modify standing and sitting behaviour and musculoskeletal symptoms during school time and physical activity during waking time? *Int J Environ Res Public Health.* (2018) 15:1668. doi: 10.3390/ijerph15081668

Interpersonal Dynamics in 2-vs-1 Contexts of Football: The Effects of Field Location and Player Roles

*Timo Laakso[1], Keith Davids[2], Jarmo Liukkonen[1] and Bruno Travassos[3]**

[1]Department of Sport Sciences, University of Jyväskylä, Jyväskylä, Finland, [2]Centre for Sports Engineering Research, Sheffield Hallam University, Sheffield, United Kingdom, [3]CreativeLab, Research Center for Sports Sciences, Health Sciences and Human Development (CIDESD), Universidade da Beira Interior, Covilhã, Portugal

***Correspondence:**
Bruno Travassos
bfrt@ubi.pt

This study analyzed the spatial-temporal interactions that sustained 2-vs-1 contexts in football at different field locations near the goal. Fifteen male players (under 15 years, age 13.2 ± 1.03 years, years of practice 4.2 ± 1.10 years), 5 defenders, 7 midfielders, and 3 attackers, participated in the study. Each participant performed a game to simulate a 2-vs-1 sub-phase as a ball carrier, second attacker, and defender at three different field locations, resulting in a total number of 142 trials. The movements of participants in each trial were recorded and digitized with TACTO software. Values of interpersonal distance between the ball carrier and defender and interpersonal angles between players and between the goal target, defender, and ball carrier were calculated. The results revealed a general main effect of field location. Generally, the middle zone revealed the lowest values of interpersonal distance and angle between players and the right zone and the highest values of interpersonal distance between players and interpersonal angle between players and the goal. Related with participants' roles, defenders revealed subtle differences as attackers on interpersonal distances and relative angles compared with midfielders and attackers. Findings supported that field location is a key constraint of players' performance and that players' role constraint performance effectiveness in football.

Keywords: football, patterns of play, affordances, effectiveness, players' roles

INTRODUCTION

Team sports have been investigated, as complex adaptive systems, with the aim of describing and explaining emergent behaviors of players from an ecological dynamics perspective. This approach requires analysis of the continuous interactions between attacking and defending players who, fundamentally, compete to gain/retain possession of the ball and move it into favorable attacking positions in critical scoring spaces in the playing area (Araújo and Davids, 2016). McGarry (2009) highlighted the dynamical nature of these continuous interactions, which can be observed at different levels of analysis from the entire competitive context to relevant game sub-phases (i.e., 1-vs-1, 2-vs-1, 3-vs-2, etc.). For this reason, a team game has been conceptualized as a complex adaptive system whose behaviors are driven or perturbed by interactions of multiple, smaller sub-systems composed of attackers and defenders interacting under constraints (Travassos et al., 2013b). For instance, research has highlighted specific contextual performance constraints that change the emergent behaviors of players and teams. These task constraints include the number of players involved (Silva et al., 2014), the field dimensions (Vilar et al., 2014a), the number of goals (Travassos et al., 2014a), or even contextual performance constraints such as game pace or match outcome (Sampaio et al., 2013).

In line with the ecological dynamics perspective, the adaptive behaviors of players and teams to constant changes in contextual constraints is a result of information exchanges among the competing and cooperating players in relation to game demands (Travassos et al., 2012; Folgado et al., 2018). That is, players and teams constantly interact to create information, make decisions, and organize actions when functioning as a team during competitive performance. This view of competitive performance in teams, in ecological dynamics, is based on the sharing of spatial-temporal information that continuously supports the utilization of individual, sub-group, and team affordances (i.e., possibilities or opportunities for action to achieve a specific performance goal) (Silva et al., 2013). For each individual, as well as collective sub-systems, evidence has revealed that affordances are sustained by variations in space-time relations defined by the co-positioning of teammates and opponents, co-variations in their displacement trajectories and their movement velocities with respect to field markings and dimensions, and the location of scoring targets like goals, baskets, and try lines, for example (Vilar et al., 2012b; Silva et al., 2013; Gesbert et al., 2017). Also, players who have different team roles usually exhibit different physical, technical, and tactical capabilities (also effectivities) during performance (Varley et al., 2017; Lovell et al., 2018) and, consequently, explore and use the space-time relations in a different way for the identification of affordances for play (Laakso et al., 2017; Baptista et al., 2018). Previous research revealed that manipulating players' roles constraint the spatial-temporal patterns of play from 1-vs-1 (Laakso et al., 2017) to 7-vs-7 (Baptista et al., 2018).

Research investigations have explored and exemplified these ideas in many different team sports including basketball (Araújo et al., 2006; Esteves et al., 2012), rugby union (Passos et al., 2008), Futsal (Travassos et al., 2012; Vilar et al., 2013b), and also in association football (Duarte et al., 2012; Clemente et al., 2013; Laakso et al., 2017).

In the context of association football, research findings have revealed that attackers need to lead the interactions in spatial-temporal relations with defenders, by promoting unpredictable changes in the values of key variables such interpersonal distance, relative angles with players and with the goal, and relative velocity to achieve successful outcomes (Schulze et al., 2018). On the other hand, defenders try to constrain attackers' actions and maintain spatial-temporal equilibrium with them to enhance sub-system stability and successfully perform (Duarte et al., 2012; Clemente et al., 2013). That is, evidence suggests how attackers vary key movement displacement parameters to de-stabilize an "unwanted" symmetrical relationship with a marking defender in a dyad. In contrast, defenders use actions to maintain system stability and prevent attackers from breaking up their temporary dyad.

As previously reported, the field location of these ongoing interactions has a substantial effect to constrain the spatial-temporal relations in attacker-defender dyadic systems (Headrick et al., 2011; Vilar et al., 2012c; Laakso et al., 2017). Variations in proximity to the goal area or in field "longitudinal corridors of play" (middle or wing zones) result in emergence of different coordination dynamics of key variables like relative distance and the angle between an attacker and defender in relation to the goal (Headrick et al., 2011; Laakso et al., 2017). Although the effects of these constraints are clear, previous studies have mainly reported their influence in 1-vs-1 sub-phases of play.

In most team games, attackers try to gain an advantage by rapidly creating a temporary numerical overload against defenders in a specific location of the field. Particularly in association football, the creation of offensive or defensive numerical superiority near the ball is directly related to successful performance in terms of attacking space behind a defensive line or in recovering the ball (Vilar et al., 2013a). Thus, the 2-vs-1 sub-phase is the minimum sub-phase of game that represents such numerical (overload) advantage to an attacking team. During this sub-phase, the ball carrier and the support attacker need to manage the spatial-temporal relations with an immediate opponent to support emergence of two possibilities for action: (s)he can dribble and face the defender in a 1-vs-1 if the defender is protecting a passing line to the second attacker or (s)he can draw the defender and pass the ball to the support attacker if a passing line emerges by the defender being drawn toward the ball dribbler. Despite its relevance for understanding the spatial-temporal changes that support the emergence of possibilities for action in overloads, little research has been conducted to observe actual competitive interactions during performance in this important sub-phase. In addition, there is a need to improve understanding of how interpersonal patterns of coordination between attackers and a defender in 2-vs-1 sub-phases are influenced by field location effects relative to the goal. A key issue is whether a defender changes co-positioning behavior, when constrained by the field location in football. Clear implications for practice could result from this study. The implications of the manipulation of the relative position of the goal target (Coutinho et al., 2018) in relation to the 2-vs-1 sub-phases or the attacker-defender participants' performance roles (Laakso et al., 2017) allow coaches to improve the design of practice tasks according to the planned goals. Also, in line with previous studies, this study will allow to identify the task constraints that coaches can stress to improve players' decision and action according to each task condition (Correia et al., 2012). Thus, the aim of this study was to analyze the adaptive behaviors of players who sustained 2-vs-1 sub-phases in football at different field locations near the goal (left, middle, and right zones on field) and manipulate participants' team performance roles (i.e., divided into roles as attackers, midfielders, and defenders). In line with previous research in 1-vs-1 sub-phases (Laakso et al., 2017), we expected to observe changes in interpersonal distances and relative angles between players and the goal at different field location with high correlations between interpersonal distances and angles for right and left zones and low correlations in middle zone. Also, it was expected changes in interpersonal distances according to participants' team performance roles as attackers or defenders on the emergent spatial-temporal patterns of interaction in the 2-vs-1 sub-phase.

MATERIALS AND METHODS

Participants

Fifteen male players (under 15 years, age 13.2 ± 1.03 years, years of practice 4.2 ± 1.10 years) participated in this study. The sample size was calculated with G*Power (Version 3.1.5.1 Institut für Experimentelle Psychologie, Düsseldorf, Germany) for an effect size of 0.7, an α of 0.05, and a power of 0.8 (1–β). The total sample size computed by this method was a minimum of 15 players with a statistical power of 82.4%.

For the purposes of analysis, with the advice of the coaching staff, the participants were categorized into their main team performance role, resulting in sub-samples of five defenders (center-backs and full-backs), seven midfielders (center midfielders, lateral midfielders), and three attackers (forwards). All players belong to one youth team competing in a national Finnish level (2016/2017 season). All participants were right-footed and played in the first team of the club. The participants participated in five training sessions per week (90 min per session) and played an official competitive match at the weekend. The club, all parents, and the participants provided prior informed and written consent for participation in the study. The study was approved by the Ethics Committee of University of Jyväskylä according to the Declaration of Helsinki.

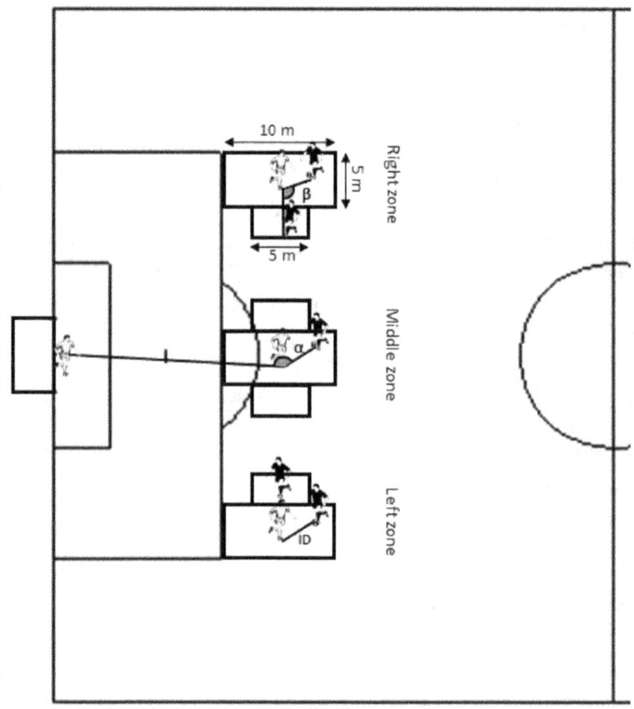

FIGURE 1 | Representation of the three areas of play (left, middle, right) of ball carrier and defender and the area of second attacker and their location in relation to the goal. α – interpersonal angle between ball carrier, defender and second attacker (IABDA); β – interpersonal angle between goal target, defender and ball carrier (IAGDB); ID – interpersonal distance between ball carrier and defender.

Task and Procedures

All players were tested during four sessions in 1 week of summer break of competitive season (July) in an artificial grass pitch. The temperature was about 17–19°. The first session was used for the players being familiarized with task conditions in all field zones, and the three next sessions were used for testing purposes. Each participant performed in a game to simulate a 2-vs-1 sub-phase as a ball carrier, second attacker, and defender at three different field locations. The 2-vs-1 sub-phases occurred in a predefined area of 10 × 5 m (Passos et al., 2008; Headrick et al., 2011) in three different field locations (Left, middle and right) under competitive performance conditions (See **Figure 1**). The task constraints included a regular size goal (2.44 m × 7.32 m) with a goalkeeper. The starting distance between attacker and defender was 3 m. When performing in the left or on the right side of the field, the second attacker was placed in the inner side of the field in order to maintain free the wing for a possible dribble. That is, when in the right-side zone of the field, the second attacker was placed to the left of ball carrier, and when in the left zone, to the right of ball carrier. In the middle zone, the second attacker was placed at the side of the first attacker's non-dominant foot. The area for the second attacker to move was 5 × 1.30 m (**Figure 1**). Before practice, all the players were informed about the rules and the goals of the tasks and encouraged to compete like in the game. The goalkeepers were also informed to act as in a competitive game. No coach feedback or encouragement was allowed during the conditions.

Before data collection, all participants engaged in a thorough warm-up routine. Each trial started when both the attacking and defending participants were ready in their starting positions and the attacking participant was requested to start the trial. As soon as the attacker moved the ball, the defender could start defending. After crossing the midline of the playing area (5 m from the end of attacking area), the attacker could dribble or pass the ball to the second attacker. The performance aim of attacking participants was to dribble past the defender and shoot to the goal or pass the ball to the second attacker who could shoot at goal. If these events occurred, the trial was over. The aim of the defender was to prevent the attackers from scoring a goal, within the laws of the game. The trial was considered over when defending participants intercepted the ball or when the ball moved outside the borders of the playing area. A regulation ball size 5 was used in all trials.

All participants performed the 2-vs-1 trials in all three zones acting as an attacker and as a defender, resulting in a total number of 142 trials. In each trial, two attacking players with the same positional roles attacking one defending player with a different positional role (e.g., Defender + Defender vs Midfielder or Midfielder + Midfielder vs Attacker). After each trial, the attacking teams and the opposition change to promote variability in pairs and roles in next trials. Any player performed two consecutive trials in the same zone nor playing with the same pair, or opponent. Participants rest about 3–4 min between trials to avoid fatigue. All trials were randomly allocated between left, middle, and right zones, comprising 50 trials in the left zone, 41 in the middle, and 51 in the right performance area. The experimental protocol allowed us to analyze the effects of participants' performance roles in attack, and the distribution of trials by role was defenders (49 trials), midfielders (45 trials), and attackers (48 trials).

Participant movements were captured by using a single digital video camera (Sony HRX-MC50E) placed 4 m above ground forming an angle of approximately 45° with the longitudinal axis of the performance area to capture participant movements during the whole experimental task. All video recordings captured the displacement trajectories of all participants without moving the camera. The movements of participants in each trial were digitized with TACTO software at 25 Hz (Fernandes and Malta, 2007; Duarte et al., 2010). The displacement trajectories of the participants and the ball were tracked using a computer mouse, by following, in every frame, a working point located between players' feet on the ground plan. After calibration of the pitch, with real measures of six control points for each zone (4 corners of the zone of play, and the two goalposts position), the x and y virtual coordinates of the players were extracted. The obtained virtual coordinates were transformed into real coordinates using the direct linear transformation method (2D-DLT) to avoid parallax error and filtered with a Butterworth low pass filter (6 Hz) to reduce the noise of the process of digitizing (Winter, 2005).

Reliability of the Digitizing Procedure

Fifteen trials were selected at random and the displacement trajectories of attackers and defenders ($n = 45$) were re-digitized after 1 month by the same experimenter. Intra-digitizer reliability values were assessed using technical error of measurement (TEM) and coefficient of reliability (R) statistics (for details see Goto and Mascie-Taylor, 2007). The intra-TEM yielded values of 0.235 m (2.25%) with a corresponding coefficient of reliability ($R = 0.991$).

Variables

According to our purposes, the interpersonal distance between the ball carrier and defender (ID) was calculated. Also, the interpersonal angles between (1) ball carrier, defender, and second attacker (IABDA) and (2) between the goal target (the center of the goal in order to maintain the reference fixed and allow a better understanding of the relationships between players and the goal), defender, and ball carrier (IAGDB) were calculated to investigate changes in interpersonal interactions between participants in the 2-vs-1 performance contexts (See **Figure 1**; Vilar et al., 2014a; Laakso et al., 2017).

Data Analysis

Descriptive statistics were reported for all performance measures recorded. Comparisons between field zones and participants' roles were assessed using standardized mean differences with 90% confidence intervals. The smallest worthwhile differences were estimated from the standardized units multiplied by 0.2 (Hopkins et al., 2009; Cumming, 2012). Effect size statistics were reported using the following ranges: trivial (0–0.19); small (0.2–0.59); moderate (0.6–1.19); large (1.2–1.99); and very large (≥2.0). Magnitudes of clear effects were considered at the following scale: 25–75%, possibly; 75–95%, likely; 95–99%, very likely; >99%, most likely (observed effects were represented by –ive and +ive directions) (Hopkins et al., 2009). Correlation values between variables were accessed through Pearson correlation using SPSS 22.0 software (IBM SPSS Inc., Chicago, USA). Thresholds for correlation coefficients (r) were: 0.30, small; 0.49, moderate; 0.69, large; 0.89, very large; and 1.00, near perfect (Hopkins et al., 2009).

RESULTS

Effects of Field Location

Analysis of ID revealed main effects for field zones. Small higher values were observed in comparisons of the left to middle zone (likely –ive). Moderate higher values were observed in comparisons of middle to right zone (very likely +ive). Unclear values were observed in comparisons of left to right zone (unclear). Generally, the middle zone revealed the lowest ID values, while the right zone revealed the highest ID values (see **Table 1** and **Figure 2**).

Analysis of IABDA revealed main effects for field zones. Moderate higher values were observed in comparisons of left to middle zone (very likely –ive). Small higher values were observed in comparisons of middle zone to right zone

TABLE 1 | Descriptive statistics and differences in means for field location and players' roles.

	(Mean ± SD)			Difference in means (d; 90% CL)		
			Field location			
Variables	**Left**	**Middle**	**Right**	**Left vs Middle**	**Left vs Right**	**Middle vs Right**
ID (meters)	3.21 ± 1.42	2.68 ± 1.49	3.67 ± 1.73	−0.35 [−0.7–0.01]	0.28 [−0.04 0.62]	0.60 [0.26 0.95]
IABDA (degrees)	121.34 ± 20.57	107.77 ± 22.28	115.94 ± 23.22	−0.63 [−0.98–0.27]	−0.24 [−0.57 0.608]	0.36 [0.01 0.07]
IAGDB (degrees)	122.9 ± 20.76	135.72 ± 23.87	140.40 ± 17.12	0.57 [0.22 0.92]	0.91 [0.58 1.24]	0.22 [−0.13 0.57]
			Players' role			
Variables	**Defenders**	**Midfielders**	**Attackers**	**Defenders vs Midfielders**	**Defenders vs Attackers**	**Midfielders vs Attackers**
ID (meters)	3.75 ± 1.81	3.30 ± 1.59	2.77 ± 1.13	−0.26 [−0.6 0.07]	−0.65 [−0.98–0.31]	−0.38 [−0.73–0.04]
IABDA (degrees)	120.83 ± 19.88	110.45 ± 19.22	114.74 ± 26.86	−0.52 [−4.7 3.62]	−0.25 [−3.69 3.18]	0.18 [−3.29 3.66]
IAGDB (degrees)	131.71 ± 20.55	136.77 ± 20.35	130.45 ± 24.07	0.24 [−3.72 4.21]	−0.06 [−3.67 3.57]	−0.28 [−3.92 3.36]

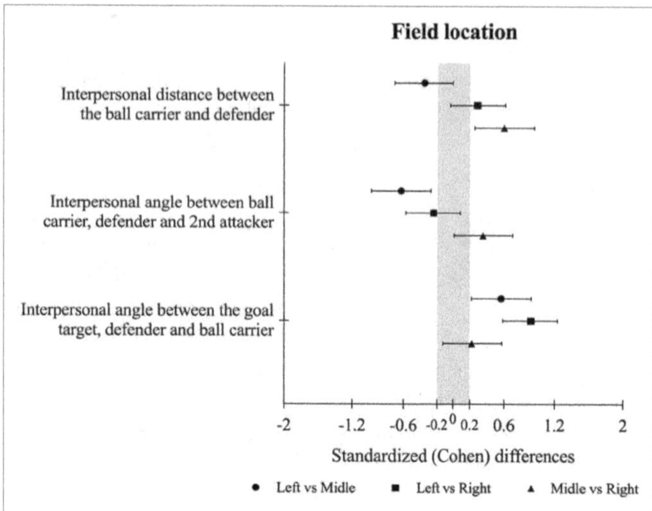

FIGURE 2 | Standardized (Cohen) differences of ID, IABDA, and IAGDB for field zones (left vs. middle vs. right).

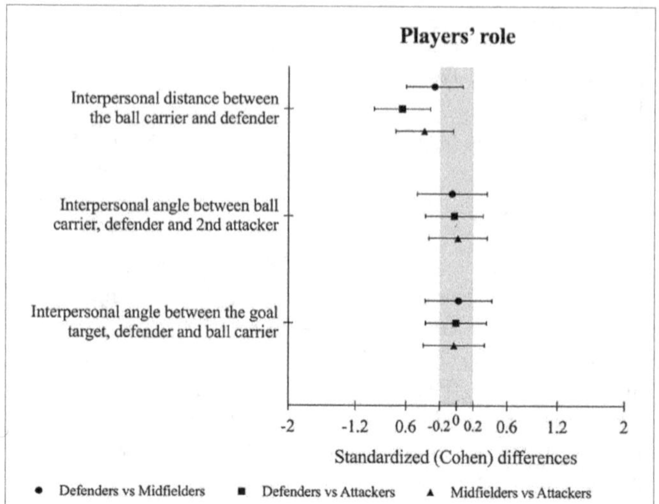

FIGURE 3 | Standardized (Cohen) differences of ID, IABDA, and IAGDB for players' role (defenders vs. midfielders vs. attackers).

(likely +ive). Unclear values were observed in comparisons of left to right zone (unclear). Generally, the left zone revealed higher values of IABDA, while the middle zone revealed lower values (see **Table 1** and **Figure 2**).

Analysis of IAGDB revealed main effects for field zones. Small lower values were observed in comparisons of left to middle zone (very likely +ive). Unclear values were observed in comparisons of middle to right zone (unclear). Moderate higher values were observed in comparisons of left to right zone (most likely +ive). Generally, the right zone revealed the higher values and the left zone revealed the lower values of IAGDB (see **Table 1** and **Figure 2**).

Analysis of relationships between ID, IABDA, and IAGDB for each field zone revealed interesting effects. In the left field zone, a large negative correlation was revealed between ID and IABDA values [r = −0.76, R^2 = 0.57 (90%CI: −0.84 to −0.64), most likely −ive], a large positive correlation between ID and IAGDB values [r = 0.72, R^2 = 0.52 (90%CI: 0.59–0.82), most likely +ive], and a moderate negative correlation between IABDA and IAGDB values [r = −0.46, R^2 = 0.21 (90%CI: −0.62 to −0.24), most likely −ive]. On the right, an unclear correlation was revealed between ID and IABDA values [r = 0.08, R^2 = 0.01 (90%CI: −0.16 to 0.31), unclear], a large negative correlation between ID and IAGDB values [r = −0.70, R^2 = 0.48 (90%CI: −0.8 to −0.55), most likely −ive], and a moderate negative correlation between IABDA and IAGDB values [r = −0.56, R^2 = 0.31 (90%CI: −0.7 to −0.37), most likely −ive]. In the middle zone, a near perfect positive correlation was revealed between ID and IABDA values [r = 0.93, R^2 = 0.87 (90%CI: 0.9 to 0.96), most likely +ive], and unclear correlations between ID and IAGDB [r = 0.15, R^2 = 0.02 (90%CI: −0.37 to 0.1), unclear] and IABDA and IAGDB values [r = 0.10, R^2 = 0.02 (90%CI: −0.14 to 0.33), unclear].

Effects of Players' Roles

Analysis of players' roles, as attacking players, revealed subtle changes in emergent interpersonal coordination tendencies (see **Table 1** and **Figure 3**). When defenders acted as attacking players, small higher values of ID were observed compared to midfielders (possibly −ive) and a moderate higher ID was observed compared to attackers (very likely −ive). Also, when midfielders acted as attacking players, small higher ID values were observed compared to attackers (possibly −ive). No other effects on IABDA and IAGDB were revealed in analysis of effects of players' roles when participants acted as attacking players (see **Table 1** and **Figure 3**). Analyses of relationships between ID, IABDA, and IAGDB for each player role were unclear.

DISCUSSION

The aim of the present study was to analyze the adaptive behaviors of players who sustained 2-vs-1 sub-phases in football at different field locations near the goal (left-, middle- and right- zones on field) and manipulate participants' team performance roles (i.e., divided into roles as attackers, midfielders, and defenders). As expected, results indicated a main effect of field location and a subtle effect of participants' roles on spatial-temporal coordination tendencies in the 2-vs-1 sub-phases. Generally, the findings reinforced effects noted in previous studies on performer interactions in football (Laakso et al., 2017).

Effect of Field Locations

Field location was confirmed as an important constraint on interpersonal coordination of players, not just in 1-vs-1 sub-phases (Headrick et al., 2011; Laakso et al., 2017) but also in 2-vs-1 sub-phases of football. As observed in performance context (Schulze et al., 2018), according to changes in field zones of performance, the relationship between values of interpersonal distances and relative angles between players and the goal revealed different relational dynamics. Analysis of interactions in the middle zone revealed lower values for ID and IABDA (near 1–10°) and medium values (near 135°) for IAGDB. These findings contrasted with data reported in previous research on performance in 1-vs-1 sub phases, in which higher values of ID and greater relative angles between players and the goal were observed in the middle zone, compared to performance in the other zones. In 2-vs-1 sub-phases, the additional teammate increases the available affordances for the ball carrier (dribbling, shooting, passing), not allowing the defender to perform as conservatively. Thus, defenders tried to cope with the increase in affordances for attackers by dividing their efforts to occupy passing lines and inhibit the emergence of dribbling/shooting lines for the ball carrier (Vilar et al., 2012c). The near perfect correlation values observed in mid zone between ID and IABDA variables reinforced such an interpretation. Similar results have been observed in previous research (Travassos et al., 2014b; Vilar et al., 2014b).

When a defending team performing with a numerical disadvantage usually adopts a zonal defense to simultaneously occupy space and close down options for the ball carrier at the same time (Travassos et al., 2014a). That is, the defenders or even the defensive team seeks to co-position themselves to mark the opponents and the space at the same time, inhibiting the emergence of the most advantageous affordances for attackers. This strategy of defenders can be explained by an attempt to adapt to the emerging informational constraints of the 2-vs-1 sub-phase, increasing the time for ball carriers to interact, that is, explore, decide, and perform actions (van Andel et al., 2017).

Observations of performance in left and right field zones revealed contrasting findings. Analysis of performance in the left zone revealed mid values for ID, higher values for IABDA, and lower values for IAGDB. In opposition, analysis of performance in the right zone revealed higher values for ID, mid values for IABDA, and higher values for IAGDB. These performance observations may be related to the fact that all the players were right-footed, constraining possibilities for the ball carrier to explore affordances for shooting or passing, consequently allowing different affordances for defenders (Paterson et al., 2016). It is worth noting that the ball carriers' preferred foot was the "outside" foot on the right field zone, providing the ball carrier with affordances to typically pass the defender on the right side. This affordance typically constrained the interactions for the defending players so that they could focus more on their alignment with the goal (IAGDB). These adaptations allowed defenders to maintain a large ID to provide an affordance for the ball carrier to dribble to the right and shoot at goal from the "outside" (with a narrow angle to the goal). The negative correlations between ID and IAGDB values support the use of this functional defensive strategy. It suggests that when the defender presses the ball carrier, he is seeking to maintain symmetry of the system with the goal to ensure that he could not shoot at goal with the preferred foot.

In contrast, in the left field zone, the starting position of the second attacking player was on the right side of the area. In this case, the ball carrier tried to open space to explore a dribble to the middle or to open a passing line to the second attacker. While this was happening, the defender sought to constrain the ball carrier to drive to the left and use the preferred foot and, simultaneously, seeking to occupy the passing line to the second attacker. These interactions were driven by increases in IABDA and decreases in IAGDB values. The emergent negative correlations between ID and IABDA and the positive correlations between ID and IAGDB supported the use of this defensive strategy. When a defender presses the ball carrier, a major aim is to cut the passing line from the ball carrier to the second attacker, increasing the value of IABDA and temporarily decreasing alignment with the goal. These dynamical interactions suggest that the exploration of affordances by attackers and defenders, during performance, was context-dependent and forged by variations in spatial-temporal relations between players (Vilar et al., 2012b; Silva et al., 2013; Gesbert et al., 2017) and their own effectivities (Silva et al., 2013; Paterson et al., 2016). Also, the findings clearly revealed how the location of the scoring target acted as a powerful constraint on emergent interpersonal spatial-temporal interactions of players and teams in football (Headrick et al., 2011; Vilar et al., 2012c; Laakso et al., 2017).

Effect of Team Roles

As expected, the participants' main performance roles constrained interpersonal coordination tendencies in the 2-vs-1 sub-phases. However, only subtle changes were revealed, particularly for defenders, compared with midfielders and attackers (Laakso et al., 2017). Compared to midfielders and attackers, defenders usually displayed different technical and tactical abilities, which constrained the identification of affordances and consequently shaped the coordination tendencies during performance (Laakso et al., 2017; Baptista et al., 2018). In this study, results revealed higher ID values for defenders, acted as attacking, compared to participants with other main performance roles. Midfielders revealed higher ID values than attackers, when acting also as attacking players. The findings suggested that the familiarity and past experience of players, acting in their main performance role or other, may influence their interaction tendencies with other participants, especially in exploiting affordances. For instance, defenders, in attack, revealed generally higher ID values than midfielders and attackers. In competition, defenders typically do not have as many opportunities to face 2-vs-1 situations near the opposite goal to achieve scoring box opportunities, as do midfielders and attackers in their team roles. Due to their typically less effective skills in attacking situations to create scoring box opportunities, defenders seek to manipulate the ball when well away from attackers. That is, defenders usually face the 2-vs-1 situations with the aim of keeping the ball possession and achieving in-depth passing opportunities, and for that, it makes sense to play with high distance from opponents to ensure secure passing lines or other options for play. In 2-vs-1 sub-phases, this lack of skill and experience may lead defenders to seek more possibilities to pass the ball to the second attacker rather than to try to dribble the defending player with the ball. These findings in contrast with previous results in a study of 1-vs-1 sub-phases show that, when defenders attack and attackers defend, lower values in interpersonal distance emerged in comparison to performance of participants with other role combinations (Laakso et al., 2017).

Our data suggest that an individual's team role is an individual constraint that can be related to performance effectiveness (Varley et al., 2017). Due to differences in performance contexts and the requisite actions, players of different team roles exploited affordances and performed differently in competition condition (Travassos et al., 2013a; Silva et al., 2014; Araújo et al., 2017). The findings signified that participants revealed different levels of effectiveness, especially the defenders in comparison to participants with other team roles.

CONCLUSIONS

Our findings supported the general idea that field location is a key constraint on interpersonal coordination tendencies in 2-vs-1 sub-phases of association football, as also observed in previous work on 1-vs-1 sub-phases (Headrick et al., 2011; Laakso et al., 2017). Taken together, these findings imply how coaches can design practice environments for team sport athletes. These findings in 2-vs-1 sub-phases suggested the need to analyze interactional dynamics of attackers and defenders in different relevant sub-phases of team games (i.e., 3-vs-2, 3-vs-3, 4-vs-3, 5-vs-5) (Laakso et al., 2017). These observations are important to understand how manipulated constraints in team games practice can change interpersonal coordination tendencies and how players explore such variations. The results also suggested that the manipulation of different field playing locations should be promoted in practice. Further research is also required to understand the dynamics of this game sub-phase during training sessions or in the game environment. That is, what is really the transfer between such spatial-temporal coordination tendencies in training and competition and how it happens at different levels of relations (from individuals to teams).

The manipulation of the relative position of the goal could highlight the behavior of defenders to effectively manage the spatial-temporal relations with opponents and constrain affordances according to the current effectivities (capacities) of players (for instance use of a preferred foot). Such manipulations have implications for specificity of practice, highlighting the importance of conditioning for footwork and management of spatial-temporal relations with opponents, which can be best attained in sub-phase practices (rather than ladder drills) because of the perception of information for action (affordances).

Despite the obtained results, some limitations should be acknowledged. In this study, only U15 players from one team were considered for analysis. Further research should be developed using larger sample of players and considering diferent ages and levels of practice to identify variations or similarities between spatial-temporal coordination tendencies. Also, independently of the age and level of practice, further studies should evaluate the technical/tactical proficiency of players and their level of fitness and maturation in order to understand the impact of individual characteristics on the spatial-temporal coordination tendencies developed in 2-vs-1 sub-phases of association football.

At the end, it was clear that changes in contextual game constraints such as relative position of the goal promote adaptive behaviors of players to perform. In line with that, coaches should constantly promote changes in the field location of 2-vs-1 sub-phases of game in order to promote the creation of new possibilities for action of players. Also, the definition of different couples of attackers and defenders according to different levels of effectivities seems to be a good constraint to create new spatial-temporal information and promote new possibilities for action of players according to their effectivities. Further research is required to understand the contribution of such manipulations to the learning process.

ETHICS STATEMENT

The club and all parents of participants provided prior informed consent for participation in the study. The study was approved by the Local Ethics Committee according to the Declaration of Helsinki.

AUTHOR CONTRIBUTIONS

TL, KD, JL, and BT participated in study design. TL and JL participated in data collection. TL, KD and BT participated in data analysis and in the first draft manuscript. All the authors participated and approved the final version of the manuscript and agree with the order of the presentation of the authors.

REFERENCES

Araújo, D., and Davids, K. (2016). Team synergies in sport: theory and measures. *Front. Psychol.* 7:1449. doi: 10.3389/fpsyg.2016.01449

Araújo, D., Davids, K., and Hristovski, R. (2006). The ecological dynamics of decision making in sport. *Psychol. Sport Exerc.* 7, 653–676. doi: 10.1016/j.psychsport.2006.07.002

Araújo, D., Hristovski, R., Seifert, L., Carvalho, J., and Davids, K. (2017). Ecological cognition: expert decision-making behaviour in sport. *Int. Rev. Sport Exerc. Psychol.* 1–25. doi: 10.1080/1750984X.2017.1349826

Baptista, J., Travassos, B., Gonçalves, B., Mourão, P., Viana, J. L., and Sampaio, J. (2018). Exploring the effects of playing formations on tactical behaviour and external workload during football small-sided games. *J. Strength Cond. Res.* doi: 10.1519/jsc.0000000000002445 [Epub ahead of print].

Clemente, F., Couceiro, M., Martins, F., Dias, G., and Mendes, R. (2013). Interpersonal dynamics: 1v1 sub-phase at sub-18 football players. *J. Hum. Kinet.* 36, 179–189. doi: 10.2478/hukin-2013-0018

Correia, V., Araújo, D., Duarte, R., Travassos, B., Passos, P., and Davids, K. (2012). Changes in practice task constraints shape decision-making behaviours of team games players. *J. Sci. Med. Sport* 15, 244–249. doi: 10.1016/j.jsams.2011.10.004

Coutinho, D., Gonçalves, B., Santos, S., Travassos, B., Wong, D. P., and Sampaio, J. (2018). Effects of the pitch configuration design on players' physical performance and movement behaviour during soccer small-sided games. *Res. Sports Med.* 27, 298–313. doi: 10.1080/15438627.2018.1544133

Cumming, G. (2012). *Understanding the new statistics: effect sizes, confidence intervals, and meta-analysis.* New York: Routledge.

Duarte, R., Araújo, D., Davids, K., Travassos, B., Gazimba, V., and Sampaio, J. (2012). Interpersonal coordination tendencies shape 1-vs-1 sub-phase performance outcomes in youth soccer. *J. Sport Sci.* 30, 871–877. doi: 10.1080/02640414.2012.675081

Duarte, R., Araújo, D., Fernandes, O., Fonseca, C., Correia, V., Gazimba, V., et al. (2010). Capturing complex human behaviors in representative sports contexts with a single camera. *Medicina* 46, 408–414.

Esteves, P., Araújo, D., Davids, K., Vilar, L., Travassos, B., and Esteves, C. (2012). Interpersonal dynamics and relative positioning to scoring target of performers in 1 vs. 1 sub-phases of team sports. *J. Sports Sci.* 30, 1285–1293. doi: 10.1080/02640414.2012.707327

Fernandes, O., and Malta, P. (2007). Techno-tactics and running distance analysis using one camera. *J. Sports Sci. Med.* 6, 204–205.

Folgado, H., Duarte, R., Marques, P., Gonçalves, B., and Sampaio, J. (2018). Exploring how movement synchronization is related to match outcome in elite professional football. *Sci. Med. Football* 2, 101–107. doi: 10.1080/24733938.2018.1431399

Gesbert, V., Durny, A., and Hauw, D. (2017). How do soccer players adjust their activity in team coordination? An enactive phenomenological analysis. *Front. Psychol.* 8:854. doi: 10.3389/fpsyg.2017.00854

Goto, R., and Mascie-Taylor, C. G. N. (2007). Precision of measurement as a component of human variation. *J. Physiol. Anthropol.* 26, 253–256. doi: 10.2114/jpa2.26.253

Headrick, J., Davids, K., Renshaw, I., Araújo, D., Passos, P., and Fernandes, O. (2011). Proximity-to-goal as a constraint on patterns of behaviour in attacker-defender dyads in team games. *J. Sport Sci.* 30, 247–253. doi: 10.1080/02640414.2011.640706

Hopkins, W., Marshall, S., Batterham, A., and Hanin, J. (2009). Progressive statistics for studies in sports medicine and exercise science. *Med. Sci. Sports Exer.* 41, 3–12. doi: 10.1249/MSS.0b013e31818cb278

Laakso, T., Travassos, B., Liukkonen, J., and Davids, K. (2017). Field location and player roles as constraints on emergent 1-vs-1 interpersonal patterns of play in football. *Hum. Mov. Sci.* 54, 347–353. doi: 10.1016/j.humov.2017.06.008

Lovell, T. W. J., Bocking, C. J., Fransen, J., Kempton, T., and Coutts, A. J. (2018). Factors affecting physical match activity and skill involvement in youth soccer. *Sci. Med. Football* 2, 58–65. doi: 10.1080/24733938.2017.1395062

McGarry, T. (2009). Applied and theoretical perspectives of performance analysis in sport: scientific issues and challenges. *Int. J. Perform. Anal. Sport* 9, 128–140. doi: 10.1080/24748668.2009.11868469

Passos, P., Araújo, D., Davids, K., Gouveia, L., Milho, J., and Serpa, S. (2008). Information-governing dynamics of attacker-defender interactions in youth rugby union. *J. Sports Sci.* 26, 1421–1429. doi: 10.1080/02640410802208986

Paterson, G., Van der Kamp, J., Bressan, E., and Savelsbergh, G. (2016). Action-specific effects on perception are grounded in affordance perception: an examination of soccer players' action choices in a free-kick task. *Int. J. Sport Pshychol.* 47, 318–334. doi: 10.7352/IJSP2016.47.318

Sampaio, J., Lago, C., Gonçalves, B., Maçãs, V. M., and Leite, N. (2013). Effects of pacing, status and unbalance in time motion variables, heart rate and tactical behaviour when playing 5-a-side football small-sided games. *J. Sci. Med. Sport* 17, 229–233. doi: 10.1016/j.jsams.2013.04.005

Schulze, E., Mendes, B., Maurício, N., Furtado, B., Cesário, N., Carriço, S., et al. (2018). Effects of positional variables on shooting outcome in elite football. *Sci. Med. Football* 2, 93–100. doi: 10.1080/24733938.2017.1383628

Silva, P., Garganta, J., Araújo, D., Davids, K., and Aguiar, P. (2013). Shared knowledge or shared affordances? Insights from an ecological dynamics approach to team coordination in sports. *Sports Med.* 43, 765–772. doi: 10.1007/s40279-013-0070-9

Silva, P., Travassos, B., Vilar, L., Aguiar, P., Davids, K., Araújo, D., et al. (2014). Numerical relations and skill level constrain co-adaptive behaviors of agents in sports teams. *PLoS One* 9:e107112. doi: 10.1371/journal.pone.0107112

Travassos, B., Araújo, D., Davids, K., O'Hara, K., Leitão, J., and Cortinhas, A. (2013a). The effect of expertise on decision making in sport – a meta-analysis. *Psychol. Sport Exerc.* 14, 211–219. doi: 10.1016/j.psychsport.2012.11.002

Travassos, B., Araújo, D., Duarte, R., and McGarry, T. (2012). Spatiotemporal coordination patterns in futsal (indoor football) are guided by informational game constraints. *Hum. Mov. Sci.* 31, 932–945. doi: 10.1016/j.humov.2011.10.004

Travassos, B., Davids, K., Araujo, D., and Esteves, P. (2013b). Performance analysis in team sports: advances from an ecological dynamics approach. *Int. J. Perform. Anal. Sport* 13, 83–95. doi: 10.1080/24748668.2013.11868633

Travassos, B., Gonçalves, B., Marcelino, R., Monteiro, R., and Sampaio, J. (2014a). How perceiving additional targets modifies teams' tactical behavior during football small-sided games. *Hum. Mov. Sci.* 38, 241–250. doi: 10.1016/j.humov.2014.10.005

Travassos, B., Vilar, L., Araújo, D., and McGarry, T. (2014b). Tactical performance changes with equal vs unequal numbers of players in small-sided football games. *Int. J. Perform. Anal. Sport* 14, 594–605. doi: 10.1080/24748668.2014.11868745

van Andel, S., Cole, M., and Peping, G. J. (2017). A systematic review on perceptual-motor calibration to changes in action capabilities. *Hum. Mov. Sci.* 51, 59–71. doi: 10.1016/j.humov.2016.11.004

Varley, M. C., Gregson, W., McMillan, K., Bonanno, D., Stafford, K., Modonutti, M., et al. (2017). Physical and technical performance of elite youth soccer players during international tournaments: influence of playing position and team success and opponent quality. *Sci. Med. Football* 1, 18–29. doi: 10.1080/02640414.2016.1230676

Vilar, L., Araújo, D., Davids, K., and Bar-Yam, Y. (2013a). Science of winning soccer: emergent pattern-forming dynamics in association football. *J. Syst. Sci. Complex.* 26, 73–84. doi: 10.1007/s11424-013-2286-z

Vilar, L., Araújo, D., Davids, K., Correia, V., and Esteves, P. T. (2013b). Spatial-temporal constraints on decision-making during shooting performance in the team sport of futsal. *J. Sports Sci.* 31, 840–846. doi: 10.1080/02640414.2012.753155

Vilar, L., Araújo, D., Davids, K., and Travassos, B. (2012b). Constraints on competitive performance of attacker–defender dyads in team sports. *J. Sport Sci.* 30, 459–469. doi: 10.1080/02640414.2011.627942

Vilar, L., Araújo, D., Davids, K., Travassos, B., Duarte, R., and Parreira, J. (2012c). Interpersonal coordination tendencies supporting the creation/prevention of goal scoring opportunities in futsal. *Eur. J. Sport Sci.* 14, 28–35. doi: 10.1080/17461391.2012.725103

Vilar, L., Duarte, R., Silva, P., Chow, J., and Davids, K. (2014a). The influence of pitch dimensions on performance during small-sided and conditioned soccer games. *J. Sports Sci.* 32, 1–9. doi: 10.1080/02640414.2014.918640

Vilar, L., Esteves, P. T., Travassos, B., Passos, P., Lago-Peñas, C., and Davids, K. (2014b). Varying numbers of players in small-sided soccer games modifies action opportunities during training. *Int. J. Sports Sci. Coach.* 9, 1007–1018. doi: 10.1260/1747-9541.9.5.1007

Winter, D. (2005). *Biomechanics and motor control of human movement.* 3rd ed. New York: John Wiley & Sons.

23

Physical Fitness and Somatic Characteristics of the Only Child

*Luis P. Rodrigues [1,2], Ricardo Franco Lima [1,2], Ana Filipa Silva [1,2,3], Filipe Manuel Clemente [1,4], Miguel Camões [1,2], Pantelis Theodoros Nikolaidis [5], Thomas Rosemann [6] and Beat Knechtle [6,7]**

[1] Escola Superior Desporto e Lazer, Instituto Politécnico de Viana do Castelo, Rua Escola Industrial e Comercial de Nun'Álvares, Viana do Castelo, Portugal, [2] Research Center in Sports Sciences Health Sciences and Human Development, CIDESD, Vila Real, Portugal, [3] N2i, Polytechnic Institute of Maia, Maia, Portugal, [4] Instituto de Telecomunicações, Delegação da Covilhã, Portugal, [5] Exercise Physiology Laboratory, Nikaia, Greece, [6] Institute of Primary Care, University of Zurich, Zurich, Switzerland, [7] Medbase St. Gallen Am Vadianplatz, St. Gallen, Switzerland

***Correspondence:**
Beat Knechtle
beat.knechtle@hispeed.ch

The purpose of this study was to examine if only child show differences on somatic growth and physical fitness compared to be a child with siblings. The participants included 542 children (boys: $N = 270$; girls: $N = 270$) between 7 and 15 years of age. Somatic growth (height, weight, body mass index) and physical fitness (handgrip strength; flexed harm hang; 60-s sit-ups; standing long jump; 10-m shuttle run and PACER test) were assessed. Variance analysis revealed significant advantages for children with siblings in the flexed arm hang ($p = 0.046$), 60-s sit-ups ($p = 0.002$), 10-m shuttle run ($p = 0.013$) and PACER ($p = 0.032$). An examination of the possible differential effect of sex on the results revealed no significance for physical fitness variables, but significant interaction were found for weight ($p = 0.004$) and body mass index ($p = 0.005$). Despite a lack of interactions between offspring and sex in physical fitness, significant differences between sexes were found in all fitness variables. In conclusion, having siblings showed to be advantageous for general physical fitness in children. This evidence may be used for future analysis and interventions in motor competence, namely considering the growing number of only children in some regions of the world.

Keywords: only child, motor competence, motor performance, human development, children

INTRODUCTION

In the European Union in 2016, almost half (47% or 31 million) of all households with children had only one child. In Portugal, there was also a tendency for single-child families to increase over the last few decades. In 1991, 44% of Portuguese households with children had only one child. This number rose to 51% in 2001, and to 55% in the last 2011 census. At the same time, the percentage of couples with three or more children has decreased (17, 11, and 8% in 1991, 2001, and 2011 respectively), and the number of couples with two children has remained at 38% (1). Surely this phenomenon of the only child, associated with the diminishing autonomy of children and young people (2), has an effect on the opportunities (affordances) for motor stimulation in these children and, consequently, on the development of their motor competence and physical fitness. For instance, solitary play, without a brother or sister, will be more sedentary, focused on individual play without movement, while the lack of autonomy will hamper children from experiencing new environments and motor challenges, with evident implications on his(her) perceive motor competence and self-confidence.

The only-child condition was widely examined in the literature throughout the 20th century and was particularly boosted by the single child policy imposed in China and by the general concern that the development of only children could be impaired by a lack of stimulation from siblings (3).

On the contrary, the expectation of an enriched family-child involvement and investment (4) within the context of only-child education and development conflicts with previously stated ideas. In an extended review from 1986, Fabo and Polit showed that English-speaking only children had more positive developmental outcomes (achievement, character, and intelligence) than their peers with siblings.

Urban Korean only children showed a greater tendency for depression (5), while Brazilian only sons were less likely to have an alcohol intoxication episode during adolescence (6).

In a recent study with 20,592 adult subjects in New Zealand, Stronge et al. (3) tested for differences in Big Six personality traits in adults and found that the ones with no siblings showed lower average levels of honesty-humility and conscientiousness and higher levels of neuroticism and openness. However, while statistically significant, these differences did not rise to the level of practical effects (3).

Physical fitness is a determinant of healthy child development, as it is related to several health outcomes and is a good summative measure of the body's ability to perform physical activity and exercise (7, 8).

Children with low levels of physical fitness (9) and motor competence are at greater risk for obesity (10).

A significantly higher likelihood of being overweight and obese has been found in only children, both in a recent systematic review and meta-analysis (11) and amongst a national sample of 43,046 children born in 2001 in Japan (12). Children with no siblings also had significantly lower levels of moderate-to-vigorous physical activity than children with siblings (13).

It is largely reported in research that environmental variables are important in influencing positive health behaviors and improving physical fitness. Several studies have revealed that birth weight, the mother's lifestyle during her pregnancy, the father's health, and the presence of siblings had the strongest influence on children's fitness (14–18). Regarding the birth order of siblings, the literature shows differences in motor development between older and younger siblings (15). These differences are probably due to the influence of older siblings on younger ones, although the authors conclude that this relationship may depend on biological characteristics.

The presence of siblings and peers seems to be a predictor of enriched motor development (19, 20). When the sibling influence is compared for sportsmen, elite athletes are more likely to be later-born children, while non-elite athletes are more likely to be the firstborn (21).

Although the number of single-child households is increasing, the consequences for child motor development have not been fully addressed in the literature. Individual pathways of change in physical fitness and growth are expected to be influenced by children's immediate environments and the presence or absence of other children in the family.

Consequently, the aim of this study is 2-fold: (i) to examine if being an only child is associated with negative differences on somatic growth and physical fitness compared to being a child with siblings and (ii) to analyze whether these differences are influenced by the child's sex. Our specific hypothesis is that only child will show detrimental differences in physical fitness and weight status.

MATERIALS AND METHODS

Sample

Participants in this study belong to the Melgaço Youth Observatory (MYO), a mixed-longitudinal growth and development project that is currently taking place at this location in the north of Portugal. A convenience sample that included all participants who entered the study between 2015 and 2019 was selected. A database was organized with data from the first year of assessment of each MYO participant, resulting in a total of 542 children (270 boys; 270 girls), aged from seven to 15 years of age (boys mean age= 10.47 ± 2.67; girls mean age=10.44 ± 2.64). Within the sample, 141 children were only child (71 boys; 70 girls) and 399 children had brothers or sisters (197 boys, 202 girls).

Procedures

The study was approved by the Scientific Council of the Polytechnic Institute of Viana do Castelo with the reference CTC-ESDL-001-2014. School directors approved the study, adult participants and the parents or tutors of underage children gave their informed consent. Children also gave verbal assent prior to data collection. All procedures were carried out in accordance with the 1964 Helsinki declaration and its later amendments.

Participants were individually interviewed by a research assistant to fill a sociodemographic questionnaire containing information about the family (parent's professional occupation, number of brothers and sisters and respective age). All somatic characteristics and physical fitness assessments were done in the same order at the laboratories of the Melgaço School of Sports and Leisure. Observers were trained in the assessment's protocols and its specifications, and each observer was responsible for only one test or measure. At least two of the three first authors of this study personally supervised all data collection.

Assessments Protocols

Somatic Measures

Somatic measurements included height and weight, which were measured with a SECA 217 stadiometer and a SECA 762 weight scale. All measurements were taken according to the International Society for the Advancement of Kinanthropometry's (22) standardized protocol.

Body mass index (BMI) was calculated using by dividing body weight (in kilograms) by height (in square meters).

Physical Fitness

Handgrip strength (HS) was tested using the handgrip dynamometer (SAEHAN, model SH5001), with individuals seated with their shoulders adducted, their elbows flexed at

90°, and their forearms in a neutral position, according to the American Society of Hand Therapists (23). In this analysis, we reported data only for the right hand, as some children of younger ages were not fully able to report their preferred hand.

Flexed arm hang (FAH) performances were assessed by noting the time the participant could hold herself with the chin above the bar, arms flexed, and using a supine grasp position. Two observers helped the child to assume the initial position, and the stopwatch counted the time between this moment and the moment the child's chin touched the bar or fell below the level of the bar. Results are recorded in tenths of seconds.

The maximum number of correct sit-ups (SU) performed in 60 s was counted. The participant started by lying down on a mat with their arms crossed across the chest and legs flexed at ~45°. An observer secured the participant's feet using two hands throughout the test. A correct sit-up was counted when the participant touched their knees with their arms kept close to the chest. The total number of correct SU is the result of the test.

Standing long jump (SLJ) performances were assessed by recording the length of a landing horizontal jump, with the participant departing from a line in the ground at a two-foot-long take-off. The result of the test was the best result of three trials. The length of the jump was measured from the departing line to the nearest point where the heels touch the ground. The results were recorded in cm.

Performances in a 10-m shuttle run (SHR) were recorded using the following protocol. Two parallel lines were marked on the floor 10 meters apart. Two blocks of wood were placed behind one of the lines opposite the starting line. On the signal "Ready? Go!" the child ran to the blocks, picked one up, ran back to the starting line, and placed the block behind the line; he then ran back and picked up the second block, which he carried back across the starting line. Two attempts were allowed, with the best time used as the result of the test.

The PACER test is a widely used progressive test where participants run back and forth at a specified pace from two lines that are 20 meters apart. The pace is externally regulated by an auditory sign (a beep) that marks the moment participants should be at each end of the course (a lap). The pace is increased every minute, and participants remain in the test until they can no longer keep up with the pace at the end of two consecutive laps. Participants were encouraged to achieve their maximal performance. When they did not, according to the observer's judgment (e.g., when showing a lack of motivation to complete the task, stopping due to injury or pain, or not showing facial flushing, sweating, hyperpnoea, or an unsteady gait), the result was not included. For children below 10 years of age, a pacing light apparatus was used throughout the testing time to assure full participation and motivation in the 20-m SRT test. The number of completed laps was recorded as the result of the test.

Maturation

Time to Peak Height Velocity (PHV) was used as a maturational index assessed according to the following equations for each sex (24):

Time to PHV Boys = −8.3971103 + (0.0070346 * decimal age * sitting height).

Time to PHV Girls = = −7.709133 + (0.0042232 * decimal age * height).

Statistics

Descriptive statistics for age groups (7–9, 10–12, 13–15 years-of-age) according to the sex and offspring condition are presented for all variables. A two factor ANCOVA full factorial model was used to test for the effects of Sex (boy or girl) and Offspring (only child or sibling) on each somatic and physical fitness variable, while adjusting for decimal age (covariate). All variables were previously tested for normality and homoscedasticity and, in accordance, the FAH and PACER data were logarithmic transformed. Residuals configurations from of the ANCOVAs were scrutinized for possible non-normal or biased configurations.

RESULTS

Descriptive results according to sex, age, and existence of siblings in the family can be found in **Table 1**.

Although no differences were found between decimal ages of boys and girls ($p = 0.521$), girls proved to be maturational advanced relative to boys (time PHV = -1.37 ± 2.19 and -2.78 ± 1.97 respectively for girls and boys; $p < 0.001$). Nonetheless no differences were found in the time to PHV between the only child and the siblings' groups ($p = 0.500$). The correlation between decimal age and maturational time to PHV was of 0.98 for boys and 0.99 for girls showing that decimal age is also a very good indicative of both chronological and biological age of the participants.

In order to understand if being an only child can result on deleterious differences on the somatic growth and physical fitness of children, a two-way ANCOVA was run for each collected variable. The main effect of interest was related to the offspring condition of being an only child compared with having other siblings in the house, but we were also interested in understanding if being a boy or a girl can affect this possible offspring effect. Since different ages were present in the sample, we used decimal age as a covariate in order to control for the age and maturation effect in the variables. The results are shown in **Table 2** below.

For all tested variables, except for BMI, Sex has proved to have a significant effect on the outcome value, as expected. Similar thing happened with Decimal Age entering as a covariate in the models, but in this case the effect was significant for all variables ($p < 0.001$ for all models).

Interaction between Offspring conditions and Sex was never significant for all physical fitness variables tested but turned out as significant for Weight and BMI, meaning that the Offspring effect on weight and BMI can be different depending on the sex of the child.

Finally, and looking for our condition of interest in this study, the Offspring condition, we can see that significant differences were found between children that are the only child in the family and the ones that have brothers and/or sisters (siblings) for most of the physical fitness variables (FAH, SU, SHR, and PACER), and for height and weight. In general, the difference found was

TABLE 1 | Number of subjects, mean, and standard deviation values for all variables according to age group, sex, and the existence of siblings in the family.

		Girls				Boys			
		Only child		Sibling		Only child		Sibling	
Variable	**Age**	***n***	**Mean SD**	***n***	**Mean SD**	***n***	**Mean SD**	***n***	**Mean SD**
Height	7–9	36	129.8 ± 6.7	110	130.3 ± 6.6	32	133.0 ± 7.3	107	130.3 ± 7.4
	10–12	19	150.6 ± 10.5	46	148.8 ± 9.4	23	147.4 ± 8.7	45	143.9 ± 6.7
	13–15	15	158.4 ± 5.5	46	158.1 ± 6.3	16	165.4 ± 5.9	45	165.6 ± 10.0
Weight	7–9	36	29.8 ± 6.9	110	30.3 ± 6.9	32	34.1 ± 10.8	107	30.5 ± 8.4
	10–12	19	43.9 ± 11.4	46	42.6 ± 9.2	23	45.0 ± 12.0	45	40.4 ± 9.9
	13–15	15	53.2 ± 8.9	46	56.8 ± 10.2	16	61.3 ± 11.3	45	55.9 ± 13.5
BMI	7–9	36	17.6 ± 3.2	110	17.7 ± 3.0	32	18.9 ± 4.3	107	17.7 ± 3.4
	10–12	19	19.1 ± 3.4	46	19.1 ± 2.8	23	20.4 ± 3.9	45	19.3 ± 3.4
	13–15	15	21.2 ± 3.4	46	22.8 ± 4.3	16	22.3 ± 3.5	45	20.2 ± 3.2
HG	7–9	36	12.3 ± 2.5	110	12.3 ± 3.0	32	13.2 ± 3.4	107	13.0 ± 3.1
	10–12	19	21.1 ± 6.0	46	19.9 ± 5.0	23	18.9 ± 6.0	45	20.5 ± 5.1
	13–15	15	24.2 ± 4.5	46	25.2 ± 3.8	16	32.6 ± 6.2	45	31.8 ± 7.4
FAH	7–9	36	7.8 ± 6.3	110	11.0 ± 10.8	32	9.0 ± 11.2	107	10.9 ± 8.3
	10–12	19	8.2 ± 8.6	46	7.3 ± 9.4	23	9.0 ± 9.2	45	16.5 ± 17.4
	13–15	15	14.1 ± 10.9	46	12.8 ± 10.2	16	37.0 ± 21.3	45	43.2 ± 24.4
SU	7–9	36	23.0 ± 9.7	110	25.2 ± 8.1	32	24.3 ± 9.0	107	26.4 ± 7.2
	10–12	19	27.9 ± 6.8	46	30.5 ± 6.8	23	29.4 ± 9.8	45	34.4 ± 8.2
	13–15	15	32.7 ± 4.0	46	33.1 ± 7.0	16	40.9 ± 8.7	45	43.5 ± 8.9
SLJ	7–9	36	108.6 ± 15.6	110	113.3 ± 17.9	32	114.7 ± 20.3	107	117.6 ± 19.0
	10–12	19	133.6 ± 23.5	46	128.6 ± 18.6	23	125.9 ± 22.2	45	139.4 ± 20.1
	13–15	15	135.5 ± 20.2	46	130.4 ± 21.3	16	179.9 ± 27.9	45	176.0 ± 24.4
SHR	7–9	36	14.5 ± 1.2	110	14.2 ± 1.2	32	14.1 ± 1.4	107	13.8 ± 1.4
	10–12	19	12.7 ± 1.0	46	12.7 ± 0.9	23	13.0 ± 1.5	45	12.2 ± 1.2
	13–15	15	12.4 ± 0.7	46	12.5 ± 1.0	16	10.7 ± 0.9	45	10.8 ± 0.8
PACER	7–9	36	22.7 ± 8.4	110	25.3 ± 9.8	32	25.8 ± 12.5	107	30.2 ± 16.0
	10–12	19	28.5 ± 12.6	46	36.6 ± 16.1	23	37.0 ± 18.8	45	41.2 ± 18.6
	13–15	15	29.6 ± 10.0	46	30.3 ± 11.4	16	66.1 ± 20.8	45	61.7 ± 18.5

TABLE 2 | Main effects for Offspring condition, Sex, and interaction between them, controlling for decimal age, for each somatic and physical variable.

	Offspring		Sex		Interaction	
	Only child (yes or no)		(boy or girl)		Sex x Offspring	
	F	*sig*	*F*	*sig*	*F*	*sig*
Somatic growth						
Height	4.062	**$p = 0.044$**	7.578	**$p = 0.006$**	1.897	$p = 0.169$
Weight	4.316	**$p = 0.038$**	6.006	**$p = 0.001$**	8.251	**$p = 0.004$**
BMI	2.414	$p = 0.121$	1.832	$p = 0.177$	7.896	**$p = 0.005$**
Physical Fitness						
Handgrip	0.025	$p = 0.873$	19.636	**$P < 0.001$**	0.178	$p = 0.673$
Flexed arm hang	3.989	**$p = 0.046$**	9.145	**$p = 0.001$**	1.579	$p = 0.209$
60 s Sit-ups	9.355	**$p = 0.002$**	21.714	**$P < 0.001$**	0.379	$p = 0.539$
Standing Long Jump	1.265	$p = 0.261$	40.907	**$P < 0.001$**	1.399	$p = 0.237$
10 m SHR	6.166	**$p = 0.013$**	35.809	**$P < 0.001$**	0.910	$p = 0.340$
PACER	4.636	**$p = 0.032$**	33.958	**$P < 0.001$**	0.075	$p = 0.784$

Decimal age was a covariate present in all statistical tests reported in the table, and showed a significant effect for all models ($p < 0.001$). Significant values ($p < 0.05$) are showed in bold.

deleterious for the only child group that always showed a worst average performance in the physical fitness tests but tend to be taller and heavier than the sibling's group (see **Figure 1**).

DISCUSSION

The aim of the present study was to understand whether being an only child can be associated with a deleterious difference on somatic growth and physical fitness between the ages of seven and fifteen, our hypothesis being that those differences will be identified in physical fitness and weight status.

Our results showed that only children were taller ($p = 0.044$) and heavier ($p = 0.038$) than children with siblings, although no differences were found in BMI ($p = 0.121$). The growth and maturity features of a child (morphological, physiological, and neuromuscular) have an important role in the development of motor performance during infancy and childhood (25). Differences in height and weight during late childhood and adolescence can be due to differences in maturational status (25–28). However, in the present case, no differences were found in maturational time at PHV (peak height velocity) between these two groups. Genetics and nutritional or environmental conditions are possible explanations for this phenomenon, but more information is needed to substantiate these allegations.

Considering weight, different profiles were observed between sexes regarding each child's condition, with boys achieving higher results in the only-child group and girls achieving higher scores in the children with siblings group. The boys' results were in line with a study conducted with Chinese children aged six to eighteen, which showed that only children were about four times more likely to be obese than children with siblings, even after controlling for sex, age, parental weight status, parental education level, household income, and urban/rural residence (29). Also, Bagley et al. (30) found that boys without siblings spent more time watching television than boys with siblings. The consequence of this was an increase in sedentary time and, in turn, an increase in body weight. On the other hand, the girls' results could be related to the fact that having a sibling has been associated with a 2-fold increase in the likelihood of adolescents viewing $\geq$ 2 h of television per day (31). Nevertheless, contradictory results were found in the same study that registered less time spent viewing television in girls with siblings compared to girls without siblings. In the same vein, the BMI results displayed a different profile regarding sex and offspring conditions, although any sex differences were registered.

After removing the effect of age, children with siblings showed better results in four of the six tested items (FAH, 60 s sit-ups, 10 m SHR, and PACER), with no differences found for the other two items (handgrip and SLJ).

Consistent with the literature [e.g., (19, 32–35)], boys performed better than girls in all physical fitness tests across all ages. In fact, studies have shown that girls outperform boys only in tasks that include mainly balancing, hopping (19, 32), and flexibility (36). Such results have been interpreted as a social rather than genetic influence in childhood, as the physical characteristics of girls and boys are very similar (37–39). During pubertal age, sexual dimorphism explains the male's advantages in most physical fitness tasks (37).

Age of the study participants ranged from pre-pubertal to pubertal ages, surely living in different motor skill development periods and maturational levels, both wich can influence physical fitness performance and be associated with sex differences. Trying to account for this question we had sex groups with similar age (10.47 $\pm$ 2.67 and 10.44 $\pm$ 2.64, respectively, for mean and standard deviation of boys and girls) in the sample. Furthermore, age groups within sexes also showed similar decimal ages (see **Table 1**) reducing the chance for impacting the main effect of interest in the study. Maturation is expected to influence physical fitness performance but, in this case, decimal age and maturational age (age at peak of height velocity) was found to be highly correlated (0.98 and 0.99, respectively, for boys and girls). Because decimal age was used as a covariate in the analysis, the results are independent for both age and maturation level. Boys and girls had the same decimal age.

Relative age or season of birth, is another known variable that seems to be associated with differences in motor competence specifically in sports, with athletes born in the first months of the year showing advantages on the long term sport's career (40). Our sample showed similar distribution of birth month between only child and non-only child by sex (Boys $\chi^2(268,11) = 10.86$, $p = 0.455$; Girls $\chi^2(272,11) = 10.65$, $p = 0.473$), showing that this characteristic did not affect our results.

Muscular fitness is an important marker of health that has been inversely and independently associated with insulin resistance, clustered cardiometabolic risk, and inflammatory proteins during childhood and adolescence (41–43). Considering the strength-related tests conducted in this study, it seems that maximal force (expressed in the HG test) showed no differences between offspring conditions, as well as the leg power test (expressed in the SLJ), in each sex. Nevertheless, in the resistance strength tests (SU and FAH), different profiles were expressed when comparing offspring conditions. In boys, those with siblings clearly demonstrated an advantage, presenting consistently higher values than only-child boys. In fact, other studies suggest that children may benefit from having siblings, especially older siblings who serve as role models, as parents tend to be over-protective of only or firstborn children (19). The same pattern was clearly observed in girls in the SU test, but in FAH, a mixed profile was expressed, with sibling girls showing higher values between 7 and 9 years of age while only child girls outperformed those with siblings in terms of physical growth. Indeed, Wrotniak et al. (44) also concluded that motor proficiency was not related among siblings, while Costa et al. (45) and Pereira et al. (46) observed that only children and firstborn siblings showed greater strength values while exhibiting worse velocity and flexibility results. Such contradictory results confirm the need to conduct more studies in this field.

SHR is commonly used to measure agility (47). In our sample, this capacity differed based on offspring conditions; however, it led to a clear difference between boys and girls. In only-child boys, the 10-m SHR times were slower, especially for those between 7 and 12 years of age. However, in children between 13 and 15 years old, this difference seemed to disappear. It should be noted that the participants in our sample live in a

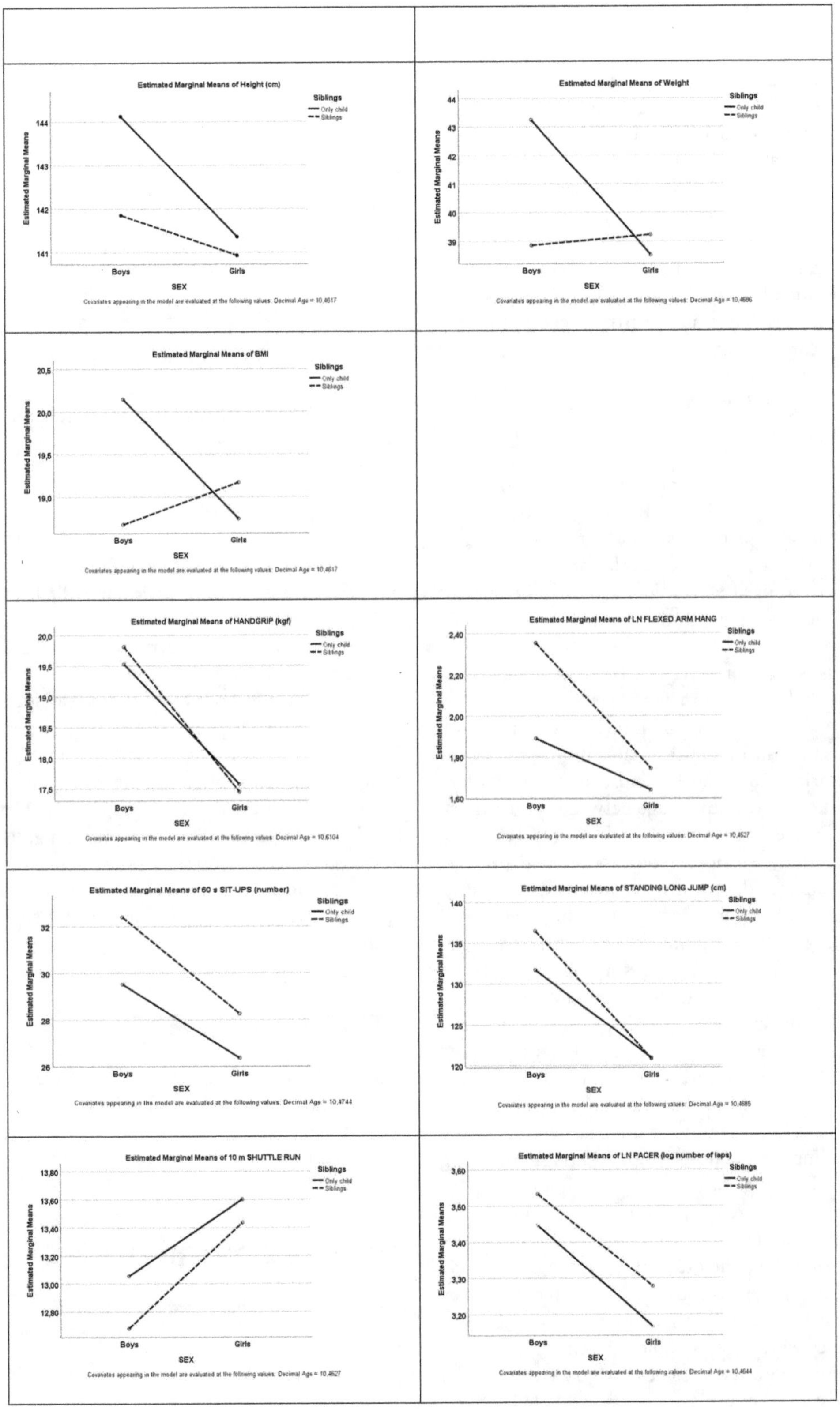

FIGURE 1 | Representation of the estimated marginal mean for somatic measures and physical fitness tests according to the number of siblings (only child or with siblings) by sex.

rural environment, which could lead only children to explore the surrounding spaces to a greater extent as they become older and more autonomous. Nevertheless, in girls, this same pattern was observed as being smoother. Only slight differences were observed for girls between 7 and 9 years of age, with the same values maintained in the older ages. Earlier stabilization in girls could be related to the maturation process, which also happens earlier in girls (generally, when they are 10–12 years old) (48).

The PACER, which is strongly associated with health, was developed as a field-based measure for estimating cardiovascular fitness (7, 49). This capacity seems to be developed further in children with siblings than in only children—for both sexes, only children showed poorer results for all age groups, except for boys between 13 and 15 years old. In fact, (50) have suggested that siblings have an unequivocal advantage in motor competence and physical fitness independent of age, sex, or birth order. This phenomenon was observed in children of both sexes of 7 to 15 years of age.

This was the first study that looked at the condition of being an only child in relation to physical fitness. In summary, our results suggest that not having brothers or sisters to play with in the family is a clear disadvantage for the development of physical fitness and highlights the need to conduct more studies in this field, especially because Portuguese statistics show that only-child families are increasing (1).

Although siblings share, on average, 50% of their genes identical-by-descent and a common family environment, they differ in their chronological age, sex, and health behaviors as well as in their physical growth, biological maturation, and motor development trajectories (28). The literature is not consistent when considering who has the advantage between the firstborn [e.g., (17, 51, 52)] or the later-born child [e.g., (15, 19, 53)], suggesting that differences in motor competence and physical fitness exist between siblings depending on birth order and sex.

Very young (preschool age and younger) siblings can spend more time interacting with each other than with any other person, including their parents (54–56). Normally, parents are more protective of an only child, which can result in restrained autonomy and less moving around physically. The only child has the parents' attention for a longer time. In this sense, the family environment seems to play an important role in the development of physical fitness.

In this study, we did not account for the sex, age difference, or the number of siblings in the household. Although including participants from different growing ages, we should keep in mind the cross-sectional nature of the study, so caution should be used when longitudinal inferences are made. Future studies should include these questions and attempt to further disentangle possible causes for the differences found. Age difference and sex of the sibling(s) relative to the child can be variables of interest to analyze in next studies with larger samples. Parenting styles can be of importance, along with the socioeconomic background of the family since there is a known association with the number of siblings. Motor competence as a foundational cornerstone for movement abilities should also be examined within the scope of only children. Longitudinal follow-ups of children, or simply to look for the association of adult's level of motor competence with their offspring condition can probably bring us a better understanding of the only-child motor development phenomena.

Our findings give support to the need for special attention of parents, educators and coaches to the only child physical fitness and somatic development. Parents should try to compensate for the lack of peers in the household by organizing more shared time with friends at home and out of it. Educators should be aware of these potential characteristics of the only child and its consequences within the children's group relationships, and act accordingly. Coaches are to understand the uniqueness of the only child to give them the opportunity to catch up on their specific motor competence whenever the case.

In this study we conclude that children with siblings show positive differences on somatic growth and physical fitness compared to the only child. This conclusion holds for both sexes and for all ages between 7 and 15 years of age.

CONCLUSIONS

The present study compared the somatic characteristics and physical fitness of only children with those of children with siblings. It revealed significantly better levels of flexed arm hang, 60-s sit-ups, 10-m shuttle run, and PACER results in children with siblings despite only children having significantly greater values of height and weight. No significant interaction was found between offspring and sex, considering physical fitness. Comparisons between sexes revealed that boys had significantly better results than girls for the handgrip strength, flexed arm hang, 60-s sit-ups, standing long jump, 10-m shuttle run, and PACER tests. Generally, our results highlight the importance of offspring in the physical fitness of children. This should be carefully considered by parents, educators and specialists who aim to analyze the contexts that may influence motor competence in the future.

ETHICS STATEMENT

The study was approved by the Scientific Council of the Polytechnic Institute of Viana do Castelo. Written informed consent to participate in this study was provided by the participants' legal guardian/next of kin.

AUTHOR CONTRIBUTIONS

All authors listed have made a substantial, direct and intellectual contribution to the work, and approved it for publication.

ACKNOWLEDGMENTS

LR work was partially supported by the Portuguese Foundation for Science and Technology, I.P., under project UID04045/2020.

REFERENCES

Atalaia S, Wall K, Cunha V, Marinho P, Ramos V, Guerreiro D, et al. Famílias nos Censos 2011: Diversidade e Mudança. Como evoluíram as famílias em Portugal: Instituto Nacional de Estatística (2013). Available online at: http://www.ine.pt/xportal/xmain?xpid=INE&xpgid=ine_destaques& DESTAQUESdest_boui=206614582&DESTAQUESmodo=2&xlang=pt

Lopes F, Cordovil R, Neto C. Children's independent mobility in Portugal: effects of urbanization degree and motorized modes of travel. *J Transport Geogr.* (2014) 41:210–9. doi: 10.1016/j.jtrangeo.2014.10.002

Stronge S, Shaver JH, Bulbulia J, Sibley CG. Only children in the 21st century: Personality differences between adults with and without siblings are very, very small. *J Res Person.* (2019) 83:103868. doi: 10.1016/j.jrp.2019.103868

Leung MCM, Zhang J. Gender preference, biased sex ratio, and parental investments in single-child households. *Rev Econ Household.* (2008) 6:91–110. doi: 10.1007/s11150-007-9026-x

Kim K, Jung SJ, Cho SMJ, Park JH, Kim HC. Perceived discrimination, depression, and the role of perceived social support as an effect modifier in Korean Young Adults. *J Prev Med Public Health.* (2019) 52:366–76. doi: 10.3961/jpmph.19.114

Tavares MB, Fuchs FC, Diligenti F, de Abreu JRP, Rohde LA, Fuchs SC. Características de comportamento do filho único vs filho primogênito e não primogênito. Braz J Psychiatry. (2004) 26:17–23. doi: 10.1590/S1516-44462004000100007

Ortega FB, Ruiz JR, Castillo MJ, Sjöström M. Physical fitness in childhood and adolescence: a powerful marker of health. *Int J Obesity.* (2008) 32:1–11. doi: 10.1038/sj.ijo.0803774

Utesch T, Dreiskamper D, Strauss B, Naul R. The development of the physical fitness construct across the childhood. *Scand J Med Sci Sports.* (2018) 28:212– 9. doi: 10.1111/sms.12889

Rodrigues LP, Leitão R, Lopes VP. Physical fitness predicts adiposity longitudinal changes over childhood and adolescence. *J Sci Med Sport.* (2013) 16:118–23. doi: 10.1016/j.jsams.2012.06.008

Rodrigues LP, Stodden, DF, Lopes, V. Development pathways of change in fitness and motor competence are related to overweight and obesity status at the end of primary school. *Sci. Med. Sport.* (2016) 19:87–92. doi: 10.1016/j.jsams.2015.01.002

Meller FO, Loret de Mola C, Assunção MCF, Schäfer AA, Dahly DL, Barros FC. Birth order and number of siblings and their association with overweight and obesity: a systematic review and meta-analysis. *Nutr Rev.* (2018) 76:117– 24. doi: 10.1093/nutrit/nux060

Ikeda N, Fuse K, Nishi N. Changes in the effects of living with no siblings or living with grandparents on overweight and obesity in children: results from a national cohort study in Japan. *PloS ONE.* (2017) 12:e0175726. doi: 10.1371/journal.pone.0175726

Kracht CL, Sisson SB. Sibling influence on children's objectively measured physical activity: a meta-analysis and systematic review. *BMJ Open Sport Exerc Med.* (2018) 4:e000405. doi: 10.1136/bmjsem-2018-000405

Ahlqvist VH, Persson M, Ortega FB, Tynelius P, Magnusson C, Berglind D. Birth weight and grip strength in young Swedish males: a longitudinal matched sibling analysis and across all body mass index ranges. *Sci Rep.* (2019) 9:1–8. doi: 10.1038/s41598-019-46200-0

Berger S, Nuzzo K. Older siblings influence younger siblings' motor development. *Infant Child Dev.* (2009) 18:238–54. doi: 10.1002/icd.571

Brophy S, Rees A, Knox G, Baker J, Thomas NE. Child fitness and father's BMI are important factors in childhood obesity: a school based cross-sectional study. *PLoS ONE.* (2012) 7:1–7. doi: 10.1371/annotation/62537085-2630-490b-b489-8dfdcc3a84fa

Lopes VP. *Desenvolvimento Motor: Indicadores Bioculturais e Somáticos do Rendimento Motor em Crianças de 5/6 Anos. Universidade Técnica de Lisboa* (1992).

Rer R, Fillon A, Thivel D, Henderson M, Barnett TA, Bigras JL, et al. *Anthropometry and physical fitness testing explain physical activity levels in children and adolescents with obesity? J Sci Med Sport.* (2019) 23:580–5. doi: 10.1016/j.jsams.2019.12.005

Krombholz H. Physical performance in relation to age, sex, birth order, social class, and sports activities of preschool children.

Percep Motor Skills. (2006) 102:477–84. doi: 10.2466/pms.102.2. 477-484 Lopes VP, Gabbard C, Rodrigues LP. Physical activity in adolescents: examining influence of the best Friend Dyad. *J Adolesc Health.* (2013) 52:752– 6. doi: 10.1016/j.jadohealth.2012.12.004

Hopwood MJ, Farrow D, MacMahon C, Baker J. Sibling dynamics and sport expertise. *Scand J Med Sci Sports.* (2015) 25:724–33. doi: 10.1111/sms. 12387

International Society for the Advancement of Kinanthropometry. *International Standards for Anthropometric Assessment.* South Africa: Potchefstroom (2001).

Fess EE. Grip strength. In: Casanova JS, editors *Clinical assessment recommendations. 2nd ed.* Chicago: American Society of Hand Therapists (1992). p. 41–5.

Moore S, Mckay H, Macdonald H, Nettlefold L, Baxter-Jones A, Cameron N, et al. Enhancing a somatic maturity prediction model. *Med Sci Sports Exerc.* (2015) 47:1755–64. doi: 10.1249/MSS.0000000000000588

Malina RM. Motor development during infancy and early childhood: Overview and suggested directions for research. *Int J Sport Health Sci.* (2004) 2:50–66. doi: 10.5432/ijshs.2.50

Ahmed M. Comparative study of well being, thought control, academic achievement and health related physical fitness of active and inac- tive adolescent school students. *Int Leisure Rev.* (2013) 2:135–56. doi: 10.6298/ILR.2013.2.2

Freitas VH. Sensitivity of physiological and psychological markers to training load intensification in volleyball players sensitivity of physiological and psychological markers to training load intensi- fication in volleyball players. *J Sports Sci Med.* (2014) 13:571–9.

Malina RM, Bouchard C, Bar-Or O. *Growth, Maturation, and Physical Activity.* 2nd ed. Champaign, IL: Human Kinetics (2004).

Min J, Xue H, Wang VH, Li M, Wang Y. Are single children more likely to be overweight or obese than those with siblings? The influence of China's one-child policy on childhood obesity. *Prev Med Rep.* (2017) 103:8–13. doi: 10.1016/j.ypmed.2017.07.018

Bagley S, Salmon J, Crawford D. Family structure and children's television viewing and physical activity. *Med Sci Sports Exerc.* (2015) 38:910–8. doi: 10.1249/01.mss.0000218132.68268.f4

Hardy LL, Baur LA, Garnett SP, Crawford D, Campbell KJ, Shrewsbury VA, et al. Family and home correlates of television viewing in 12–13 year old adolescents: The Nepean Study. *Int J Behav Nutr Phys Activity.* (2006) 3:24. doi: 10.1186/1479-5868-3-24

Esteves CM, Freitas DL, Gouveia ÉR, Lopes VP. Coordenação e habilidades motoras. Associação com o crescimento físico humano, atividade física e fatores de envolvimento. In *Crescer com saúde na Região Autónoma da Madeira.* Funchal: Universidade da Madeira e Universidade do Porto (2013). p. 63–85.

Guedes DP, Guedes JERP. Crescimento e desempenho motor em escolares do município de Londrina, Paraná, Brasil. *Cadernos Saúde Públ.* (1993) 9:S58–70. doi: 10.1590/S0102-311X1993000500007

Martín-Matillas M, Valadés D, Hernández-Hernández E, Olea-Serrano F, Sjöström M, Delgado-Fernández M, et al. Anthropometric, body composition and somatotype characteristics of elite female volleyball players from the highest Spanish league. *J Sports Sci.* (2014) 32:137–48. doi: 10.1080/02640414.2013.809472

Ortega FB, Artero EG, Ruiz JR, España-Romero V, Jiménez-Pavón D, Vicente-Rodriguez G, et al. Physical fitness levels among European adolescents: The HELENA study. *Br J Sports Med.* (2011) 45:20–9. doi: 10.1136/bjsm.2009.062679

Pereira S, Katzmarzyk PT, Gomes TN, Chaves RN, Santos FK, Santos D, et al. Multilevel modelling of somatotype components: the portuguese sibling study on growth, fitness, lifestyle and health. *Ann Human Biol.* (2016) 44:316–24. doi: 10.1080/03014460.2016.1243727

Malina M. Motor development duritng childhood and adolescence. In Thomas JR, editor. *Physical Growth and Maturation.* Minneapolis: Burgess (1984). p. 2–26.

Manios Y, Kafatos A, Kodrington C. Gender differences in physical fitness in young children in Crete. *J Sports Med Phys Fitn.* (1999) 39:24–30.

Thomas JR, French KE. Gender differences across age in motor performance: a meta-analysis. *Psychol Bull.* (1985) 98:260–82. doi: 10.1037/0033-2909.98.2.260

Delorme N, Boiché J, Raspaud M. Relative age effect in female sport: a diachronic examination of soccer players. *Scand J Med Sci Sports.* (2010) 20:509–515. doi: 10.1111/j.1600-0838.2009.00979.x

Artero EG, Lee D, Lavie CJ, España-Romero V, Sui X, Church TS, et al. Effects of muscular strength on cardiovascular risk factors and prognosis. *J Cardiopulm Rehabil Prev.* (2012) 32:351–8. doi: 10.1097/HCR.0b013e3182642688

Cohen DD, Gómez-Arbeláez D, Camacho PA, Pinzon S, Hormiga C, Trejos-Suarez J, et al. Low muscle strength is associated with metabolic risk factors in Colombian children: the ACFIES study. *PLoS ONE.* (2014) 9:e93150. doi: 10.1371/journal.pone.0093150

Steene-Johannessen J, Kolle E, Andersen LB, Anderssen SA. Adiposity, aerobic fitness, muscle fitness, and markers of inflammation in children. *Med Sci Sports Exerc.* (2013) 45:714–21. doi: 10.1249/MSS.0b013e318279707a

Wrotniak B, Salvy S, Lazarus L, Epstein L. Motor proficiency relationships among siblings. *Percept Motor Skills*. (2009) 108:112–20. doi: 10.2466/pms.108.1.112-120

da Costa YP, Cirilo de Sousa MDS, da Silva JCG, de Araújo JP, Neto GR, Batista GR. Technical and tactical performance indicators based on the outcome of the set in the school volleyball. *Motricidade*. (2017) 13:34–40. doi: 10.6063/motricidade,.12935

Pereira S, Katzmarzyk PT, Hedeker D, Maia J. Profile resemblance in health-related markers: The portuguese sibling study on growth, fitness, lifestyle, and health. *Int J Environ Res Public Health*. (2018) 15:1–14. doi: 10.3390/ijerph15122799

Deane RS, Chow JW, Tillman AD, Fournier KA. Effect of hip flexor training on sprint, shuttle run, and vertical jump performance. *J Strength Condit Res*. (2005) 19:615–21. doi: 10.1519/00124278-200508000-00022

Witkowski K, Piepiora P, Migasiewicz J, Maslinski J, Salachna A. Physical fitness, developmental age and somatic development of youth Greco-Roman wrestlers and school youth aged 13-14 years. *Sci Mart Arts Extreme Sports*. (2018) 14:63–74.

Lang JJ, Belanger K, Poitras V, Janssen I, Tomkinson GR, Tremblay MS. Systematic review of the relationship between 20m shuttle run performance and health indicators among children and youth. *J Sci Med Sport*. (2018) 21:383–97. doi: 10.1016/j.jsams.2017.08.002

Rodrigues LP, Lima R, Silva A, Camões M. A importância dos irmãos no desenvolvimento da competência motora e aptidão física. In: Rodrigues P, Rebolo A, Vieira F, Dias A, Silva L, editor. *Estudos em Desenvolvimento Motor da Criança* (Piaget Editions). Almada: Horizontes Pedagógicos (2018). p. 57–79.

Price J. Parent-child quality time does birth order matter? *J Human Resour*. (2008) 43:240–65. doi: 10.1353/jhr.2008.0023

Barclay K, Myrskylä M. Birth order and physical fitness in early adulthood: Evidence from Swedish military conscription data. *Soc Sci Med*. (2014) 123:141–8. doi: 10.1016/j.socscimed.2014. 11.007

Sundström M, Duvander AE. Gender division of childcare and the sharing of parental leave among new parents in Sweden. *Eur Sociol Rev*. (2002) 18:433–47. doi: 10.1093/esr/18.4.433

Abramovitch R, Corter CM, Lando B. Sibling interaction in the home. *Child Dev*. (1979) 50:997–1003. doi: 10.2307/1129325

Kraemer WJ, Comstock B, Clark JE, Dunn-Lewis C. Athlete needs analysis. In: Hoffman J, editor. *NSCA's Guide to Program Design*. Champain, IL: Human Kinetics (2012). p. 10–26.

McHale SM, Updegraff KA, Helms-Erikson H, Crouter AC. Sibling influences on gender development in middle childhood and early adolescence: a longitudinal study. *Dev Psychol Am Psychol Assoc*. (2001) 37:115–25. doi: 10.1037/0012-1649.37.1.115

24

Strategies for Maintaining the Coach–Analyst Relationship within Professional Football Utilizing the COMPASS Model

Michael Bateman* and Gareth Jones

School of Sport and Exercise Science, University of Worcester, Worcester, United Kingdom

Correspondence:
Michael Bateman
m.bateman@worc.ac.uk

There is a considerable body of research by that has investigated the coach–athlete relationship in sport. However, given the multi-disciplinary nature of modern elite coaching, there is a scarcity of research focusing on the relationship between coaches and other members of the coaching and support team. This study examined the perceptions of six elite professional football analyst's relationships with their respective coaches. Semi structured interviews utilizing the COMPASS Framework were conducted focusing on Conflict, Openness, Motivation, Preventative Strategies, Assurance, Support, and Social Networks. The results verified that the COMPASS Model of relationship maintenance was applicable to this dyad. Content analysis indicated that there was 215 raw data units comprising of 16 higher order themes across the model which was further broken down into 29 lower order themes. All aspects of the model were found to contribute toward a positively maintained relationship. Having an open relationship underpinned by honesty and being able to provide an opinion was seen as the highest rated attribute that was closely followed by supporting the coach by understanding their requirements for successful coaching practice. Not meeting the coach's expectations was found to cause conflict and was further highlighted by an inductive analysis that revealed the existence of a relationship that is fundamentally dictated by the coach. Implications of this investigation are that professionals which support elite performers need to set out clear expectations of working practice and hierarchies in order to minimize the chance of internal conflict that can impact on the service levels received by the performer.

Keywords: sports performance analysis, relationship maintenance, elite sport, soccer, coach, analysts, power relationships

INTRODUCTION

O'Donoghue (2010) showcased that performance analysis has become a validated support structure for coaches and athletes and although there is a body of research which investigates the role of the analyst (Bampouras et al., 2012; Wright et al., 2013) and the perceptions of performance analysis within the coaching process (Francis and Jones, 2014; Wright et al., 2016), there is a scarcity of information surrounding the way coaches create, interact and maintain working relationships with performance analysts (Wright et al., 2013). The relationship between the analyst and coach has however, been shown to be so important that coaches would attempt to recruit analysts that they have worked with in previous roles when they gain new employment (Reid et al., 2004; Butterworth and Turner, 2014; Huggan et al., 2015).

Whilst research has identified that elite coaches are supported by a large group of support staff, collaborating data and observations for the benefit of the athletes (Reid et al., 2004; Gustafsson et al., 2008; Bampouras et al., 2012; Clement and Arvinen-Barrow, 2013; Wagstaff et al., 2015), research investigating the relationships present within this group has focused primarily around the coach and athlete (Poczwardowski et al., 2002; Jowett, 2003; Lafrenière et al., 2008; Adie and Jowett, 2010). It has been shown that the emotions, cognitions and behaviors of the persons within this dyad have been shown to be central in developing meaningful relationships (Jowett and Ntoumanis, 2004). Research has also been conducted around the maintenance of relationships, including the conceptualization of the COMPASS Model and Coach–Athlete Relationship Maintenance Questionnaire (CARM-Q) validation process (Rhind and Jowett, 2010, 2012) which has provided valuable insights of coaches within typical dyads in sport.

Jowett and colleagues have employed a number of methodological approaches for the expansive array of research into the coach–athlete relationship. They have mainly centered around the use of questionnaires for model validation purposes (Jowett and Chaundy, 2004; Jowett and Clark-Carter, 2006; Lafrenière et al., 2008; Olympiou et al., 2008; Jowett, 2009; Adie and Jowett, 2010; Jowett et al., 2012b; Rhind and Jowett, 2012; Yang and Jowett, 2013) and interviews for exploratory investigations (Jowett and Meek, 2000; Jowett, 2003; Jowett and Cockerill, 2003; Rhind and Jowett, 2010; Jowett et al., 2012a; Jowett and Carpenter, 2015). All interviews adopted a semi structured format utilizing open ended questions and prompts where required to elicit deeper insight (Patton, 2002). This pattern was followed regardless of the sample size being small (n = 2) (Jowett, 2003) or large (n = 30) (Jowett and Carpenter, 2015). Of those studies to undertake interviews, the selection criteria for inclusion ranged from a minimum 6-month coach–athlete relationship (Jowett et al., 2012a; Jowett and Carpenter, 2015) to 4 years (Jowett and Cockerill, 2003). Jowett and Cockerill's (2003) research only interviewed athletes. This enabled free expression of the athletes, without worry of their coaches' involvement or retort (McKenna and Mutrie, 2003). Rhind and Jowett (2010) recruited unconnected coaches and athletes as previous studies had shown this amplified the range and scope of the data to make it more generalizable in the wider sporting context.

Whilst most interviews were conducted in person, Jowett et al. (2012a) utilized telephone interviews for data collection as the data had not been shown to produce significantly different data to interviews in person (Sweet, 2002). The authors did concede that the format may have limited the expression of experiences and impacted on the perception of the information. Content analysis (Weber, 1990) was used extensively (Jowett and Meek, 2000; Jowett, 2003; Jowett and Cockerill, 2003; Rhind and Jowett, 2010; Jowett et al., 2012a) to categorize the data points into a hierarchy of responses and determine a frequency analysis and is well documented as a common approach for sports psychology studies (Côté et al., 1993). This type of processing was found to highlight prominent themes across responses from all participants (Rhind and Jowett, 2010).

Jowett and Meek (2000) investigated the constructs of closeness, co-orientation and complementarity (3C's) when interviewing four atypical dyads (married couples who also held a coach–athlete relationship) and identified that the coach–athlete relationship was interdependent. Closeness referred to the emotions of the dyad and the affective elements of the coach–athlete relationship were reflected in mutual feelings of trust and respect. Co-orientation was reflective of the quality of the coach–athlete relationship that was highlighted through the thoughts and perspectives of the dyad where mutual empathetic feelings suggested a more effective relationship. Complementarity considered the interactions and co-operative behaviors of the coach and athlete. Where corresponding behaviors were elicited, an increase in the strength of the relationship was perceived. Interdependence is characterized in the coach–athlete dyad by the high levels of closeness, co-orientation and complementarity creating a mutually beneficial relationship at an affective, cognitive and behavioral level (Jowett et al., 2012a). Although the qualitative method provided a rich source of information, useful in advancing the scope of knowledge in the area, including the web of interactions that crossed the 3C's, the small sample size and use of atypical participants meant that there was a need for a more quantitative study using greater sample size to create generalizable results (Jowett and Meek, 2000). Further validation of the interactive aspects of the 3C's was explored via interviews with 12 elite Olympic medalists where connections between the C's were uncovered, although the causality could not be confirmed (Jowett and Cockerill, 2003). They did establish that the relationships contained attributes including, but not limited to, respect, trust, and clear roles. Inconsistencies in the data collection method (some interviews and some written responses to questions) may have impacted upon the validity of the results. The findings were however, suggested to be integral in the initial construct of the Coach–Athlete Relationship Questionnaire (CART-Q) (Jowett and Ntoumanis, 2004) where co-orientation (+1C) was validated as commitment and that has been used as the basis for various empirical research (Jowett, 2009; Rhind and Jowett, 2010; Yang and Jowett, 2013). The conceptualization of the 3+1C's model (Jowett, 2007) to include co-orientation which measured how accurately the coach/athlete was able to understand how the other was feeling, thinking and behaving. This led to the requirement for better understanding of how these relationships use strategies including conflict management and socializing to keep a dyad in a specific way (Dindia and Canary, 1993).

Keeping a relationship in a stable state using effective maintenance strategies, facilitated long term, satisfying relationships (Canary and Stafford, 1994, p. 4). Rhind and Jowett (2010) investigated how coaches and athletes used such approaches to preserve a steady coach–athlete environment. The authors based the categorization of themes for their research on previous work into romantic relationship maintenance (Stafford and Canary, 1991; Canary and Stafford, 1994) and led to the conceptualization of the COMPASS model. The original categories were: Conflict management (proactive and reactive), openness (discussing feelings), motivation (effort, motivate the other, fun and demonstrations), positivity (adaptability, fairness and external pressure), advice (sport focused, reward feedback and constructive criticism), support (assurance, Sport specific, personal), and social networks (socializing and shared networks).

The "COMPASS" model complemented the 3+1C's model and was proposed as a method to understand and manage the complex dynamics of the coach–athlete dyad. The authors also identified the potential for the COMPASS model to be transferable to other interpersonal sporting relationships (Rhind and Jowett, 2010). This body of work was further validated by Rhind and Jowett (2012) with the development of the CARM-Q. The authors found some inconsistencies of the COMPASS model after an exploratory factor analysis had identified highly related subscales (Stafford et al., 2000). Positivity was replaced by Preventative Strategies as positivity was found across various subscales of other categories and Advice was replaced by Assurance to differentiate between support and openness which was validated by Study 2 in the paper.

Research within sport has investigated the domineering power exerted by coaches over their athletes (Johns and Johns, 2000; Cushion and Jones, 2006; Rylander, 2016). A number of theories have contributed to a large body of research on power within social psychology that have often been influenced by the seminal work of French and Raven (1959). Their 5 stage model of interpersonal influence depicted the bases of power which were identified as expert, referent, legitimate, coercive and reward. Rylander (2016) interpreted these for research within the coach–athlete setting and defined expert power as the coaches knowledge which the athlete requires or values. Referent power was based around the coach being identified as a role model or somebody that they could relate to creating reciprocal behavioral and actions. Legitimate power was shown as the recognition within society that the athlete was expected to be comply with their direction. Coercive and reward power were seen as the ability of the coach to discipline or reward athlete behavior based on conformity or outcome. This model has undergone several amendments (Raven, 1965, 1992, 1999) over time and have come under some scrutiny (Patchen, 1974; Carson et al., 1993; Yukl, 2006) although the original model is still considered to be applicable for contemporary research (Groom et al., 2012). Cushion and Jones (2006) found that players within a professional football academy were hegemonized by the historical culture which had existed within the industry for years. The social control elicited by a coach has been further investigated (Purdy et al., 2008; Purdy and Jones, 2011) in adult sport and is perceived to be more transient with the idea of power being negotiable between the coach and athlete depending on the circumstance (Poczwardowski et al., 2002; Cushion et al., 2003; Purdy et al., 2008). Jones (2006) also argued that the coach perceived that they were required to interact socially with other contextual stakeholders such as technical staff to maintain their status of power. This is in accordance with Giddens (1984) conceptualization of power that showed the subservient parties had the ability to change the balance of power relationships through social interactions. This was further validated by Purdy et al. (2008) when the athletes showed resistance in addition to compliance and co-operation to a coach in turmoil (Locke, 1985).

The concept of the power dynamic struggles between asymmetrical relationships is well documented and as a result of hierarchical relationships (Cushion et al., 2003; Jones et al., 2009). However, it was suggested that a strong relationship identified through the 3+1C's model (Jowett, 2007) could negate the conflict that has often been associated with this type of dyad which would result in the coach often looking to teach and guide the protégé (Jowett et al., 2012a). McCalla and Fitzpatrick (2016) argued that although micro-politics are prevalent within high performance teams, when a synergy exists between the value of each contributing facet, and the experts of each field work within their remit, the potential of the staff can contribute to harmonious working environments. However, if the boundaries become blurred, then anxiety and confusion could develop (Frost et al., 2005).

Wright et al. (2013) examined 48 completed questionnaires from performance analysts and found that 89.4% of participants stated that the relationship between the coach and analyst was "Very Important." They discovered that analysts were consulted to varying degrees within professional football but very rarely led feedback sessions. They summarized that this was due to a number of factors including coaches trust in the analyst, but suggested further investigation was required. They also spoke of the negotiations around the design of analytical processes and defining measures of successful performance. This collaborative workflow contradict the results of Bampouras et al. (2012). Whilst they acknowledged the relationship was instrumental for analytical system success, the perception was that the analyst was responsible for purely collecting the information as directed by the coach. This idea of an unbalanced power relationship has been further supported by Huggan et al. (2015) when an analyst considered the value of the role and their own self-esteem due to the dominance of the coach in the applied setting.

Sarmento et al. (2015) provided evidence of the numerous benefits and attributes that analysts brought to a technical team. However, of the six coaches interviewed, only one coach had access to a full-time analyst which suggests other coaches may have based this opinion on beliefs or past experiences, rather than current circumstance. Huggan et al. (2015) had first hand narrative evidence from a Performance Analyst which reported the participant placed an emphasis on creating strong working relationships with cooperative and supportive colleagues. Manzanares et al. (2014) concluded that bridging the gap between the scientific analysis and the practical coaching process would be mutually beneficial and would only serve to enhance the development of athletes performance. The authors acknowledged the workload and resources required by the analysts within elite sport that was required to support the needs of the coach to make reliable technical and tactical appraisals of performance. Fernandez-Echeverria et al. (2017) have criticized the lack of studies which consider how the analyst is utilized by coaches within the coaching process. These suggestions have been highlighted in football, particularly as the role of a dedicated performance analyst is now a necessity in the current staffing structure (Reeves and Roberts, 2013).

As performance analysts have become more integral to the coaching and feedback process, Hughes (2004) indicated that analysis has interjected into the coach–athlete relationship. They found that the addition of another stakeholder in the process (gathering and analyzing data) allowed greater information share which is instrumental in developing teams. For this to be a successful working relationship, mutual trust and respect must be observed for all parties (Francis and Jones, 2014).

The research outlined above has provided evidence that the quality of the relationships coaches have with their athletes, and their ability to maintain them at a good level, has a correlation with the success that the athletes are able to attain. This coupled with the literature that identifies the performance analyst to be a key component in the coaching process justifies the need to examine the relationship of the coach and the performance analyst to investigate if maintenance strategies are transferable across to this dyad. There is limited research into the relationships between coaches and members of their sports science support staff, so this paper will aim to fill a gap within the literature that can further enhance the coaching process and expand the knowledge base within performance analysis and coaching. The aim of the study is to investigate the relationship between the coach and performance analyst within professional football. Specifically, the research is looking to confirm behaviors that relate to maintenance strategies within this dyad.

Aim 1. Investigate the main components of maintaining the coach–analyst relationship.

Aim 2. Determine if the conceptualized coach–athlete COMPASS model is adaptable to the coach–analyst relationship.

Aim 3. Understand any other pertinent trends which arise from the data.

MATERIALS AND METHODS

Participants

Expert purposive sampling was employed to enlist six current first team performance analysts working full time in professional football clubs in England. By stipulating first team analysts, the researcher was able to gain understanding from participants with significant experiences which hoped to enrich the data provided thorough insight into coach analyst relationships at the highest levels of professional sport (Simonton, 1999; Jowett and Cockerill, 2003). They were also required to have maintained a current or past coach analyst relationship for a minimum of 6 months (Jowett et al., 2012a,b; Jowett and Carpenter, 2015). The selected contributors were recruited personally due to pre-existing relationships with the researcher who had a previous career within the industry. Participants received an information pack which clarified the aims of the study, included an information sheet about the underlying 3+1C's model and an informed consent sheet.

The six participants ranged in age from 25 to 37 years with a mean age of 30.3 years (±4.88 years) and had an average of 8.16 years (±3.2 years) experience working as a performance analyst within professional football. Five out of the six interviewees had worked for four professional teams and the sixth had worked for two teams during their nine years' experience. The participants current coach analyst relationships ranged between 3 and 24 months (mean = 10.3 ± 7.5 months). The shortest dyadic working relationship encountered during the analyst's careers was acknowledged as 21 days by A3 who was also involved in the longest continuous relationship (5 years). The average for the shortest relationship was 84 days (±46 days) and 30 months (±17.69) for the longest relationship.

Procedures

Ethical approval was granted by the University of Worcester's ethics and research governance committee to undertake this study. Written and voluntary informed consent was obtained from all participants within the study. The interview questions were validated through a pilot interview with an experienced performance analyst (greater than 10 years' experience) to assist in identifying any epistemological concerns (Kim, 2010). This initial authentication process resulted in the addition of one question to the schedule to improve the balance of the questions being asked.

The interviews were conducted via telephone (O'Donoghue, 2010, p. 39; Jowett et al., 2012a). This style of data collection negated any restrictions on participation based on the analyst location and has been validated as useful for shorter, focused interviews with busy people (Miller, 1995). The duration of the interviews lasted between 21 min, 14 s and 50 min, 25 s. Semi structured, open ended questions were used with prompts where required based on the conceptualized COMPASS model, the validation of the categories via the CARM-Q framework (Rhind and Jowett, 2010, 2012) and the 3+1C's framework (Jowett, 2007). The interview was split into three parts; an introductory section to build rapport with the interviewees and collect demographic information (Kvale and Brinkmann, 2009, pp. 123–125). Secondly, the main section of the interview asked four questions pertaining to the analyst's perceptions and experiences of relationship maintenance strategies (**Supplementary Data Sheet 1**). Finally, the participants were offered an opportunity to provide any further information they deemed pertinent to the investigation.

An independent coder who had experience of both the applied Performance Analyst role (3 years) and theoretical Academic role (2 years) was employed to assess the raw data units obtained from interview one to ensure the results were not biased via the researcher's knowledge or experiences (Woods and Thatcher, 2009; Jones et al., 2014). Fifty-seven deductive data units and forty inductive data units were investigated and categorized by the coder which resulted the re-categorization of two units.

Owing to the researchers 10 years' experience of working within professional football, knowledge of all participants annulled the need to spend time *in situ* building rapport with the analysts. This closeness and prior knowledge of the industry could have led to personal bias, so the researcher practiced bracketing of their opinion through the pilot study and continued this during the main study (Tufford and Newman,

2010). Transcripts of all interviews were sent to the respective interviewee to confirm the accuracy of their account. All participants had their data anonymized whereby each interviewee was referred to as A1–A6 and where names were referred to, pseudonyms were used where required to hide the true identity of those involved.

Data Analysis

Content analysis was used to systematically discover themes within the data (Weber, 1990, p. 41). After reviewing the interview transcriptions, a deductive content analysis identified themes and sub themes based upon previous research (Rhind and Jowett, 2010, 2012). An inductive approach was also used to identify themes previously not recorded (Rubin and Rubin, 1995; Elo and Kyngäs, 2008). 215 meaningful units were found in the deductive analysis and 142 units were created through the inductive analysis. All units were highlighted and catergorised accordingly.

RESULTS AND DISCUSSION

"COMPASS Model" in the Coach–Analyst Relationship

The coded results showed (**Table 1**) that raw data units were divulged for all seven themes within the amended "COMPASS Model" (Rhind and Jowett, 2010, 2012). All six analysts provided insights regarding six of the seven themes yielding varying levels of raw data units ranging between 6 and 18.1% of the total raw units. In percentage contribution order, the results were; Support (18.1%), Preventative Strategies (16.3%), Motivation and Social Networks (14.5%), Conflict Management (11.2%), and Assurance (6%). of the total raw data, Openness provided statements by five out of six participants although it had the highest total number of raw data units of any of the themes commanding 19.5% of the total number of units.

Conflict Management

Conflict management was responsible for the reactive elements of maintaining relationships. This is in contrast to Rhind and Jowett (2010) as the pro-active statements were later considered to be their own category (Rhind and Jowett, 2012). It correlated the findings of the subcategory "Consequences of Unmet Expectations" with nine observations (4.2%). These ranged from not allowing conflict to affect the relationship by A1 who stated:

> "*if I overstepped the mark, he would either let it go, or he would pull you up on it but it wouldn't ever be a negative thing*"

Through to severe consequences that ended the association for A3:

> "*When you stop being part of a group, or the group I suppose, then I found myself out the door with my p45 so you know, there's cause and effect*"

Five of the six interviewees reported attempts to diffuse conflicts once they had arisen to enable the relationship to be maintained. These predominately focused around confronting the issue:

> "*if you do have an issue, that it's not just kind of brushed under the carpet, it's raised in the right way, communicated in the right way and its dealt with at the appropriate time*" (A6: 8 of 15 data units in this sub category)

Or trying to provide solutions with various statements beginning in this manner:

> "*Now I tried to resolve this...*" (A3)

> "*I think there was smaller things in place where I'd try and get round it...*" (A2)

> "*I ended up realising that all I had to do...*" (A5)

The attempts to resolve the situations through co-operative acts was in correlation with the findings of Rhind and Jowett (2010). This was also confirmed by Jowett (2003) who found that if either member of the dyad was unwilling to try and understand the source of the conflict, then the relationship could not be restored to its previously successful state. This studies results suggest the analysts were able to engage in these conversations although the threat of being dismissed due to conflict was still evident from two analysts.

Openness

Openness contained two of the three sub categories that were also reported by Rhind and Jowett (2010). Other awareness (understanding how the coach is feeling) was not conveyed although 42 units highlighting both non-sport communication (8.8%) and talk about anything (10.7%) themes were present. The two main subcategories to emerge from non-sport communicating were honesty and trust which centered around discussion of topics that were still work related (Rhind and Jowett, 2010). Examples were provided by A4, A5, and A6 respectively:

> "*have that honesty and openness between the both of you to try and improve what you're doing*"

> "*But in terms of having conversations that I know, they wouldn't want to leave them four walls, you've obviously been in plenty of them, and I guess that's a good sign, that you're trusted and accepted*"

> "*I think the key things trust between the two, the coach and the analyst. So, they've got to be able to have two way trust in each other so the coach can trust that the analyst is giving them good information and the analyst trusts that the coach is going to use it and use it the correct way*"

For the analyst, the thought of being trusted and respected was paramount in maintaining open relationships with the coach. This perception of closeness (Jowett and Meek, 2000) was imperative for the analyst to feel they were deemed competent by the coach (Jowett and Cockerill, 2003) and has been shown to differentiate between harmonious and non-harmonious relationships (Canary and Stafford, 1994; Francis and Jones, 2014). These findings built upon Wright et al.'s (2013) call for more research into the trust between the coach and analyst.

TABLE 1 | Summary of the results from the COMPASS Model.

	Frequencies				Frequencies				Frequencies		
Compass model	***n***	**%**	**Analysts**	**Higher order**	***n***	**%**	**Analysts**	**Lower order**	***n***	**%**	**Analysts**
Conflict management	24	11.2	6/6	Reactive	24	11.2	6/6	Consequences of unmet expectations	9	4.2	4/6
								Diffusion of conflict	15	7.0	5/6
Openness	42	19.5	5/6	Non-sport communication	19	8.8	5/6	Honesty	14	6.5	5/6
								Trust	5	2.3	3/6
				Talk about anything	23	10.7	5/6	Approachability	13	6.0	3/6
								Providing your opinion	10	4.7	5/6
Motivation	31	14.4	6/6	Effort	7	3.3	3/6	Commitment to the coach	6	2.8	3/6
								Positivity	1	0.5	1/6
				Fun	4	1.9	2/6	Humor	4	1.9	2/6
				Motivate the other	9	4.2	5/6	Togetherness	6	2.8	3/6
								Multidisciplinary team togetherness	3	1.4	2/6
				Show ability	11	5.1	4/6	Hard work	11	5.1	4/6
Preventative strategies	35	16.3	6/6	Avoiding conflict	14	6.5	6/6	Awareness of coach expectations	5	2.3	3/6
								Submissive avoidance	9	4.2	4/6
				Relationship continuity	8	3.7	5/6	Establishing early understanding	4	1.9	4/6
								Judging dyadic preferences	4	1.9	3/6
				Respecting boundaries	13	6.0	4/6	Respecting others	11	5.1	4/6
								Solution based opinion	2	0.9	1/6
Assurance	13	6.0	6/6	Constructive feedback	1	0.5	1/6	Advice	1	0.5	1/1
				Sport communication	12	5.6	6/6	Relationship building phase	4	1.9	3/6
								Providing analytical expertise	8	3.7	5/6
Support	39	18.1	6/6	Person support	10	4.7	3/6	Mutual respect	4	1.9	2/6
								Unconditional support	6	2.8	2/6
				Sport support	29	13.5	6/6	Communication	5	2.3	4/6
								Understanding coach requirements	24	11.2	5/6
Social networks	31	14.4	6/6	Socialization	4	1.9	1/6	Maintaining previous relationships	4	1.9	1/6
				Shared network	27	12.6	6/6	Casual interactions	10	4.7	5/6
								Obligatory socialization	7	3.3	3/6
								Socialization through sport	10	4.7	4/6
Total	215	100.0		Total	215	100.0		Total	215	100.0	

The present results may have been found due to the length of the dyadic relationships which were not reported within the Wright study.

"Approachability" and "Providing Your Opinion" materialized within the "Talk About Anything" sub category although the overriding premise still surrounded work-based conversations. A6 talked extensively (6 of 13 units) about approachability and examples included:

> *"if you've got a good relationship with someone, regardless of if you agree with them. I mean, it can go both ways. You can get on with someone personally but not agree with them professionally, or the other way around, but as long as you've got at least one of those relationships, you can be, you can have that conversation"*

> *"it's important you get to know the coach as well as you can on an individual work level and how they like information"*

This correlated with the results from Rhind and Jowett (2010) and was further underpinned by the "Openness" facet of Stafford and Canary's (1991) work.

Motivation

Unlike the findings of Rhind and Jowett (2010), Motivation was not the most frequently discussed form of relationship maintenance, although it was mentioned by 100% of participants. It provided 14.4% of the total units and was catergorised into effort, fun, motivate the other and show ability in line with previous literature (Rhind and Jowett, 2010). Effort suggested a commitment to the coach and was highlighted by the following quotes:

> *"So results affect you more and you're more willing to go the extra mile. For example, we lost a game earlier in the season and I was up until... I stayed up until. I think it was like 5 o clock in the morning after that night game, changing this match report because I was motivated to help and make things better."*

> *"I think sometimes the best relationships, you probably are willing to do the extra that you might not if you didn't have that relationship with the coach"*

Motivate the other resulted in quotes that alluded to togetherness of the multidisciplinary team as well as the specific dyad in question. A2 and A4 spoke enthusiastically about this subject:

> *"He knows it's not just always all about him. And that there's he has a team of staff and he wants to keep them happy, he wants you to want to work for him"*

> *"empowered straight away if someone is going to be willing to listen to your opinions based on your analysis that you've done. Umm, so yeah, very empowered, very valued from that interaction"*

The following quotes regarding the requirement of the analyst to work hard in order to show ability was mirrored by 4 out of the 6 analysts interviewed.

> *"if you keep performing as they asked or above, then they get more faith in you, they'll give you more respect, more pressure, and then you'll build a better relationship"*

> *"standards remain really high, so the quality of the work you're producing is still of the standard that's required that I think that helps maintain that relationship along the way"*

Akin to the findings of Huggan et al. (2015), the analyst's willingness to provide extra effort based upon the perceived strength of the relationship was also demonstrated. Their findings also allied to the suggestions that portraying motivation also created more supportive colleagues, leading to stronger relationships (Huggan et al., 2015).

Preventative Strategies

This dimension was considered important by all participants and provided 16.3% of the total raw units. The sub categories were made up of "Avoiding Conflict," "Respecting Boundaries" (respecting others role and responsibility within the team) and "Relationship Continuity" (through establishing early understanding and judging dyadic preferences. The relative contribution to these results suggest that the requirement to be separate from Conflict Management was justified (Rhind and Jowett, 2012).

By establishing early understanding of the coaches' methods, it was perceived that the analyst could adapt their work to suit the preferences of the manager. A4 summarized this by stating:

> *"Is to very quickly understand what they require and kind of, shape your work to that because if you don't, I think that's when you start to encounter problems"*

3 of 6 interviewees built upon this, suggesting that by having the ability to judge the preferences and character of the coach, they could then ensure the relationship strength was maintained. A3 stressed this by saying:

> *"I think you have to get a read on people and rather than chase people round stadiums and pitches with a laptop you need to know when to, when to speak, when you're allowed to speak, and when to say nothing"*

The concept of respecting boundaries continued the closely associated themes with 5.1% of the data units acknowledging that:

> *"Really clear guidelines and like, a real good understanding of what was required from both sides"* (A4)

was key to the success of the relationship. By establishing rules, not only did the relationship reduce the possible conflict scenarios, but also allows for greater motivation from both parties (Jowett and Carpenter, 2015).

Avoiding conflict was subdivided into two themes. "Awareness of Coach Expectations" and "Submissive Avoidance" both showed aspects of the micro-politics associated within this type of dyadic relationship. A2 talked about coach expectations of the analyst:

> *"I think delivering, delivering results so like, getting stuff ready or like hitting deadlines etc. – if the coach or manager has asked you for something for a certain time, ya know, have you delivered on time. If you're failing to deliver then they'll stop asking you for things, that relationships gunna break down"*

And A3 spoke around submissive avoidance in order to maintain parity within the relationship:

> *"So they say, we might do a meeting, and then you know that they won't, but you have do it anyway, just in case you do have to do it"*

These outcomes add to the current literature surrounding the requirement for the performance analyst to be subordinate to the coach in order for relationships to be maintained (Bampouras et al., 2012; Huggan et al., 2015).

Assurance

Assurance was an adaptation from the original COMPASS Model (Rhind and Jowett, 2010) after it replaced "Advice" but it was responsible for the lowest collection of data units, registering just 6% of the total findings. It was however, supported by all participants of the study and primarily revolved around sport communication (12 of 13 total units). Similarly to Preventative Strategies, an emphasis was placed upon the building phase of the relationships to cement the status of the relationship, but data units suggested that they would provide assurances of how they could impact on the success of the athletes rather than being submissive. A6 and A1 supposed:

> *"I think probably try and at the very start, in terms of getting an understanding of what they want, and try just to say look this is, this is how I think this could be better"*

> *"once that relationship starts building up they will start asking you more and more questions regarding more tactical side of things. So once I had built that relationship up, they were asking me, and I felt open enough to suggest ideas of how meetings could be led and how we can engage players more and how we can get players to get more out of the meetings"*

It was suggested that providing analytical expertise would have a positive effect on the relationship with the coach. A3 and A4 recalled:

> *"And he'll walk in the next day and you have the successful and unsuccessful crosses broken down and you'll say, ya know, just based on what you said to the other coaches, here's some bits and pieces and he might show that back to the lads"*

> *"quite a lot of our discussion around the pre match was normally verbal, rather than documents if you like so, we would sit an brief the manager on kinda, how we were going to play or how the opposition play"*

There was consensus with previous findings that show how the analyst's skill-set and alternative viewpoint allowed for greater opportunities for athletes to improve (Hughes, 2004; Francis and Jones, 2014; Huggan et al., 2015).

Support

Three of the analysts referenced the personal support that they felt was important within the coach–athlete dyad. A4 provided 3 of the 4 units for this subcategory and suggested:

> *"I think respect, kind of a mutual respect between the two is very important"*

This was contradicted, primary by A1 and A2 who believed they were required to give their unconditional support to the coach, as in A2's words:

> *"the gaffer is the one at the top, with the decision making. He's got the final say on everything, but he's got to have his own staff, and he's got to have staff that want to work for him"*

This challenges the findings of Jowett and Cockerill (2003), who perceived that interpersonal relationships were ineffective if the coaches support and knowledge were deemed inadequate by the athlete.

Sport Support was supported with 29 data units (13.5% of the total recorded) from 6 out of 6 analysts'. The majority (24) of these focused around understanding the coaches' requirements. A3 suggested that part of the responsibility lay with the analyst when they said:

> *"you should almost be able to anticipate what the coach wants"*

Whereas A6 had experienced coaches that prescribed the support they required explicitly.

> *"I've worked with coaches that, they know exactly what they want, and they don't really want to deviate from that so it's a case of this is what you're going to do, this is how you're going to do it, that's it!"*

These conflicting viewpoints of the participant have been shown to be important for maintaining relationships as the coach and analyst may need to show leading roles in addition to support roles in certain circumstances throughout the lifespan of the relationship (Jowett et al., 2012a; Yang and Jowett, 2013).

Social Networks

Socialization (the social interaction which only included the two members of the dyad) was only alluded to by A1. The 4 (1.9%) examples they provided related to maintaining previous relationships with coaches they are not currently working with:

> *"13 of my 14 managers I get on with, still got my back, pick up the phone to them now and speak to them now"*

> *"But in a positive way, I've been asked to work for previous managers on a few occasions and I've had to decline. But I think that shows they value me, and my honesty and my relationship with them"*

This was in stark distinction to previous research which found that 21 of 25 data units were focused upon socializing solely with the coach (Rhind and Jowett, 2010). The participants were mainly sub elite and individual sport focused so may not have been involved within such large sporting environments that employed numerous technical and coaching staff. By showing that maintaining relationship with coaches they were not currently working with professionally, the analyst was able to provide future opportunities for employment within a dyad they perceived as strong and could therefore lead to greater job satisfaction and motivation (Butterworth and Turner, 2014; Huggan et al., 2015).

The remaining units (27–12.6%) were focused around shared networks and were cited by all six analysts. This sub category was further divided into three themes of "Casual

Interactions" (non-sport or work-related activities), "Obligatory Socialization" (situations where attendance was mandatory such as end of season awards, or team meals during away travel) and "Socialization Through Sport" (both within work and outside work). A4 defined their interactions with the coach as compulsory:

> *"There was always a work kind of emphasis on those kind of... You know, if it was a meal or a get together, it was always kind of work related"*

This was in stark contrast to 5 of 6 analysts, including A2, who provided positive examples of casual interactions with the coach:

> *"it just gives you that sort of extra, you get to know more about the person, it's not just always a working relationship. You get to learn a bit more outside which then helps your working relationship"*

Socialization through sport, especially within the confines of the working environment was discussed optimistically on 10 occasions by 4 of the analysts. A6 talked about head tennis matches with staff:

> *"the court opens up and it's a good interaction for staff from different departments, not just coach and analyst but it gets you the opportunity to kind of have a bit of, a bit of fun, a bit of a laughter, a bit of joking around, a bit of competition and you kind of see how the coach reacts in different ways"*

This correlates with findings that social interaction could have positive correlations on the dyad in addition to wider relationships (Jowett and Chaundy, 2004; Rhind and Jowett, 2010). Huggan et al. (2015) also concluded that the social interactions created greater co-operation within the coach–analyst relationship.

Power Relationships in the Coach–Analyst Relationship

The inductive content analysis provided 142 raw data units related to power relationships and micro-politics (**Table 2**). Whilst there was data units that aligned to previous research (French and Raven, 1959), especially coercive power:

> "the managers great but ya know, he still the manager and he's still the one that's gunna sack ya at the end of the day" (A3)

> "the managers more inclined to get rid of you because you don't have a connection and relationship with him" (A1)

And legitimate power:

> "whatever he says in fine. Don't feel as if you can say, ya know, why don't we try this instead? I listen to whatever he says, and whether I like it not, you go away and do it which I guess is the point of the manager, but at the same time, my expertise is in analysis. That's where my expertise lies and I might know more than them, I might know better way to do things but I don't feel as though I can bring that up because I don't feel as though they're going to want to hear it or they'll shoot me down" (A2)

> "I said about just listening and producing exactly what they want rather than what you want to do" (A1)

TABLE 2 | Summary of results of Power Relationships in the Coach–Analyst Relationship.

Theme	Hierarchical	Task focused	Social	Total
Authority	**37**	**53**	**5**	**95**
%	26.1	37.3	3.5	66.9
No of analysts	5/6	6/6	4/6	6/6
Equality	**11**	**19**	**17**	**47**
%	7.7	13.4	12.0	33.1
No of analysts	5/6	6/6	4/6	6/6
Total	**48**	**72**	**22**	**142**
%	33.8	50.7	15.5	
No of analysts	6/6	6/6	5/6	

It was felt the data suggested a very specific type of relationships that was governed by three main higher order themes. These original themes were identified as Hierarchical (thoughts and feelings, non-specific), Task Focused (work related tasks and activities) and Social (non-work related). 66.9% of the points allied to an authoritarian approach whereby the coach was controlling of the relationship. All six analysts provided responses which represented both an authoritarian (Coach dictates) and an equal (where responsibility or behaviors are on a matched level). This was in connection with prior empirical evidence around compliance and co-orientation (Locke, 1985; Purdy et al., 2008).

Hierarchical Theme

The following two quotes denoted how the behavior of analyst was dictated by the coach:

> *"Be respectful, that's difficult sometimes when you're feeling down and your struggling for motivation. At the end of the day, he's the manager of the football club. Whether he deserves respect or not, you have to give it him because that the nature of the industry we're in"* (A1)

> *"I think a lot of the time, the coach analyst relationship, if one of you is wrong, the analyst has to take it and go ok, well I guess I'm wrong"* (A5)

This form of compliance was responsible for 26.1% of the inductive results and was in-keeping with the findings of Cushion and Jones (2006) and Purdy and Jones (2011). The analysts perceived themselves to be in a similar predicament to the athletes, in that any rebellion against the coaches, may jeopardize their future career within elite sport. In contradiction to these findings, a desire for a more equal relationship was alluded to by just 7.7% of the units suggesting that the coach does command power over the analysts within the workplace.

Task Focused Theme

The greatest number of comments were recorded in the Task Focused Authority group and offered 37.3% of the total units analyzed. Comments were recorded from all 6 analyst's and suggested that most work processes and analysis that was undertaken was controlled by the coach. A2 summarized this section by stating:

"I listen to whatever he says, and whether I like it not, you go away and do it which I guess is the point of the manager, but at the same time, my expertise is in analysis. That's where my expertise lies and I might know more than them, I might know better way to do things but I don't feel as though I can bring that up because I don't feel as though they're going to want to hear it or they'll shoot me down"

Although sometimes begrudgingly, the analysts showed that they entered into a consented coach dominated scenario which led to a legitimate power relationship (Cushion and Jones, 2006). This category helps to unearth some of the intricacies' of how the analyst is deployed by coaches within professional football which was considered to be previously sparse (Fernandez-Echeverria et al., 2017).

In repost, A4 provided examples of equality with one particular coach which was perceived by visiting coaches as usual. They suggested that under this coach:

"it would be very much open and for example, developing a game plan for the weekend. He might say, Oh, I want to play this formation, I would say well, if we play that formation, this might, these are the problems we might encounter. You know, have you thought about doing this?"

Giddens (1984) argued that within any structure, the persons within must sanction power being exerted over them for that power to be successful. Therefore, if both parties have an alternative mindset, this may lead to a different relationship that deserves further scrutiny.

Social Theme

The social theme was the only category which provided greater responses surrounding equality (12%) than authoritative behaviors (3.5%). Just five comments were recorded, which centered around financial authority and humor. A5 said:

"have a good sense of humor between you, you're more than happy to take the stick, more than you're probably giving it, I think it's quite important"

Purdy et al. (2008) found that the use of humor and banter between coaches and athletes was often used to instill a belief of influence over the other. They also found that in accordance with Giddens (1984), social interactions were used to change the balance of power and this was validated by the current study with comments being expressed to support this argument:

"they're great exercise because the manager stops being the manager and becomes the person that you're sat in the pub with" (A3).

CONCLUSION

This study outlines that the COMPASS Model, developed through research into the coach–athlete relationship, is transferable across dyads within sport with only minor alterations based upon the roles and responsibilities of analysts. The strategies suggested for maintaining the relationship are centered around the analyst understanding the requirements of the coach to support their needs. By employing a hard working ethos, underpinned by honesty and being approachable, the analysts perceive that the relationship can be productive. The results also highlight the need to employ strategies to prevent conflict occurring as it can lead to the breakdown of relationships if not dealt with swiftly and utilizing the aforementioned behaviors. The respondents also found that socialization through sport and casual interactions was a positive contributor of healthy relationships as it balances the *status quo* of the relationship. This was highlighted by an inductive analysis has also that showcased the existence of authoritative coach behavior's that, whilst not always appreciated by the analyst, often serve to provide the rules that govern relationships.

The results offer aspiring performance analysts insight into the working relationships within first team elite football environments. This is often perceived as an inaccessible environment due to the secretive nature of professional football and as such, it offers relatively unreported insight. This provides clarity for behaviors which may shape the success and ability of analysts to maintain close working relationships that have been shown to correlate to increased technical and tactical insights for opportunities to improve performance outputs. This paper also provides coaches with knowledge of the perceptions of the performance analyst within this working relationship and how their actions may have a positive or negative effect on the analysts view of the dyad. This may enable coaches to consider their behavior to maintain or enhance their relationships with the analyst and other sport science support staff.

Although the underlying research that developed the COMPASS Model acknowledged the transferability of the conceptualization, only interviewing one half of the investigated dyad may have had an impact on the generalizability of the results. Future studies should look to interview both the coach and analyst to better understand the perspectives and meta perspectives of both persons as the coach would likely have a different portrayal of events. Whilst the use of telephone interviews was justified due to geographical locations of the participants, the inability to view the non-verbal cues of the analyst's may have caused the researcher to impact upon the flow of conversation.

As this study has investigated a previously unreported area, it should serve as a basis for future research and not be considered conclusive on the subject. Further studies may wish to consider if similar results are found in academy football relationships or across different sports. The identification of power within the relationship may serve as a foundation for future exploration of this phenomena within other relationships within coaches and technical staff within elite sport so that we may provide academia with insight from the applied world.

ETHICS STATEMENT

This study was carried out in accordance with the recommendations of the University of Worcester with written informed consent from all subjects. All subjects gave written informed consent in accordance with the Declaration of Helsinki. The protocol was approved by the University of Worcester.

AUTHOR CONTRIBUTIONS

MB organized the data collection and analysis, and provided the draft one. GJ read and edited necessary revisions to the manuscript. Both the authors contributed to the conception and design of the work, and confirmed the version was ready for submission.

ACKNOWLEDGMENTS

The authors acknowledge the valuable contribution of the study participants for the rich data they provided. The authors also acknowledge the feedback from Kelvin Beeching for his support to the authors with the project.

REFERENCES

Adie, J. W., and Jowett, S. (2010). Meta-perceptions of the coach-athlete relationship, achievement goals, and intrinsic motivation among sport participants. *J. Appl. Soc. Psychol.* 40, 2750–2773. doi: 10.1111/j.1559-1816.2010.00679.x

Bampouras, T. M., Cronin, C., and Miller, P. K. (2012). Performance analytic processes in elite sport practice: an exploratory investigation of the perspectives of a sport scientist, coach and athlete. *Int. J. Perf. Anal. Sport* 12, 468–483. doi: 10.1080/24748668.2012.11868611

Butterworth, A. D., and Turner, D. J. (2014). Becoming a performance analyst: autoethnographic reflections on agency, and facilitated transformational growth. *Reflect. Pract.* 15, 552–562. doi: 10.1080/14623943.2014.900014

Canary, D. J., and Stafford, L. (1994). *Maintaining Relationships Through Strategic and Routine Interaction. in Communication and Relational Maintenance.* San Diego, CA: Academic Press.

Carson, P., Carson, K., and Roe, W. (1993). Social power bases: a meta-analytic examination of interrelationships and outcomes. *J. Appl. Soc. Psychol.* 23, 1150–1169. doi: 10.1111/j.1559-1816.1993.tb01026.x

Côté, J., Salmela, J. H., Baria, A., and Russell, S. J. (1993). Organizing and interpreting unstructured qualitative data. *Sport Psychol.* 7, 127–137. doi: 10.1123/tsp.7.2.127

Clement, D., and Arvinen-Barrow, M. (2013). "Sport medicine team influences in psychological rehabilitation: A multidisciplinary approach," in *The Psychology of Sport Injury and Rehabilitation*, eds M. Arvinen-Barrow and N. Walker (New York, NY: Routledge/Taylor and Francis Group), 156–170.

Cushion, C., and Jones, R. L. (2006). Power, discourse, and symbolic violence in professional youth soccer: the case of albion football club. *Sociol. Sport J.* 23, 142–161. doi: 10.1123/ssj.23.2.142

Cushion, C. J., Armour, K. M., Jones, R. L., Cushion, C. J., Armour, K. M., Coach, R. L. J., et al. (2003). Coach education and continuing professional development: experience and learning to coach. *Quest* 55, 215–230. doi: 10.1080/00336297.2003.10491800

Dindia, K., and Canary, D. J. (1993). Definitions and theoretical perspectives on maintaining relationships. *J. Soc. Pers. Relatsh.* 10, 163–173. doi: 10.1177/026540759301000201

Elo, S., and Kyngäs, H. (2008). The qualitative content analysis process. *J. Adv. Nurs.* 62, 107–115. doi: 10.1111/j.1365-2648.2007.04569.x

Fernandez-Echeverria, C., Mesquita, I., González-Silva, J., Claver, F., and Perla Moreno, M. (2017). Match analysis within the coaching process: a critical tool to improve coach efficacy. *Int. J. Perf. Anal. Sport* 17, 149–163. doi: 10.1080/24748668.2017.1304073

Francis, J., and Jones, G. (2014). Elite rugby union players perceptions of performance analysis. *Int. J. Perf. Anal. Sport* 14, 188–207. doi: 10.1080/24748668.2014.11868714

French, J., and Raven, B. (1959). "The bases of social power," in *Studies in Social Power*, ed. D. Cartwright (Ann Arbor, MI: Institute for Social Research), 150–167.

Frost, N., Robinson, M., and Anning, A. (2005). Social workers in multidisciplinary teams: issues and dilemmas for professional practice. *Child Fam. Soc. Work* 10, 187–196. doi: 10.1111/j.1365-2206.2005.00370.x

Giddens, A. (1984). *The Constitution of Society: Outline of the Theory of Structuration.* Berkeley, CA: University of California Press.

Groom, R., Cushion, C., and Nelson, L. (2012). Analysing coach-athlete 'talk in interaction' within the delivery of video-based performance feedback in elite youth soccer. *Q. Res. Sport Exerc. Health* 4, 439–458. doi: 10.1080/2159676X.2012.693525

Gustafsson, H., Holmberg, H. C., and Hassmen, P. (2008). An elite endurance athleteŠs recovery from underperformance aided by a multidisciplinary sport science support team. *Eur. J. Sport Sci.* 8, 267–276. doi: 10.1080/17461390802195652

Huggan, R., Nelson, L., and Potrac, P. (2015). Developing micropolitical literacy in professional soccer: a performance analyst's tale. *Q. Res. Sport Exerc. Health* 7, 504–520. doi: 10.1080/2159676X.2014.949832

Hughes, M. (2004). Performance analysis - a 2004 perspective. *Int. J. Perf. Anal. Sport* 4, 103–109. doi: 10.1080/24748668.2004.11868296

Johns, D. P., and Johns, J. S. (2000). Surveillance, subjectivism and technologies of power: an analysis of the discursive practice of high-performance sport. *Int. Rev. Sociol. Sport* 35, 219–234. doi: 10.1177/101269000035002006

Jones, G. W., Høigaard, R., and Peters, D. M. (2014). Just going through the motions: a qualitative exploration of athlete perceptions of social loafing in training and competition contexts — implications for team sport coaches. *Int. J. Sports Sci. Coach.* 9, 1067–1082. doi: 10.1260/1747-9541.9.5.1067

Jones, R. (2006). *Dilemmas, Maintaining "Face," and Paranoia An Average Coaching Life.* Thousand Oaks, CA: Sage.

Jones, R. L., Harris, R., and Miles, A. (2009). Mentoring in sports coaching: a review of the literature. *Phys. Educ. Sport Pedagogy* 14, 267–284. doi: 10.1080/17408980801976569

Jowett, S. (2003). When the honeymoon is over. a case study of a coach-athlete dyad in crisis. *Sport Psychol.* 17, 444–460. doi: 10.1123/tsp.17.4.444

Jowett, S. (2007). "Interdependence analysis and the 3+1Cs in the coach-athlete relationship," in *Social Psychology in Sport*, eds S. Jowette, and D. Lavallee (Champaign, IL: Human Kinetics).

Jowett, S. (2009). Factor structure and criterion-related validity of the metaperspective version of the coach-athlete relationship questionnaire (CART-Q). *Group Dyn.* 13, 163–177. doi: 10.1037/a0014998

Jowett, S., and Carpenter, P. (2015). The concept of rules in the coach-athlete relationship. *Sports Coach. Rev.* 4, 1–23. doi: 10.1080/21640629.2015.1106145

Jowett, S., and Chaundy, V. (2004). An investigation into the impact of coach leadership and coach-athlete relationship on group cohesion. *Group Dyn.* 8, 302–311. doi: 10.1037/1089-2699.8.4.302

Jowett, S., and Clark-Carter, D. (2006). Perceptions of empathic accuracy and assumed similarity in the coach-athlete relationship. *Br. J. Soc. Psychol.* 45, 617–637. doi: 10.1348/014466605X58609

Jowett, S., and Cockerill, I. M. (2003). Olympic medallists' perspective of the althlete-coach relationship. *Psychol. Sport Exerc.* 4, 313–331. doi: 10.1016/S1469-0292(02)00011-0

Jowett, S., Kanakoglou, K., and Passmore, J. (2012a). The application of the 3+1Cs relationship model in executive coaching. *Consul. Psychol. J.* 64, 183–197. doi: 10.1037/a0030316

Jowett, S., Yang, X., and Lorimer, R. (2012b). The role of personality, empathy, and satisfaction with instruction within the context of the coach-athlete relationship. *Int. J. Coach. Sci.* 6, 3–20.

Jowett, S., and Meek, J. (2000). The coach-athlete relationship in married couples. *Sport Psychol.* 14, 157–175. doi: 10.1123/tsp.14.2.157

Jowett, S., and Ntoumanis, N. (2004). The coach–athlete relationship questionnaire (CART-Q): development and initial validation. *Scand. J. Med. Sci. Sports* 14, 245–257. doi: 10.1111/j.1600-0838.2003.00338.x

Kim, Y. (2010). The pilot study in qualitative inquiry. *Q. Soc. Work* 10, 190–206. doi: 10.1177/1473325010362001

Kvale, S., and Brinkmann, S. (2009). *InterViews: Learning the Craft of Qualitative Research Interviewing.* Thousand Oaks, CA: Sage.

Lafrenière, M.-A. K., Jowett, S., Vallerand, R. J., Donahue, E. G., and Lorimer, R. (2008). Passion in sport: on the quality of the coach–athlete relationship. *J. Sport Exerc. Psychol.* 30, 541–560. doi: 10.1123/jsep.30.5.541

Locke, L. (1985). "Research and the improvement of teaching: the professor as the problem," in *Myths, models and methods in sport pedagogy*, eds M. Barrette, G. Feingold, R. Rees, and R. Pieron (Champaign, IL: Human Kinetics), 1–26.

Manzanares, P., Palao, J., and Ortega, E. (2014). The coach's perception of the performance of game actions in training sessions. a case study in volleyball. *Int. J. Perf. Anal. Sport* 14, 894–906. doi: 10.1080/24748668.2014.11868766

McCalla, T., and Fitzpatrick, S. (2016). Integrating sport psychology within a high-performance team: potential stak. *J. Sport Psychol. Act.* 7, 33–42. doi: 10.1080/21520704.2015.1123208

McKenna, J., and Mutrie, N. (2003). Emphasizing quality in qualitative papers. *J. Sports Sci.* 21, 955–958. doi: 10.1080/02640410310001641359

Miller, C. (1995). In-depth interviewing by telephone: some practical considerations. *Eval. Res. Educ.* 9, 29–38. doi: 10.1080/09500799509533370

O'Donoghue, P. (2010). *Research Methods for Sports Performance Analysis.* Abingdon: Routledge.

Olympiou, A., Jowett, S., and Duda, J. L. (2008). The psychological interface between the coach-created motivational climate and the coach-athlete relationship in team sports. *Sport Psychol.* 22, 423–438. doi: 10.1123/tsp.22.4.423

Patchen, M. (1974). The locus and basis of influence on organizational decisions. *Organ. Behav. Hum. Perf.* 11, 195–221. doi: 10.1016/0030-5073(74)90014-2

Patton, M. Q. (2002). *Qualitative Research & Evaluation Methods.* Thousand Oaks, CA: Sage.

Poczwardowski, A., Barott, J. E., and Henschen, K. P. (2002). The athlete and coach: their relationship and its meaning. results of an interpretive study. *Int. J. Sport Psychol.* 33, 116–140.

Purdy, L., Potrac, P., and Jones, R. (2008). Power, consent and resistance: an autoethnography of competitive rowing. *Sport Educ. Soc.* 13, 319–336. doi: 10.1080/13573320802200693

Purdy, L. G., and Jones, R. L. (2011). Choppy waters: elite rowers' perceptions of coaching. *Soc. Sport J.* 28, 329–346. doi: 10.1123/ssj.28.3.329

Raven, B. (1965). "Social influence and power," in *Current Studies in Social Psychology*, eds I. Steiner, and M. Fishbein (New York, NY: Holt McDougal), 371–382.

Raven, B. (1992). A power/interaction model of interpersonal influence: french and raven thirty years later. *J. Soc. Behav. Pers.* 7, 217–244.

Raven, B. (1999). Kurt Lewin address: influence, power, religion, and the mechanisms of social control. *J. Soc. Issues* 55, 161–186. doi: 10.1111/0022-4537.00111

Reeves, M. J., and Roberts, S. J. (2013). Perceptions of performance analysis in elite youth football. *Int. J. Perf. Anal. Sport* 13, 200–211. doi: 10.1080/24748668.2013.11868642

Reid, C., Stewart, E., and Thorne, G. (2004). Multidisciplinary sport science teams in elite sport: Comprehensive servicing or conflict and confusion? *Sport Psychol.* 18, 204–217. doi: 10.1123/tsp.18.2.204

Rhind, D. J. A., and Jowett, S. (2010). Relationship maintenance strategies in the coach-athlete relationship: the development of the COMPASS model. *J. Appl. Sport Psychol.* 22, 106–121. doi: 10.1080/10413200903474472

Rhind, D. J. A., and Jowett, S. (2012). Development of the coach-athlete relationship maintenance questionnaire (CARM-Q). *Int. J. Sports Sci. Coach.* 7, 121–137. doi: 10.1260/1747-9541.7.1.121

Rubin, H. J., and Rubin, I. (1995). *Qualitative Interviewing: the Art of Hearing Data.* Thousand Oaks, CA: SAGE Publications.

Rylander, P. (2016). Coaches' bases of power and coaching effectiveness in team sports. *Int Sports Coach. J.* 3, 128–144. doi: 10.1123/iscj.2015-0046

Sarmento, H., Bradley, P., and Travassos, B. (2015). The transition from match analysis to intervention: optimising the coaching process in elite futsal. *Int. J. Perf. Anal. Sport* 15, 471–488. doi: 10.1080/24748668.2015.11868807

Simonton, D. K. (1999). Significant samples: the psychological study of eminent individuals. *Psychol. Methods* 4, 425–451. doi: 10.1037/1082-989X.4.4.425

Stafford, L., and Canary, D. J. (1991). Maintenance strategies and romantic relationship type, gender and relational characteristics. *J. Soc. Pers. Relatsh.* 8, 217–242. doi: 10.1177/0265407591082004

Stafford, L., Dainton, M., and Haas, S. (2000). Measuring routine and strategic relational maintenance: scale revision, sex versus gender roles, and the prediction of relational characteristics. *Commun. Monogr.* 67, 306–323. doi: 10.1080/03637750009376512

Sweet, L. (2002). Telephone interviewing: is it compatible with interpretive phenomenological research? *Contemp. Nur.* 12, 58–63. doi: 10.5172/conu.12.1.58

Tufford, L., and Newman, P. (2010). Bracketing in qualitative research. *Q. Soc. Work* 11, 80–96. doi: 10.1177/1473325010368316

Wagstaff, C. R. D., Gilmore, S., and Thelwell, R. C. (2015). Sport medicine and sport science practitioners' experiences of organizational change. *Scand. J. Med. Sci. Sports* 25, 685–698. doi: 10.1111/sms.12340

Weber, R. (1990). *Basic Content Analysis*, 2nd Edn. Thousand Oaks, CA: Sage.

Woods, B., and Thatcher, J. (2009). A qualitative exploration of substitutes' experiences in soccer. *Sport Psychol.* 23, 451–469. doi: 10.1123/tsp.23.4.451

Wright, C., Atkins, S., Jones, B., and Todd, J. (2013). The role of performance analysts within the coaching process: performance analysts survey "the role of performance analysts in elite football club settings.". *Int. J. Perf. Anal. Sport* 13, 240–261. doi: 10.1080/24748668.2013.11868645

Wright, C., Carling, C., Lawlor, C., and Collins, D. (2016). Elite football player engagement with performance analysis. *Int. J. Perf. Anal. Sport* 16, 1007–1032. doi: 10.1080/24748668.2016.11868945

Yang, S. X., and Jowett, S. (2013). Conceptual and measurement issues of the complementarity dimension of the coach-athlete relationship across cultures. *Psychol. Sport Exerc.* 14, 830–841. doi: 10.1016/j.psychsport.2013.06.003

Yukl, G. (2006). *Leadership in Organizations*, 6th Edn. Upper Saddle River, NJ: Pearson Education.

25

Relationship between Sport Expertise and Postural Skills

*Thierry Paillard**

Laboratoire Mouvement, Equilibre, Performance et Santé (UPRES EA 4445), Département STAPS, Université de Pau et des Pays de l'Adour, Tarbes, France

***Correspondence:**
Thierry Paillard
thierry.paillard@univ-pau.fr

The review addresses the relationship between sport expertise (i.e., sport competition level), postural performance (amount of motion of the center of mass/of pressure of foot or ability to preserve body balance), and postural strategy (geometric organization of different body segments as well as neurobiological involvement of organism). Since the conditions of postural evaluation are likely to influence results, the aim is to compare athletes at different competition levels in ecological postural conditions (specific postural conditions related to the sport practiced) and non-ecological postural conditions (decontextualized postural conditions in relation to the sport practiced). Evidence suggests that the most successful athletes in terms of sport competition level have the best postural performance both in ecological and non-ecological postural conditions. However, in non-ecological conditions, the postural tasks should be preferentially challenging or relatively close to the sport practice stance. Moreover, the most successful athletes also have more elaborate postural strategies compared with athletes at lower competition level. Mechanistic explanations as well as conceptual models are proposed to explain the role of different factors influencing the relationship between sport expertise and postural performance and strategy.

Keywords: balance, posture, postural control, sport, expertise, postural performance

INTRODUCTION

An expert athlete can be defined as a specialist in a particular sport who is able to achieve high levels of motor skills related to the sport practiced. His/her expertise requires the expression of physical qualities related to biomechanical (e.g., muscle strength, power, and segmental mobility), bioenergetic (energy supply), and/or bio-informational (information taking, reaction time, and response accuracy) aspects that are skillfully exploited in order to accomplish efficient motor command and control. In fact, his/her motor expression achieves maximal efficiency for minimal effort. The motor expression is based on phases of movement and balance whatever the sport practiced (i.e., any kind of sport technique carried out), however complex it may be. Indeed, a motor activity as basic as walking includes phases of monopedal and bipedal balance as well as phases of movement (swing) at the lower limb level (Bessou et al., 1988).

When movement is described in terms of efficiency or aestheticism in the sports community (by athletes, trainers, and the media), balance is rarely taken into account in the commentary/analysis of performance (Masseglia, 2011). However, movement and balance are intimately linked and inseparable when analyzing performance for most sport activities since no sport technique movement is (efficiently) achievable without an efficient body balance (Paillard,

2017a). Indeed, the slightest segmental movement engenders the displacement of the center of mass (COM), which means that movement potentially generates body imbalance which needs to be restored to avoid falling (Paillard, 2017b). Hence, during the sport practice, movement is continuous which compels the athlete to continually restore his/her balance through compensatory postural adjustments. In expert athletes, postural regulation is even anticipated before the onset of movement by anticipatory postural adjustments (Paillard, 2017a).

Before running, jumping, throwing, or any kind of motor action, each athlete must be able to maintain his/her balance (i.e., maintenance of the vertical projection of his/her center of mass above the base of support) and his/her posture (i.e., position of different body segments) in static condition (the base of support does not deform or move) or dynamic condition (the base of support is deformed and/or displaced) in order to not only resist falling but also to act efficiently (Paillard and Noe, 2015). An expert athlete showing high motor skills (e.g., in terms of accuracy, precision, agility, and velocity) in the expression of his/her motricity necessarily needs high postural skills (i.e., high ability to maintain balance in different postures when stationary or moving in the most economical way possible), particularly in the specific positions related to his/her sport (Asseman et al., 2008). Hence, evidence suggests that the skill level related to movement should be associated to the skill level related to balance in athletes. More precisely, there should be a relationship between sport expertise and postural skills for a given attainment level in a particular sport.

However, even if postural skills are fundamental to the use of motor skills, no proof of a direct relationship (i.e., the greater the sport competition level, the better postural skills; or better athletes also have better postural skills) has been established to date (Paillard, 2014, 2017a). It is not yet established that there is a close relationship between the motor expertise level (often analyzed through the sport competition level, e.g., amateur, local, regional, national, sub-elite, professional, international, and elite) and the postural skill level within the same sport, excluding comparison between different sports since each sport develops specific postural abilities (Paillard, 2014). Although a number of observational studies have analyzed this relationship, the resulting data are still subject to question. Hrysomallis (2011) carried out a significant review dealing with balance ability and athletic performance on the basis of quantitative analysis of postural skills (i.e., displacement of the center of foot of pressure – COP). However, the comparison of postural conditions related, or not related, to the sport practiced, i.e., ecological (specific postural condition) versus non-ecological (decontextualized postural condition) conditions, was not considered, although this seem likely to influence the relationship between the motor expertise level and the postural skills level. Indeed, in ecological condition, such as gymnasts executing handstands or rifle shooters accomplishing shooting while measuring the displacements of their COP, the possible relationship between motor (sport) expertise and postural skills could be strong since the amplitude of body sway (in stationary situations) is a criterion of performance in gymnastics (depending on the evaluation of judges) and the body segmental movements can be transmitted to the rifle barrel at the moment of shooting which are likely to affect performance (accuracy of shot) in rifle shooting. By comparison, in non-ecological or decontextualized postural conditions, such as for instance, bipedal quiet stance, for all kinds of athletes, this relationship between motor expertise and postural skills could be weaker or nonexistent, since there would not necessarily be any interaction between them. Moreover, qualitative data of postural skills could also deepen the knowledge relating to the relationship between the motor expertise level and the postural skills level by analyzing and describing how postural skills are organized in relation to the mechanical (geometric organization of different body segments) and neurophysiological (neurobiological involvement of organism) aspects.

The refinement of the method of analysis of the relationship between sport expertise and postural skills, based on the postural conditions in the sports studied supplemented by qualitative data of postural skills, could improve the analysis of sport performance and the elaboration of sport training. The present work therefore aims to provide an overview of the relationship between sports expertise and postural skills by identifying new mechanistic explanations.

METHODS FOR STUDYING THE RELATIONSHIP BETWEEN MOTOR EXPERTISE AND POSTURAL SKILLS

Postural regulation is considered in the present manuscript as a motor action that involves taking information (sensory functions), processing this information, and command of action (central integration and command) as well as motor execution (motor function). It relies on neurophysiological components (the neural loops involved as well as their sensory receptors), cognitive function relative to body representation in space (cortical regulation), and motor function (muscle command). In this context, posture and balance are regulated on the basis of reference values (position and orientation of the segments that serve as a reference frame for perception and action with respect to the environment) and internal representation of the body (also named body representation in space or postural body scheme) (**Figure 1**). Actions require matching multisensory inputs regulating orientation and stabilization of body segments with anticipated and compensated postural adjustments (postural responses and motor programs) (Massion, 1994). In order to analyze the influence of these different components in the regulation of posture and balance, quantitative and qualitative measures are required.

Quantitative and Qualitative Analyses

In each postural condition, postural skills can be quantified to assess postural performance not only by measuring the movement of the COM, the COP, and body segments but also by measuring electromyographic activities and evaluations of the contribution of different sensory information (i.e., visual, vestibular, proprioceptive, and cutaneous) in the participation of postural regulation. Postural skills can also be considered

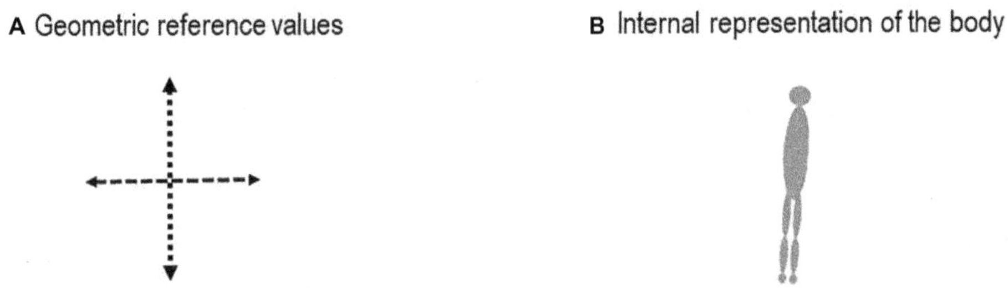

FIGURE 1 | Posture and balance are regulated on the basis of reference values [**(A)**: geometric position and orientation of the segments that serve as a reference frame for perception and action with respect to the environment, i.e., knowledge of the orientation of the body axis and verticality] and internal representation of the body [**(B)**: also named body representation in space or postural body scheme].

qualitatively to assess postural strategy by analyzing and describing how postural balance is organized in relation to the mechanical and neurophysiological aspects (Paillard and Noe, 2015). Postural performance combined with postural strategy is the main component of postural skills.

Postural Performance and Strategy

In static condition, postural performance can be equated to the ability to minimize body sway (i.e., displacements of the COM – or displacements of the whole body – and/or displacements of the COP – or variation of the moment around the ankle) in conventional postural conditions (e.g., bipedal quiet stance). It can also refer to the ability to maintain body balance in challenging postural conditions with small bases of support (e.g., a stance classed as a handstand, monopedal stance) to avoid falling or/and postural imbalance (Paillard and Noe, 2015). In dynamic condition, postural performance can be equated to the ability to maintain body balance in changing postural conditions (e.g., displacement of pedal supports and displacement of the base of support), as well as in external mechanical changes (e.g., fast horizontal accelerations of the ground surface, unexpected percussion, or pushing a large body segment requiring postural reactions) in order to avoid falling (Paillard and Noe, 2015). Postural strategy can be defined on the basis of the spatial and temporal organization of different body segments as well as the extent and order of recruitment of different muscles activated. The different sensory inputs involved in postural regulation as well as the relative importance of different sensory information and/or the preferential involvement of different neuronal loops can also contribute to postural strategy.

Methodological Caution

Movement can be characterized by whole body displacements or body segmental displacements in space. These displacements involve large and small accelerations and decelerations over large and small amplitudes. Body segments can alternate phases of long displacements with phases more or less stationary. During phases of long displacements, postural skills are used particularly in dynamic condition while during stationary phases postural skills are mainly used in static conditions but both phases follow each other continually. Hence, the separate analysis of movement and balance is mechanically very complex. As mentioned above, movement and balance are intimately linked and inseparable when analyzing motor expertise (e.g., performance) for many sports.

Evaluation Conditions

For a given sport, motor expertise could greatly depend on postural skills while postural skills could also depend on motor expertise. Both skills can be reciprocally influenced but it is difficult to determine precisely the influence of each one, particularly in a very mobile sport (constant and long displacements). As part of mobile sports, the analysis of the relationship between motor expertise (e.g., performance) and postural skills cannot be directly quantified since balance and dynamic movement are almost inextricable. Hence, one can only attempt to correlate/associate postural skills with motor skills through separate tests evaluating each of the two skills. In this case, the evaluation of postural skills can only be undertaken in non-ecological conditions, i.e., in a decontextualized environment in relation to the sport practice. However, for a static or low mobility sport activity (no significant displacements), the postural skills and motor expertise can be simultaneously quantified. In this case, the evaluation of postural skills can be made in ecological conditions, i.e., during the sport practice (contextualized environment).

Knowing that each sport develops specific postural skills (Paillard, 2014), the study of the relationship between sport expertise and postural skills should only include young adult athletes (in order to avoid the effects related to age, i.e., development in children and involution in aged subjects) who practice the same sport. Sport experts are elite athletes compared to sub-elite, amateur, or recreational athletes, who are not considered as sport experts but as non-elite athletes.

POSTURAL PERFORMANCE AND SPORT PERFORMANCE

The quantitative analysis of postural skills helps to define the postural performance of athletes while their sport performance is established through their sport competition level. Since postural performance can be studied in ecological and non-ecological postural conditions (specific condition versus non-specific or decontextualized condition) in relation to the considered sport, it is worth studying the relationship between postural performance and sport performance in these two postural conditions.

Ecological Postural Conditions

In ecological conditions, athlete's postural skills are evaluated during their practice of the sport (e.g., rifle shooting, recurve archery) or during the execution of specific motor skills (e.g., handstand posture in gymnasts, juggling in jugglers). With sports such as rifle shooting and recurve archery, one could naturally think that body sway at the moment of shooting would affect its accuracy. Hence, it seems relevant to evaluate the relationship between sport performance and postural performance during shooting. It was observed that the best elite rifle shooters and archers also had the best postural performance (Ball et al., 2003; Musa et al., 2018). By holding their rifles with their arms, rifle shooters create a trunk-head-arms block that must be well interlocked to limit the movements of the rifle and to enable the best possible shooting score (Bermejo et al., 2015). Hence, Ball et al.'s result is not surprising since body sway (evaluated through displacement of COP) is likely to be transmitted to the motion of the gun and aim point and is thus likely to affect shooting performance. The average magnitude of displacement of COP would be smaller before high shooting scores than before low shooting scores (Konttinen et al., 1999). Obviously, shooting accuracy depends on body sway while the ability to keep the gun stable is a sine qua none condition for high shooting performance (Mononen et al., 2007). Indeed, the reduction of body sway alone is not a guarantee for improving shooting performance if it is not (necessarily) associated to minimal movement of the gun barrel (Konttinen et al., 1999). This explains why postural performance would have a limited direct influence on shooting score (in terms of variance of shooting score) but would have a real but indirect influence on shooting score through the ability to hold more stably (Ihalainen et al., 2016, 2018). This principle was corroborated by Ko et al. (2018) who showed that the amount of the COP and pistol motion was lower for skilled pistol shooters than novice shooters. Postural regulation was better coordinated with arm movements to minimize the motion of the pistol in skilled shooters than in novice shooters (Ko et al., 2017).

Moreover, the postural performance level would reflect the sport performance level of rifle shooters since international level rifle shooters were more stable than national level shooters who were more stable than amateur shooters (Era et al., 1996). These authors specified that elite shooters were able to reduce their body sway in the last few seconds just before shooting while amateur shooters kept their body sway pattern during the same time. Moreover, expert shooters limit/control movement in the medio-lateral direction more than shooters without experience (Niinimaa and McAvoy, 1983). In fact, international shooters were able to reduce medio-lateral movements more throughout the test period and antero-posterior movements more during the last few seconds before shooting than national shooters (Ihalainen et al., 2016). COP measurements carried out 1 s prior to arrow release and 0.5 s post-arrow release with elite archery shooters confirmed that reduced postural sway was a predictor of higher scoring shots (Spratford and Campbell, 2017).

Ecological postural tasks performed in dynamic condition (i.e., in movement) such as ball juggling tasks are also of use to study the relationship between motor performance and postural performance using simultaneous measures. Expert jugglers showed better postural performance than intermediate jugglers which corroborated the idea that juggling skills are associated with body sway (Rodrigues et al., 2016). In addition, these authors observed that expert jugglers were less affected by the reduction of the basis of support during juggling tasks than intermediate jugglers. Moreover, the execution of gymnastic tasks by expert and non-expert gymnasts while measuring body sway with force platform can increase our understanding of this subject. The handstand and monopedal stance (but not the bipedal quiet stance) differentiates postural performance between expert gymnasts and non-expert gymnasts (Asseman et al., 2005, 2008; Marcolin et al., 2019). These authors reported that the more the postural tasks are specific and difficult, the more the athletes' postural performance can be related to their competition level. Other works corroborate this principle since dance-like postural tasks have made it possible to discriminate expert dancers from intermediate dancers while this was not possible though static postural tasks (Munzert et al., 2018). Paillard et al. (2011) observed that surfers at national and international competition levels were distinguished from surfers at local competition level when using dynamic postural tasks carried out on an unstable support (very close to the postural condition implied by surfing) but not when using static postural tasks completed on a stable support.

Evidence suggests that in ecological postural condition there is a relationship between postural performance and sport performance.

Non-ecological Postural Conditions

For non-ecological postural tasks such as bipedal quiet stance or any other postural stance decontextualized in relation to the sport considered, the relationship considered was largely studied through a number of sport activities whether mobile or immobile. In an immobile sport activity, without holding a rifle and without specific clothing (i.e., non-ecological condition), elite shooters (competition shooters) had better postural performance than non-elite (military) shooters in visual and nonvisual conditions (Aalto et al., 1990). In mobile sports, there would be also a relationship between sport performance and postural performance in athletes practicing different activities such as soccer, gymnastics, golf, baseball, and stand-up paddle board (Paillard et al., 2006, 2007b, 2011; Paillard and Noe, 2006; Sell et al., 2007; Asseman et al., 2008; Butler et al., 2016; Schram et al., 2016; Jadczak et al., 2018; Pau et al., 2018). However, for a given sport, it is not always possible to distinguish the athletes' postural performance according to their competition levels in the standard postural conditions (e.g., bipedal quiet stance) often used by experimenters (Paillard et al., 2002; Asseman et al., 2004). Similarly, in static and non-specific conditions (i.e., non-ecological conditions), expert judokas and surfers did not exhibit better postural performance than non-expert judokas and surfers (Paillard et al., 2002; Chapman et al., 2008). In fact, postural tasks too simple and easy make it difficult to discriminate between the competition levels of athletes in terms of postural performance.

Nevertheless, in response to unexpected external disturbances, elite female ice hockey players showed shorter recovery period of COM and smaller body sway than non-athletes (Kim et al., 2018). Golfers and runners demonstrated faster onset of trunk muscle activation and higher muscle activation amplitudes in response to sudden trunk loading disturbances when compared to control subjects (Glofcheskie and Brown, 2017). Young soccer players at national level displayed faster and more efficient postural stabilization after a forward jump than young soccer players at regional level (Pau et al., 2018). On the basis of specific and difficult postural tasks, one can wonder whether the relationship between sport performance and postural performance is found in postural disturbance conditions particularly when activating, naturally or artificially, the sensory functions of athletes. As part of vestibular stimulation induced by several and successive body rotations related to dance figures, the COP displacements of elite dancers were smaller than those of amateur dancers and control subjects (Hopper et al., 2014). As part of artificial sensory manipulations at the level of plantar cutaneous (cooling the feet) and myotatic proprioceptive (electrically stimulating the lower limb musculature and blockage of cervical segment) information, professional soccer players who initially exhibited better postural performance (non-manipulated postural condition) than amateur soccer players also showed smaller COP displacements in the manipulated condition (Paillard et al., 2007b). Evidence suggests that whatever the postural condition - i.e., with or without disturbance - the most successful athletes (competition level) also display better postural performance.

Moreover, the conditions of practice of some sports are likely to impact negatively postural performance when they are intensively practiced (i.e., frequent practices). Indeed, at the end of a sports season, skiers competing at a national level showed worse postural performance than skiers competing at a regional level (Noé and Paillard, 2005). On the basis of data mentioned above, this result is contradictory since Noé and Paillard (2005) postulated that this phenomenon occurred because of the effects of wearing ski boots during frequent training sessions. Ski boots of Alpine skiing are rigid and limit/reduce ankle movement, so in the long run the frequent wearing of such ski boots would adversely affect proprioception and postural performance. Since national skiers spent more time at training than regional skiers, this would explain why their postural performance was worse than regional skiers at the end of sport season (Noé and Paillard, 2005).

In non-ecological postural conditions, the relationship between sport performance and postural performance is not systematically observed in athletes and requires caution in the methods of analysis.

Summary

According to the current literature, the ecological postural condition turns out to be more appropriate to investigate the relationship between sport performance and postural performance. In non-ecological postural conditions, this relationship would assuredly be preserved only in two conditions. First, the postural tasks used for the evaluation should be sufficiently specific and difficult in relation to the sport considered, and second, material conditions of sport practice should not affect proprioception.

POSTURAL STRATEGY AND SPORT PERFORMANCE

By describing postural strategy, i.e., how postural regulation is organized in relation to the mechanical and neurophysiological aspects (cf. the sub-section "Postural Performance and Strategy"), it turns out to be possible to compare expert or elite athletes with non-expert or non-elite athletes and to specify the differences between them from a postural view point.

Ecological Postural Conditions

Postural strategy between expert athletes and non-expert athletes can be differentiated through biomechanical and neurophysiological analyses which focus on input of information (sensory functions), processing this information, and commanding action (central integration) as well as motor action (motor function).

Shooting and juggling tasks are well suited to our study framework since it is relatively easy to simultaneously evaluated motor performance and postural performance. Elite shooters gave less importance to visual cues and more importance to proprioceptive and vestibular cues than non-elite shooters (Aalto et al., 1990). In shooting conditions, the vision is devoted only to targeting and does not contribute to control of posture (Aalto et al., 1990). In this case, the reduction of the contribution of visual information in postural regulation is compensated for by greater contributions of proprioceptive and vestibular information (Aalto et al., 1990) which enables elite shooters to dedicate more resources to the main motor task (i.e., shooting) especially for controlling the rifle movement and pressing its trigger (Konttinen et al., 1999). Moreover, expert jugglers were less dependent on foveal vision than intermediate jugglers who moved their gaze around a larger visual area. This suggests that intermediate jugglers were searching spatially for the balls which would be associated with an increase of body sway (Rodrigues et al., 2016).

Konttinen et al. (1999) found that non-elite rifle shooters more actively controlled their posture (cerebral and muscle activities) during shooting than elite rifle shooters. Intermediate jugglers displayed a higher level of attention and prioritized the manipulation task rather than postural regulation, increasing body sway differently from expert jugglers, who were able to deal better with both the manipulation task and postural regulation (Rodrigues et al., 2016). A lower cognitive load for expert jugglers would use their resources less which could explain why they were less affected than intermediate jugglers since their adaptation capacities remained greater (Rodrigues et al., 2016). Moreover, high level biathletes would present better central integration of sensory cues and/or better filtering of erroneous cues than lower level biathletes (Simoneau et al., 1996). According to these authors, higher level biathletes would also detect the discrepancy between the actual posture and the desired posture more quickly while they would demonstrate better motor coordination and motor responses earlier than lower level biathletes.

In ecological postural conditions, on the basis of the data above, elite and non-elite shooters, biathletes, and jugglers would implement different postural strategies to regulate their posture.

Non-ecological Postural Conditions

Biomechanical and neurophysiological analyses also highlighted differences in terms of postural strategies between elite and non-elite athletes in non-ecological postural conditions.

With decontextualized postural tasks in relation to the sports considered (e.g., bipedal stance), biomechanical data obtained with accelerometric measures showed that the number of mobilized body segments decreased as the sport level increased in judokas (Mesure and Crémieux, 1996). Moreover, with greater gymnastic skills, acceleration time series were less variable and more stable (Lamoth et al., 2009). This suggests that the best athletes in terms of sport level could proceed by slight (local) postural adjustments while the other athletes would undertake more global postural strategies as part of pure postural tasks. However, as part of more complex locomotor tasks (e.g., narrow and wide beam-walking) rather than pure postural tasks, Sawers et al. (2015) observed that expert ballet dancers used multiple motor modules for executing a biomechanical function whereas novice dancers executed such functions with a single motor module. Taken together, these results emphasize that the postural adjustment strategy between experts and non-experts could depend on the context of the motor task. Experts would have more flexibility in achieving motor goals thanks to a larger motor repertoire which would be useful under challenging conditions (Sawers et al., 2015). In turn, as part of easy or reflex postural conditions experts could operate through slight postural adjustments. Moreover, postural strategies could be more automatic in expert athletes (Lamoth et al., 2009; Sawers et al., 2015; Michalska et al., 2018) while they would be more actively controlled in non-expert athletes.

Neurophysiological data indicate that gymnast and soccer player experts made better use of vestibular inputs, probably through a better central integration, than gymnast and soccer player non-experts (Bringoux et al., 2000; Paillard et al., 2006). In expert athletes, a greater contribution of vestibular information would reduce the contribution of proprioception especially as part of easy and simple postural tasks. In this case, the proprioceptive function would be saved and would offer supplementary resources for carrying out more challenging postural tasks. Hence, expert athletes would have additional abilities to cope with destabilizing motor tasks (Paillard et al., 2006). By comparison, in non-expert athletes, as part of easy and simple postural tasks, the lower contribution of vestibular information would result in a greater contribution of proprioception which would already be fully exploited. Thus, the contribution of proprioception in postural regulation could not increase as the difficulty of the postural task increased and would not make it possible to cope with particularly challenging and destabilizing postural tasks (Paillard et al., 2006). Evidence suggests that the contribution of vestibular and proprioceptive inputs increases in postural regulation as the competition level is raised. In this context, it would be logical that the contribution of visual cues diminishes.

Indeed, the contribution of visual information is reduced as the sport competition level increased in surfers and soccer players (Paillard et al., 2006, 2011; Paillard and Noé, 2006; Chapman et al., 2008). The lower visual dependence in elite soccer players in comparison with sub-elite soccer players enables elite soccer players to devote their gaze more to processing the information that stems from the game (Paillard and Noé, 2006; Paillard et al., 2006; Zouita Ben Moussa et al., 2012). Sub-elite soccer players being more visually-dependent than elite soccer players would have less resources to devote to the game actions. Indeed, the analysis of movements of the ball and the team partners and opponents is essential in soccer in order to implement cooperative or opposition strategies. For a given soccer player, the time required to take in visual information needed to perform his/her own motor actions (i.e., balance, movement, displacement, control of the ball) reduces the time available for analyzing the game (Paillard and Noé, 2006). For instance, the control of the ball with the feet involves looking down which limits the observation time of the environment.

Moreover, it turns out that the less the visual contribution, the more the proprioception contribution in postural regulation by athletes. This phenomenon is particularly observed as part of the sport expertise (e.g., Paillard and Noé, 2006). Expert surfers shifted sensorimotor dominance from vision to proprioception (Chapman et al., 2008). Postural regulation achieved on the basis of low visual dependence would facilitate the technical expression and motor skills. This would explain why the visual dependence is lower in expert surfers than in non-expert surfers. Expert surfers would divert their visual contribution from postural regulation mainly to processing the relevant information about environmental factors such as height and shape of waves. As observed previously by Asseman et al. (2005) with elite and sub-elite gymnasts, Paillard et al. (2011) indicated that the difference in visual dependence between elite surfers and sub-elite surfers increased as the difficulty of the postural task increased (e.g., bipedal vs. monopedal, stable support vs. unstable support; upright vs. handstand postures).

It is however important to note that certain physical activities such as dancing develop postural and motor strategies which are more visually-dependent (related to the fact that the environment is stable) than most other activities such team sports or sliding sports as mentioned above (Michalska et al., 2018). This is why the contribution of visual information does not decrease as the expertise level is increased in dancers. The suppression of visual cues would penalize expert dancers more than non-expert dancers (Paillard, 2017a). The physical activities practiced in a stable environment and an unmoving space, such as dance sports, remain exceptions since generally in an unstable environment and/or space, the contribution of visual information decreases as the expert level is increased. Overall, sport skill-specific expertise impacts sensory integration for spatial referencing and postural skills (Thalassinos et al., 2018).

Moreover, the expertise level would also influence the motor command of the postural function. Kim et al. (2018) observed that non-athletes displayed more co-activation of the ankle plantar flexors and dorsiflexors while elite female ice hockey players showed low co-activation strategy of agonist and antagonist in ankle and neck extensors. Sawers et al. (2015) also found less muscle co-activation and greater efficiency in muscle output in expert ballet dancers than in novice dancers (no dance or gymnastic training).

In non-ecological postural conditions, the different sensory and motor resources are exploited differently in expert and non-expert athletes for regulating posture.

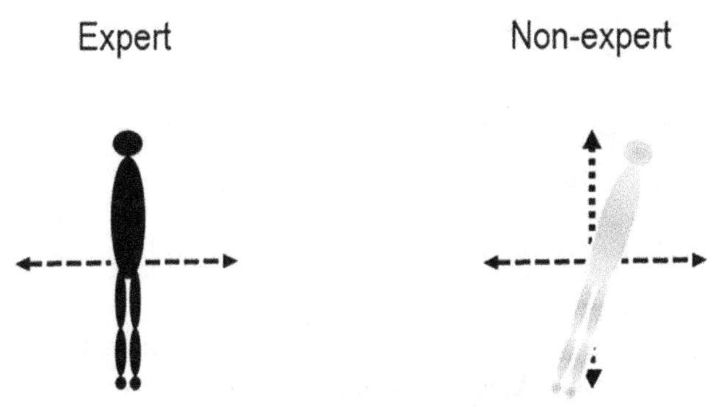

FIGURE 2 | Comparison of abilities to regulate posture and balance between sportive non-experts and sportive experts. Experts would have a better knowledge of the orientation of the body axis and verticality as well as a more accuracy internal body representation than non-experts.

Summary

Overall, for both ecological and non-ecological postural tasks, expert and non-expert athletes deploy different postural strategies whether for basic or challenging postural tasks.

POSTURAL SKILLS AND INDIVIDUAL NATURAL PREDISPOSITIONS

It is known that motor performance depends on training (quantitative and qualitative aspects) as well as individual natural predispositions (psychological and physiological qualities adapted to the specific aspects of a given sport). While it is also known that training influences postural skills of athletes (Paillard, 2017a), little is known about the influence of individual natural predispositions on postural skills and this deserves to be studied.

If the individual natural predispositions can affect postural skills, they could act on the sensory, central and/or motor components of the postural function. At the sensory level, the proprioception emanating from lower and upper limbs would be more accurate in elite athletes than in sub-elite athletes independent of the amount of training (i.e., the number of years of practice) for different sports such as badminton, soccer, swimming (Han et al., 2015a). According to these authors, this result illustrates that the amount of training would not impact proprioception but individual predispositions would determine its accuracy. Even if caution is due, one can postulate that the amount of training would not be fundamental to the proprioception output.

At the level of the central component of the postural function, Paillard et al. (2006) inferred that elite soccer players had a better knowledge of the orientation of body axis and verticality than sub-elite soccer players (**Figure 2**). This could mean more accurate internal body representation and subjective verticality in elite soccer players than in sub-elite soccer players. In addition, the reaction time (total reaction time and premotor reaction time) to sport-specific visual stimuli was shorter in elite taekwondo practitioners than in sub-elite taekwondo practitioners (Chung and Ng, 2012). Hence, these authors highlighted that the speed of perception would be faster to discriminate relevant cues in motor actions of opponents (especially sport-specific postures) in the elites taekwondo practitioners than in sub-elite practitioners.

At the level of motor output of the postural function, Barbado et al. (2016) reported higher trunk extensor muscle strength in elite judokas than in sub-elite judokas. On the basis of postural data, Paillard and Noé (2006) concluded that the tone of the posterior leg muscles would be greater in elite soccer players than in sub-elite soccer players. Moreover, the neuromuscular excitability threshold of the quadriceps muscles was lower in the elite taekwondo practitioners than in sub-elite taekwondo practitioners (Chung and Ng, 2012). As it is accepted that the higher the muscle excitability, the better the muscle contractility, these authors stated that the motor output of the postural function would be naturally better in elite taekwondo practitioners than in sub-elite taekwondo practitioners.

On the basis of the data above, it can be assumed that individual predispositions influence postural skills. Hence, one can wonder whether the individual postural potential can be improved thanks to sport training.

INDIVIDUAL POSTURAL TRAINABILITY

The athlete's potential to increase his/her postural skills following training can be defined by the term "postural trainability". The postural skills can initially (naturally) be low or high in athletes but with increased experience whatever their initial level (low or high), some athletes continue to progress while others stagnate. Hence, the postural trainability differs between athletes. On the basis of these practical observations that emanate from coaches (unpublished data) regardless of the initial natural predispositions, the individual trainability is more or less great and it is difficult to identify the subjects who can make great progress and those who cannot. According to current knowledge, whether for trainers (coaches) or scientists, individual trainability is difficult to estimate prospectively (predict) for a sports career. Future research works should explore individual postural trainability on the basis of interventional studies since the current literature is relatively devoid of useful data likely to advance the training and selection plans of young athletes.

TRANSFER BETWEEN POSTURAL SKILLS AND MOTOR SKILLS

Another problem that presents itself to trainers is that the influence of postural skills on sport performance is currently still unknown. One can observe that the most successful athletes (in relation to the competition level) have the best postural skills but one does not know if those with the best postural skills are always the most successful athletes. Although there are relationships between postural skills and technical skills (dribbles, passes, shots) as well as running speeds (including accelerating, stopping) in small-sided soccer games (Edis et al., 2016, 2017), currently, the transfer of postural skills toward motor skills remains to be explored through sport training. As far as is known, there is no evidence that improvement in postural skills would enhance motor skills.

In turn, particular training leads to specific postural regulation induced by the acquisition of specific new motor skills due to the practice of the specific movements (Paillard et al., 2007a). This would support the idea that each learned new technique is associated with new postural adaptation/skills. However, if a transfer of motor skills toward postural skills occurs, it would be limited to very close movements in terms of posture/position compared to those practiced in training and competition (Paillard et al., 2017a). If it is not a skills transfer, the acquisition of new postural skills would be integrated into new motor skills which would mean that motor skills and postural skills are indissociable.

The state of the current literature suggests that studies should be undertaken in order to unravel the possible reciprocal influences between postural skills and motor (sport) skills. These works could also show that there is not any dependence between these two skills which would be surprising from a theoretical point of view, on the basis of current knowledges.

CONCLUSION

Evidence suggests that the most successful athletes in term of sport competition level have the best postural performance both in ecological and non-ecological postural conditions. However, in non-ecological condition, postural tasks should be preferentially challenging or relatively close to the sport practice stance. The relationship between sport performance and postural performance is not systematic when the postural conditions are remote from those of the sport practice. Moreover, the most successful athletes also have more elaborate postural strategies compared with athletes at lower competition levels. Sports experts would also show better natural postural predispositions than sports non-experts. Currently, it is known that motor skills could greatly depend on postural skills while postural skills could also depend on motor skills. Both skills influence each other but it is difficult to determine precisely the influence of one over the other either for ecological and non-ecological postural tasks, even if the current assumption is that the influence of motor skills toward postural skills would probably be stronger than the reverse influence. Future studies should unravel the concepts involved thus enabling sports trainers (coaches) to improve their intervention and to refine their training programs for athletes as well as enabling physicians to enhance their preventive and therapeutic strategies.

AUTHOR CONTRIBUTIONS

The author confirms being the sole contributor of this work and has approved it for publication.

REFERENCES

Aalto, H., Pyykkö, I., Ilmarinen, R., Kähkönen, E., and Starck, J. (1990). Postural stability in shooters. *ORL J. Otorhinolaryngol Relat. Spec.* 52, 232–238.

Asseman, F., Caron, O., and Crémieux, J. (2004). Is there a transfer of postural ability from specific to unspecific postures in elite gymnasts? *Neurosci. Lett.* 358, 83–86.

Asseman, F., Caron, O., and Crémieux, J. (2005). Effects of the removal of vision on body sway during different postures in elite gymnasts. *Int. J. Sports Med.* 26, 116–119.

Asseman, F. B., Caron, O., and Crémieux, J. (2008). Are there specific conditions for which expertise in gymnastics could have an effect on postural control and performance? *Gait Posture* 27, 76–81.

Ball, K. A., Best, R. J., and Wrigley, T. V. (2003). Body sway, aim point fluctuation and performance in rifle shooters: inter- and intra-individual analysis. *J. Sports Sci.* 21, 559–566.

Barbado, D., Lopez-Valenciano, A., Juan-Recio, C., Montero-Carretero, C., van Dieën, J. H., and Vera-Garcia, F. J. (2016). Trunk stability, trunk strength and sport performance level in judo. *PLoS One* 11:e0156267. doi: 10.1371/journal.pone.0156267

Bermejo, J. L., García-Massó, X., Gomis, M., Noé, F., Huertas, F., Pablos, C., et al. (2015). The difficulty of postural tasks amplifies the effects of fatigue on postural stability. *Eur. J. Appl. Physiol.* 115, 489–495.

Bessou, P., Dupui, P., Montoya, R., and Pagès, B. (1988). Simultaneous recording of longitudinal displacements of both feet during human walking. *J. Physiol.* 83, 102–110.

Bringoux, L., Marin, L., Nougier, V., Barraud, P. A., and Raphel, C. (2000). Effects of gymnastics expertise on the perception of body orientation in the pitch dimension. *J. Vestib. Res.* 10, 251–258.

Butler, R. J., Bullock, G., Arnold, T., Plisky, P., and Queen, R. (2016). Competition-level differences on the lower quarter Y-balance test in baseball players. *J. Athl. Train.* 51, 997–1002.

Chapman, D. W., Needham, K. J., Allison, G., Lay, B., and Edwards, D. J. (2008). Effects of experience within a dynamic environment on postural control. *Br. J. Sports Med.* 42, 16–21.

Chung, P., and Ng, G. (2012). Taekwondo training improves the neuromotor excitability and reaction of large and small muscles. *Phys. Ther. Sport* 13, 163–169.

Edis, Ç., Vural, F., and Vurgun, H. (2016). The importance of postural control in relation to technical abilities in small-sided soccer games. *J. Hum. Kinet.* 53, 51–61.

Edis, C., Vural, F., and Vurgun, H. (2017). Does running performance in small-sided games have a relation with postural control in youth soccer players. *Turk. J. Sport Exerc.* 19, 83–91.

Era, P., Konttinen, N., Mehto, P., Saarela, P., and Lyytinen, H. (1996). Postural stability and skilled performance – a study on top-level and naive rifle shooters. *J. Biomech.* 29, 301–306.

Glofcheskie, G. O., and Brown, S. H. (2017). Athletic background is related to superior trunk proprioceptive ability, postural control, and neuromuscular responses to sudden perturbations. *Hum. Mov. Sci.* 52, 74–83.

Han, J., Waddington, G., Anson, J., and Adams, R. (2015a). Level of competitive success achieved by elite athletes and multi-joint proprioceptive ability. *J. Sci. Med. Sport* 18, 77–81. doi: 10.1016/j.jsams.2013.11.013

Hopper, D. M., Grisbrook, T. L., Newnham, P. J., and Edwards, D. J. (2014). The effects of vestibular stimulation and fatigue on postural control in classical ballet dancers. *J. Dance Med. Sci.* 18, 67–73.

Hrysomallis, C. (2011). Balance ability and athletic performance. *Sports Med.* 41, 221–232.

Ihalainen, S., Kuitunen, S., Mononen, K., and Linnamo, V. (2016). Determinants of elite-level air rifle shooting performance. *Scand. J. Med. Sci. Sports* 26, 266–274.

Ihalainen, S., Laaksonen, M. S., Kuitunen, S., Leppävuori, A., Mikkola, J., Lindinger, S. J., et al. (2018). Technical determinants of biathlon standing shooting performance before and after race simulation. *Scand. J. Med. Sci. Sports* 28, 1700–1707.

Jadczak, L., Grygorowicz, M., Dzudziński, W., and Śliwowski, R. (2018). Comparison of static and dynamic balance at different levels of sport competition in professional and junior elite soccer players. *J. Strength Cond. Res.* doi: 10.1519/JSC.0000000000002476 [Epub ahead of print].

Kim, M., Kim, Y., Kim, H., and Yoon, B. (2018). Specific muscle synergies in national elite female ice hockey players in response to unexpected external perturbation. *J. Sports Sci.* 36, 319–325. doi: 10.1080/02640414.2017.1306090

Ko, J. H., Han, D. W., and Newell, K. M. (2017). Skill level constrains the coordination of posture and upper-limb movement in a pistol-aiming task. *Hum. Mov. Sci.* 55, 255–263.

Ko, J. H., Han, D. W., and Newell, K. M. (2018). Skill level changes the coordination and variability of standing posture and movement in a pistol-aiming task. *J. Sports Sci.* 36, 809–816. doi: 10.1080/02640414.2017.1343490

Konttinen, N., Lyytinen, H., and Era, P. (1999). Brain slow potentials and postural sway behavior during sharpshooting performance. *J. Mot. Behav.* 31, 11–20.

Lamoth, C. J., van Lummel, R. C., and Beek, P. J. (2009). Athletic skill level is reflected in body sway: a test case for accelometry in combination with stochastic dynamics. *Gait Posture* 29, 546–551.

Marcolin, G., Rizzato, A., Zuanon, J., Bosco, G., and Paoli, A. (2019). Expertise level influences postural balance control in young gymnasts. *J. Sports Med. Phys. Fitness.* 59, 593–599. doi: 10.23736/S0022-4707.18.08014-3

Masseglia, D. (2011). "Technologie et performance sportive" *La chimie et le sport* eds. M.-T. Dinh-Audouin, R. A. Jacquesy, D. Olivier, and P. Frankish (Les Ulis, France: EDP Sciences), 99–110.

Massion, J. (1994). Postural control system. *Curr. Opin. Neurobiol.* 4, 877–887.

Mesure, S., and Crémieux, J. (1996). "L'entraînement de judo se traduit-il par l'utilisation de nouvelles stratégies sensori-motrices dans le contrôle postural?" in *Arts martiaux et sports de combats*. eds. Y. Kerlirzin, and G. Fouquet (Paris: Cahiers de l'INSEP 12-13), 77–83.

Michalska, J., Kamieniarz, A., Fredyk, A., Bacik, B., Juras, G., and Słomka, K. J. (2018). Effect of expertise in ballet dance on static and functional balance. *Gait Posture* 64, 68–74.

Mononen, K., Konttinen, N., Viitasalo, J., and Era, P. (2007). Relationship between postural balance, rifle stability and shooting accuracy among novice rifle shooters. *Scand. J. Med. Sci. Sports* 17, 180–185.

Munzert, J., Müller, J., Joch, M., and Reiser, M. (2018). Specificity of postural control: comparing expert and intermediate dancers. *J. Mot. Behav.* 23, 1–13. doi: 10.1080/00222895.2018.1468310 [Epub ahead of print].

Musa, R. M., Abdulla, M. R., Juahir, H., Maliki, A. B. H. M., Mat-Rasid, S. M., Kosni, N. A., et al. (2018). A multidimensional analysis of physiological and mechanical variables among archers of different levels of expertise. *J. Fund. Appl. Sci.* 10, 18–32. doi: 10.4314/jfas.v10i1s.2

Niinimaa, V., and McAvoy, T. (1983). Influence of exercise on body sway in the standing rifle shooting position. *Can. J. Appl. Sport Sci.* 8, 30–33.

Noé, F., and Paillard, T. (2005). Is postural control affected by expertise in alpine skiing? *Br. J. Sports Med.* 39, 835–837.

Paillard, T. (2014). Sport-specific balance develops specific postural skills. *Sports Med.* 44, 1019–1020.

Paillard, T. (2017a). Plasticity of the postural function to sport and/or motor experience. *Neurosci. Biobehav. Rev.* 72, 129–152. doi: 10.1016/j.neubiorev.2016.11.015

Paillard, T. (2017b). Relationship between muscle function, muscle typology and postural performance according to different postural conditions in young and older adults. *Front. Physiol.* 8:585. doi: 10.3389/fphys.2017.00585. eCollection 2017

Paillard, T., Bizid, R., and Dupui, P. (2007b). Do sensorial manipulations affect subjects differently depending on their postural abilities? *Br. J. Sports Med.* 41, 435–438. doi: 10.1136/bjsm.2006.032904

Paillard, T., Costes-Salon, C., Lafont, C., and Dupui, P. (2002). Are there differences in postural regulation according to the level of competition in judoists? *Br. J. Sports Med.* 36, 304–305.

Paillard, T., Margnes, E., Portet, M., and Breucq, A. (2011). Postural ability reflects the athletic skill level of surfers. *Eur. J. Appl. Physiol.* 111, 1619–1623.

Paillard, T., Montoya, R., and Dupui, P. (2007a). Postural adaptations specific to preferred throwing techniques practiced by competition-level judoists. *J. Electromyogr. Kinesiol.* 17, 241–244. doi: 10.1016/j.jelekin.2006.01.006

Paillard, T., and Noé, F. (2006). Effect of expertise and visual contribution on postural control in soccer. *Scand. J. Med. Sci. Sports* 16, 345–348.

Paillard, T., and Noe, F. (2015). Techniques and methods for testing the postural function in healthy and pathological subjects. *Biomed. Res. Int.* 2015:891390. doi: 10.1155/2015/891390

Paillard, T., Noé, F., Rivière, T., Marion, V., Montoya, R., and Dupui, P. (2006). Postural performance and strategy in the unipedal stance of soccer players at different levels of competition. *J. Athl. Train.* 41, 172–176.

Pau, M., Porta, M., Arippa, F., Pilloni, G., Sorrentino, M., Carta, M., et al. (2018). Dynamic postural stability, is associated with competitive level, in youth league soccer players. *Phys. Ther. Sports* 35, 36–41. doi: 10.1016/j.ptsp.2018.11.002

Rodrigues, S. T., Polastri, P. F., Gotardi, G. C., Aguiar, S. A., Mesaros, M. R., Pestana, M. B., et al. (2016). Postural control during cascade ball juggling: effects of expertise and base of support. *Percept. Mot. Skills* 123, 279–294.

Sawers, A., Allen, J. L., and Ting, L. H. (2015). Long-term training modifies the modular structure and organization of walking balance control. *J. Neurophysiol.* 114, 3359–3373.

Schram, B., Hing, W., and Climstein, M. (2016). Profiling the sport of stand-up paddle boarding. *J. Sports Sci.* 34, 937–944. doi: 10.1080/02640414.2015.1079331

Sell, T. C., Tsai, Y. S., Smoliga, J. M., Myers, J. B., and Lephart, S. M. (2007). Strength, flexibility, and balance characteristics of highly proficient golfers. *J. Strength Cond. Res.* 21, 1166–1171.

Simoneau, M., Bard, C., Fleury, M., Teasdale, N., and Boulay, M. R. (1996). Les effets de l'activation métabolique sur la stabilité posturale et la précision de tir chez les biathlètes de niveau élite et intermédiaires. *Sci. Mot.* 29, 22–29.

Spratford, W., and Campbell, R. (2017). Postural stability, clicker reaction time and bow draw force predict performance in elite recurve archery. *Eur. J. Sport Sci.* 17, 539–545.

Thalassinos, M., Fotiadis, G., Arabatzi, F., Isableu, B., and Hatzitaki, V. (2018). Sport skill-specific expertise biases sensory integration for spatial referencing and postural control. *J. Mot. Behav.* 50, 426–435. doi: 10.1080/00222895.2017.1363704

Zouita Ben Moussa, A., Zouita, S., Dziri, C., and Ben Salah, F. Z. (2012). Postural control in Tunisian soccer players. *Sci. Sports* 27, 54–56.

The Validity and Reliability of Live Football Match Statistics from Champdas Master Match Analysis System

Bingnan Gong[1,2], Yixiong Cui[3*], Yang Gai[2], Qing Yi[2] and Miguel-Ángel Gómez[2]

[1] China Football College, Beijing Sport University, Beijing, China, [2] Facultad de Ciencias de la Actividad Física y del Deporte, Universidad Politécnica de Madrid, Madrid, Spain, [3] AI Sports Engineering Lab, School of Sports Engineering, Beijing Sport University, Beijing, China

***Correspondence:**
Yixiong Cui
cuiyixiong@bsu.edu.cn

The aim of the present study was to investigate the validity of match variables and the reliability of *Champdas Master System* used by trained operators in live association football match. Twenty professional football coaches voluntarily participated in the validation of match variables used in the System. Four well-trained operators divided into two groups that independently analyzed a match of Spanish La Liga. The Aiken's V averaged at 0.84 ± 0.03 and 0.85 ± 0.03 for the validation of indicators. The high Kappa values (Operator 1: 0.92, 0.90; Operator 2: 0.91, 0.88), high intra-class correlation coefficients (varied from 0.93 to 1.00), and low typical errors (varied from 0.01 to 0.34) between the first and second data collection represented a high level of intra-operator reliability. The Kappa values for the inter-operator reliability of were 0.97 and 0.89. The intra-class correlation coefficients and typical errors ranged from 0.90 to 1.00 and ranged from 0.01 to 0.24 for two independent operators within two data collections. The results suggest that the *Champdas Master system* can be used validly and reliably to gather live football match statistics by well-trained operators. Therefore, the data obtained by the company can be used by coaches, managers, researchers and performance analysts as valid match statistics from players and teams during their professional tasks and investigations.

Keywords: performance analysis, reliability, validity, football, match statistics

INTRODUCTION

Sport performance analysis during actual competition is one of the main sources of information that are beneficial for the training and coaching process (Sampaio and Leite, 2013). In essence, coaches and athletes could be provided with information of interest that is difficult to be detected throughout their subjective perception, and then refine their training planning and improve athlete's performance purposefully (Hughes and Franks, 2015). Within its domain, the analysis of technical and tactical performance has captured substantial research interest in either individual sports (Reid et al., 2016; Cui et al., 2019), or team sports (Zhang et al., 2018; Zhou et al., 2018), where a set of performance indicators that contains relevant information about players and teams' match performance during competition have been established and collected via observational approaches (Hughes and Bartlett, 2002; Lames and McGarry, 2007; Hughes and Franks, 2015). Fundamentally, it is mainly based on systematic observation, understood as an organized recording and quantification of sport behaviors in their natural context (O'Donoghue and Mayes, 2013; Sampaio and Leite, 2013). To achieve this purpose, both a well-designed notational system and valid, precise and objective performance indicators are required so that technical-tactical aspects of match performance could be easily gathered and used for the subsequent analysis and practical applications (Bradley et al., 2007; Carling et al., 2007; O'Donoghue, 2007).

Therefore, as a prerequisite for any performance analysis research that uses novel system or instrument, the repeatability and accuracy of this new tool, and the validity of performance indicators used should be validated, before collecting and analyzing players and teams' performances (O'Donoghue, 2014; Chacón-Moscoso et al., 2018). Despite that currently there are some automatic player tracking system available for performance analysis, most of observational studies or practices in sport field are still done with computerized notational systems where performance analysts are required to manually code sport performance indicators with predetermined short-cut keys (Bradley et al., 2007; Hizan et al., 2010; Liu et al., 2013; Beato et al., 2018). From a theoretical and applied perspective, a performance indicator should help to explain the match outcome; and thus advance understanding, providing for meaningful insights of game behavior (O'Donoghue, 2009). The use of precise operational definitions and the validity of performance indicators are related to reliability of data collection in performance analysis and therefore have a strong impact on the correct interpretation of match performances (McGarry, 2009).

Validity is generally referred to as the ability of a measurement tool to reflect what it is designed to measure (Atkinson and Nevill, 1998), and usually for performance analysis instrument, it can be determined through expert coaches' opinions in each sports category (Hraste et al., 2008; Cupples and O'Connor, 2011; Larkin et al., 2016; Torres-Luque et al., 2018). For instance, Larkin et al. (2016) validated a coding instrument of assessing movement awareness and technical skills for soccer players with a panel of nine experts. Similarly, with the review and confirmation of eleven experts, Torres-Luque et al. (2018) validated an observational instrument for analyzing the technical-tactical match performance in tennis. Further, the reliability of a sport notational system is as important as its validity (Hayen et al., 2007). It refers to the reproducibility of values of a test, assay or other measurement in repeated trials on the same individuals (intra-observer reliability) (O'Donoghue, 2009), and repeatability over different observers (inter-observer reliability) (Hopkins, 2000). Sports notational system may be limited in reliability due to manual errors, observer's inexperience, number of observers (Beato et al., 2018) so that its results will mislead coaches or performance analysts to make poor decisions about training and match preparation.

In recent years, the development of semi-automatic match analysis systems in elite football has enhanced the accessibility to match information related to match events and movements (Carling et al., 2007; Mackenzie and Cushion, 2013). And as a result, performance directors, coaches and researchers frequently utilize these systems to gain insights into football match performance. Concurrently, the accuracy and reliability of some widely used systems from various commercial football match statistics providers have been validated and verified, such as AMISCO® system (Carling et al., 2008; Zubillaga et al., 2009; Lago et al., 2010; Dellal et al., 2011; Castellano et al., 2014), PROZONE Sports Ltd.® (Bradley et al., 2007, 2011; Castellano et al., 2014), SportsCode (Hughes, 2004; Reed and Hughes, 2006; O'Donoghue and Holmes, 2014), OPTA Sportsdata (Oberstone, 2009, 2010, 2011; Liu et al., 2013), SICS (Rampinini et al., 2009; Osgnach et al., 2010; Beato and Jamil, 2017), Dartfish (Eltoukhy et al., 2012; Padulo et al., 2015; Larkin et al., 2016; Li et al., 2016), and Nacsports (Clear et al., 2017). Indeed, these systems have presented both coder-friendly operating platform and high reliability in measuring technical-tactical performance indicators. Yet, there remain some limitations concerning the above-mentioned studies and measures. Most of them only studies the test-retest reliability of these systems, not considering the content validity of performance events or indicators included. Besides, some systems were mainly focused on the successful or unsuccessful outcome of technical performance events, such as shoots, dribbles, crosses (Larkin et al., 2016), so that tactical information related to pass directions and network is not able to be gathered, which helps to understand complex match characteristics of this invasion sport and becomes one of the recent research topics for football investigators (Gonçalves et al., 2017; Pollard, 2019; Praça et al., 2019).

In comparison with the previous existing systems, *Champdas Master System*, a semi-automatic match analysis system developed by the Champion Technology Co., Ltd., (a leading Chinese sport data company founded in 2004), has been employed to provide match data services for the majority of professional teams from Chinese Football Super League (first division) and Chinese Football Association China League (second division), China National Youth Super League (U13–U19 divisions), China Men's National Team, clubs from Korean K-league (first division). Meanwhile, the company has also been cooperating with major Chinese online sport video media (PPTV), by collecting, storing, analyzing and visualizing professional football match data of the first leagues in Korea, Spain and United Kingdom (first leagues) during online match broadcasting. In a word, most of match reports and analyses provided by the system are widely used by Asian professional football clubs, coaches, media, and governing organizations. Furthermore, what stands the system out is that it not only allows for common match performance indicators as its peers do, but also includes a more complex classification of players' passing directions, which is seldom found in other systems. As noted above, passing behaviors reveal great extent of tactical information about football, because some teams try to create opportunities by long direct passes, whereas other teams are characterized by possession-style type of play (Larkin et al., 2016; Goes et al., 2019). Players are most likely more successful when passing the ball backward or sideways than attempting forward passes, but the latter has been regarded as a key performance indicator when evaluating penetration of offensive actions and assessing players' performance (Goes et al., 2019). However, given a wide range of professional leagues, clients and audience it serves, little is known about whether match performance indicators used in the *Champdas Master System* are valid and the live match data collecting process is reliable among its trained operators.

Consequently, it is imperative to execute a thorough validity and reliability analysis of the system, so that its statistics would be trustworthy for research, coaching and broadcasting purposes. Therefore, the present study was aimed: (i) to identify the validity of match performance variables used by *Champdas Master System*; (ii) to verify the intra- and inter-operator reliability of *Champdas Master System* used by well-trained operators to collect match statistics in live association football match.

MATERIALS AND METHODS

Validity of Performance Variables Used by *Champdas Master System*

At the first stage of the study, a panel of experts constituted by 20 coaches or assistant coaches from China, Spain, Portugal, Germany, and Ireland voluntarily participated and completed the questionnaire that was aimed to validate the performance variables used in *Champdas Master System*. The inclusion criteria of the coaches were as follows: (i) Having coached professional teams of a level equivalent to the first and second divisions in Asian Football Confederation (AFC) or Union of European Football Associations (UEFA) or coached in a semi-professional level, equivalent to AFC or UEFA third division; and (ii) Owning coach licenses equivalent or higher than AFC-B or UEFA-A level. The participating coaches had an average coaching experience of 13.3 ± 7.1 years, and among twenty of them, five had UEFA-Pro license, five had UEFA-A license, nine had AFC-A license and one had AFC-B license. Prior to the filling of questionnaire and sign the voluntary informed consent, the study purpose and the anonymously academic use of their answers were explained to each coach.

Performance Variables and Operational Definitions

The questionnaire was based on performance variables used by *Champdas Master System* and they were divided into three domains: (i) Attacking-related performance; (ii) Passing-related performance, and (iii) Defending-and-Goalkeeper-related performance. The criterion of selecting these variables were mainly based on two categories of existing literature, namely, studies that examined the validity of other match analysis systems and analyzed variables (Valter et al., 2006; Bradley et al., 2007; Liu et al., 2013; Castellano et al., 2014; Beato et al., 2018); and studies that focused on tactical patterns and passing behaviors of football players (Rein et al., 2017; Goes et al., 2019; Pollard, 2019). Within all variables, the inclusion of two variables should be highlighted. First of all, considering the width of the pitch and different pitch paths (left, center, and right) and their actual usefulness in interpreting offensive behaviors (Sgrò et al., 2017), we included the "attacking shift" as a performance variable, revealing a quick ball transition from side to side. This corroborates with the findings of Rein et al. (2017) in that more successful teams could increase space control in the attacking zone through passing, creating defensive disadvantages for the opposing teams. Secondly, passing directions were established calculating the angles from current passes to the next events in relation to the sideline and attacking direction (see **Figure 1**; Serpiello et al., 2017; Goes et al., 2019).

Attacking-Related Performance

Attacking shift

The situation takes place in midfield or attacking third where the attacking players take the initiative to transfer the ball from one sideway to the other (done with no more than three passes), for creating better attacking space.

Enter into attacking third

(Pitch is divided into three zones, including attacking third, middle third and defending third. Enter into offensive zone means entering into attacking third). It includes the following conditions: (1) After players enter into the attacking third, a transition of ball possession is realized (including possession gained by defensive actions or opponent's turnover); (2) A dead ball occurs.

Dribble

A dribble is an attempt by a player to beat an opponent in possession of the ball. A successful dribble means the player beats the defender while retaining possession; unsuccessful ones are where the dribbler is tackled.

Shot

An attempt to score a goal, made with any (legal) part of the body, either on or off target. The outcomes of shot could be: goal, shot on target, shot off target, blocked shot, post.

Shot on target

The definition of a "shot on target" or a "shot on goal" (SOG) is goal or any shot attempt to goal, which required intervention to stop it going in or resulted in a goal if left unblocked.

Possession gained

The total number of possession regained by active defending (tackle, interception), or by passive recovery (ball cleared by the opponents).

Aerial Duel

Aerial Duel can be also called as heading duel. Two players competing for a ball in the air, for it to be an aerial both players must jump and challenge each other in the air and have both feet off the ground. The player who wins the duel gets the Aerial Won, and the player who doesn't get an Aerial Lost.

Passing-Related Performance

Pass

Any pass attempted from one player to another. Excluding free kicks, corners, throw-ins, and goal kicks.

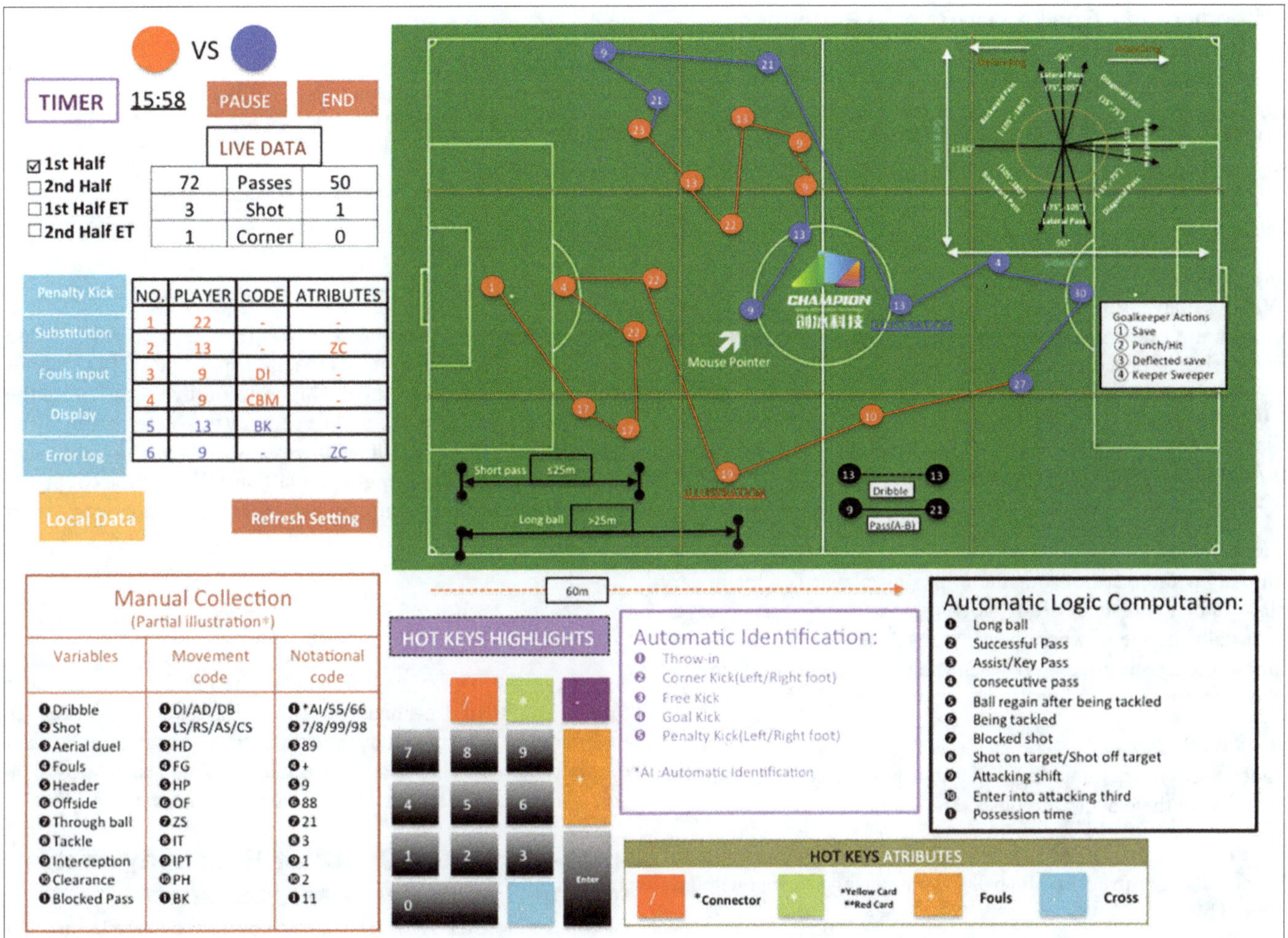

FIGURE 1 | Illustration of *Champdas Master System* operation interface diagram.

Successful pass
Any pass successfully reached from one player to another. Excluding free kicks, corners, throw-ins, and goal kicks.

Forward pass
Forward pass (The angle between pass direction and the parallel of sideline is $<15°$).

Through ball
Ball passed through the last line of defense.

Lateral pass
The lateral pass to the left or right (the angle between pass direction and the parallel of goal line $\leq 15°$).

Diagonal pass
The pass with the angle between pass direction and the parallel of sideline is $\{(15°, 75°), (105°, 165°)\}$.

Backward pass
The pass with the angle between backward pass route and side line $\leq 75°$.

Long pass
The distance of pass >25 m.

Short pass
The distance of pass ≤ 25 m.

Assist
The final pass or cross leading to goal-scoring.

Consecutive pass
The total number of passes that a team realizes without losing ball possession or causing a dead ball.

Key pass
The final pass or cross leading to the recipient of the ball that attempts to make a goal, but fails.

Cross
Any pass that delivers the ball into the penalty area by the attacking team, from lateral areas of the attacking third (not played inside of the penalty area).

Defending-and-Goalkeeper-Related Performance

Tackle

When the opposing player is in possession of the ball, but has no intention to pass, the defending player acts dispossessing the ball. A tackle won is given during following conditions: when a player makes a tackle and possession is retained by either himself or one of his teammates; when the tackle results in the ball leaving the field of play.

Interception

When a player intercepts any pass event between opposition players and prevents the ball reaching its target. Note: Defending player should be close to the receiver.

Clearance

Player under pressure gets the ball clear of the danger zone or/and out of play. If the ball is intentionally played into another teammate, it is not considered as a clearance, but a pass.

Blocked pass

Similar to interception but the opposing player is already very close to ball and successfully block the pass from passing player. It usually happens when player consciously or unconsciously blocks the pass immediately when the ball is attempted from one player to another.

Blocked shot

A defensive block, blocking a shot going on target. This must be awarded to the player who blocks the shot.

Save

The goalkeeper prevents the ball from entering the goal with any part of his body.

Punch

The goalkeeper punches/hits any ball played into the box.

Deflected save

When goalkeeper saves a shot, but does not catch the ball.

Keeper sweeper

When the goalkeeper runs out from the goal line to either intercept a pass or close down an attacking player.

Questionnaire Design and Quantitative Evaluation

In order to make sure that variables were precisely defined and validly represented certain aspect match behavior (O'Donoghue, 2007), the questionnaire was designed to quantitatively evaluate: (i) the level of correct definitions of the performance variables, and (ii) the level of variable pertinence to match behaviors. This evaluation was comprised of a scale from 1 to 10, and an example of the questionnaire is presented in **Table 1**. There was no time limit to complete the questionnaire and the average time the coaches used to fill out the questionnaire was 20 min.

Afterward, their answers were collected and analyzed to calculate the content validity for each variable. To achieve this, the Aiken's V coefficient of each item and its respective 95% confidence interval were used (Aiken, 1980; Penfield et al., 2004).

TABLE 1 | Illustration of questionnaire sent to experts.

Dribble
(1) Definition: A dribble is an attempt by a player to beat an opponent in possession of the ball. A successful dribble means the player beats the defender while retaining possession; unsuccessful ones are where the dribbler is tackled
Poorly defined 1-2-3-4-5-6-7-8-9-10 **Correctly defined**
(2) Pertinence: Does this variable seem pertinent to the match performance?
None 1-2-3-4-5-6-7-8-9-10 **Maximum**

The magnitude of this coefficient was from 0 to 1, with 1 being the greatest possible magnitude that indicates a perfect agreement among the judges regarding the highest validity score "10" of the contents evaluated in the scale. An item was determined to be valid if its Aiken's V coefficient exceeds the exact critical value calculated by the following formula that takes into account the number of judges and items in the questionnaire sample was used (Aiken, 1985):

$$\bar{V} = 0.5 + \left(z\ .2\sqrt{\frac{3mn(c-1)}{c+1}} \right)$$

where z is the level of significance, m the number of items that the experts should evaluate, n is the number of expert judges that participate in the study, and c the maximum value that can evaluate an item. The exact critical value was then calculated to be 0.52 via the formula at a statistical significance level of $p < 0.05$.

Intra- and Inter-Operator Reliability Test for the *Champdas Master System*

Champdas Master System is a computerized match analysis system developed by Champion Technology Co., Ltd., to generate live match statistics for professional association football matches. Any performance analyst using the System has to firstly go through a rigorous learning process to get comprehensively familiarized with the definitions of all match actions or events, live coding mode, hot-keys, on-screen manual positioning with mouse, and movement characteristics (see the illustration in **Figure 1**). Later, they are required to practice the learned knowledge and skills within various trial matches so as to be capable of collecting formal live match statistics.

Main data capture mode combines hot-keys of keyboard and on-screen positioning to represent events and labels. The on-screen positioning functions by using mouse markings on a scaled-down version of football pitch, which is employed for tracking players. The movements of mouse and codes correspond to the actual actions performed by players in the actual match.

Event buttons/labels represent match events that are to be recorded over the course the match. Some events may have multiple levels of information, so that some short-cut keys or combination of keys recording different aspects of the same event are used and synchronized by the system.

Two categories of data source are automatically input into the system once manually coding match events. The first category includes corner, free kick and throw-in, etc., events that can be automatically identified given the marking locations on the simulated pitch; the other category is composed of long ball, successful pass, consecutive pass, attacking shift, etc., actions that can be automatically and logically generated from the relationship of players and pitch zones. The corresponding time of the event is also recorded automatically once an event is notated. Meanwhile, the marked event locations would be later integrated to generate additional tactical performance information.

Live Data Collection and Sampled Match

To test the system reliability, four well-trained operators (experience = 1.5, 1.5, 2, and 2 years) from Champion Technology Co., Ltd., collected twice (with an interval of 2 weeks) the match data of the 19th round of Spanish La Liga Santander between Real Madrid and Villarreal contested in January 13, 2018 (Live broadcast from a conventional TV coverage). The number of match used and the coding procedure followed the routine of previous studies that validated similar systems (Bradley et al., 2007; Choi et al., 2007; Liu et al., 2013; Beato et al., 2018).

The operators were separated into two groups and observed the match independently. To be capable of formally operating the system, new operators should take part in a training process that consists of five parts: (i) definition learning, (ii) actions coding, (iii) practice in test server, (iv) played-match coding, and (v) live match coding (Champion Technology Co., Ltd., 2018). Normally, during months of training process, new operators were required to get familiar with all match actions, events and corresponding codes, and gradually develop the accuracy and proficiency in data collection. During the live match coding, there was only one principal operator from each group who was in charge of coding all match events. While the other was responsible for checking the completeness of whole dataset, amending any major inconsistence of statistics wherever needed, and then the final report was usually regarded as one-operator work. Therefore, in the current study, Operator 1 and Operator 2 were used to represent each coding group. A total of 27 players were observed, which included 22 starters, 5 substitutes, and 2 goalkeepers. The data collection was officially authorized and supported by Champion Technology Co., Ltd., and the institutional ethics committee from the Technical University of Madrid approved the study.

After the data collection, the raw data were output into Microsoft Excel with their corresponding timeline. As there were large differences in players' action counts due to different on-field time, the agreement of match actions and events coded by independent operators was analyzed by considering the same three number of groups used during validation stage: (i) attacking related actions: dribble won, dribble lost, corner, attacking shift, possession gained, free kick, goal, header, shot, shot on target, shot off target, shot saved, throw-in, offside, and enter into attacking third; (ii) passing-related actions: pass, successful pass, forward pass, through ball, lateral pass, diagonal pass, backward pass, long pass, short pass, assist, consecutive pass, key pass, and cross; and (iii) defending and goalkeeper related actions: blocked pass, blocked shot, clearance, interception, tackle won, tackle lost, aerial won, aerial lost, yellow card, keeper sweeper, save, punch, and deflected save.

Statistical Analysis

The intra- and inter-operator reliability of collected match statistics were determined using weighted *Kappa* statistic (Altman, 1990; O'Donoghue, 2010), mean, change in the mean, standardized typical error (TE) and intra-class correlation (ICC) (Hopkins, 2000). The *kappa* statistic was interpreted according to Altman's evaluation scheme (Altman, 1990): $\kappa \leq 0.2$ poor agreement; $0.2 \leq \kappa < 0.4$ fair agreement; $0.4 \leq \kappa < 0.6$ moderate agreement; $0.6 \leq \kappa < 0.8$ good agreement; $\kappa \geq 0.8$ very good agreement. The value of standardized typical error should be doubled and the thresholds for the levels of disagreement are as follow: < 0.20 trivial; 0.21–0.60 small; 0.61–1.20 moderate; 1.21–2.00 large; 2.01–4.00 very large; >4.00 extremely large (Hopkins, 2000; Smith and Hopkins, 2011). The mean, change in the mean and standardized TE and ICC were calculated using the spreadsheet developed by Hopkins (2000).

RESULTS

Based on the evaluation of twenty professional coaches over 31 variables, the result of Aiken's V averaged at 0.84 ± 0.03 for the degree of variable pertinence to match performance and 0.85 ± 0.03 for the correct definition of variable, showing high values in relation to content validity of all variables (see **Table 2**).

Table 3 showed that there were in total 5,430 events agreed by two independent operators within two collections for Real Madrid, and 4,065 for Villarreal. Comparing intra-operator data collections between the first and second collection, the average time difference of event-coding was 0.91 ± 0.94 s for Operator 1 and 0.81 ± 0.88 s for Operator 2, respectively. While average time difference was 0.89 ± 0.88 s between Operator 1 and Operator 2 for inter-operator data collections. Details can be seen from **Figures 2, 3**. The *Kappa* statistics for the events of two teams were 0.97 and 0.89, showing a very good agreement between independent operators.

Table 4 showed that there were in total 2,619 events agreed by Operator 1 within two collections for Real Madrid, and 1,948 for Villarreal. The Kappa values for the events of two teams were 0.91 and 0.93. While **Table 4** showed that there were in total 2,781 events agreed by Operator 2 within two collections for Real Madrid, and 1,953 for Villarreal. The Kappa values for the events of two teams were 0.91 and 0.87. These results demonstrated a very good intra-operator agreement (see **Supplementary Tables 1–4**).

Table 5 shows that the intra-class correlation coefficients (ICC) ranged from 0.98 to 1.00 and the standardized typical errors (TE) varied from 0.01 to 0.15 for different groups of match actions coded by the same operator within two data collections, showing very good intra-operator reliability. The ICC ranged from 0.93 to 1.00, and TE varied from 0.01 to 0.29 for different match actions coded by different operators within two data collections, showing high level of inter-operator reliability. Furthermore, an empirical comparison was made

TABLE 2 | Evaluation by 20 expert judges of the pertinence and definition of performance variables.

	Pertinence to match performance			Correct definition of variable		
	Mean (SD)	**Aiken's V**	**95% CL**	**Mean (SD)**	**Aiken's V**	**95% CL**
Attacking shift	8.3 (1.4)	0.81	0.806–0.815	8.2 (1.6)	0.79	0.789–0.799
Enter into attacking third	8.5 (1.6)	0.83	0.823–0.832	8.4 (1.7)	0.82	0.817–0.826
Possession time	8.9 (1.8)	0.87	0.868–0.875	9.1 (1.6)	0.89	0.89–0.897
Dribble	8.5 (1.8)	0.83	0.823–0.831	8.7 (1.5)	0.85	0.845–0.854
Shot	9.3 (1.2)	0.92	0.918–0.925	9.4 (1.0)	0.93	0.929–0.936
Shot on target	9.0 (1.4)	0.88	0.878–0.887	9.0 (1.3)	0.88	0.878–0.887
Possession gained	9.0 (1.3)	0.89	0.884–0.892	9.1 (1.1)	0.90	0.895–0.903
Aerial Duel	8.5 (2.0)	0.83	0.823–0.831	8.6 (1.7)	0.84	0.84–0.848
Pass	8.5 (2.8)	0.83	0.824–0.831	8.8 (2.4)	0.87	0.863–0.869
Successful pass	8.6 (2.5)	0.84	0.841–0.847	8.7 (2.4)	0.86	0.852–0.858
Forward pass	9.0 (1.6)	0.88	0.879–0.887	9.1 (1.4)	0.89	0.89–0.898
Through ball	8.4 (2.4)	0.82	0.818–0.825	8.6 (2.3)	0.84	0.835–0.842
Lateral pass	8.7 (1.7)	0.85	0.845–0.854	8.7 (1.6)	0.86	0.851–0.859
Diagonal pass	8.7 (1.7)	0.85	0.845–0.854	8.7 (1.5)	0.86	0.851–0.859
Backward pass	8.5 (1.8)	0.83	0.823–0.831	8.7 (1.6)	0.85	0.845–0.854
Long pass	8.7 (1.8)	0.85	0.845–0.853	8.8 (1.7)	0.86	0.856–0.865
Short pass	8.8 (1.9)	0.87	0.862–0.87	9.0 (1.6)	0.88	0.879–0.886
Assist	8.9 (2.5)	0.87	0.869–0.875	8.9 (2.4)	0.88	0.874–0.88
Consecutive pass	8.5 (2.5)	0.83	0.824–0.831	8.5 (2.4)	0.83	0.829–0.836
Key pass	8.5 (2.5)	0.83	0.83–0.836	8.6 (2.4)	0.84	0.841–0.847
Cross	8.4 (1.5)	0.82	0.817–0.826	8.5 (1.5)	0.83	0.828–0.837
Tackle	8.5 (1.5)	0.83	0.823–0.832	8.5 (1.4)	0.83	0.828–0.837
Interception	8.9 (1.1)	0.87	0.867–0.876	9.0 (0.9)	0.89	0.883–0.893
Clearance	8.8 (1.5)	0.87	0.862–0.87	8.9 (1.3)	0.88	0.873–0.881
Ball regain after being tackled	8.3 (2.5)	0.81	0.807–0.814	8.5 (2.3)	0.83	0.829–0.836
Blocked pass	8.3 (2.4)	0.81	0.807–0.814	8.5 (2.2)	0.83	0.824–0.831
Blocked shot	8.7 (2.3)	0.85	0.846–0.853	8.7 (2.4)	0.85	0.846–0.853
Save	8.6 (2.4)	0.84	0.835–0.842	8.6 (2.3)	0.84	0.84–0.847
Punch	8.3 (2.7)	0.81	0.802–0.808	8.5 (2.4)	0.83	0.829–0.836
Deflected save	8.4 (2.3)	0.82	0.818–0.825	8.6 (2.3)	0.84	0.835–0.842
Keeper sweeper	8.6 (2.4)	0.84	0.835–0.842	8.6 (2.3)	0.84	0.84–0.847

between match statistics provided by OPTA Sports[1] and Operator 1 and 2 from Champdas Master System, concerning the same match events that both systems comprise (see **Table 6**). It is shown that generally both operators demonstrated an acceptable agreement with OPTA in all compared variables, expect for a slight discrepancy in short passes.

[1]http://www.whoscored.com

TABLE 3 | Number of events coded by different operators during two data collections.

	Agreement	Operator 1		Operator 2		*Kappa*
		Total	**Disagreed**	**Total**	**Disagreed**	
Real Madrid	5,430	5,518	88	5,519	89	0.97
Villarreal	4,065	4,393	328	4,391	326	0.89

All event numbers presented in the table are sum of two data collections.

DISCUSSION

This study has examined the validity and the inter- and intra-operator reliability of *Champdas Master System* operated by different well-trained operators, who were unaware of study purpose. The validation process of this system is important for scientific acknowledgment and credibility. From professional football coaches' evaluation, match variables included in the system had high levels of content validity. Operators separately coded more than 4,000 events in each data collection, which was higher than the values from previous studies applying other systems such as Prozone, OPTA and Digital.Stadium (Bradley et al., 2007; Liu et al., 2013; Beato et al., 2018). Moreover, results reported in this study showed that *Champdas Master System* had high levels of absolute and relative reliability. This reveals that the system is capable of measuring football match events reliably and provide more technical-tactical performance details than its peer systems.

Operator 2 (columns); Operator 1 (rows)

Real Madrid	Foul	DW	DL	Corner	AS	Goal kick	PG	Free Kick	Goal	Header	Shot	SO	ST	SS	Throw-in	Offside	EAT	Pass	SP	FP	TB	LP	DP	BP	Long	Short	Assist	CP	KP	Cross	BP	BS	Clearance	Interception	TW	TL	AW	AL	YC	KS	Save	Punch	DS	None	Total
Foul	22																																											0	22
DW		14											1																						1									5	21
DL			7																																									5	12
Corner				22																																								0	22
AS					7																									1														0	8
Goal kick						10																																						1	11
PG							85			1																				1					5									0	92
Free Kick								26																																				0	26
Goal									0																																			0	0
Header										40																								4			2							0	46
Shot											54																																	0	54
SO												21																																0	21
ST													14																															0	14
SS														19																														0	19
Throw-in															38																													0	38
Offside																6																												0	6
EAT																	160																											15	175
Pass																		1243																										0	1243
SP																			1046																									0	1046
FP																				81																								0	81
TB																					2																							0	2
LP																						176	2																					0	178
DP																							471												1									0	472
BP																								315																				0	315
Long					5																				44	3																		0	52
Short																										994																		0	994
Assist																											0																	0	0
CP																										4		219																5	228
KP																													50															0	50
Cross																														80														0	80
BP																															5													0	5
BS																																6												0	6
Clearance																										3							16	2										0	21
Interception																																		23	1									0	24
TW																																			35									0	35
TL																																				33								0	33
AW										7																											17							0	24
AL										8																												18						5	31
YC																																							4					0	4
KS																																								1				0	1
Save																																									4			0	4
Punch																																										2		0	2
DS																																											0	0	0
None	1	8	3	0	0	0	6	0	0	0	0	0	0	0	0	0	0	4	2	1	0	0	1	0	0	0	0	0	0	2	1	0	0	1	5	2	0		0	0	0	0	0		37
Total	23	22	10	22	12	10	91	26	0	56	54	21	15	19	38	6	160	1247	1048	82	2	176	474	315	44	1004	0	219	50	84	6	6	16	30	48	35	19	18	4	1	4	2	0	36	5555

FIGURE 2 | Frequency of Real Madrid's events recorded by the two independent operators in two collections. DW, dribble won; DL, dribble lost; AS, attacking shift; PG, possession gained; SO, shots off target; ST, shot on target; SS, shot saved; EAT, enter into attacking third; SP, successful pass; FP, forward pass; TB, through ball; LP, lateral pass; DP, diagonal pass; BP, backward pass; CP, consecutive pass; KP, key pass; BP, blocked pass; BS, blocked shot; TW, tackle won; TL, tackle lost; AW, aerial won; AL, aerial lost; YC, yellow card; KS, keeper sweeper; DS, deflected save.

Operator 2 (columns); Operator 1 (rows)

Villarreal	Foul	DW	DL	Corner	AS	Goal kick	PG	Free Kick	Goal	Header	Shot	SO	ST	SS	Throw-in	Offside	EAT	Pass	SP	FP	TB	LP	DP	BP	Long	Short	Assist	CP	KP	Cross	BP	BS	Clearance	Interception	TW	TL	AW	AL	YC	KS	Save	Punch	DS	None	Total
Foul	22																																											0	22
DW		13	1																																									6	20
DL			8																																									3	11
Corner				0																																								0	0
AS					2																																							0	2
Goal kick						24																																						0	24
PG							76			2																					1		1	1	2									12	95
Free Kick								28																																				0	28
Goal									1																																			0	1
Header			1				1			59																											2							4	67
Shot											18																																	0	18
SO												6																																0	6
ST													4																															0	4
SS														6																														0	6
Throw-in															22																													0	22
Offside																2																												0	2
EAT																	100																											0	100
Pass																		908																										0	908
SP																			758																									0	758
FP																				77			25																					8	110
TB																					3																							0	3
LP																						86	24	15																				5	130
DP																				26		30	311	2																				9	378
BP																						18	3	262																				10	293
Long																									74																			6	80
Short																										807																		21	828
Assist																											1																	0	1
CP																												130																0	130
KP																													13	1														0	14
Cross																														12														0	12
BP							1																								45		1	1										2	50
BS																																17	1											0	18
Clearance							6			2																					2		55	5										11	81
Interception																															1			10	1									5	17
TW							2																												21									4	27
TL																															1					31								7	39
AW										10																											18	4						2	34
AL										3																							1				1	9						11	25
YC																																							2					0	2
KS																																								0				2	2
Save																																									14			0	14
Punch																																										10		0	10
DS																																											0	0	0
None	0	8	3	0	0	0	11	0	0	5	0	0	0	0	0	0	0	0	0	0	1	8	17	8	5	26	0	0	0	0	7	0	4	3	3	12	1	5	0	0	0	0	0		127
Total	22	21	13	0	2	24	97	28	1	81	18	6	4	6	22	2	100	908	758	103	4	142	380	287	79	833	1	130	13	13	57	17	63	20	27	43	22	18	2	0	14	10	0	128	4519

FIGURE 3 | Frequency of Real Madrid's events recorded by the two independent operators in two collections. DW, dribble won; DL, dribble lost; AS, attacking shift; PG, possession gained; SO, shots off target; ST, shot on target; SS, shot saved; EAT, enter into attacking third; SP, successful pass; FP, forward pass; TB, through ball; LP, lateral pass; DP, diagonal pass; BP, backward pass; CP, consecutive pass; KP, key pass; BP, blocked pass; BS, blocked shot; TW, tackle won; TL, tackle lost; AW, aerial won; AL, aerial lost; YC, yellow card; KS, keeper sweeper; DS, deflected save.

A practical measure with high validity must have high reliability in the meantime. While a measure with high reliability may have low validity. But only the valid and reliable performance indicators can be reliable used in sports performance profiling (O'Donoghue, 2007; McGarry et al., 2013). Therefore, the study initially examined the validity of performance indicators by evaluating experts' opinions according to the previous literature (Trniniæ et al., 2000; Hraste et al., 2008; Larkin et al., 2016). Based on the high values of Aiken's V calculated for twenty professional coaches' responses to the pertinence (0.84 ± 0.03) and definition

TABLE 4 | Agreement of team events coded by intra-operators.

		Agreement	First data collection		Second data collection		Kappa value
			Total	Disagreed	Total	Disagreed	
Operator 1	Real Madrid	2,619	2,769	150	2,782	163	0.91
	Villarreal	1,948	2,049	101	2,045	97	0.93
Operator 2	Real Madrid	2,781	2,959	178	2,980	199	0.91
	Villarreal	1,953	2,124	171	2,136	183	0.87

TABLE 5 | Intra-operator and inter-operator reliability of match actions coded within two data collection.

		Real Madrid				Villarreal			
	Variables	Mean (SD)	Change in the mean (CL)	Standardized typical error	ICC	Mean (SD)	Change in the mean (CL)	Standardized typical error	ICC
Operator 1 (1st vs. 2nd)	Attacking	17(21)	−4.4(5.4)	0.03	1.00	12(15)	−0.4(1.0)	0.09	0.99
	Passing	182(219)	1.6(1.5)	0.01	1.00	128(161)	−0.1(1.6)	0.01	1.00
	Defending and goalkeeper	7.4(6.9)	−0.4(0.8)	0.14	0.99	12(11)	−0.3(1.0)	0.07	0.99
	All actions	64(142)	0.14(0.49)	0.01	1.00	48(102)	−0.35(0.50)	0.01	1.00
Operator 2 (1st vs. 2nd)	Attacking	17(19)	−0.3(1.0)	0.07	1.00	13(16)	0.0(0.5)	0.05	1.00
	Passing	182(221)	2.3(1.9)	0.01	1.00	129(163)	0.8(2.1)	0.02	1.00
	Defending and goalkeeper	7.2(7.5)	0.40(0.90)	0.15	0.98	10.8(9.7)	−0.1(1.0)	0.14	0.99
	All actions	64(142)	0.70(0.64)	0.01	1.00	48(103)	0.21(0.58)	0.02	1.00
Operator 1vs. Operator 2	Attacking	34(40)	−0.1(2.5)	0.08	0.99	25(31)	0.8(1.4)	0.06	1.00
	Passing	364(441)	0.4(3.0)	0.01	1.00	257(323)	1.4(2.9)	0.01	1.00
	Defending and goalkeeper	14(14)	−0.4(3.3)	0.29	0.93	22(20)	−2.4(3.9)	0.24	0.95
	All actions	128(285)	−0.05(1.31)	0.01	1.00	95(206)	0.05(1.57)	0.02	1.00

1st, First data collection; 2nd, second data collection; CL, 95% confidence limits; ICC, intra-class correlation.

TABLE 6 | Match events provided by OPTA Sports and *Champdas Master System*.

Variables	OPTA	Real Madrid				OPTA	Villarreal			
		Champdas Master System					***Champdas Master System***			
		Operator 1-1st	Operator 1-2nd	Operator 2-1st	Operator 2-2nd		Operator 1-1st	Operator 1-2nd	Operator 2-1st	Operator 2-2nd
Shots	28	27	27	26	28	10	9	9	8	8
Shots on target	7	7	7	7	7	4	2	2	2	2
Goals	0	0	0	0	0	1	1	1	1	1
Pass success %	89%	84%	84%	84%	84%	84%	83%	84%	84%	83%
Aerial duel success	45%	43%	44%	44%	48%	55%	57%	56%	61%	59%
Dribbles won	8	12	9	10	12	7	11	8	9	12
Tackles	19	19	16	25	23	14	13	13	14	15
Passes	650	620	623	621	626	467	455	453	455	459
Crosses	44	40	40	41	43	7	6	6	6	7
Through balls	0	1	1	1	1	2	1	2	2	2
Short passes	574	495	499	589	592	393	357	356	414	421

1st and 2nd stand for the first and second match data collections.

(0.85 ± 0.03) of match variables, it was revealed that the variables comprised in the system have appropriate operational definitions and are able to represent match events and player actions during data gathering and analysis.

As previously argued, valid operational definition is not sufficient to guarantee a reliable observation, because it is frequent that human error affects the repeatability of the data. (Williams and O'Donoghue, 2006; O'Donoghue, 2007; Beato et al., 2018). Therefore, the current study verified that after rigorous training and large quantity of practice using *Champdas Master System*, operators could achieve high intra- and inter-operator reliability when coding live football match events, and the data provided were reliable, which was supported by the high Kappa values, high intra-class correlation coefficients and low standardized typical errors. The findings were similar to the previously tested Prozone MatchViewer System (Bradley et al., 2007), OPTA Client System (Liu et al., 2013), and Data.Stadium System (Beato et al., 2018). This suggests that the semi-automatic operation errors in collection with the system were extremely limited. Besides, it should be noted that former research focused on the measurements of typical technical-tactical variables that were mainly notated via shortcut keys (Liu et al., 2013). Nonetheless, compared with its counterparts, the current system is operated via both shortcut keys and mouse clicking on a simulated pitch. On the account, the system not only produces more data related to attacking and passing behaviors, but also effectively provides tactical information, considering pitch zones where match performance took place. This allows more comprehensive technical-tactical match statistics for performance analysis and broadcasting purposes.

However, there were several limitations that should addressed. First of all, more matches may be needed to test the generalization of the system and operator reliability. Additionally, it is admitted that occasions of discrepancy existed in some match actions related to passing directions, short/long pass. This phenomenon happens when comparing OPTA Sport and *Champdas Master System*, as well as assessing intra- and inter operators reliability. This may be explained from two perspectives. Primarily, the inconsistence between OPTA Sport and *Champdas Master System* in short pass might be caused by different definition of the length. This is supported by the similar total number of passes both systems recorded in the current match. Moreover, after a round of retrospection with participating operators, we were informed that the disagreements in determining the lengths and directions of passes mainly originated from plotting errors and entry errors. These types of errors were due to the manual marking discrepancy when operating on the miniaturized on-scree pitch. For example, for the passing direction related variables, the system would automatically recognize a pass as lateral pass even if a player made a forward pass (the angle between pass direction and the parallel of sideline is $< 15°$) to his teammate who is located at the left front of him. Therefore, if operators could not observe or notate properly similar pass directions on the screen as what are actually taking place on the field, disagreements in passing categories would occur. In fact, this issue was also reported in ProZone MatchViewer system (Bradley et al., 2007; Castellano et al., 2014) and Trakperformance system (Burgess et al., 2006; Edgecomb and Norton, 2006; Carling et al., 2008), which used a similar approach. Furthermore, operator's observation would be affected while gathering data from live TV coverage, as Tenga and Albin (Tenga, 2010) found that camera angles, image sizes and feature film could be blurry when accurate event location is expected. Consequently, more precision problems appear especially when operators are notating positions, distances and angles related match events.

In a word, the largest technical problem was that operators had difficulty in consistently plotting the X/Y coordinates of the events on the miniaturized pitch. In light of these issues, it is suggested that simplification in passing directions be considered. Instead of including diagonal pass (**Figure 1**), four types of categories could be established with angle interval of 90° (Goes et al., 2019): forward, left and right sideways, and backward. Meanwhile, automatic player tracking instruments should be further developed and integrated in the data collection process so that operators could avoid subjective determination of directions, lengths and outcomes of passes (Beato and Jamil, 2017). Nonetheless, the current results show that the match statistics could be deemed acceptable so long as operators undergo adequate training and practice in maneuvering the system and identifying specific match events.

The quality of data provided plays a prominent role in performance analysis, sport coaching, media reporting, and scientific research (O'Donoghue, 2009, 2014; O'Donoghue et al., 2017). The study reveals a high level of validity and reliability using *Champdas Master System* to measure live football match statistics. From a theoretical and practical perspective, coaches, sport scientists, and media could benefit from the application of the system to gain reliable technical-tactical performance information. Additionally, future studies could evaluate the generalization of system with a larger sample in similar or distinct leagues, as well as under distinct light conditions.

CONCLUSION

The analysis of football expert panel opinions evidenced the validity of tactical and technical match performance variables from *Champdas Master system*. Moreover, high Kappa values, high intra-class correlation coefficients and low standardized typical errors demonstrated a high level of intra- and inter-operator reliability using the *system* to collect sampled match events. Although, slight discrepancy was shown in the identification of players' passing directions, our results suggest that the *Champdas Master system* can be used validly and reliably to collect live football match statistics by well-trained operators. The system and statistics generated could be trustworthy for coaching, academic research and media report.

ETHICS STATEMENT

We state clearly that written informed consent was obtained from the participants of all phases of the study, and the study was approved by the Ethics Committee of the Technical University of Madrid.

AUTHOR CONTRIBUTIONS

M-ÁG, BG, and YC designed the experiments. YC, YG, and QY performed the statistical analysis. BG wrote and revised the manuscript. M-ÁG supervised the design and reviewed the manuscript. All authors have made a substantial and direct contribution to manuscript, and approved the final version of the manuscript.

REFERENCES

Aiken, L. R. (1980). Content validity and reliability of single items or questionnaires. *Educ. Psychol. Meas.* 40, 955–959. doi: 10.1177/001316448004000419

Aiken, L. R. (1985). Three coefficients for analyzing the reliability and validity of ratings. *Educ. Psychol. Meas.* 45, 131–142. doi: 10.1177/0013164485451012

Altman, D. G. (1990). *Practical Statistics for Medical Research*. Boca Raton, FL: CRC press.

Atkinson, G., and Nevill, A. M. (1998). Statistical methods for assessing measurement error (reliability) in variables relevant to sports medicine. *Sports Med.* 26, 217–238. doi: 10.2165/00007256-199826040-00002

Beato, M., and Jamil, M. (2017). Intra-system reliability of SICS: video-tracking system (Digital. Stadium®) for performance analysis in football. *J. Sports Med. Phys. Fit.* 58, 831–836.

Beato, M., Jamil, M., and Devereux, G. (2018). The reliability of technical and tactical tagging analysis conducted by a semi-automatic video-tracking system (Digital.Stadium®) in soccer. *J. Hum. Kinet.* 62, 103–110. doi: 10.1515/hukin-2017-0162

Bradley, P., O'Donoghue, P., Wooster, B., and Tordoff, P. (2007). The reliability of ProZone MatchViewer: a video-based technical performance analysis system. *Int. J. Perform. Anal. Sport* 7, 117–129. doi: 10.1080/24748668.2007.11868415

Bradley, P. S., Carling, C., Archer, D., Roberts, J., Dodds, A., Di Mascio, M., et al. (2011). The effect of playing formation on high-intensity running and technical profiles in English FA Premier League soccer matches. *J. Sports Sci.* 29, 821–830. doi: 10.1080/02640414.2011.561868

Burgess, D., Naughton, G., and Norton, K. I. (2006). Profile of movement demands of national football players in Australia. *J. Sci. Med. Sport* 9, 334–341. doi: 10.1016/j.jsams.2006.01.005

Carling, C., Bloomfield, J., Nelsen, L., and Reilly, T. (2008). The role of motion analysis in elite soccer. *Sports Med.* 38, 839–862. doi: 10.2165/00007256-200838100-00004

Carling, C., Reilly, T., and Williams, A. M. (2007). *Handbook of Soccer Match Analysis: A Systematic Approach to Improving Performance*. Abingdon: Routledge.

Castellano, J., Alvarez-Pastor, D., and Bradley, P. S. (2014). Evaluation of research using computerised tracking systems (Amisco® and Prozone®) to analyse physical performance in elite soccer: a systematic review. *Sports Med.* 44, 701–712. doi: 10.1007/s40279-014-0144-3

Chacón-Moscoso, S., Sanduvete-Chaves, S., Anguera, M. T., Losada, J. L., Portell, M., and Lozano-Lozano, J. A. (2018). Preliminary checklist for reporting observational studies in sports areas: content validity. *Front. Psychol.* 9:291. doi: 10.3389/fpsyg.2018.00291

Champion Technology Co., Ltd. (2018). *Champdas Master System Training Manual 3.0."*. Baton Rouge, LA: Champion Technology Co., Ltd.

Choi, H., O'Donoghue, P., and Hughes, M. (2007). An investigation of inter-operator reliability tests for real-time analysis system. *Int. J. Perform. Anal. Sport* 7, 49–61. doi: 10.1080/24748668.2007.11868387

Clear, C., Hughes, M., and Martin, D. (2017). Attacking profiles in elite hurling. *Int. J. Perform. Anal. Sport* 17, 319–333. doi: 10.1080/24748668.2017.1338074

Cui, Y., Gómez, M. -Á, Gonçalves, B., and Sampaio, J. (2019). Clustering tennis players' anthropometric and individual features helps to reveal performance fingerprints. *Eur. J. Sport Sci.* 1–13. doi: 10.1080/17461391.2019.1577494

Cupples, B., and O'Connor, D. (2011). The development of position-specific performance indicators in elite youth rugby league: a coach's perspective. *Int. J. Sports Sci. Coach.* 6, 125–141. doi: 10.1260/1747-9541.6.1.125

Dellal, A., Chamari, K., Wong, D. P., Ahmaidi, S., Keller, D., Barros, R., et al. (2011). Comparison of physical and technical performance in European soccer match-play: FA premier league and La Liga. *Eur. J. Sport Sci.* 11, 51–59. doi: 10.1080/17461391.2010.481334

Edgecomb, S. J., and Norton, K. I. (2006). Comparison of global positioning and computer-based tracking systems for measuring player movement distance during Australian football. *J. Sci. Med. Sport* 9, 25–32. doi: 10.1016/j.jsams.2006.01.003

Eltoukhy, M., Asfour, S., Thompson, C., and Latta, L. (2012). Evaluation of the performance of digital video analysis of human motion: Dartfish tracking system. *IJSER* 3, 1–6.

Goes, F. R., Kempe, M., Meerhoff, L. A., and Lemmink, K. A. (2019). Not every pass can be an assist: a data-driven model to measure pass effectiveness in professional soccer matches. *Big Data* 7, 57–70. doi: 10.1089/big.2018.0067

Gonçalves, B., Coutinho, D., Santos, S., Lago-Penas, C., Jiménez, S., and Sampaio, J. (2017). Exploring team passing networks and player movement dynamics in youth association football. *PLoS One* 12:e0171156. doi: 10.1371/journal.pone.0171156

Hayen, A., Dennis, R. J., and Finch, C. F. (2007). Determining the intra-and inter-observer reliability of screening tools used in sports injury research. *J. Sci. Med. Sport* 10, 201–210. doi: 10.1016/j.jsams.2006.09.002

Hizan, H., Whipp, P. R., and Reid, M. (2010). Validation of match notation (A coding system) in tennis. *J. Quant. Anal. Sports* 6, 1–13.

Hopkins, W. G. (2000). Measures of reliability in sports medicine and science. *Sports Med.* 30, 1–15. doi: 10.2165/00007256-200030010-00001

Hraste, M., Dizdar, D., and Trniniæ, V. (2008). Experts opinion about system of the performance evaluation criteria weighted per positons in the water polo game. *Coll. Antropol.* 32, 851–861.

Hughes, M. (2004). Performance analysis–a 2004 perspective. *Int. J. Perform. Anal. Sport* 4, 103–109. doi: 10.1080/24748668.2004.11868296

Hughes, M., and Franks, I. (2015). *Essentials of Performance Analysis in Sport*. London: Routledge.

Hughes, M. D., and Bartlett, R. M. (2002). The use of performance indicators in performance analysis. *J. Sports Sci.* 20, 739–754. doi: 10.1080/026404102320675602

Lago, C., Casais, L., Dominguez, E., and Sampaio, J. (2010). The effects of situational variables on distance covered at various speeds in elite soccer. *Eur. J. Sport Sci.* 10, 103–109. doi: 10.1080/17461390903273994

Lames, M., and McGarry, T. (2007). On the search for reliable performance indicators in game sports. *Int. J. Perform. Anal. Sport* 7, 62–79. doi: 10.1080/24748668.2007.11868388

Larkin, P., O'Connor, D., and Williams, A. M. (2016). Establishing validity and reliability of a movement awareness and technical skill (MATS) analysis instrument in soccer. *Int. J. Perform. Anal. Sport* 16, 191–202. doi: 10.1080/24748668.2016.11868880

Li, Y., Alexander, M., Glazebrook, C., and Leiter, J. (2016). Quantifying inter-segmental coordination during the instep soccer kicks. *Int. J. Exerc. Sci.* 9, 646.

Liu, H., Hopkins, W., Gómez, A. M., and Molinuevo, S. J. (2013). Inter-operator reliability of live football match statistics from OPTA Sportsdata. *Int. J. Perform. Anal. Sport* 13, 803–821. doi: 10.1080/24748668.2013.11868690

Mackenzie, R., and Cushion, C. (2013). Performance analysis in football: a critical review and implications for future research. *J. Sports Sci.* 31, 639–676. doi: 10.1080/02640414.2012.746720

McGarry, T. (2009). Applied and theoretical perspectives of performance analysis in sport: scientific issues and challenges. *Int. J. Perform. Anal. Sport* 9, 128–140. doi: 10.1080/24748668.2009.11868469

McGarry, T., O'Donoghue, P., de Eira Sampaio, A. J., and Sampaio, J. (2013).). *Routledge Handbook of Sports Performance Analysis*. Abingdon: Routledge.

Oberstone, J. (2009). Differentiating the top English premier league football clubs from the rest of the pack: Identifying the keys to success. *J. Quant. Anal. Sports* 5, 1–29.

Oberstone, J. (2010). Comparing English premier league goalkeepers: identifying the pitch actions that differentiate the best from the rest. *J. Quant. Anal. Sports* 6:9.

Oberstone, J. (2011). Comparing team performance of the English premier league, Serie A, and La Liga for the 2008-2009 season. *J. Quant. Anal. Sports* 7:2.

O'Donoghue, P. (2007). Reliability issues in performance analysis. *Int. J. Perform. Anal. Sport* 7, 35–48. doi: 10.1080/24748668.2007.11868386

O'Donoghue, P. (2009). *Research Methods for Sports Performance Analysis*. Abingdon: Routledge.

O'Donoghue, P. (2010). "Measurement issues in performance analysis," in *Research Methods for Sports Performance Analysis*. ed. P. O'Donoghue (Abingdon: Routledge), 149–177.

O'Donoghue, P. (2014). *An Introduction to Performance Analysis of Sport*. Abingdon: Routledge.

O'Donoghue, P., and Holmes, L. (2014). *Data Analysis in Sport.* Abingdon: Routledge.

O'Donoghue, P., Holmes, L., and Robinson, G. (2017). *Doing a Research Project in Sport Performance Analysis.* Abingdon: Routledge.

O'Donoghue, P., and Mayes, A. (2013). "Performance analysis, feedback and communication in coaching," in *Routledge Handbook of Sports Performance Analysis.* eds T. McGarry, P. O'Donoghue, and J. Sampaio (Abingdon: Routledge), 155–164.

Osgnach, C., Poser, S., Bernardini, R., Rinaldo, R., and Di Prampero, P. E. (2010). Energy cost and metabolic power in elite soccer: a new match analysis approach. *Med. Sci. Sports Exerc.* 42, 170–178. doi: 10.1249/MSS.0b013e3181ae5cfd

Padulo, J., Haddad, M., Ardigo, L., Chamari, K., and Pizzolato, F. (2015). High frequency performance analysis of professional soccer goalkeepers: a pilot study. *J. Sports Med. Phys. Fit.* 55, 557–562.

Penfield, R. D., Peter, R., and Giacobbi, J. (2004). Applying a score confidence interval to aiken's item content-relevance index. *Meas. Phys. Educ. Exerc. Sci.* 8, 213–225. doi: 10.1207/s15327841mpee0804_3

Pollard, R. (2019). Invalid interpretation of passing sequence data to assess team performance in football: repairing the tarnished legacy of charles reep. *Open Sports Sci. J.* 12, 17–21. doi: 10.2174/1875399x01912010017

Praça, G. M., Lima, B. B., Bredt, S. D. G. T., Sousa, R. B. E., Clemente, F. M., and Andrade, A. G. P. D. (2019). Influence of match status on players' prominence and teams' network properties During 2018 FIFA World Cup. *Front. Psychol.* 10:695. doi: 10.3389/fpsyg.2019.00695

Rampinini, E., Impellizzeri, F. M., Castagna, C., Coutts, A. J., and Wisløff, U. (2009). Technical performance during soccer matches of the Italian Serie A league: effect of fatigue and competitive level. *J. Sci. Med. Sport* 12, 227–233. doi: 10.1016/j.jsams.2007.10.002

Reed, D., and Hughes, M. (2006). An exploration of team sport as a dynamical system. *Int. J. Perform. Anal. Sport* 6, 114–125. doi: 10.1080/24748668.2006.11868377

Reid, M., Morgan, S., and Whiteside, D. (2016). Matchplay characteristics of Grand Slam tennis: implications for training and conditioning. *J. Sports Sci.* 34, 1791–1798. doi: 10.1080/02640414.2016.1139161

Rein, R., Raabe, D., and Memmert, D. (2017). "Which pass is better?" Novel approaches to assess passing effectiveness in elite soccer. *Hum. Move. Sci.* 55(Suppl. C), 172–181. doi: 10.1016/j.humov.2017.07.010

Sampaio, J., and Leite, N. (2013). "Performance indicators in game sports," in *Routledge Handbook of Sports Performance Analysis*, eds T. McGarry, P. O'Donoghue, and J. Sampaio (Abingdon: Routledge), 115–126.

Serpiello, F. R., Cox, A., Oppici, L., Hopkins, W. G., and Varley, M. C. (2017). The Loughborough Soccer passing test has impractical criterion validity in elite youth football. *Sci. Med. Football* 1, 60–64. doi: 10.1080/02640414.2016.1254810

Sgrò, F., Aiello, F., Casella, A., and Lipoma, M. (2017). The effects of match-playing aspects and situational variables on achieving score-box possessions in Euro 2012 Football Championship. *J. Hum. Sport Exerc.* 12, 58–72. doi: 10.14198/jhse.2017.121.05

Smith, T. B., and Hopkins, W. G. (2011). Variability and predictability of finals times of elite rowers. *Med. Sci. Sports Exerc.* 43, 2155–2160. doi: 10.1249/MSS.0b013e31821d3f8e

Tenga, A. (2010). *Reliability and Validity of Match Performance Analysis in Soccer: A Multidimensional Qualitative Evaluation of Opponent Interaction.* Ph. D thesis. Oslo: Norwegian School of Sports Sciences.

Torres-Luque, G., Fernández-García, ÁI., Cabello-Manrique, D., Giménez-Egido, J. M., and Ortega-Toro, E. (2018). Design and validation of an observational instrument for the technical-tactical actions in singles Tennis. *Front. Psychol.* 9:2418. doi: 10.3389/fpsyg.2018.02418

Trniniæ, S., Dizdar, D., and Dežman, B. (2000). Empirical verification of the weighted system of criteria for the elite basketball players quality evaluation. *Coll. Antropol.* 24, 443–465.

Valter, D. S., Adam, C., Barry, M., and Marco, C. (2006). Validation of Prozone®: a new video-based performance analysis system. *Int. J. Perform. Anal. Sport* 6, 108–119. doi: 10.1080/24748668.2006.11868359

Williams, L., and O'Donoghue, P. (2006). Defensive strategies used by international netball teams. *Perform. Anal. Sport* 7, 474–479.

Zhang, S., Lorenzo, A., Zhou, C., Cui, Y., Gonçalves, B., and Angel Gómez, M. (2018). Performance profiles and opposition interaction during game-play in elite basketball: evidences from National Basketball Association. *Int. J. Perform. Anal. Sport* 19, 28–48. doi: 10.1080/24748668.2018.1555738

Zhou, C., Zhang, S., Lorenzo Calvo, A., and Cui, Y. (2018). Chinese soccer association super league, 2012–2017: key performance indicators in balance games. *Int. J. Perform. Anal. Sport* 18, 645–656. doi: 10.1080/24748668.2018.1509254

Zubillaga, A., Gorospe, G., Hernandez, A., and Blanco, A. (2009). "Comparative analysis of the high-intensity activity of soccer players in top level competition," in *Science and Football VI*, eds H. Reilly and F. Korkusuz (Milton Park: Taylor & Francis Group), 182–185.

27

Post-Activation Potentiation: Effects of Different Conditioning Intensities on Measures of Physical Fitness in Male Young Professional Soccer Players

Cristina Petisco[1], Rodrigo Ramirez-Campillo[1,2], Daniel Hernández[1], Oliver Gonzalo-Skok[1,3], Fabio Y. Nakamura[1,4,5] and Javier Sanchez-Sanchez[1]*

[1] Research Group Planning and Assessment of Training and Athletic Performance, Pontifical University of Salamanca, Salamanca, Spain, [2] Laboratory of Human Performance, Research Nucleus in Health, Physical Activity and Sport, Department of Physical Activity Sciences, Universidad de Los Lagos, Osorno, Chile, [3] Faculty of Health Sciences, University of San Jorge, Zaragoza, Spain, [4] College of Healthcare Sciences, James Cook University, Townsville, QLD, Australia, [5] Department of Medicine and Aging Sciences, "G. d'Annunzio" University of Chieti-Pescara, Chieti, Italy

***Correspondence:**
Javier Sanchez-Sanchez
jsanchezsa@upsa.es

The aim of this study was to compare the effects of different warm-up conditioning intensities on the physical fitness (i.e., post-activation potentiation -PAP), of professional male field soccer players. Athletes (n = 10; age: 21.6 ± 3.2 years) completed a control warm-up and warm-ups aimed to induce PAP, in random and counterbalanced order. After control and experimental warm-up sessions participants completed a triple hop test with the dominant (H3Jd) and a non-dominant (H3Jnd) leg, a squat jump (SJ), a countermovement jump (CMJ), a change of direction ability (COD) test, a repeated sprint with a COD (RSCOD) test and a linear 30-m sprint test (S-30). The control warm-up (WU) protocol was designed according to athlete's regular warm-up practice. The experimental warm-ups included the same exercises as the WU, with addition of one set of half-back squats for 10 repetitions at 60%, 5 repetitions at 80%, and 1 repetition at 100% of 1RM (60%-1RM, 80%-1RM and 100%-1RM, respectively.) Threshold values for Cohen's effect sizes (ES) were calculated and used for group's comparison. Likely to most likely improvements were shown in H3Jd (*ES* = 0.52), H3Jnd (*ES* = 0.51), COD (*ES* = 0.38), fasted sprint (RSCODb) (*ES* = 0.58) and the total time of all sprints (RSCODt) (*ES* = 0.99) only after the 80%-1RM protocol in comparison to the WU. Conversely, 100%-1RM and 60%-1RM protocols, compared to WU, induced possibly to most likely poorer performance in all jumps, COD and RSCODb (*ES* = −0.07 to −1.03 and *ES* = −0.48 to −0.91, respectively). Possibly to most likely improvements were shown in all jumps, COD, RSCODb and RSCODt after the 80%-1RM warm-up protocol in comparison to the 100%-1RM and 60%-1RM warm-up protocols (*ES* = 0.35 to 2.15 and *ES* = 0.61 to 1.46, respectively). A moderate warm-up intensity (i.e., 80%-1RM back squat) may induce greater PAP, including improvements in jumping, repeated and non-repeated change of direction speed in male soccer players.

Keywords: plyometric, speed, fatigue, warm-up, soccer

INTRODUCTION

Aside from the total distance covered, performing high-intensity actions repeatedly during a match is a key feature of soccer (Stølen et al., 2005). During a competitive match, soccer players may perform ~1400 short-duration maximal or near maximal intensity activities, including sprints, change of directions (COD), tackling, accelerations, decelerations, jumps, among others (Iaia et al., 2009). Although training programs may improve such performance actions at long-term, short-term (or acute) improvements may also be induced by warm-up activities, a method routinely used by athletes, coaches and strength and conditioning specialists to improve muscle force and power involved in athletic performance during competition (Evetovich et al., 2015).

A large amount of research regarding the effects of a warm-up on human performance have been conducted (Rahimi, 2014; Barnes et al., 2015; González-Mohíno et al., 2018). There is a general consensus pointing the benefits of a warm-up on subsequent performance (Lockie et al., 2017). However, the optimal warm-up strategy for soccer players before a match is not well established (Hammami et al., 2018). Most soccer-related warm-up strategies involved static and dynamic stretching, neuromuscular activities, and short-duration high-intensity activities (Zois et al., 2011). Regarding the latter, they may induce post-activation potentiation (PAP) (Evetovich et al., 2015).

The PAP is a phenomenon in which neuromuscular performance characteristics are enhanced after intense contractile stimulation (Hodgson et al., 2005). The PAP in humans may be induced by isometric maximum voluntary contraction (Hamada et al., 2000), high-intensity resistance stimulus (McBride et al., 2005), and plyometric exercise (Turner et al., 2015). Although the existing research tends to reveal inconsistent findings (Moir et al., 2009), some studies has shown that performing muscular contractions under near-maximal load conditions improves subsequent performance during movements requiring large muscular power outputs of the stimulated muscle groups (Hodgson et al., 2005). However, there is little research regarding the effects of heavy resistance exercise on subsequent performance in soccer (Hammami et al., 2018). Some authors indicated that heavy resistance exercise may improve subsequent jump and COD (Zois et al., 2011), repeated sprints (Low et al., 2015; Sanchez-Sanchez et al., 2018) and single linear sprint (McBride et al., 2005; Tillin and Cooke, 2009).

The exact mechanism responsible for this PAP response remains uncertain (Lockie et al., 2017). Chemical, neuromuscular and mechanical changes may occur that temporarily aid the contractile properties of muscle tissue (Sale, 2004). One common PAP mechanism theory indicates the phosphorylation of myosin light chains resulting from the initial muscle activity, which would turn the actin and myosin molecules more sensitive to calcium ($Ca2+$) availability (Tillin and Bishop, 2009). Also it is speculated that PAP can increase the excitability of motoneurons (Hodgson et al., 2005) and enhancement of neural output by recruitment of faster motor units (Hamada et al., 2000; Sale, 2004). Moreover, it was also reported that pre-loading may increase muscle stiffness (Moir et al., 2009). Previous studies have suggested that PAP responses might be dependent on individual characteristics (Sanchez-Sanchez et al., 2018). For instance, stronger subjects exhibited a greater PAP response when compared with weaker counterparts (Seitz and Haff, 2016). In contrast, other studies concluded that performance after a PAP inducing activity was not related to training status (McBride et al., 2005). Furthermore, it has been proposed that the PAP may be related to the type of muscle fiber being activated (Wilson et al., 2013), with a higher proportion of fast fibers being related to greater PAP effect (Sole et al., 2013).

Therefore, in order to maximize PAP, these factors (e.g., training status) should be taken into account together with the load used during the warm-up (Lockie et al., 2017). McBride et al. (2005), for example, demonstrated that 1 set of 3 repetitions at 90% of one repetition maximum (1RM) significantly improve sprint time performance, whilst 1 set of 3 repetitions at 30%-1RM did not. In the same context, a previous study conducted with male soccer players showed that in order to induce optimal running speed enhancements, it is necessary to set the intensity of the warm-up protocol with loads ≥80%-1RM (Rahimi, 2014).

The competition rules require the physical trainers to finish the warm-up 15–20 min before the start to the matches. The PAP could be used between the end of the warm up and the start of the game, to maintain the level of activation in the players (Russell et al., 2014). Although greater loads have been recommended to induce PAP in strength and power tasks (McBride et al., 2005; Rahimi, 2014), its practical application in soccer is difficult. This is because of the limited time-frame separating the end of the warm-up and the start of a soccer match which is not sufficient to include multiple sets (Russell et al., 2014). Therefore, the aim of this study was to compare the effects of different warm-up conditioning intensities on physical fitness (i.e., PAP), of professional male field soccer players.

MATERIALS AND METHODS

Participants

Professional male soccer players (n = 10; age: 21.6 ± 3.2 years, body height: 177.9 ± 4.3 cm, and body mass: 69.5 ± 3.1 kg) with ≥6-years of training and competition experience were recruited for the study. Their regular training schedule involved four training sessions plus a competitive match per week in the Spanish second division "B." All participants: (1) were field players (four defenders, four midfielders and two forward), (2) were free of injuries in the last 3-months, (3) had regularly trained and competed in the past 6-months and (4) haven't got any lower extremity surgery in the past 2-years. Soccer players signed an informed consent before starting the data collection. The protocol was approved by the Ethics Committee of the Pontifical University of Salamanca (Annex III, Act 13/2/2019) and conformed to the latest version of the Declaration of Helsinki.

Procedures

The experiments were conducted during the competitive period of the season 2018. The control and experimental warm-up sessions were completed in a random, counterbalanced order, completed in a period of 3-weeks. The tests during control and experimental sessions were completed in the same order, between 15:00 and 20:00 h, at an indoor venue, with the same sports clothes and by the same investigator, who was blinded to the group allocation of the participants. To avoid the effects of fatigue on testing results, participants completed the control and the experimental warm-up sessions no less than 48 h after the last training/competition session. Each intervention was applied twice, making the tests in the following order. After control and experimental warm-up sessions participants completed measure in day 1: triple hop test with dominant (H3Jd) and non-dominant (H3Jnd) leg, squat jump (SJ) and repeated sprint with COD (RSCOD); measure in day 2: linear 30-m sprint test (S-30), countermovement jump (CMJ), COD test. The recovery between tests was 1 min. Participants were asked to attend each session under an adequate feeding and hydration state. The testing protocols were performed in the facilities where athletes usually train and compete.

Familiarization and Maximal Dynamic Strength Test

During a 120 min familiarization session, athletes simulated the warm-up protocols and completed a maximal dynamic strength test (1RM) in order to assess the specific loads to be used during PAP warm-up sessions. The maximal dynamic strength was assessed through the half back squat exercise using the Smith machine (MultipowerPeroga®, Murcia, Spain), with the barbell constrained to move along the vertical axis. The 1RM test was preceded by a 5-minutes low-intensity run in which the heart rate not exceed at 140 b·min^{-1} (Polar RS800CX, Electro Oy, Kempele, Finland), and by 5 and 3 half back squat repetitions at an estimated 50% and 70% 1RM, respectively. In the initial position the barbell was at shoulder-level, feet at shoulder-width distance, and knee and hips in full extension. Adhesive marks were added to the floor and the barbell to assure consistency in the hands and feet position during testing. In addition, a wooden seat with adjustable heights was placed behind the subjects to keep bar displacement and knee angle (~90° knee angle) constant on each half back squat attempt. The 1RM load was defined as the maximum weight that could be lifted once using the proper exercise technique through a full range of motion (Okuno et al., 2013). A 3-minutes rest interval was adopted between attempts, and the subjects had up to five attempts to obtain their 1RM.

Jumping Test

Athletes completed the H3Jd and H3Jnd (Noyes et al., 1991). Participants take maximal jumps forward as far as possible on the testing leg and land on two legs during the final jump. At the end of each horizontal jump attempt, athletes maintained the landing position for a brief moment. Soccer players also completed the CMJ and SJ tests following previous suggestions (Maulder et al., 2015), with minimal flexion of the trunk during take-off. Jumping was measured with a contact mat (Globus Ergo System®, Codogné, Italy). In all jumps, the hands were used freely, except during the SJ and CMJ, where athletes positioned arms akimbo. Athletes performed two maximal trials for each test with 1-minute of rest in between. The best value achieved was selected for analysis.

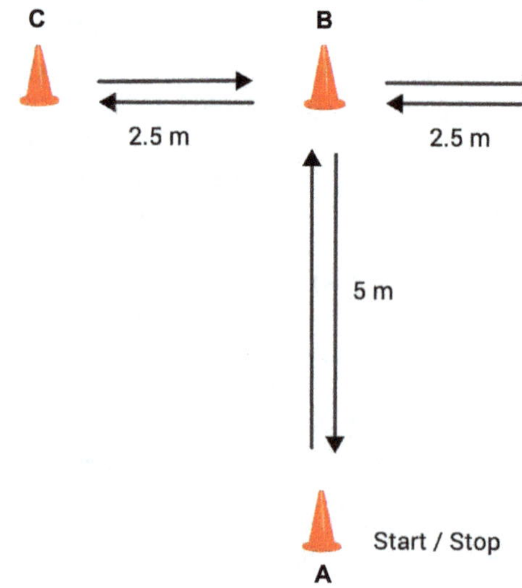

FIGURE 1 | Change of direction ability test.

Change of Direction Ability Test

Athletes also completed a modified *t*-test (Sassi et al., 2009) to evaluate COD. A photocell gate system (Witty, Microgate®, Italy) was used to record the time. The players performed the test using the same directives as the traditional test, although they were not required to move laterally or face forward (**Figure 1**). The players had to touch the top of the cones instead of its base. The displacement followed this route: AB displacement, at his own discretion, each subject sprinted forward to cone B and touched the top of the cone with the right hand; BC displacement, facing forward the participant shuffled to the left to cone C and touched the top of the cone with the left hand; CD displacement, the soccer player then shuffled to the right to cone D and touched its top; DB displacement, the players shuffled back to the left to cone B and touched its top; BA displacement, the players moved backward as quickly as possible and returned to line A. Players performed two maximal trials, with 1-minute of rest in between. The best value achieved was selected for analysis.

Linear 30-m Sprint Test

For maximal sprinting physical fitness assessment, athletes completed a S-30 sprint. The S-30 involved single maximal-effort sprints from a stationary start. Players initiated the sprint at their own discretion, positioning the foot 0.5-m behind the start line. Thirty-meter linear sprint performance was assessed using a double-beam photocell system (Witty, Microgate®, Italy). Athletes performed two maximal trials, with 1-minute of rest in between. The best value achieved was selected for analysis.

Repeated Sprint With COD Test

In addition to the linear sprint, athletes completed a RSCOD test. The RSCOD test included 6 sprints, with a passive recovery period of 20-seconds in between (Okuno et al., 2013). Each sprint involved 15-m of linear sprint, a COD of 180°, and another 15-m linear sprint [15-m + 15-m (COD−180°)]. Times were recorded

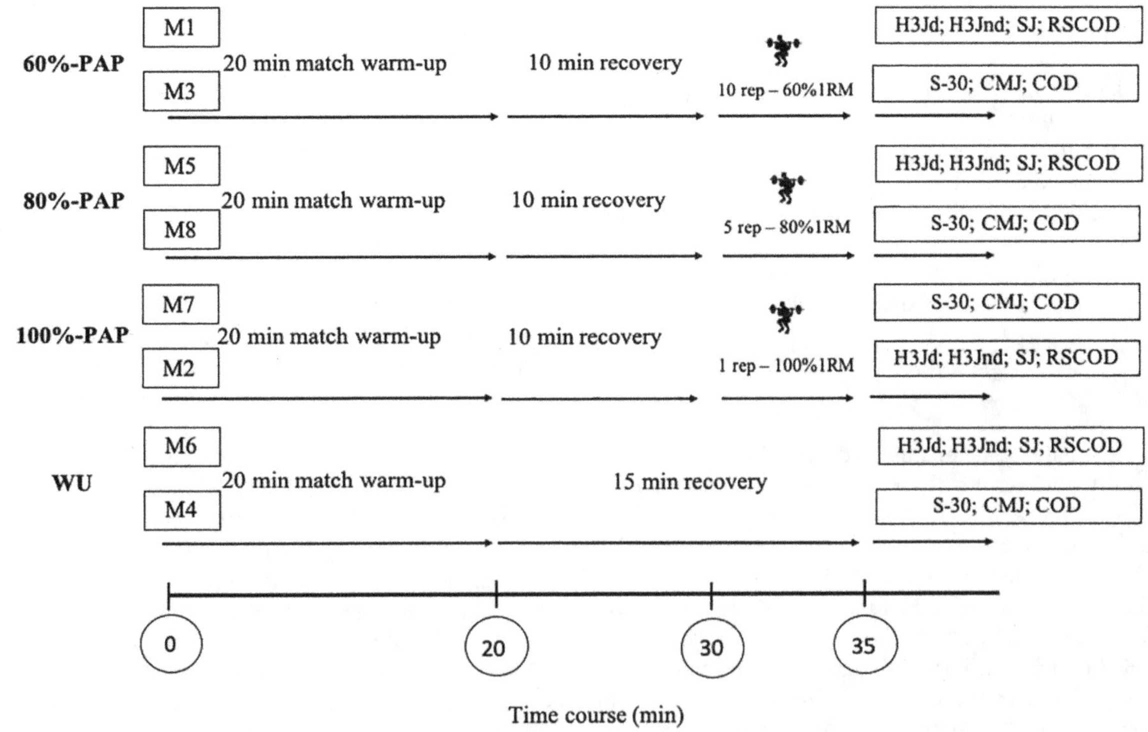

FIGURE 2 | Overview of the cross-over experimental design, indicating the control and three different warm-up conditions. The 15-minutes recovery period was included during control condition. The 10-minutes plus 5-minutes recovery period were included during PAP protocols, to simulate match conditions. The tests were divided at two measurement (M) day corresponding to each protocols. 60%-1RM, 80%-1RM, and 100%-1RM refer to match warm-up post-activation potentiation (PAP) protocols at 60, 80 and 100% of 1RM, respectively; WU, match warm-up protocol; M, measurement; H3Jd, triple hop test with dominant leg; H3Jnd, triple hop test with non-dominant leg; SJ, squat jump test; RSCOD, repeated sprint with change of direction test; S-30, linear 30-m sprint test; CMJ, countermovement jump test; COD, change of direction ability test.

with a double-beam photocell system (Witty, Microgate®, Italy). Athletes received verbal encouragement during the test. The players were verbally and visually informed to assume the starting position 0.5-m behind the starting line 6-seconds before each sprint. Also a 3-seconds countdown was visually provided with a light panel (Microgate®, Italy) that informed of the start of the next sprint. The fastest sprint (RSCODb) and the total time of all sprints (RSCODt) were retained for further analyses.

Warm-Up Protocols

The overview of warm-up protocols is presented in **Figure 2**. A control warm-up protocol (WU) was designed according to athlete's regular warm-up practices. The WU included 7-minutes of general warm-up [i.e., continuous moderate-intensity ($\leq$10 km/h^{-1}) running; general main-joint movements (mobility of upper and lower extremities; proprioceptive drills [landings with dominant and non-dominant leg after low-intensity frontal and lateral jumps)], 3-minutes of specific warm-up [i.e., elastic-bands resisted drills and ballistic drills (lateral and frontal movements on 5-m and simulations of ball shots wearing an elastic on the ankles or knees)], 5-minutes of ball drills (i.e., basic technical drills with a partner), and 5-minutes of small-sided games (i.e., 5vs5 in a 30 × 20-m size pitch). After the WU athletes rested passively for 15-minutes before testing, as it happens in a competition match. The experimental PAP warm-ups included the same exercises as the WU, with the addition (10-minutes after the end of WU) of one set of half back squats at 60, 80, or 100% of 1RM for a total of 10 repetitions (60%-1RM), 5 repetitions (80%-1RM), or 1 repetition (100%-1RM), respectively. All repetitions were performed at maximal voluntary concentric velocity. After each PAP load, athletes rested passively for 5-minutes before the H3JD, H3Jnd (measure in day 1) and S-30 tests (measure in day 2), 6-minutes before the SJ (measure in day 1) and CMJ tests (measure in day 2), and 8-minutes before the RSCOD (measure in day 1) and COD (measure in day 2), respectively.

Statistical Analyses

Data is presented as mean ± standard deviation (SD). All data were first log-transformed to reduce biases arising from non-uniformity error. The standardized difference or effect size [ES, 90% confidence limits (CL)] in the selected variables was calculated. Threshold values for Cohen's *ES* statistics were >0.2 (small), >0.6 (moderate), and >1.2 (large) (Hopkins et al., 2009). For within-group comparisons, the chances that the differences in performance were better/greater [i.e., greater than the smallest worthwhile change (0.2 multiplied by the between-subject standard deviation, based on Cohen's *d* principle)], similar, or worse/smaller were calculated. Quantitative chances (QC) of beneficial/better, similar/trivial, or detrimental/poorer effect were assessed qualitatively as follows: <1%, almost certainly not; >1–5%, very unlikely; >5–25%, unlikely; >25–75%, possible; >75–95%, likely; >95–99%, very likely; and >99%, most likely (Hopkins et al., 2009). If the chance that the true value is >25% beneficial and >0.5% chance that it is harmful, the clinically effect was considered as unclear. However, the clinical inference was declared as beneficial when odds ratio of benefit/harm was >66% (Hopkins et al., 2009). A specific Excel spreadsheet from sportsci.org was used to examine the within-group (between PAP protocols) (xPostOnlyCrossover.xls) comparisons.

RESULTS

The mean 1RM half-squat for this study was 114.3 ± 15.0 kg. **Table 1** shows the results for each test after each warm-up protocol.

Comparisons between the control warm-up and the PAP warm-ups are indicated in **Table 2**. Likely to most likely improvements were shown in H3Jd, H3Jnd, COD, RSCODb, and RSCODt only after the 80%-1RM protocol in comparison to WU. Furthermore, a possibly greater enhancement was found in RSCODt after the 60%-1RM protocol compared to WU. Conversely, 100%-1RM and 60%-1RM protocols induced possible to most likely poorer performance in the H3Jd, H3Jnd, SJ, CMJ, COD, and RSCODb in comparison to WU. Similarly, a likely poorer S-30 performance was observed after 100%-1RM compared to WU.

Comparisons between the PAP warm-up protocols are indicated in **Table 3**. Possibly to most likely improvements were shown in H3Jd, H3Jnd, SJ, CMJ, COD, RSCODb, and RSCODt after the 80%-1RM warm-up protocol in comparison to the 100%-1RM and 60%-1RM warm-up protocols. In addition, a possible better performance was achieved in the S-30 after the 80%-1RM warm-up compared to the 100%-1RM warm-up, while the 60%-1RM warm-up induced possible and very likely better S-30 performance in comparison to the 80%-1RM and 100%-1RM warm-up protocols, respectively. Finally, better performance in H3Jd (possible), H3Jnd (likely) and SJ (likely) were observed after 100%-1RM warm-up compared to 60%-1RM warm-up, whereas better performance in RSCODb (possible), RSCODt (likely), and S-30 (very likely) were observed after the 60%-1RM warm-up compared to the 100%-1RM warm-up.

TABLE 1 | Physical performance of soccer players after different warm-up protocols.

	WU	100%-1RM	80%-1RM	60%-1RM
H3Jd (m)	6.53 ± 0.34	6.40 ± 0.36	6.73 ± 0.41	6.26 ± 0.49
H3Jnd (m)	6.57 ± 0.26	6.56 ± 0.43	6.71 ± 0.36	6.32 ± 0.39
SJ (cm)	37.4 ± 4.9	36.7 ± 4.9	38.8 ± 4.7	34.5 ± 5.4
CMJ (cm)	39.8 ± 3.2	38.6 ± 5.3	40.7 ± 4.7	38.4 ± 3.2
COD (s)	7.23 ± 0.27	7.39 ± 0.38	7.12 ± 0.26	7.38 ± 0.33
RSCODb (s)	5.77 ± 0.15	5.94 ± 0.11	5.67 ± 0.13	5.89 ± 0.21
RSCODt (s)	35.7 ± 0.65	35.8 ± 0.62	35.0 ± 0.67	35.5 ± 0.70
S-30 (s)	4.05 ± 0.23	4.13 ± 0.23	4.09 ± 0.28	4.04 ± 0.23

H3Jd and H3Jnd, triple hop test with dominant and non-dominant leg, respectively, SJ, squat jump; CMJ, countermovement jump; COD, change of direction ability test; RSCODb and RSCODt, repeated sprint with change of direction best and total times, respectively, S-30, linear 30-m sprint test. WU, control warm-up protocol; 100%-1RM, 80%-1RM, and 60%-1RM, PAP warm-up protocols at 60, 80, and 100% of one repetition maximum in half-squat.

DISCUSSION

The aim of this study was to compare the effects of different conditioning intensities on the physical fitness (i.e., PAP) of professional male field soccer players. Main results indicate improvements in jumping, single and repeated COD speed after the 80%-1RM protocol in comparison to WU. Moreover, better jumping, as well as single and repeated COD speed improvements were observed after the 80%-1RM compared to the 60%-1RM and 100%-1RM protocols. Therefore, a moderate intensity (i.e., 80%-1RM) appears to be more effective than low (i.e., 60%-1RM) and maximal (i.e., 100%-1RM) warm-up strategies to induce greater PAP, including greater jumping, single and repeated COD speed in male soccer players.

Regarding jumping performance, likely to most likely improvements were shown in H3Jd and H3Jnd only after the 80%-1RM protocol in comparison to WU. Moreover, possibly to most likely improvements were shown in H3Jd, H3Jnd, SJ, and CMJ test after the 80%-1RM warm-up protocol in comparison to the 100%-1RM and 60%-1RM warm-up protocols. Improvements in jumping performance after loaded squat PAP protocols have been previously observed in male athletes from team-sports such as rugby, volleyball and soccer (Gouvêa et al., 2013), and may be explained by several neuro-mechanical short-term adaptations (e.g., increased muscle-tendon stiffness) (Tillin and Cooke, 2009). Moreover, the PAP effects depend on the balance between fatigue and neuromuscular potentiation (Tillin and Bishop, 2009), which in turn depends on the load-related intensity used (Sale, 2004). In the current study, a load of moderate-intensity (i.e., 80%-1RM) induced greater jumping performance improvements compared with loads of lower (i.e., 60%-1RM) or greater (i.e., 100%-1RM) intensity, agreeing with previous studies that found greater PAP effects after loads of intermediate intensity (Gouvêa et al., 2013). Of note, the greater PAP effect after intermediate-intensity loads may be particularly important when PAP actions are performed with the intention of maximizing movement velocity, leading to the recruitment of fast-twitch muscle fibers, which is considered a key factor to induce PAP (Turner et al., 2015). This improvement in jumping performance after loaded squats have been observed even after 6 h from the PAP warm-up (Saez-Saez de Villarreal et al., 2007). In addition, is important to note that soccer players' characteristics may affect the PAP magnitude (Sanchez-Sanchez et al., 2018), thus current results should be interpreted considering the high training level of the soccer players.

The results indicate likely improvements in the COD after the 80%-1RM protocol in comparison to WU, and likely poorer performance after the 100%-1RM and 60%-1RM protocols. Current outcomes are difficult to compare with previous findings,

TABLE 2 | Comparisons of soccer player's physical performance after a traditional (control) warm-up versus three different warm-up conditions.

	% (CL90%)	ES (CL90%)	Chances	Outcome
WU vs. 100%-1RM				
H3Jd	−2.0 (−4.4; 0.5)	−0.35 (−0.79; 0.08)	2/24/73%	Possibly
H3Jnd	−0.3 (−2.7; 2.2)	−0.07 (−0.65; 0.52)	21/44/34%	Possibly
SJ	−2.0 (−8.1; 4.5)	−0.15 (−0.61; 0.32)	10/48/42%	Possibly
CMJ	−3.5 (−8.7; 1.9)	−0.41 (−1.04; 0.21)	5/22/73%	Possibly
COD	−2.1 (−4.4; 0.2)	−0.50 (−1.04; 0.04)	2/14/83%	Likely
RSCODb	−3.0 (−3.9; −2.1)	−1.03 (−1.32; −0.73)	0/0/100%	Most Likely
RSCODt	−0.3 (−0.5; −0.1)	−0.14 (−0.25; −0.03)	0/83/17%	Likely trivial
S-30	−1.7 (−2.2; −1.2)	−0.28 (−0.36; −0.20)	0/5/95%	Likely
WU vs. 80%-1RM				
H3Jd	3.0 (0.7; 5.3)	0.52 (0.13; 0.91)	92/8/0%	Likely
H3Jnd	2.2 (0.2; 4.2)	0.51 (0.05; 0.97)	88/11/1%	Likely
SJ	3.8 (−3.0; 11.1)	0.27 (−0.22; 0.76)	60/34/6%	Unclear
CMJ	2.0 (−2.6; 6.7)	0.22 (−0.30; 0.75)	53/38/9%	Unclear
COD	1.6 (−0.4; 3.5)	0.38 (−0.09; 0.86)	75/22/2%	Likely
RSCODb	1.6 (0.5; 2.8)	0.58 (0.16; 1.00)	93/6/0%	Likely
RSCODt	2.0 (1.2; 2.7)	0.99 (0.60; 1.38)	100/0/0%	Most Likely
S-30	−0.9 (−3.7; 1.7)	−0.15 (−0.60; 0.29)	9/49/42%	Unclear
WU vs. 60%-1RM				
H3Jd	−4.3 (−5.8; −2.7)	−0.77 (−1.06; −0.48)	0/0/100%	Most Likely
H3Jnd	−3.8 (−6.0; −1.6)	−0.91 (−1.46; −0.37)	0/2/98%	Very Likely
SJ	−8.0 (−11.8; −4.0)	−0.60 (−0.91; −0.30)	0/2/98%	Very Likely
CMJ	−3.5 (−5.0; −1.9)	−0.40 (−0.59; −0.22)	0/3/97%	Very Likely
COD	−2.0 (−3.3; −0.7)	−0.48 (−0.80; −0.17)	0/6/93%	Likely
RSCODb	−2.1 (−3.7; −0.4)	−0.72 (−1.28; −0.15)	1/6/94%	Likely
RSCODt	0.5 (−0.1; 1.1)	0.26 (−0.03; 0.56)	65/34/1%	Possibly
S-30	0.2 (0.1; 0.4)	0.04 (0.01; 0.07)	0/100/0%	Most Likely trivial

To avoid a misinterpretation of the results, positive results indicate a better performance in favor of the PAP warm-up protocol, while negative results show a better performance in favor of the control warm-up protocol. CL, confidence limits; ES, effect size; PAP, post-activation potentiation; H3Jd and H3Jnd, triple hop test with dominant and non-dominant leg, respectively; SJ, squat jump; CMJ, countermovement jump; COD, change of direction ability test; RSCODb and RSCODt, repeated sprint with change of direction best and total times, respectively; S-30, linear 30-m sprint test. WU, Control warm-up protocol; 100%-1RM, 80%-1RM, and 60%-1RM, post-activation potentiation warm-up protocols at 60, 80, and 100% of one repetition maximum in half-squat.

given the limited literature related to COD performance and PAP (Lockie et al., 2017). However, two previous studies observed improvements in COD performance after warm-up actions that included loaded exercises (Zois et al., 2011; Sole et al., 2013), and the improvement may be related to acute increase of reactive strength (Sole et al., 2013). Reactive strength is the ability to quickly change from the eccentric to the concentric phase during a stretch-shortening cycle muscle action (Young et al., 1998). In this sense, a greater reactive strength may help to improve the ability to perform sudden stops and to accelerate from there (Spiteri et al., 2013), hence improving COD speed (Sheppard and Young, 2006). Of note, a greater PAP effect (i.e., greater COD performance) was observed after the 80%-1RM versus the 60%-1RM, since the load used in the 80%-1RM may help to maximize the acceleration phase of the COD action (McBride et al., 2005), implicating a better use of the stretch-shortening cycle in the deceleration-acceleration transition of the COD movement. However, the 100%-1RM did not maximize COD performance. In this sense, the PAP effect may not proportionally depend on the load used (i.e., the higher the better), but other factors also may modulate the effect, such as the muscle fiber type, athletes' performance level, exercise type, time interval between the conditioning stimulus and the performance testing, among others (Sanchez-Sanchez et al., 2018). In fact, it has been suggested that there are PAP responders that may benefit from exercises designed to induce PAP, whereas others may not respond (Evetovich et al., 2015).

Regarding the RSCOD test, likely and most likely improvements were found in RSCODb and RSCODt with 80%-1RM in comparison to WU, respectively. Improvements in RSCOD performance after loaded back half-squat PAP protocols have been previously observed in elite male handball (Okuno et al., 2013) and soccer players (Sanchez-Sanchez et al., 2018). The 80%-1RM may improve neuromuscular capacity (Hodgson et al., 2005), allowing an increase in athlete's power (Tillin and Bishop, 2009), thus better ability to repeat sprints (Glaister, 2005). Although warm-ups delivered to induce PAP may increase RSCOD performance, the load used must be applied with caution. Heavy loads (>90% 1RM), with recovery times of 8-minutes, may allow improvements in the total time and sprint time in a repeated sprint test (Low et al., 2015). However, the use of a heavier load (i.e., 100%-1RM protocol)

TABLE 3 | Comparisons of soccer player's physical performance after three different warm-up conditions.

	% (CL90%)	ES (CL90%)	Chances	Outcome
100%-1RM vs. 80%-1RM				
H3Jd	5.1 (3.7; 6.5)	0.79 (0.58; 1.00)	100/0/0%	Most Likely
H3Jnd	2.5 (1.1; 3.9)	0.35 (0.15; 0.55)	90/10/0%	Likely
SJ	5.9 (3.3; 8.7)	0.40 (0.22; 0.57)	96/4/0%	Very Likely
CMJ	5.7 (2.5; 9.1)	0.38 (0.16; 0.59)	92/8/0%	Likely
COD	3.6 (1.4; 5.7)	0.65 (0.25; 1.04)	97/3/0%	Very Likely
RSCODb	4.5 (3.6; 5.4)	2.15 (1.70; 2.59)	100/0/0%	Most Likely
RSCODt	2.3 (1.6; 2.9)	1.21 (0.84; 1.57)	100/0/0%	Most Likely
S-30	0.8 (−2.1; 3.5)	0.13 (−0.36; 0.63)	41/47/12%	Possibly
100%-1RM vs. 60%-1RM				
H3Jd	−2.3 (−5.6; 1.1)	−0.37 (−0.92; 0.17)	4/24/71%	Possibly
H3Jnd	−3.5 (−6.8; −0.1)	−0.51 (−1.01; −0.01)	1/13/86%	Likely
SJ	−6.1 (−11.8; 0.0)	−0.43 (−0.86; 0.00)	1/16/83%	Likely
CMJ	0.1 (−5.7; 6.2)	0.01 (−0.39; 0.40)	20/62/18%	Possibly trivial
COD	0.1 (−2.4; 2.5)	0.01 (−0.43; 0.46)	23/57/20%	Possibly trivial
RSCODb	0.9 (−0.9; 2.7)	0.41 (−0.44; 1.26)	67/22/11%	Possibly
RSCODt	0.8 (0.2; 1.5)	0.43 (0.08; 0.78)	87/12/0%	Likely
S-30	1.9 (1.4; 2.4)	0.34 (0.25; 0.43)	99/1/0%	Very Likely
60%-1RM vs. 80%-1RM				
H3Jd	7.6 (4.3; 10.9)	0.88 (0.51; 1.24)	100/0/0%	Most Likely
H3Jnd	6.2 (3.1; 9.4)	0.90 (0.45; 1.34)	99/1/0%	Very Likely
SJ	12.9 (5.8; 20.3)	0.72 (0.34; 1.11)	98/2/0%	Very Likely
CMJ	5.6 (0.3; 11.2)	0.61 (0.04; 1.18)	89/10/1%	Likely
COD	3.6 (1.5; 5.9)	0.87 (0.36; 1.39)	98/2/0%	Very Likely
RSCODb	3.8 (1.6; 6.0)	1.46 (0.64; 2.29)	99/1/0%	Very Likely
RSCODt	1.5 (0.6; 2.4)	0.69 (0.27; 1.10)	97/3/0%	Very Likely
S-30	−1.2 (−3.8; 1.6)	−0.16 (−0.53; 0.21)	5/52/42%	Possibly

To avoid a misinterpretation of the results, positive results denote a better performance in favor of the PAP warm-up protocol indicated at the right, while negative results denote a better performance in favor of the PAP warm-up protocol indicated at the left. CL, confidence limits; ES, effect size; PAP, post-activation potentiation; H3Jd and H3Jnd, triple hop test with dominant and non-dominant leg, respectively; SJ, squat jump; CMJ, countermovement jump; COD, change of direction ability test; RSCODb and RSCODt, repeated sprint with change of direction best and total times, respectively; S-30, linear 30-m sprint test. WU, control warm-up protocol; 100%-1RM, 80%-1RM, and 60%-1RM, PAP warm-up protocols at 60, 80, and 100% of one repetition maximum in half-squat.

may induce most likely poorer performance in the RSCODb in comparison to a WU, even when 8-minutes of rest are allowed. Although potentiation and fatigue coexist, the 100%-1RM protocol may have induced fatigue to a greater extent than its PAP effect, potentially due to decreased release of calcium from the sarcoplasmic reticulum, leading to reduced calcium concentration in the myoplasm (Rassier and MacIntosh, 2000). In this sense, to optimally induce PAP, the load used must be selected accurately in male soccer players (Hammami et al., 2018). Although previous studies analyzed the effect of PAP warm-ups on RSCOD (Sanchez-Sanchez et al., 2018), this is the first study that compared the effects of three different loaded protocols on RSCOD performance, a key fitness specific-trait for soccer (Schimpchen et al., 2015), which determines match physical performance (Rampinini et al., 2007) and differentiates between competitive levels (Rampinini et al., 2009). Therefore, current findings may help practitioners to optimally prepare players before a match.

No changes in S-30 performance was observed after the 60%-1RM and the 80%-1RM compared to WU. No effects in sprint time after heavy loaded squat PAP protocols have been previously observed in soccer players (Tillin and Cooke, 2009). In contrast, the positive effects of heavy-load squats was obtained at distances of 10 to 40-m (McBride et al., 2005; Chatzopoulos et al., 2007; Rahimi, 2014). The mechanisms that underlie the effects of PAP warm-ups using loaded exercises on sprint performance have not been clarified (McBride et al., 2005). Maximal sprint velocity (i.e., distances >30 m) may depend on the force of the extensor muscles of the hip in order to re-incorporate the leg in the swing phase and thus maintain an adequate stride length (Weyand et al., 2000). Although the muscle force may be increased through a PAP warm-up, inducing an increased muscle stiffness (Moir et al., 2009), based on previous research, it was speculated that the PAP should be related to the volume of the pre-load (Evetovich et al., 2015). The PAP has traditionally been induced through the use of multiple sets of heavy isotonic resistance exercise (Wilson et al., 2013), but in this study only one set of 60%-1RM and 80%-1RM was applied. From a practical perspective, given the timeframe separating the end of the warm-up and the start of a soccer match, there is no time to include multiple sets (Russell et al., 2014). On the other hand, a likely poorer performance after 100%-1RM compared to WU was observed. It is possible that the recovery time used in the present study (i.e., 5-minutes) was not enough to elicit a significant PAP effect after the 100%-1RM in some players. Considering that fatigue and potentiation co-exist (Rassier and MacIntosh, 2000), shorter rest intervals may increase fatigue (Tillin and Cooke, 2009). In this sense, <4 min of rest after a PAP warm-up of 5-RM did not induce an increase in sprint performance (Tillin and Cooke, 2009). However, 5 min of rest after a PAP warm-up, as used in the current study, seems to be adequate in order to reload phosphocreatine stores (Chatzopoulos et al., 2007). Still, this did not explain the lack of improvements or even poorer sprinting capability after the 100%-1RM strategy used in the current study. It has been suggested that in order to improve sprinting performance, the potential effect of heavier PAP protocols, including load scheme and rest time, should be prescribed on an individual basis (Mola et al., 2014).

Using an 80%-1RM protocol could be an effective strategy to enhance the physical performance of elite male soccer player, with potential implications for a better performance, especially at the beginning of games. Coaches should carefully consider the recovery time between the PAP application and the start of a match in order to reduce the risk of fatigue. Moreover, although in the current study an 80%-1RM protocol induced greater mean improvements in the physical performance of soccer players, PAP protocols should be elaborated considering athlete's individual characteristics.

Potential limitations of the current study are related to the lack of physiological and biochemical measurements, in order to further understand the underlying factors related with the observed PAP phenomenon. The limited number of subjects involved in the current study could be recognized as an additional limitation, in line with the use of magnitude-based inferences (MBI). Such statistical approach has been criticized as may induce a greater risk of type I error (Sainani, 2018). On the other side, its use have been strongly supported in sport science studies (Batterham and Hopkins, 2019). Future studies should strive to elucidate if current results may be transferred to competition scenarios, analyzing performance indices during a match, such as covered distance at high-intensity, accelerations, among others short-term high-intensity actions. In addition, future studies may analyse the potential interfering effect (if any) of repeated physical fitness test (i.e., H3JD, SJ) performed on the same testing session and its role on PAP after warm-ups using different 1RM back-squat intensities.

CONCLUSION

In conclusion, a moderate intensity (i.e., 80%-1RM back squat) may induce greater improvements (i.e., PAP effect) in jumping, repeated COD speed and non-repeated COD speed in elite level male soccer players when compared to low (60%-1RM) and high (100%-1RM) intensity warm-up protocols.

ETHICS STATEMENT

This study was carried out in accordance with the recommendations of "Ethics Committee, Pontifical University of Salamanca" with written informed consent from all subjects. All subjects gave written informed consent in accordance with the Declaration of Helsinki. The protocol was approved by the "Ethics Committee, Pontifical University of Salamanca (Annex III, Act 13/2/2019)."

AUTHOR CONTRIBUTIONS

CP, RR-C, and JS-S designed the work. CP, DH, and JS-S acquired the data. CP, FN, RR-C, JS-S, and OG-S analyzed and interpreted of data. All authors drafted the manuscript, critically revised the manuscript and approved the final version of the manuscript to be published. CP, RR-C, FN, and JS-S agreed to be accountable for all aspects of the work in ensuring that questions related to the accuracy or integrity of any part of the work were appropriately investigated and resolved.

REFERENCES

Barnes, K. R., Hopkins, W. G., McGuigan, M. R., and Kilding, A. E. (2015). Warm-up with a weighted vest improves running performance via leg stiffness and running economy. *J. Sci. Med. Sport* 18, 103–108. doi: 10.1016/j.jsams.2013.12.005

Batterham, A., and Hopkins, W. (2019). The problems with "The Problem with 'Magnitude-Based Inference'". *Med. Sci. Sports Exerc.* 51:599.

Chatzopoulos, D. E., Michailidis, C. J., Giannakos, A. K., Alexiou, K. C., Patikas, D. A., Antonopoulos, C. B., et al. (2007). Postactivation potentiation effects after heavy resistance exercise on running speed. *J. Strength Cond. Res.* 21, 1278–1281. doi: 10.1519%2F00124278-200711000-00051

Evetovich, T. K., Conley, D. S., and McCawley, P. F. (2015). Postactivation potentiation enhances upper- and lower-body athletic performance in collegiate male and remale athletes. *J. Strength Cond. Res.* 29, 336–342. doi: 10.1519/JSC.0000000000000728

Glaister, M. (2005). Multiple sprint work: physiological responses, mechanisms of fatigue and the influence of aerobic fitness. *Sport Med.* 35, 757–777. doi: 10.2165%2F00007256-200535090-00003

González-Mohíno, F., Martín, R., Juárez Santos-García, D., Fidel, P. A., de Asís-Fernández, F., Yustres, I., et al. (2018). Effects of high-intensity warm-ups on running performance. *Int. J. Sports Med.* 39, 426–432. doi: 10.1055/s-0044-102132

Gouvêa, A. L., Fernandes, I. A., César, E. P., Silva, W. A. B., and Gomes, P. S. C. (2013). The effects of rest intervals on jumping performance: a meta-analysis on post-activation potentiation studies. *J. Sports Sci.* 31, 459–467. doi: 10.1080/02640414.2012.738924

Hamada, T., Sale, D. G., MacDougall, J. D., and Tarnopolsky, M. A. (2000). Postactivation potentiation, fiber type, and twitch contraction time in human knee extensor muscles. *J. Appl. Physiol.* 88, 2131–2137. doi: 10.1152%2Fjappl.2000.88.6.2131

Hammami, A., Zois, J., Slimani, M., Russel, M., and Bouhlel, E. (2018). The efficacy, and characteristics, of warm-up and re-warm-up practices in soccer players: a systematic review. *J. Sports Med. Phys. Fitness* 58, 135–149. doi: 10.23736/S0022-4707.16.06806-7

Hodgson, M., Docherty, D., and Robbins, D. (2005). Post-activation potentiation: underlying physiology and implications for motor performance. *Sport Med.* 35, 585–595. doi: 10.2165%2F00007256-200535070-00004

Hopkins, W. G., Marshall, S. W., Batterham, A. M., and Hanin, J. (2009). Progressive statistics for studies in sports medicine and exercise science. *Med. Sci. Sports Exerc.* 41, 3–13.

Iaia, F. M., Rampinini, E., and Bangsbo, J. (2009). High-intensity training in football. *Int. J. Sports Physiol. Perform.* 4, 291–306.

Lockie, R. G., Lazar, A., Davis, D. L., and Moreno, M. R. (2017). Effects of postactivation potentiation on linear and change-of-direction speed: analysis of the current literature and applications for the strength and conditioning coach. *Strength Cond. J.* 40, 75–91.

Low, D., Harsley, P., Shaw, M., and Peart, D. (2015). The effect of heavy resistance exercise on repeated sprint performance in youth athletes. *J. Sports Sci.* 33, 1028–1034. doi: 10.1080/02640414.2014.979857

Maulder, P., Cronin, J., Maulder, P., and Cronin, J. (2015). Horizontal and vertical jump assessment: reliability, symmetry, discriminative and predictive ability discriminative and predictive ability. *Phys. Ther. Sport* 6, 74–82. doi: 10.1016%2Fj.ptsp.2005.01.001

McBride, J. M., Nimphius, S., and Erickson, T. M. (2005). The acute effects of heavy-load squats and loaded countermovement jumps on sprint performance. *J. Strength Cond. Res.* 19, 893–897. doi: 10.1519%2F00124278-200511000-00029

Moir, G. L., Dale, J. R., and Dietrich, W. W. (2009). The acute effects of heavy back squats on machanical variables during a series of bilateral hops. *J. Strength Cond. Res.* 23, 1118–1124. doi: 10.1519/JSC.0b013e31819166c2

Mola, J. N., Bruce-Low, S. S., and Burnet, S. J. (2014). Optimal recovery time for postactivation potentiation in professional soccer players. *J. Strength Cond. Res.* 28, 1529–1537. doi: 10.1519/JSC.0000000000000313

Noyes, F. R., Barber, S. D., and Mangine, R. E. (1991). Abnormal lower limb symmetry determined by functional hop tests after anterior cruciate ligament rupture. *Am. J. Sports Med.* 19, 513–518. doi: 10.1177%2F036354659101900518

Okuno, N. M., Tricoli, V., Silva, S. B., Bertuzzi, R., Moreira, A., and Kiss, M. (2013). Postactivation potentiation on repeated-sprint ability in elite handball players. *J. Strength Cond. Res.* 27, 662–668. doi: 10.1519/JSC.0b013e31825bb582

Rahimi, R. (2014). The acute effects of heavy versus light-load squats on sprint performance. *Phys. Educ. Sport* 5, 163–169.

Rampinini, E., Couts, A. J., Castagna, C., Sassi, R., and Impellizzeri, F. M. (2007). Variation in top level soccer match performance. *Int. J. Sports Med.* 28, 1018–1024. doi: 10.1055%2Fs-2007-965158

Rampinini, E., Sassi, A., Morelli, A., Mazzoni, S., Fanchini, M., and Coutts, A. J. (2009). Repeated-sprint ability in professional and amateur soccer players. *Appl. Physiol. Nutr. Metab.* 34, 1048–1054. doi: 10.1139/H09-111

Rassier, D. E., and MacIntosh, B. R. (2000). Coexistence of potentiation and fatigue in skeletal muscle. *Braz. J. Med. Biol. Res.* 33, 499–508. doi: 10.1590%2Fs0100-879x2000000500003

Russell, M., Cook, C. J., and Kilduff, L. P. (2014). "Match day strategies to enhance the physical and technical performance of rugby players," in *The Science of Rugby*, eds C. Twist and P. Worsfold (London: Routledge), 97–114.

Saez-Saez de Villarreal, E., Gonzalez-Badillo, J. J., and Izquierdo, M. (2007). Optimal warm-up stimuli of muscle activation to enhance short and long-term acute jumping performance. *Eur. J. Appl. Physiol.* 100, 393–401. doi: 10.1007%2Fs00421-007-0440-9

Sainani, K. L. (2018). The problem with "Magnitude-based Inference". *Med. Sci. Sports Exerc.* 50, 2166–2176. doi: 10.1249%2Fmss.0000000000001645

Sale, D. (2004). Postactivation potentiation: role in performance. *Br. J. Sports Med.* 38, 386–387. doi: 10.1136%2Fbjsm.2002.003392

Sanchez-Sanchez, J., Rodríguez-Fernández, A., Petisco, C., Ramirez-Campillo, R., and Nakamura, F. Y. (2018). Effects of different post-activation potentiation warm-ups on repeated sprint ability in soccer players from different competitive levels. *J. Hum. Kinet.* 61, 189–197. doi: 10.1515/hukin-2017-0131

Sassi, R. H., Dardouri, W., Yahmed, M. H., Gmada, N., Mahfoudhi, M. E., and Gharbi, Z. (2009). Relative and absolute reliability of a modified agility T-test and its relationship with vertical jump and straight sprint. *J. Strength Cond. Res.* 23, 1644–1651. doi: 10.1519/JSC.0b013e3181b425d2

Schimpchen, J., Skorski, S., Nopp, S., and Meyer, T. (2015). Are "classical" tests of repeated-sprint ability in football externally valid? A new approach to determine in-game sprinting behaviour in elite football players. *J. Sports Sci.* 34, 519–526. doi: 10.1080/02640414.2015.1112023

Seitz, L. B., and Haff, G. G. (2016). Factors modulating post-activation potentiation of jump, sprint, throw, and upper-body ballistic performances: a systematic review with meta-analysis. *Sport Med.* 46, 231–240. doi: 10.1007/s40279-015-0415-7

Sheppard, J. M., and Young, W. B. (2006). Agility literature review: classifications, training and testing. *J. Sports Sci.* 24, 919–932. doi: 10.1080%2F02640410500457109

Sole, C. J., Moir, G. L., Davis, S. E., and Witmer, C. A. (2013). Mechanical analysis of the acute effects of a heavy resistance exercise warm-up on agility performance in court-sport athletes. *J. Hum. Kinet.* 39, 147–156. doi: 10.2478/hukin-2013-0077

Spiteri, T., Cochrane, J. L., Hart, N. H., Haff, G. G., and Nimphius, S. (2013). Effect of strength on plant foot kinetics and kinematics during a change of direction task. *Eur. J. Sport Sci.* 13, 646–652. doi: 10.1080/17461391.2013.774053

Stølen, T., Chamari, K., Castagna, C., and Wisløff, U. (2005). Physiology of soccer. *Sport Med.* 35, 501–536.

Tillin, K. A., and Cooke, C. (2009). The effects of postactivation potentiation on sprint and jump performance of male academy soccer players. *J. Strength Cond. Res.* 23, 1960–1967. doi: 10.1519/JSC.0b013e3181b8666e

Tillin, N. A., and Bishop, D. (2009). Factors modulating post-activation potentiation and its effect on performance of subsequent explosive activities. *Sport Med.* 39, 147–166. doi: 10.2165/00007256-200939020-00004

Turner, A. P., Bellhouse, S., Kilduff, L. P., and Russell, M. (2015). Post-activation potentiation of sprint acceleration performance using plyometric exercise. *J. Strength Cond. Res.* 29, 343–350. doi: 10.1519%2Fjsc.0000000000000647

Weyand, P. G., Sternlight, D. B., Bellizzi, M. J., and Wright, S. (2000). Faster top running speeds are achieved with greater ground forces not more rapid leg movements. *J. Appl. Physiol.* 89, 1991–1999. doi: 10.1152%2Fjappl.2000.89.5.1991

Wilson, J. M., Duncan, N. M., Marin, P. J., Brown, L. E., Loenneke, J. P., Wilson, S., et al. (2013). Meta-Analysis of postactivation potentiation and power: effects of conditioning activity, volume, gender, rest periods, and training status. *J. Strength Cond. Res.* 27, 854–859. doi: 10.1519/JSC.0b013e31825c2bdb

Young, W. B., Jenner, A., and Griffiths, K. (1998). Acute enhancement of power performance from heavy load squats. *J. Strength Cond. Res.* 12, 82–84. doi: 10.1519%2F00124278-199805000-00004

Zois, J., Bishop, D. J., Ball, K., and Aughey, R. J. (2011). High-intensity warm-ups elicit superior performance to a current soccer warm-up routine. *J. Sci. Med. Sport* 14, 522–528. doi: 10.1016/j.jsams.2011.03.012

Permissions

All chapters in this book were first published by Frontiers; hereby published with permission under the Creative Commons Attribution License or equivalent. Every chapter published in this book has been scrutinized by our experts. Their significance has been extensively debated. The topics covered herein carry significant findings which will fuel the growth of the discipline. They may even be implemented as practical applications or may be referred to as a beginning point for another development.

The contributors of this book come from diverse backgrounds, making this book a truly international effort. This book will bring forth new frontiers with its revolutionizing research information and detailed analysis of the nascent developments around the world.

We would like to thank all the contributing authors for lending their expertise to make the book truly unique. They have played a crucial role in the development of this book. Without their invaluable contributions this book wouldn't have been possible. They have made vital efforts to compile up to date information on the varied aspects of this subject to make this book a valuable addition to the collection of many professionals and students.

This book was conceptualized with the vision of imparting up-to-date information and advanced data in this field. To ensure the same, a matchless editorial board was set up. Every individual on the board went through rigorous rounds of assessment to prove their worth. After which they invested a large part of their time researching and compiling the most relevant data for our readers.

The editorial board has been involved in producing this book since its inception. They have spent rigorous hours researching and exploring the diverse topics which have resulted in the successful publishing of this book. They have passed on their knowledge of decades through this book. To expedite this challenging task, the publisher supported the team at every step. A small team of assistant editors was also appointed to further simplify the editing procedure and attain best results for the readers.

Apart from the editorial board, the designing team has also invested a significant amount of their time in understanding the subject and creating the most relevant covers. They scrutinized every image to scout for the most suitable representation of the subject and create an appropriate cover for the book.

The publishing team has been an ardent support to the editorial, designing and production team. Their endless efforts to recruit the best for this project, has resulted in the accomplishment of this book. They are a veteran in the field of academics and their pool of knowledge is as vast as their experience in printing. Their expertise and guidance has proved useful at every step. Their uncompromising quality standards have made this book an exceptional effort. Their encouragement from time to time has been an inspiration for everyone.

The publisher and the editorial board hope that this book will prove to be a valuable piece of knowledge for researchers, students, practitioners and scholars across the globe.

List of Contributors

Žan Luca Potočnik, Gregor Jurak and Gregor Starc
Laboratory for Physical and Motor Development Diagnosis, Faculty of Sport, University of Ljubljana, Ljubljana, Slovenia

Jonathan D. Connor, Anthony S. Leicht and Kenji Doma
Sport and Exercise Science, James Cook University, Townsville, QLD, Australia

David L. Mann
Department of Human Movement Sciences, Vrije Universiteit Amsterdam, Amsterdam, Netherlands

Miguel-Angel Gomez
Faculty of Physical Activity and Sports Sciences, Polytechnic University of Madrid, Madrid, Spain

Manou Anselma, Anniek van Berkum, Mai J. M. Chinapaw and Teatske M. Altenburg
Amsterdam UMC, Vrije Universiteit Amsterdam, Department of Public and Occupational Health, Amsterdam Public Health Research Institute, Amsterdam, Netherlands

Dorine C. M. Collard
Mulier Instituut, Utrecht, Netherlands

Jos W. R. Twisk
Amsterdam UMC, Vrije Universiteit Amsterdam, Department of Epidemiology and Biostatistics, Amsterdam Public Health Research Institute, Amsterdam, Netherlands

Cameron Donkin, Ranel Venter and Wilbur Kraak
Department of Sport Science, Stellenbosch University, Stellenbosch, South Africa

Derik Coetzee
Department of Sport and Exercise Sciences, University of the Free State, Bloemfontein, South Africa

Annika Frahsa and Ansgar Thiel
Institute of Sport Science, University of Tüebingen, Tuebingen, Germany
Interfaculty Research Institute for Sport and Physical Activity, University of Tüebingen, Tuebingen, Germany

Thadeu Gasparetto
Department of Management, National Research University Higher School of Economics, Saint Petersburg, Russia

Cornel Nesseler
Business School, Norwegian University of Science and Technology, Trondheim, Norway

Claudia Niessner, Steffen C. E. Schmidt, Alexander Woll and Klaus Bös
Institute of Sport and Sport Science, Karlsruhe Institute of Technology, Karlsruhe, Germany

Till Utesch
Department of Pedagogical Assessment and Potential Development, Institute of Educational Sciences, University of Münster, Münster, Germany

Anke Hanssen-Doose and Annette Worth
Institute of Movement and Sport, University of Education, Karlsruhe, Germany

Doris Oriwol
Institute of Sport and Sport Science, Karlsruhe Institute of Technology, Karlsruhe, Germany
Institute of Movement and Sport, University of Education, Karlsruhe, Germany

Enrique Colino, Jorge Garcia-Unanue, Manuel Leon and Leonor Gallardo
IGOID Research Group, University of Castilla–La Mancha, Toledo, Spain

Javier Sanchez-Sanchez
Faculty of Sport Sciences, Universidad Europea de Madrid, Madrid, Spain
Research Group Planning and Assessment of Training and Athletic Performance, Pontifical University of Salamanca, Salamanca, Spain

Jose Luis Felipe and Archit Navandar
Faculty of Sport Sciences, Universidad Europea de Madrid, Madrid, Spain

Javier Calvo-Monera
Nothingbutnet S.L., Valencia, Spain

María Jose Carvalho
Faculdade de Desporto da Universidade do Porto, Porto, Portugal

Lisa Baumgartner, Tanja Postler, Renate Oberhoffer-Fritz and Thorsten Schulz
TUM Department of Sport and Health Sciences, Institute of Preventive Pediatrics, Technical University of Munich, Munich, Germany

Christine Graf and Nina Ferrari
Institute of Movement and Neurosciences, German Sport University Cologne, Cologne, Germany

Bernhard Haller
Institute of Medical Informatics, Statistics and Epidemiology, Technical University of Munich, Munich, Germany

Elena Sierra-Palmeiro and Marta Bobo-Arce
Department of Physical Education and Sports, Faculty of Sports Science and Physical Education, University of A Coruña, A Coruña, Spain

Alexandra Pérez-Ferreirós and María A. Fernández-Villarino
Department of Especial Teaching, Faculty of Education and Sports Sciences, University of Vigo, Pontevedra, Spain

Susanne Kobel, Christine Laemmle, Olivia Wartha and Juergen Michael Steinacker
Division of Sports and Rehabilitation Medicine, Department of Internal Medicine, University Hospital Ulm, Ulm, Germany

Lea Henle and Bertram Szagun
Faculty Social Work, Health & Nursing, University of Applied Sciences Ravensburg-Weingarten, Weingarten, Germany

Corrado Lupo, Gennaro Boccia, Alexandru Nicolae Ungureanu and Paolo Riccardo Brustio
NeuroMuscularFunction Research Group, School of Exercise & Sport Sciences, Department of Medical Sciences, University of Turin, Turin, Italy

Riccardo Frati and Roberto Marocco
School of Exercise & Sport Sciences, SUISM, University of Turin, Turin, Italy

Vedrana Sember, Marjeta Kovač and Shawnda A. Morrison
Laboratory for the Diagnostics of Somatic and Motor Development, Faculty of Sport, University of Ljubljana, Ljubljana, Slovenia

Sergio J. Ibáñez, Sergio Gonzalez-Espinosa and Javier García-Rubio
Faculty of Sport Science, University of Extremadura, Cáceres, Spain

Sergio Martinez-Fernández
Faculty of Sport Science, University of Extremadura, Cáceres, Spain
Cáceres Club Baloncesto, Cáceres, Spain

Sebastián Feu
Faculty of Education, University of Extremadura, Badajoz, Spain

Yansong Li and Chunhua Zhang
School of Kinesiology, Shanghai University of Sport, Shanghai, China

Xue Xia
School of Psychology, Shanghai University of Sport, Shanghai, China

Fanying Meng
Institute of Physical Education, Huzhou University, Huzhou, China

José A. Navia and Jesús Aceituno
Facultad de Ciencias de la Actividad Física y del Deporte, Departamento de Ciencias Sociales, de la Actividad Física y del Ocio, Universidad Politécnica de Madrid, Madrid, Spain

John van der Kamp
Faculty of Behavioral and Movement Sciences, Department of Human Movement Sciences, Vrije Universiteit Amsterdam, Amsterdam, Netherlands
Research Centre for Exercise, School and Sport, Windesheim University of Applied Sciences, Zwolle, Netherlands

Carlos Avilés
Facultad de Educación, Departamento de Didáctica de las Lenguas, Artes y Educación Física, Universidad Complutense de Madrid, Madrid, Spain

Arvid Kuritz
Department of Sport Science, University of Konstanz, Konstanz, Germany

Christoph Mall, Melina Schnitzius and Filip Mess
Department of Sport and Health Sciences, Technical University of Munich, Munich, Germany

Aurelio Olmedilla
Department of Personality, Evaluation and Psychological Treatment, University of Murcia, Murcia, Spain

Roberto Ruiz-Barquín
Department of Developmental and Educational Psychology, Autonomous University of Madrid, Madrid, Spain

Francisco Javier Ponseti
Department of Pedagogy, University of the Balearic Islands, Mallorca, Spain

Francisco Javier Robles-Palazón
Department of Physical Activity and Sport, University of Murcia, Murcia, Spain

Alexandre García-Mas
Department of Psychology, University of the Balearic Islands, Mallorca, Spain

Pedro Antonio Sánchez-Miguel, Miguel Angel Tapia-Serrano and Mikel Vaquero-Solís
Faculty of Teaching Training, University of Extremadura, Cáceres, Spain

Patxi León-Guereño
Faculty of Psychology and Education, University of Deusto, Donostia-San Sebastian, Spain

David Hortigüela-Alcalá
Department of Specific Didactics, Faculty of Education, University of Burgos, Burgos, Spain

Miguel A. López-Gajardo
Faculty of Sports Sciences, University of Extremadura, Cáceres, Spain

Inmaculada Yustres and José María González-Ravé
Department of Physical Activity and Sport Sciences, University of Castilla-La Mancha, Toledo, Spain

Jesús Santos del Cerro
Department of Statistics, University of Castilla-La Mancha, Toledo, Spain

Fernando González-Mohíno
Department of Physical Activity and Sport Sciences, University of Castilla-La Mancha, Toledo, Spain Departamento de Educación, Facultad de Educación y Lenguas, Universidad Nebrija, Madrid, Spain

Michael Peyrebrune
Department of Exercise and Health Sciences, School of Sport, Exercise and Health Sciences, Loughborough University, Leicestershire, United Kingdom

Ole Sprengeler and Antje Hebestreit
Department of Epidemiological Methods and Etiologic Research, Leibniz Institute for Prevention Research and Epidemiology - BIPS, Bremen, Germany

Hannah Gohres
School of Public Health, Bielefeld University, Bielefeld, Germany

Jens Bucksch
Department of Sociological and Human Sciences, Heidelberg University of Education, Heidelberg, Germany

Christoph Buck
Department of Biometry and Data Management, Leibniz Institute for Prevention Research and Epidemiology - BIPS, Bremen, Germany

Timo Laakso and Jarmo Liukkonen
Department of Sport Sciences, University of Jyväskylä, Jyväskylä, Finland

Keith Davids
Centre for Sports Engineering Research, Sheffield Hallam University, Sheffield, United Kingdom

Bruno Travassos
CreativeLab, Research Center for Sports Sciences, Health Sciences and Human Development (CIDESD), Universidade da Beira Interior, Covilhã, Portugal

Luis P. Rodrigues, Ricardo Franco Lima and Miguel Camões
Escola Superior Desporto e Lazer, Instituto Politécnico de Viana do Castelo, Rua Escola Industrial e Comercial de Nun'Álvares, Viana do Castelo, Portugal Research Center in Sports Sciences Health Sciences and Human Development, CIDESD, Vila Real, Portugal

Ana Filipa Silva
Escola Superior Desporto e Lazer, Instituto Politécnico de Viana do Castelo, Rua Escola Industrial e Comercial de Nun'Álvares, Viana do Castelo, Portugal Research Center in Sports Sciences Health Sciences and Human Development, CIDESD, Vila Real, Portugal N2i, Polytechnic Institute of Maia, Maia, Portugal

Filipe Manuel Clemente
Escola Superior Desporto e Lazer, Instituto Politécnico de Viana do Castelo, Rua Escola Industrial e Comercial de Nun'Álvares, Viana do Castelo, Portugal
Instituto de Telecomunicações, Delegação da Covilhã, Portugal

Pantelis Theodoros Nikolaidis
Exercise Physiology Laboratory, Nikaia, Greece

Thomas Rosemann
Institute of Primary Care, University of Zurich, Zurich, Switzerland

Beat Knechtle
Institute of Primary Care, University of Zurich, Zurich, Switzerland
Medbase St. Gallen Am Vadianplatz, St. Gallen, Switzerland

Michael Bateman and Gareth Jones
School of Sport and Exercise Science, University of Worcester, Worcester, United Kingdom

Thierry Paillard
Laboratoire Mouvement, Equilibre, Performance et Santé (UPRES EA 4445), Département STAPS, Université de Pau et des Pays de l'Adour, Tarbes, France

Bingnan Gong
China Football College, Beijing Sport University, Beijing, China
Facultad de Ciencias de la Actividad Física y del Deporte, Universidad Politécnica de Madrid, Madrid, Spain

Yang Gai, Qing Yi and Miguel-Ángel Gómez
Facultad de Ciencias de la Actividad Física y del Deporte, Universidad Politécnica de Madrid, Madrid, Spain

Yixiong Cui
AI Sports Engineering Lab, School of Sports Engineering, Beijing Sport University, Beijing, China

Cristina Petisco and Daniel Hernández
Research Group Planning and Assessment of Training and Athletic Performance, Pontifical University of Salamanca, Salamanca, Spain

Rodrigo Ramirez-Campillo
Research Group Planning and Assessment of Training and Athletic Performance, Pontifical University of Salamanca, Salamanca, Spain
Laboratory of Human Performance, Research Nucleus in Health, Physical Activity and Sport, Department of Physical Activity Sciences, Universidad de Los Lagos, Osorno, Chile

Oliver Gonzalo-Skok
Research Group Planning and Assessment of Training and Athletic Performance, Pontifical University of Salamanca, Salamanca, Spain
Faculty of Health Sciences, University of San Jorge, Zaragoza, Spain

Fabio Y. Nakamura
Research Group Planning and Assessment of Training and Athletic Performance, Pontifical University of Salamanca, Salamanca, Spain
College of Healthcare Sciences, James Cook University, Townsville, QLD, Australia
Department of Medicine and Aging Sciences, "G. d'Annunzio" University of Chieti-Pescara, Chieti, Italy

Index

www.ingramcontent.com/pod-product-compliance
Lightning Source LLC
LaVergne TN
LVHW080930210926
848485LV00004B/769

Dietary Fibers: Nutritional Function in Health and Disease